ALFRED BENZON SYMPOSIUM 12

GABA-Neurotransmitters

GABA-NEURO-TRANSMITTERS

PHARMACOCHEMICAL, BIOCHEMICAL AND PHARMACOLOGICAL ASPECTS

Proceedings of the Alfred Benzon Symposium 12
held at the premises of The Royal Danish
Academy of Sciences and Letters,
Copenhagen 21–25 May 1978

EDITED BY

POVL KROGSGAARD-LARSEN
JØRGEN SCHEEL-KRÜGER
HELMER KOFOD

Published by
Munksgaard, Copenhagen

In North and South America:
Academic Press, New York

In Japan:
Nankodo, Tokyo

SCANDINAVIAN UNIVERSITY BOOKS
DENMARK MUNKSGAARD *Copenhagen*
NORWAY UNIVERSITETSFORLAGET *Oslo, Bergen, Tromsø*
SWEDEN ESSELTE STUDIUM *Stockholm, Gothenburg, Lund*

Printed in Denmark by P. J. Schmidts Bogtrykkeri, Vojens
ISBN 87-16-2903-8
ISBN 0105-3639

Published simultaneously in the U.S.A. by Academic Press Inc.
ISBN 0-12-426730-0
LCCN: 79-50013

and in Japan by Nankodo Company Ltd.

Contents

II GABA Receptors and Structure-Activity Studies on GABA Agonists and Inhibitors of GABA-T and GABA Uptake

III Clinical Conditions Relevant for a Therapy with GABA-ergic Drugs and Mode of Action of Anticonvulsive Drugs

List of Participants

N.-E. ANDÉN
Department of Pharmacology
University of Göteborg
S-400 33 Göteborg 33
Sweden

J. ARNT
Department of Pharmacology
Royal Danish School of Pharmacy
Universitetsparken 2
DK-2100 Copenhagen Ø
Denmark

G. BARTHOLINI
Synthelabo
Department of Research and Development
58, Rue de la Glacière
F-75013 Paris
France

H. BITTIGER
Department Forschung
Ciba-Geigy AG
CH-4002 Basel
Switzerland

L. BREHM
Department of Chemistry BC
Royal Danish School of Pharmacy
Universitetsparken 2
DK-2100 Copenhagen Ø
Denmark

F. CATTABENI
Institute of Pharmacology & Pharmacognosy
University of Milan
Via A. del Sarto 21
I-20129 Milan
Italy

T. N. CHASE
National Institute of Neurological and
Communicative Disorders and Stroke
National Institutes of Health
Bethesda, Maryland 20014
U.S.A.

A. R. COOLS
Department of Pharmacology
University of Nijmegen
Geert Grooteplein Noord 21
Nijmegen
The Netherlands

E. COSTA
Laboratory of Preclinic Pharmacology
National Institute of Mental Health
Saint Elisabeth's Hospital
WAW Building
Washington, D.C. 20032
U.S.A.

J. T. COYLE
Department of Pharmacology and Psychiatry
John Hopkins University
School of Medicine
725 North Wolfe St.
Baltimore, Maryland 21205
U.S.A

D. R. CURTIS
Department of Pharmacology
Australian National University
P.O. Box 334
Canberra City, A.C.T. 2601
Australia

A. DELINI-STULA
Department Forschung, Division Pharma
Ciba-Geigy AG
CH-4002 Basel
Switzerland

G. DI CHIARA
Institutes of Pharmacology
University of Cagliari
I-09100 Cagliari
Italy

A. DRAY
Department of Physiology and Pharmacology
Duke University, Medical Center
Durham, North Carolina 27710
U.S.A.

S. J. ENNA
Departments of Pharmacology, Neurobiology and Anatomy
University of Texas Medical School at Houston
P.O. Box 20708
Houston, Texas 77025
U.S.A.

K. FUXE
Department of Histology
Karolinska Instituttet
S-104 01 Stockholm 60
Sweden

A. GUIDOTTI
Division of Special Mental Health Research, IRP, NIMH
WAW Building
Saint Elisabeth's Hospital
Washington, D.C. 20032
U.S.A.

W. E. HAEFELY
Pharmaceutical Research Department
F. Hoffman-La Roche & Co. Ltd.
Grenzacherstr. 124
CH-4002 Basel
Switzerland

L. L. IVERSEN
MRC Neurochemical Pharmacology Unit
Department of Pharmacology
Medical School, Hills Road
Cambridge CB2 2QD
England

G. A. R. JOHNSTON
Department of Pharmacology
Australian National University
P.O. Box 334
Canberra City, A.C.T. 2601
Australia

H. KOFOD
Department of Chemistry BC
Royal Danish School of Pharmacy
Universitetsparken 2
DK-2100 Copenhagen Ø
Denmark

P. KROGSGAARD-LARSEN
Department of Chemistry BC
Royal Danish School of Pharmacy
Universitetsparken 2
DK-2100 Copenhagen Ø
Denmark

K. G. LLOYD
Department of Neuropharmacology
Synthelabo
31, Av. P. V. Couturier
F-92220 Bagneux
France

G. MAGELUND
Sct. Hans Mental Hospital
Department of Psychopharmacology
Department E
DK-4000 Roskilde
Denmark

C. D. Marsden
University Department of Neurology
Institute of Psychiatry
De Crespigny Park
Denmark Hill
London SE5 8AF
England

E. G. McGeer
Kinsmen Laboratory of Neurological Research
Division of Neurological Sciences
University of British Columbia
Vancouver 8
British Columbia
Canada V6T 1W5

B. S. Meldrum
University Department of Neurology
Institute of Psychiatry
De Crespigny Park
Denmark Hill
London SE5 8AF
England

B. W. Metcalf
Centre de Recherche Merrell International
16, Rue d'Ankara
F-67084 Strasbourg Cedex
France

I. Munkvad
Sct. Hans Mental Hospital
Department E
DK-4000 Roskilde
Denmark

E. E. Müller
Department of Pharmacology
University of Milan
Via Vanvitelli 32
I-20129 Milan
Italy

I. Møller-Nielsen
Department of Pharmacology and Toxicology
Lundbeck & Co. A/S
Ottiliavej 7–9
DK-2500 Valby
Denmark

R. W. Olsen
Department of Biochemistry
University of California
Riverside
California 92502
U.S.A.

M. G. Palfreyman
Centre de Recherche Merrell International
16, Rue d'Ankara
F-67084 Strasbourg
France

R. R. Rando
Department of Pharmacology
Harvard Medical School
Seeley G. Mudd Building
250, Longwood Avenue
Boston, Massachusetts 02115
U.S.A.

E. Roberts
Center for Advanced Study
in the Behavioral Science
202, Junipero Serra Boulevard
Stanford, California 94305
U.S.A.

J. Scheel-Krüger
Sct. Hans Mental Hospital
Department of Psychopharmacology
Department E
DK-4000 Roskilde
Denmark

A. SCHOUSBOE
Department of Biochemistry A
Panum Institute
Blegdamsvej 3c
DK-2200 Copenhagen N
Denmark

I. WALAAS
Norwegian Defence Research
Establishment
Division of Toxicology
N-2007 Kjeller
Norway

J. R. WALTERS
National Institute of Neurological and
Communicative Disorders and Stroke
National Institutes of Health
Bethesda, Maryland 20014
U.S.A.

L. C. WEAVER
University of Minnesota
College of Pharmacy
115, Appleby Hall
128, Pleasant St. S.E.
Minneapolis, Minnesota 55455
U.S.A.

Preface

γ-Aminobutyric acid (GABA) is now widely accepted as a central nervous system transmitter and is generally considered to be the principal inhibitory brain transmitter. The last international GABA symposium took place 3 years ago. The workshop held in February, 1975 in California, was published by E. Roberts, T. N. Chase and D. B. Tower, under the title *GABA in Nervous System Function* in 1976.

The field of GABA and our state of knowledge of this amino acid is currently within a phase of nearly explosive development. The organizing committe has felt that the time was fully mature for the next conference on GABA in order to summarize the comprehensive research during the intervening period, and hopefully to stimulate the development of new directions in future GABA research.

The present Alfred Benzon Symposium entitled *GABA-Neurotransmitters* took place in Copenhagen in May 1978. Traditionally the Alfred Benzon Symposia include a maximum of 40 active participants. Consequently all aspects of the present GABA research could not be covered, and it was decided to focus on the following aspects for an up-to-date discussion: The clinical conditions appropriate for treatment with GABA-ergic drugs, the design and development of specific GABA receptor agonists, inhibitors of the GABA uptake and metabolizing processes, mapping of neuronal pathways and interaction of GABA neurons with other neurotransmitter systems, and development of new animal models relevant for testing GABA-ergic drugs.

The present status and knowledge of the role of GABA in normal brain function or various pathological brain diseases is still far from being completely understood. It is however realized that GABA participates in human motor coordination, endocrine function and higher integrative cortical function.

There is thus a malfunction of GABA in Huntington's Chorea and parkinsonism, possibly also in epilepsy, spasticity, schizophrenia, and drug-induced tardive dyskinesia. GABA function probably also changes during normal aging. However, there are still no reports available on the effects and efficiency of a prolonged pharmacotherapeutic treatment in the human clinic with *specific* and potent GABA-ergic drugs. This research field seems now in the very initial and early state of development, which may open a potential new area in psychopharmacology.

It was also the intention of this meeting to discuss the significance of GABA in the mechanism of action of a large series of various drugs already available in the human clinic, and which among other actions have been shown to facilitate GABA neurotransmission: the benzodiazepines, barbiturates, diphenylhydantoines, sodium valproate, baclofen, ethanol, and some antipsychotic neuroleptic drugs.

It is our hope that this symposium published in the present book will form the framework for fruitful interdisciplinary integration and stimulate future collaboratory research on GABA among biochemists, chemists, clinicians and pharmacologists.

Povl Krogsgaard-Larsen and Jørgen Scheel-Krüger

Chapter I
GABA, Neurotransmitter Role, Localization, and Interaction with Other Transmitter Systems

Gabergic Transmission in the Mammalian Central Nervous System

D. R. Curtis

Since this symposium is concerned with virtually all aspects of GABA as a mammalian central transmitter, especially in relation to the possibility of designing chemotherapeutic measures for restoring defective transmission processes at GABA-mediated (gabergic) synapses which may underlie certain human neurological defects, it is appropriate to outline the central pathways for which there is acceptable evidence that GABA is the transmitter. In view of the ever-increasing amount of information becoming available regarding the significance of this amino acid as an inhibitory transmitter, the types of evidence which establish transmitter function can be reviewed only in very broad terms. Central GABA-mediated pathways will then be tabulated and general rather than specific references will be provided. A number of recent reviews provide more detailed information (Curtis & Johnston 1974a, Krnjević 1974, Curtis 1975, 1978, Johnston 1976, 1978, DeFeudis 1975, Roberts *et al.* 1976, Levy 1977, Fonnum 1978).

GABA AS A TRANSMITTER

It is convenient to discuss the evidence for gabergic transmission under the subheadings A-E listed below, and to provide references in Table 1 for these types of information within various regions of the nervous system. Few investigations other than those of a biochemical nature have been carried out on the human brain, but the same gabergic pathways seem likely to occur in human beings as have been proposed to occur in the cat and laboratory rodents.

(A) *Synthesis and Storage in Presynaptic Terminals*

Consideration of GABA as a central transmitter originated from its presence in

Department of Pharmacology, John Curtin School of Medical Research, Canberra City, A. C. T. 2601, Australia.

"GABA-NEUROTRANSMITTERS", Alfred Benzon Symposium 12, Munksgaard 1978

vertebrate brain tissue (Roberts & Frankel 1950), and investigations of the gross distribution of GABA, GAD and GABA-T have been of prime significance in establishing the importance of this amino acid. More specific and detailed information has been provided using refined microdissection and micro-analytical techniques (Otsuka & Miyata 1972, Fonnum 1972a), particularly in association with operative or developmental lesions of central pathways (Storm-Mathison 1977); such studies providing, for example, a measure of the amounts of GABA and GAD within synaptic terminals (Fonnum & Walberg 1973). In both the spinal cord and cuneate nucleus depletion of GABA by the administration of agents which inhibit GAD leads to a reduction of GABA-mediated inhibitions (Levy 1977). The convulsant effects of these agents may also be related to the reduced amount of GABA available for synaptic release in these and other regions.

Increasing use is being made of cytochemical techniques, including the autoradiographic localization of labelled GABA within synaptic terminals after *in vivo* or *in vitro* uptake (Iversen *et al.* 1975), and particularly the immunohisto-chemical visualization of GAD as an indicator of synaptic sites of GABA synthesis (Wood *et al.* 1976).

(B) *Synaptic Release of GABA*

In view of the problems involved in demonstrating *in vivo* the synaptic release of any central transmitter, it is not surprising that few studies have shown that impulses in a putative gabergic pathway release GABA (Obata 1976). Although a calcium-dependent release of GABA can be induced *in vitro* from tissue slices or synaptosomes by electrical "stimulation" or elevated potassium concentration, this release is difficult to relate to that occurring synaptically *in vivo*, except perhaps where the degeneration of a pathway does or does not influence the release *in vitro* from slices prepared from the appropriate region of the CNS (Nadler *et al.* 1977).

(C) *Postsynaptic Action of GABA*

Microelectrophoretic methods have established two central actions of GABA and close analogues: *hyperpolarization* of neurones produced by an increase in membrane permeability to chloride (and possibly also potassium) ions which appears identical to the permeability increase induced at inhibitory synapses and also by 'glycine-like' amino acids (Curtis & Johnston 1974a), and *depolarization* of primary afferent terminals which, although also possibly associated with an increased permeability to chloride ions, is not produced by 'glycine-like' amino acids (Levy 1977, Curtis 1978).

These effects establish a relationship between GABA and postsynaptic (hyperpolarizing) inhibition, and also between GABA and presynaptic inhibition. The former required additional use of specific antagonists of the action of GABA to exclude the involvement of 'glycine-like' amino acids as transmitters; the latter is almost certainly associated with axo-axonic synapses on primary afferent terminals, depolarization resulting in a reduced output of excitatory transmitter by impulses in primary afferent fibres (Levy 1977, Curtis 1978). In the spinal cord and dorsal column nuclei both postsynaptic hyperpolarizing and presynaptic depolarizing actions of GABA appear to contribute to the relatively long latency and prolonged inhibition of interneurones, motoneurones and relay neurones produced by impulses in segmental, intersegmental, ascending and descending afferent fibres.

Under *in vitro* conditions, GABA binds in a sodium-independent fashion to synaptic membrane fractions of mammalian brain at sites which can be distinguished by substrate specificity from those associated with the sodium-dependent membrane transport of this and related amino acids (DeFeudis 1977, Olsen *et al.* 1978). The former sites are presumably receptors associated with the postsynaptic action of GABA, especially as there is a competitive interaction between GABA and (+)-bicuculline methochloride (Peck *et al.* 1973, Enna *et al.* 1977, Möhler & Okada 1977). Although such studies of binding provide a relatively simple technical means for establishing the kinetics of, and structural requirements for, interaction of compounds with GABA receptor sites under a variety of *in vitro* conditions, the distinction between agonists and antagonists of GABA transmitter action *in vivo* is not readily apparent, and this type of investigation has hitherto been of minimal significance to either identification of gabergic pathways or the mechanisms of GABA-mediated inhibition.

(D) *Postsynaptic Antagonists of GABA*

Since the postsynaptic effects of 'glycine-like' and 'GABA-like' amino acids appear identical, specific antagonists of these two classes of inhibitory amino acid have been required to distinguish glycine- from GABA-mediated synaptic processes. Inhibitions sensitive to low concentrations of strychnine are generally regarded as being mediated by a 'glycine-like' amino acid, whereas (+)-bicuculline methochloride, (+)-bicuculline and picrotoxinin block both the hyperpolarizing effect of GABA-like amino acids on neurones and the

Table I
Gaba mediated inhibitions

Region	*Types of inhibition*	*Key references*
Cerebral cortex	Stellate cell inhibition of Pyramidal cells	A – Otsuka *et al.* 1971
		C – Dreifuss *et al.* 1969
		D – Curtis & Felix 1971, Sillito 1977
		E – Hokfelt & Ljungdahl 1972
Retina	Amacrine and horizontal cell transmitters	A–E – Neal 1976
Olfactory bulb	Granule and periglomerular cell inhibition of mitral cells	A – Graham 1973, Ribak *et al.* 1977, Ramon-Moliner 1977
		C,D – McLennan 1971, Nicoll 1971
Hippocampal formation	Basket cell inhibition of pyramidal cells.	A – Ben-Ari *et al.* 1976, Storm-Mathisen 1977
		B – Nadler *et al.* 1977
	Recurrent inhibition of septal neurones	C,D – Curtis *et al.* 1970b, McLennan & Miller 1974, DeFrance *et al.* 1975
		E – Storm-Mathisen 1977
Cerebellum	Basket cell inhibition of Purkinje cells.	A – Otsuka *et al.* 1971, McLaughlin *et al.* 1974, Roffler-Tarlov & Sidman 1978
	Golgi cell inhibition of granule cells.	B – Obata 1976
		C – Kawamura & Provini 1970, Siggins *et al.* 1971
	Purkinje cell inhibition of deep nuclei	D – Curtis & Felix 1971, Bisti *et al.* 1971, Kawaguchi & Ono 1973
		E – Hokfelt & Ljungdahl 1972, Schon & Iversen 1972, Wilkin *et al.* 1974
Thalamus	Recurrent inhibition of thalamo-cortical relay neurones (ventro-basal and lateral geniculate nucleus)	C,D – Curtis & Tebēcis 1972, Morgan *et al.* 1976
Hypothalamus	Intrahypothalamic inter-neurones	A – Tappaz & Brownstein 1977
Basal ganglia	Inhibition by intra-caudate, strio-nigral, strio-pallidal, strio-entopeduncular neurones	A – Ribak *et al.* 1976, Brownstein *et al.* 1977, Fonnum *et al.* 1978
		C,D – Feltz, 1971, Precht & Yoshida 1971, Crossman *et al.* 1973, Obata & Yoshida 1973, Bernadi *et al.* 1976, Dray *et al.* 1976, Spehlmann *et al.* 1977
		E – Iversen *et al.* 1975
Red Nucleus	Inhibition from cerebral cortex	C,D – Altmann *et al.* 1976

Table I
Gaba mediated inhibitions

Region	*Types of inhibition*	*Key references*
Vestibular nuclei	Purkinje cell inhibition of lateral and superior nucleus neurones	A – Otsuka & Miyata 1972, Fonnum & Walberg 1973, Okada & Schimada 1976 B – Obata 1976 C,D – Obata *et al.* 1970, Curtis *et al.* 1970a, Bruggencate & Engberg 1971, Fukuda *et al.* 1972, Precht *et al.* 1973b
Cranial motonuclei	Vestibular inhibition of oculomotor neurones. Prolonged inhibition of masseter and hypoglossal motoneurones	A – Otsuka & Miyata 1972, Fonnum 1972b, Precht *et al.* 1973a, Roffler-Tarlov & Tarlov 1975 C,D – Obata & Highstein 1970, Precht *et al.* 1973a, Highstein 1973b See Curtis & Johnston 1974a
Dorsal column nuclei	Prolonged inhibition of relay neurones by pyramidal and afferent volleys. Depolarization of afferent terminals	A,B – Levy 1977 C,D – Kelly & Renaud 1973, Levy 1977
Spinal cord	Prolonged inhibition of interneurones, motor-neurones and Renshaw cells. Depolarization of primary afferent terminals	A – Otsuka & Konishi 1976, Barber *et al.* 1978 C – Curtis *et al.* 1968, Krnjević *et al.* 1977a D – Curtis *et al.* 1971, Game & Lodge 1975, Krnjevic *et al.* 1977b, Levy 1977 Ljungdahl & Hokfelt 1973

depolarization of primary afferent terminals (Curtis & Johnston 1974a,b, Curtis 1978). The selectivity of these two classes of antagonists must be determined for the particular type of neurone under investigation, and GABA is frequently accepted as the most probable transmitter when a synaptic process can be reduced or suppressed by bicuculline but is not affected by strychnine.

Binding studies suggest that whereas bicuculline may be a competitive antagonist at GABA receptors (Möhler & Okada 1977), picrotoxinin may interfere with GABA-activated ionophores (Olsen *et al.* 1978).

(E) *Inactivation of Synaptically Released GABA*
In view of the predominantly intracellular location of GABA-metabolizing enzymes, important factors in the clearance of synaptically released GABA from the extracellular environment appear to be diffusion and carrier-mediated cellular uptake into neurones, terminals and glial cells (Martin 1976). Both low- and high-affinity transport mechanisms have been described: the former may be more significant when subsynaptic concentrations of GABA are relatively high immediately after synaptic release, whereas the latter is more important for maintaining very low extracellular concentrations of the amino acid.

Under *in vitro* conditions a number of compounds inhibit GABA uptake, and the receptor sites differ from those associated with the postsynaptic action of GABA (Krogsgaard-Larsen 1978). Furthermore these substances, particularly (+)-2,4-diaminobutyric acid, (-)-nipecotic acid, guvacine and arecaidine, selectively enhance and prolong the effects of micro-electrophoretic GABA *in vivo.* None, however, influence the time course of synaptic action at synapses for which GABA is accepted as the transmitter (see Lodge *et al.* 1977). In order to demonstrate the importance *in vivo* of GABA uptake, inhibitors are presumably required which are not also substrates for the carrier processes. Although the inhibition of inactivation processes has so far not contributed to the identification of GABA as a transmitter, considerable use has been made of the uptake of radiolabelled GABA into terminals as an indication of gabergic function (Iversen *et al.* 1975).

One important characteristic of GABA-mediated inhibitions is the enhancement and prolongation by anaesthetics, especially by the barbiturates which also similarly influence the effect of microelectrophoretic GABA but not that of glycine (Lodge & Curtis 1978). This action may involve the ionophores activated by the interaction of GABA with postsynaptic receptors, rather than either these receptors *per se* or those associated with uptake processes. The benzodiazepines may have a similar mode of action.

CONCLUSION

This has been a very broadly based survey of the transmitter role of GABA in the mammalian central nervous system. Numerous key references have been omitted, but the importance of this amino acid should be readily apparent from the inhibitions listed in the table. Other substances, of course, require consideration as transmitters vital to the proper functioning of the brain (see

Krnjević 1974), but GABA can rightly be claimed as the major central inhibitory transmitter on the basis of its involvement at virtually all levels of the mammalian neuraxis.

Defects of GABA-mediated synaptic transmission may thus underlie neurological disorders, such as epilepsy and various extrapyramidal syndromes, and psychiatric disturbances. Even if the involvement of GABA synapses be a secondary event rather than a primary cause of disease, clinical benefit may follow the use of agents which, based on knowledge of the synthesis, action and inactivation of GABA, act specifically in relation to this amino acid. Although the actions of substances found to be therapeutically effective, such as the benzodiazepines, barbiturates, butyrophenones and some anticonvulsants, are probably related to gabergic synapses (Johnston 1978), the development of these has not been based on an understanding of the molecular aspects of gabergic transmission. It will thus be important to study the different types of GABA receptors in various regions of the human brain, both normal and diseased, especially those sites associated with the postsynaptic action and inactivation of this inhibitory transmitter.

Major problems which can be anticipated to limit such a chemotherapeutic approach are blood-brain barriers to agents acting at GABA receptors and the clinically undesirable modification of gabergic transmission at relatively normal synapses by an agent required to act predominantly in relation to a particular defective pathway. Defective gabergic transmission, especially if resulting from a partial loss of certain gabergic neurones, may be more susceptible than normally functioning synapses to chemical modification if the defect is associated with alterations in GABA-related enzymes, transport processes, or even in the sensitivity of neurones to this amino acid. Denervation hypersensitivity, however, has yet to be convincingly demonstrated *in vivo* for any central transmitter.

REFERENCES

Altmann, H., Bruggencate, G. ten, Pickelmann, P. & Steinberg, R. (1976) Effects of GABA, glycine, picrotoxin and bicuculline methochloride on rubrospinal neurones in cat. *Brain Res.* 111, 337–345.

Barber, R. P., Vaughn, J. E., Saito, K., McLaughlin, B. J. & Roberts, E. (1978) GABAergic terminals are presynaptic to primary afferent terminals in the substantia gelatinosa of the rat spinal cord. *Brain Res.* 141, 35–55.

Ben-Ari, Y., Kanazawa, I. & Sigmond, R. E. (1976) Regional distribution of glutamate decarboxylase and GABA within the amygdaloid complex and stria terminalis system of the rat. *J. Neurochem.* 26, 1279–1283.

Bernardi, G., Marciani, M. G., Morocutti, C. & Giacomini, P. (1976) The action of picrotoxin and bicuculline on rat caudate neurons inhibited by GABA. *Brain Res.* 102, 379–384.

Bisti, S., Iosif, G., Marchesi, G. F. & Strata, P. (1971) Pharmacological properties of inhibitions in the cerebellar cortex. *Exp. Brain Res.* 14, 24–37.

Brownstein, M. H., Mroz, E. A., Tappaz, M. L. & Leeman, S. E. (1977) On the origin of substance P and glutamic acid decarboxylase (GAD) in the substantia nigra. *Brain Res.* 135, 315–323.

Bruggencate, G. ten, & Engberg, I. (1971) Iontophoretic studies in Deiters' nucleus of the inhibitory actions of GABA and related amino acids and the interactions of strychnine and picrotoxin. *Brain Res.* 25, 431–448.

Crossman, A. R., Walker, R. J. & Woodruff, G. N. (1973) Picrotoxin antagonism of γ-aminobutyric acid inhibitory response and synaptic inhibition in the rat substantia nigra. *Br. J. Pharmac.* 49, 696–698.

Curtis, D. R. (1975) Gamma-aminobutyric and glutamic acids as mammalian central transmitters. In: *Metabolic Compartmentation and Neurotransmission,* ed. Berl, S., Clarke, D. D. & Schneider, D. pp. 11–36. Plenum Press, New York.

Curtis, D. R. (1978) Pre- and non-synaptic activities of GABA and related amino acids in the mammalian nervous system. In: *Amino Acids as Chemical Transmitters,* ed. Fonnum, F. pp. 55–86. Plenum Press, New York.

Curtis, D. R., Duggan, A. W. & Felix, D. (1970a) GABA and inhibition of Deiters' neurones. *Brain Res.* 23, 117–120.

Curtis, D. R., Duggan, A. W., Felix, D. & Johnston, G. A. R. (1971) Bicuculline, an antagonist of GABA and synaptic inhibition in the spinal cord. *Brain Res.* 32, 69–96.

Curtis, D. R. & Felix D. (1971) The effect of bicuculline upon synaptic inhibition in the cerebral and cerebellar cortices of the cat. *Brain Res.* 34, 301–321.

Curtis, D. R., Felix, D. & McLennan, H. (1970b) GABA and hippocampal inhibition. *Br. J. Pharmac.* 40, 881–883.

Curtis, D. R., Hösli, L., Johnston, G. A. R. & Johnston, I. H. (1968) The hyperpolarization of spinal motoneurones by glycine and related amino acids. *Exp. Brain Res.* 5, 235–258.

Curtis, D. R. & Johnston, G. A. R. (1974a) Amino acid transmitters in the mammalian central nervous system. *Ergebn. Physiol.* 69, 97–188.

Curtis, D. R. & Johnston, G. A. R. (1974b) Convulsant alkaloids. In: *Neuropoisons*, vol. 2, ed. Simpson, L. L. & Curtis, D. R. pp. 207–248. Plenum Press, New York.

Curtis, D. R. & Tebēcis, A. K. (1972) Bicuculline and thalamic inhibition. Exp. Brain Res. 16, 210–218.

DeFeudis, F. V. (1975) Amino acids as central neurotransmitters. *Ann. Rev. Pharmac.* 15, 105–130.

DeFeudis, F. V. (1977) GABA-receptors in the vertebrate nervous system. *Prog. Neurobiol.* 9, 123–145.

DeFrance, J. F., Yoshihara, H., McCrea, R. A. & Kitai, S. T. (1975) Pharmacology of the inhibition in the lateral septal region. *Exp. Neurol.* 48, 502–523.

Dray, A., Gonye, T. J. & Oakley, N. R. (1976) Caudate stimulation and the substantia nigra activity in the rat. *J. Physiol.* (Lond). 259, 825–849.

Dreifuss, J. J., Kelly, J. S. & Krnjević, K. (1969) Cortical inhibition and γ-aminobutyric acid. *Exp. Brain Res.* 9, 137–154.

Enna, S. J., Collins, J. F. & Snyder, S. H. (1977) Stereospecificity and structure-activity requirements of GABA receptor binding in rat brain. *Brain Res.* 124, 185–190.

Feltz, P. (1971) γ-Aminobutyric acid and a caudato-nigral inhibition. *Can. J. Physiol. Pharmac.* 49, 1114–1115.

Fonnum, F. (1972a) Application of microchemical analysis and subcellular fractionation techniques to the study of neurotransmitters in discrete areas of mammalian brain. *Adv. Biochem. Psycopharmac.* 6, 75–88.

Fonnum, F. (1972b) Localization of cholinergic and γ-aminobutyric acid containing pathways in brain. In: *Metabolic Compartmentation in the Brain,* ed. Balazs, R. & Cremer, J. pp. 243–255. Macmillan, London.

Fonnum, F. ed. (1978) *Amino Acids as Chemical Transmitters.* Plenum Pres, New York.

Fonnum, F., Gottesfeld, Z. & Grofova, I. (1978) Distribution of glutamate decarboxylase, choline acetyltransferase and aromatic amino acid decarboxylase in the basal ganglia of normal and operated rats. Evidence for striatopallidal, striatoentopeduncular and striatonigral GABAergic fibres. *Brain Res.* 143, 125–138.

Fonnum, F. & Walberg, R. (1973) An estimation of the concentration of γ-aminobutyric acid and glutamate decarboxylase in the inhibitory Purkinje axon terminals in the cat. *Brain Res.* 54, 115–127.

Fukuda, J., Highstein, S. M. & Ito, M. (1972) Cerebellar inhibitory control of the vestibulo-ocular reflex investigated in rabbit IIIrd nucleus. *Exp. Brain Res.* 14, 511-526.

Game, C. J. A. & Lodge, D. (1975) The pharmacology of the inhibition of dorsal horn neurones by impulses in myelinated cutaneous afferents in the cat. *Exp. Brain Res.* 23, 75–84.

Graham, L. T. Jr. (1973) Distribution of glutamic acid decarboxylase activity and GABA content in the olfactory bulb. *Life Sci. Oxford* 12, 443–447.

Highstein, S. M. (1973) Synaptic linkage in the vestibulo-ocular and cerebello-vestibular pathways to the VIth nucleus in the rabbit. *Exp. Brain Res.* 17, 301–314.

Hökfelt, T. & Ljungdahl, Å. (1972) Autoradiographic identification of cerebral and cerebellar cortical neurons accumulating labelled gamma-aminobutyric acid (^{3}H-GABA). *Exp. Brain Res.* 14, 354–362.

Iversen, L. L., Dick, F., Kelly, J. S. & Schon, F. (1975) Uptake and localization of transmitter amino acids in the nervous system. In: *Metabolic Compartmentation and Neurotransmission,* ed. Berl, S. Clarke, D. D. & Schneider, D. pp. 65–89. Plenum Press, New York.

Johnston, G. A. R. (1976) Physiologic pharmacology of GABA and its antagonists in the vertebrate nervous system. In: *GABA in Nervous System Function,* ed. Roberts, E., Chase, T. N. & Tower, D. B. pp. 395–411. Raven Press, New York.

Johnston, G. A. R. (1978) Neuropharmacology of amino acid inhibitory transmitters. *Ann. Rev. Pharmac.* 18, 269–289.

Kawaguchi, S. & Ono, T. (1973) Bicuculline and picrotoxin sensitive inhibition in interpositus neurones of cat. *Brain Res.* 58, 260–265.

Kawamura, H. & Provini, L. (1970) Depression of cerebellar Purkinje cells by microiontophoretic application of GABA and related amino acids. *Brain Res.* 24, 293–304.

Kelly, J. S. & Renaud, L. P. (1973) On the pharmacology of ascending, descending and recurrent postsynaptic inhibition of the cuneo-thalamic relay cells in the cat. *Br. J. Pharmac.* 48, 396–408.

Krnjević, K. (1974) Chemical nature of synaptic transmission in vertebrates. *Physiol. Rev.* 54, 418–540.

Krnjević, K., Puil, E. & Werman, R. (1977a) GABA and glycine actions on spinal motoneurones. *Can. J. Physiol. Pharmac.* 55, 658–669.

Krnjević, K., Puil, E. & Werman, R. (1977b) Bicuculline, benzyl penicillin and inhibitory amino acids in the spinal cord of the cat. *Can. J. Physiol. Pharmac.* 55, 670–680.

Krogsgaard-Larsen, P. (1978) GABA agonists and uptake inhibitors of restricted conformations: structure-activity relations. In: *Amino Acids as Chemical Transmitters,* ed. Fonnum, F. pp. Plenum

Press, New York.

Levy, R. A. (1977) The role of GABA in primary afferent depolarization. *Prog. Neurobiol.* 9, 211–267.

Ljungdahl, Å. & Hökfelt, T. (1973) Autoradiographic uptake patterns of [^{3}H] GABA and [^{3}H] glycine in central nervous tissues with special reference to the cat spinal cord. *Brain Res.* 62, 587–595.

Lodge, D. & Curtis, D. R. (1978) Time course of GABA and glycine actions on cat spinal neurones: effect of pentobarbitone. *Neurosci. Lett.* 8, 125–129.

Lodge, D., Johnston, G. A. R., Curtis, D. R. & Brand, S. J. (1977) Effects of the *Areca* nut constituents arecaidine and guvacine on the action of GABA in the cat central nervous system. *Brain Res.* 136, 513–522.

McLaughlin, B. J., Wood, J. G., Saito, K., Barber, R., Vaughn, J. E., Roberts, E. & Wu, J–Y. (1974) The fine structural localization of glutamate decarboxylase in synaptic terminals of rodent cerebellum. *Brain Res.* 76, 377–391.

McLennan, H. (1971) The pharmacology of inhibition of mitral cells in the olfactory bulb. *Brain Res.* 29, 177–184.

McLennan, H. & Miller, J. J. (1974) γ-Aminobutyric acid and inhibition in the septal nuclei of the rat. *J. Physiol. (Lond).* 237, 625–633.

Martin, D. L. (1976) Carrier-mediated transport and removal of GABA from synaptic regions. In: *GABA in Nervous System Function,* ed. Roberts, E., Chase, T. N. & Tower, D. B. pp. 347–386. Raven Press, New York.

Möhler, H. & Okada, T. (1977) GABA receptor binding with ^{3}H(+)bicuculline-methiodide in rat CNS. *Nature, Lond.* 267, 65–67.

Morgan, R., Sillito, A. M. & Wolstencroft, J. H. (1976) The use of pharmacological agents to investigate inhibition in the lateral geniculate nucleus. In: *Drugs and Central Synaptic Transmission,* ed. Bradley, P. B. & Dhawan, B. N. pp. 263–271. Macmillan, London.

Nadler, J. V., White, W. F., Vaca, K. W. & Cotman, C. W. (1977) Calcium-dependent γ-aminobutyrate release by interneurons of rat hippocampal regions: lesion-induced plasticity. *Brain Res.* 131, 241–258.

Neal, M. J. (1976) Amino acid transmitter substances in the vertebrate retina. *Gen. Pharmac.* 7, 321–332.

Nicoll, R. A. (1971) Pharmacological evidence for GABA as the transmitter in granule cell inhibition in the olfactory bulb. *Brain Res.* 35, 137–149.

Obata, K. (1976) Release of GABA into the fourth ventricle. In: *GABA in Nervous System Function,* ed. Roberts, E., Chase, T. N. & Tower, D. B. pp. 251–254. Raven Press, New York.

Obata, K. & Highstein, S. M. (1970) Blocking by picrotoxin of both vestibular inhibition and GABA action on rabbit oculomotor neurones. *Brain Res.* 18, 538–541.

Obata, K., Takeda, K. & Shinozaki, H. (1970) Further study on pharmacological properties of the cerebellar-induced inhibition of Deiters neurones. *Exp. Brain Res.* 11, 327–342.

Obata, K. & Yoshida, M. (1973) Caudate-evoked inhibition and actions of GABA and other substances on cat pallidal neurons. *Brain Res.* 64, 455–459.

Okada, Y. & Shimada, C. (1976) Gamma-aminobutyric acid (GABA) concentration in a single neuron – localization of GABA in Deiters' neuron. *Brain Res.* 107, 658–662.

Olsen, R. W., Greenlee, D., Van Ness, P. & Ticku, M. K. (1978) Studies on the gamma-aminobutyric acid receptor/ionophore proteins in mammalian brain. In: *Amino Acids as Chemical Transmitters,* ed. Fonnum, F. pp. Plenum Press, New York.

Otsuka, M. & Konishi, S. (1976) GABA in the spinal cord. In: *GABA in Nervous System Function,* ed.

Roberts, E., Chase, T. N. & Tower, D. B. pp. 197–202. Raven Press, New York.

Otsuka, M. & Miyata, Y. (1972) Application of enzymatic cycling to the measurement of gamma-aminobutyric acid in single neurons of the mammalian central nervous system. *Adv. Biochem. Psychopharmac.* 6, 61–74.

Otsuka, M., Obata, K., Miyata, Y. & Tanaka, Y. (1971) Measurement of γ-aminobutyric acid in isolated nerve cells of cat central nervous system. *J. Neurochem.* 18, 287–295.

Peck, E. J. Jr., Schaeffer, J. M. & Clark. J. H. (1973) γ-Aminobutyric acid, bicuculline, and post-synaptic binding sites. *Biochem. biophys. Res. Commun.* 52, 394–400.

Precht, W., Baker, R. & Okada, Y. (1973a) Evidence for GABA as the synaptic transmitter of the inhibitory vestibulo-ocular pathway. *Exp. Brain Res.* 18, 415–428.

Precht, W., Schwindt, P. C. & Baker, R. (1973b) Removal of vestibular commissural inhibition by antagonists of GABA and glycine. *Brain Res.* 62, 222–226.

Precht, W. & Yoshida, M. (1971) Blockage of caudate-evoked inhibition of neurons in the substantia nigra by picrotoxin. *Brain Res.* 32, 229–233.

Ramon-Moliner, E. (1977) The reciprocal synapses of the olfactory bulb: questioning the evidence. *Brain Res.* 128, 1–20.

Ribak, C. E., Vaughn, J. E., Saito, K., Barber, R. & Roberts, E. (1976) Immunocytochemical localization of glutamate decarboxylase in rat substantia nigra. *Brain Res.* 116, 287–298.

Ribak, C. E., Vaughn, J. E., Saito, K., Barber, R. & Roberts, E. (1977) Glutamate decarboxylase localization in neurons of the olfactory bulb. *Brain Res.* 126, 1–18.

Roberts, E., Chase, T. N. & Tower, D. B. eds. (1976) *GABA in Nervous System Function,* Raven Press, New York.

Roberts, E. & Frankel, S. (1950) γ Aminobutyric acid in brain. Its formation from glutamic acid. *J. biol. Chem.* 187, 55–63.

Roffler-Tarlov, S. & Sidman, R. L. (1978) Concentrations of glutamic acid in cerebellar cortex and deep nuclei of normal mice and weaver, staggerer and nervous mutants. *Brain Res.* 142, 269–283.

Roffler-Tarlov, S. & Tarlov, E. (1975) Studies of suspected neurotransmitters in the vestibuloocular pathways. *Brain Res.* 95, 383–394.

Schon, F. & Iversen, L. L. (1972) Selective accumulation of [^{3}H]- GABA by stellate cells in rat cerebellar *in vivo. Brain Res.* 42, 503–507.

Siggins, G. R., Oliver, A. P., Hoffer, B. J. & Bloom, F. E. (1971) Cyclic adenosine monophosphate and norepinephrine: effects on transmembrane properties of cerebellar Purkinje cells. *Science, N. Y.* 171, 192–194.

Sillito, A. M. (1977) Inhibitory processes underlying the directional specificity of simple, complex and hypercomplex cells in the cat's visual cortex. *J. Physiol. (Lond).* 271, 699–720.

Spehlmann, R., Norcross, K. & Grimmer, E. J. (1977) GABA in the caudate nucleus: a possible synaptic transmitter of interneurones. *Experientia* 33, 623–625.

Storm-Mathisen, J. (1977) Localization of transmitter candidates in the brain: the hippocampal formation as a model. *Prog. Neurobiol.* 8, 119–181.

Tappaz, M. L. & Brownstein, M. J. (1977) Origin of glutamate decarboxylase (GAD)-containing cells in discrete hypothalamic nuclei. *Brain Res.* 132, 95–106.

Wilkin, G., Wilson, J. E., Balazs, R., Schon, F. & Kelly, J. S. (1974) How selective is high affinity uptake of GABA into inhibitory nerve terminals? *Nature, Lond.* 252, 397–399.

Wood, J. G., McLaughlin, B. J. & Vaughn, J. E. (1976) Immunocytochemical localization of GAD in electron microscopic preparations of rodent CNS. In: *GABA in Nervous System Function, ed. Roberts, E., Chase, T. N. & Tower, D. B. pp. 133–148. Raven Press, New York.*

New Directions in GABA Research I: Immunocytochemical Studies of GABA Neurons

Eugene Roberts

There now is a vast literature dealing with GABA function and metabolism. I will not make an attempt to summarize it here in the short space allowed, since this has been done in a number of recent books and reviews. Instead, I will deal with some of the work currently going on in our laboratories in which we are attempting to delineate the rôle of GABA neurons in information processing in the vertebrate nervous system. One of our major areas of concern is that dealing with the localization of GABA-releasing neurons.

The demonstration that a synapse is a GABA-releasing one is not sufficient evidence to identify it unequivocally as an inhibitory synapse. Supporting physiological evidence always is necessary for such a functional assignment to be made. However in almost all instances adequately studied to date the overall effects of GABA, where GABA synapses have been proven to exist, have been found to be inhibitory either at pre- or postsynaptic sites. GABA typically produces an increase in membrane permeability to Cl^- ions that can be measured as an increase in membrane conductance. It is in this way that this naturally occurring transmitter can counteract the depolarizing action of exitatory processes to maintain the polarization of a cell at an equilibrium level near that of its resting value, acting essentially as a chemical voltage clamp. In most

* Division of Neurosciences, City of Hope National Medical Center, Duarte, Ca., USA.

This work was supported in part by USPHS Grants NS01615 and NS12116 from the National Institute of Neurological and Communicative Disorders and Stroke, and Grant MH22438 awarded by the National Institute of Mental Health, DHEW. This paper was written while the author was a Fellow at the Center for Advanced Study in the Behavioral Sciences, Stanford, and supported in part by grant BNS-76-22943 from the National Science Foundation.

instances studied, GABA has been shown to exert a hyperpolarizing or inhibitory effect via the above mechanism. However, when there are relatively high intracellular Cl^- concentrations, GABA can produce a decrease in membrane potential or depolarization, a mechanism probably involved in presynaptic inhibition.

The importance of detailed physiological analysis employing suitable intracellular recording techniques in ascribing functional roles to GABA neurons and in studies of GABA agonists and antagonists cannot be overemphasized. Although there often is a close relationship between the generator potential and frequency of firing, it is well known that a variety of chemical and physical changes can produce a dissociation or uncoupling between the two. Therefore, mechanisms of actions of substances on membranes cannot be established definitively from experiments in which only their effects on firing rates of neurons are determined.

IDENTIFYING GABA-RELEASING NEURONS IN REGIONS OF THE VERTEBRATE CNS

Until quite recently the localization of GABA neurons have been inferred by correlating microchemical, electrophysiological, and iontophoretic studies with what was known of the cytoarchitecture of specific regions of brain and spinal cord. A commonly used approach has been to study a particular biochemical variable in whole brain or in anatomically defined regions of brain or spinal cord. Analyses of GABA contents and GAD activities have been performed in almost all identifiable brain structures and in the spinal cord. Some studies have combined biochemical analyses with lesioning procedures in correlating specific neural degenerations with losses of GAD and GABA. Several examples of this approach have been reported at this conference. The distributions of the components of the GABA system also have been studied extensively by subcellular fractionation techniques in preparations from whole brain or selected regions. Although highly informative and necessary for range-finding, interpretation of results from the above types of analyses at the cellular level suffer from the lack of definition attributable to the presence of myriad cells of different types in any dissected region; and it is difficult to make definitive conclusions about specific synaptic connectivities from them. Individual cell bodies of large neurons, such as Purkinje and Deiters' cells, and even portions thereof, have been dissected out and subjected to microanalyses. In the latter instances it is not always possible to ensure absence of contaminating presynaptic endings from other neurons or of glial cell constituents, and therefore, their contribution to a particular measured chemical variable. The technical difficulties involved in the latter type of work usually preclude the study of large numbers of neurons in this manner.

The above approaches have not made it possible to obtain a definitive understanding of how GABA neurons might participate in information processing in different parts of the vertebrate CNS. Direct visualization of GABA neurons and nerve endings at histological and cytological levels was necessary. The purification of mouse brain glutamate decarboxylase (GAD), the enzyme that catalyzes the formation of GABA from glutamic acid, and the preparation of antibodies to it now has provided a means for the direct visualization of GABA neurons and their endings at the light and electron microscopic levels through the use of immunocytochemical peroxidase labeling procedures. The basic strategy employed by us, the chronology of its achievement, and the names of the participating scientists are shown in Table I. Many appropriate citations to pertinent literature can be found in the references cited. The publications listed also can be consulted for relevant technical details. GABA neurons have been found to form axodendritic, axosomatic, axoaxonic,

---

Fig. 1. Electron micrographs of various types of synaptic junctions formed by presynaptic terminals which contain glutamate decarboxylase (GAD), the enzyme that synthesizes the neurotransmitter γ-aminobutyric acid (GABA). All specimens were obtained from rat CNS. (a) Axodendritic synapses in the substantia nigra. Two axon terminals (T_1 and T_2) filled with electron opaque, GAD-positive reaction product are shown to synapse with a dendritic shaft (D) in the pars reticulata. One of the terminals (T_1) forms an asymmetric synaptic junction (arrow), while the other terminal (T_2) forms a symmetric synapse (arrow). ×44,000. (b) An axoaxonal synapse in the cerebral cortex. A GAD-positive axon terminal (T) is shown forming a symmetric synapse (arrow) with an axon initial segment identified by a dense undercoating of the axolemma (arrow heads) and a fasciculation of microtubules (e.g. asterisk). ×20.000.

(c) An axosomatic synapse in the dorsal horn of the spinal cord. A probable synaptic junction (arrow) is shown between a GAD-positive terminal (T) and a neuron (N) in the substantia gelatinosa. X 26,000. (d) An axoaxonal synapse in the dorsal horn of the spinal cord. A synaptic junction (white arrow) is shown between the GAD-positive presynaptic terminal (T_1) and another synaptic terminal (T) which is not GAD-positive. In addition, T_2 is the presynaptic component of another synaptic junction (black arrow) with a dendrite (D). X 38.000. (e) Dendrodendritic synapses in the glomerular layer of the olfactory bulb. Two GAD-positive gemmules (D_1, D_2) from dendrites of periglomerular neurons form synapses with a mitral/tufted dendritic shaft (D_3). One gemmule (D_1 appears to form a reciprocal synapse and the other gemmule (D_2) appears to be presynaptic only. x 54,000. Directions of synaptic transmission are indicated by arrows in a-e. Electron micrographs provided by R. P. Barber, B. J. McLaughlin, C. E. Ribak, and J. E. Vaughn.

and dendrodendritic synapses in the various regions of the rat CNS studied to date, which include spinal cord, cerebellum, cortex, hippocampus, olfactory bulb, retina, substantia nigra, and striatum. In Fig. 1 are shown electron

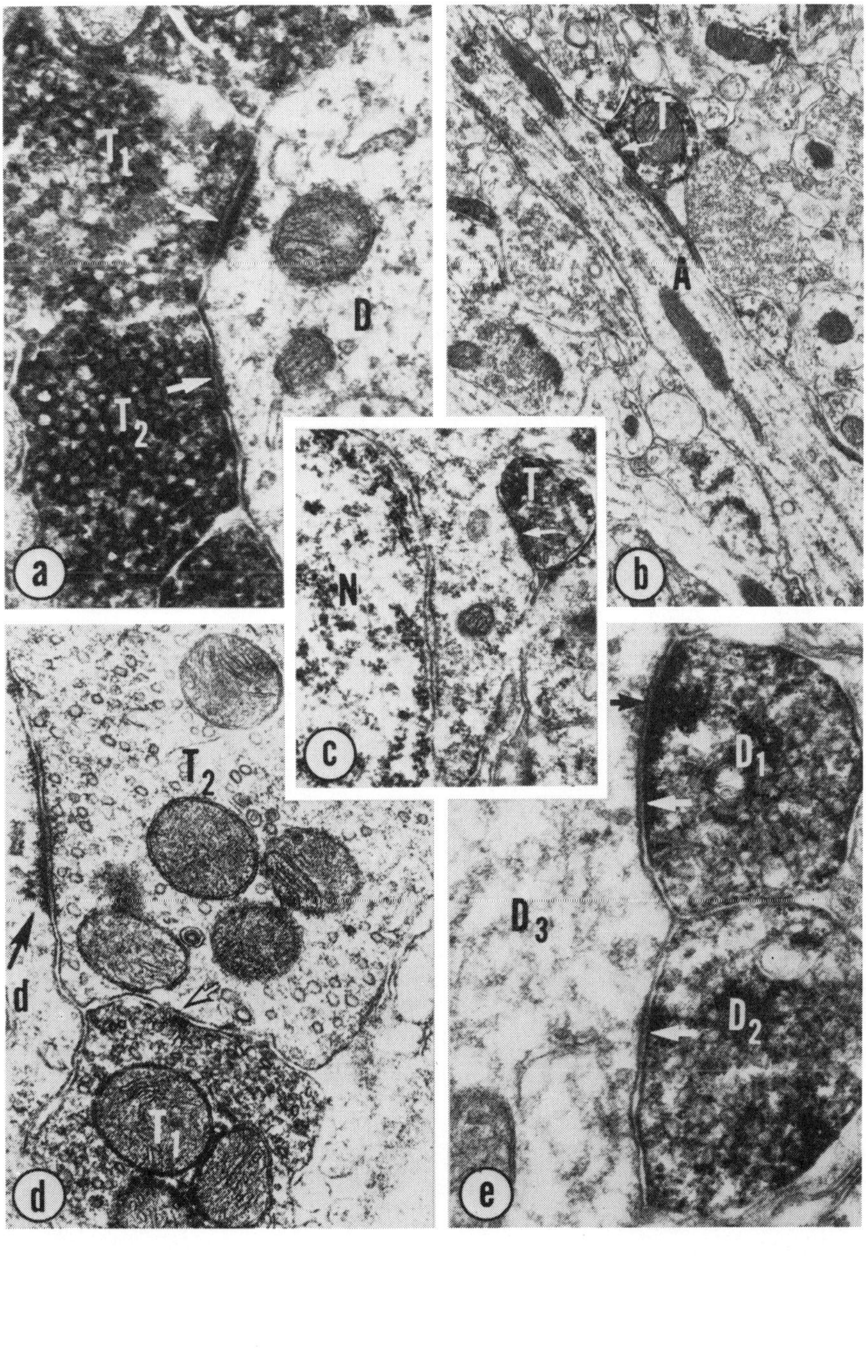

micrographs of various types of synaptic junctions formed by presynaptic terminals containing GAD. In almost all instances several, if not all, of these types of GABA synapses are found in close proximity to each other.

Only a few of the salient findings in the several regions of rat brain studied to date will be mentioned below.

Cerebellum

The cerebellum has been by far the most favorable first site for investigation of possible substances which may mediate the activity of neurons with inhibitory functions because more extensive correlative neuroanatomical and neurophysiological analyses have been made of the cerebellum than of any other structure in the vertebrate brain.

Even our first comprehensive biochemical laminar analyses of the GABA system *suggested* the possibility that all of the inhibitory cells of the cerebellum (Purkinje, basket, stellate and Golgi) might use GABA as transmitter. Subsequently, evidence was adduced for the occurrence of both GAD and GABA in high concentrations in the deep cerebellar nuclei, where the Purkinje cell axons terminate. Electrophysiological and pharmacological studies suggested strongly that Purkinje cell terminals might liberate GABA as transmitter. Our first application of the immunoperoxidase technique at the light level showed an intense punctuate deposition of reaction product around the Purkinje cells and around the neurons of the deep cerebellar nuclei, cells known to receive an inhibitory synaptic input from the Purkinje cells, suggesting the impingement of many nerve terminals containing GAD upon these neuronal surfaces (Saito *et al.* 1974). At the electron microscopic level GAD appeared to be highly localized in certain synaptic terminals in close association with the membranes of synaptic vesicles and mitochondria, but not within these organelles (McLaughlin *et al.* 1974). GAD-positive terminals, presumably largely from Purkinje cells, were seen on the somata and proximal dendrites of neurons in the deep cerebellar nuclei. Similarly, terminals presumably arising form basket, stellate and Golgi type II cells also were strongly positive for the enzyme. Thus, all of the cerebellar cortical cells known to be inhibitory were shown probably to use GABA as transmitter. Direct injections of colchicine into the cerebellar cortex, disrupting axoplasmic transport, made it possible to demonstrate that the proximal dendrites and somata of Purkinje and Golgi type II neurons and the somata of basket and stellate cells contained detectable accumulations of GAD-positive reaction product (Ribak *et al.* 1978). The

Table I
Immunocytochemistry of GABA-Related Enzymes

Steps along the way	Date	References
1. Purification and Properties		
GAD		
Purification and characterization of glutamate decarboxylase from mouse brain	1973	Wu, Matsuda & Roberts
Electrophoresis of glutamic acid decarboxylase from mouse brain in sodium dodecyl sulfate polyacrylamide gels	1973	Matsuda, Wu & Roberts
Properties of brain L-glutamate decarboxylase: inhibition studies	1974	Wu & Roberts
GABA-T		
Purification and characterization of the 4-aminobutyrate-2-ketoglutarate transaminase from mouse brain	1973	Schousboe, Wu & Roberts
Subunit structure and kinetic properties of 4-aminobutyrate-2-ketoglutarate transaminase purified from mouse brain	1974	Schousboe, Wu & Roberts
Summary		
Purification, characterization, and kinetic studies of GAD and GABA-T from mouse brain	1976	Wu
2. Immunological Studies		
GAD		
Immunochemical studies on glutamic decarboxylase from mouse brain	1973	Matsuda, Wu & Roberts
Immunochemical comparisons of vertebrate glutamic acid decarboxylase	1974	Saito, Wu, Matsuda & Roberts
Immunochemical studies of brain glutamate decarboxylase and GABA-transaminase of six inbred strain of mice	1974	Wong, Schousboe, Saito, Wu & Roberts
GABA-T		
Some immunochemical properties and species specificity of GABA-*α*-ketoglutarate	1974	Saito, Schousboe, Wu & Roberts
Summary		
Immunochemical studies of glutamate decarboxylase and GABA-*α*-ketoglutarate transaminase	1976	Saito
3. Immunocytochemical Approaches		
GAD		
Immunohistochemical localization of glutamate decarboxylase in rat cerebellum	1974	Saito, Barber, Wu, Matsuda, Roberts & Vaughn
The fine structural localization of glutamate decarboxylase in synaptic terminals of rodent cerebellum	1974	McLaughlin, Wood, Saito, Barber, Vaughn, Roberts & Wu

Table I

Steps along the way	Date	References
The fine structural localization of glutamate decarboxylase in developing axonal processes and presynaptic terminals of rodent cerebellum	1975	McLaughlin, Wood, Saito, Roberts & Wu
Immunocytochemical localization of glutamate decarboxylase in rat spinal cord	1975	McLaughlin, Barber, Saito, Roberts & Wu
Immunocytochemical localization of glutamate decarboxylase in the substantia nigra of the rat	1976	Ribak, Vaughn, Saito & Barber
Immunocytochemical localization of glutamate decarboxylase in rat substantia nigra	1976	Ribak, Vaughn, Saito, Barber & Roberts
Immunocytochemical localization of glutamate decarboxylase (GAD) in the olfactory bulb	1976	Ribak, Vaughn & Saito
Glutamate decarboxylase (GAD) localization in neurons of the olfactory bulb	1977	Ribak, Vaughn, Saito, Barber & Roberts
Immunocytochemical localization of GAD in somata and dendrites of GABA-ergic neurons following colchicine treatment	1976	Ribak & Vaughn
The immunocytochemical localization of GAD within stellate neurons of rat visual cortex	1977	Ribak
Immunocytochemical localization of glutamic acid decarboxylase in neuronal somata following colchicine inhibition of axonal transport	1978	Ribak, Vaughn & Saito
GABAergic terminals are presynaptic to primary afferent terminals in the substantia gelatinosa of the rat spinal cord	1978	Barber, Vaughn, Saito, McLaughlin & Roberts
Immunocytochemical localization of GAD in electron microscopic preparations of rodent CNS	1976	Wood, McLaughlin & Vaughn
Aspinous and sparsely-spinous stellate neurons contain glutamic acid decarboxylase in the visual cortex of rats	1978	Ribak
Immunocytochemical identification of GABAergic neurons in rat retina	1978	Vaughn, Barber, Saito, Roberts & Famiglietti
Immunocytochemical localization of glutamic acid decarboxylase (GAD) in the rat corpus striatum	1978	Ribak

Table I

Steps along the way	Date	References
GABAergic axon terminals decrease at experimental seizure foci in monkey cerebral cortex	1978	Ribak, Harris, Anderson, Vaughn & Roberts
GABA-T		
See Wood *et al.* (24)		
Summaries		
Light microscopic visualization of GAD and GABA-T in immunocytochemical preparations of rodent CNS	1976	Barber & Saito
Immunochemistry of the GABA system – a novel approach to an old transmitter	1976	Roberts
Immunocytochemical identification of GABAergic neurons	1977	Saito, Roberts & Barber
Rôles of GABA neurons in information processing in the vertebrate CNS	1978	Roberts

GAD-positive reaction product was concentrated around the cisternae of the Golgi apparatus and was not seen in nuclei or nucleoli. The latter observations are beginning to forge the necessary link between the presence of GAD in the terminals of all of the known inhibitory neurons in the cerebellar cortex and the synthesis and transport of the enzyme in these cells to sites of functional import.

In the developing rat cerebellum, GAD was present in growing neurites in close association with small vesicles prior to the time the neurites make protosynaptic contacts; differentiation of these contacts coincided with the sequestration of GAD into synaptic terminals (McLaughlin *et al.* 1975). It appears that the initial signal for GAD synthesis predates the establishment of contacts between pre- and postsynaptic elements of a developing synapse. One would like to know whether the same is true for GABA receptor-ionophore complexes or whether contact between GAD-containing nerve endings and the postsynaptic membranes must take place prior to the synthesis of the individual components and the organization of these complexes.

Spinal Cord

Light microscopic localization of GAD in the rat lumbosacral spinal cord showed heavy, punctate GAD-positive reaction product in the dorsal horn laminae I–III (McLaughlin *et al.* 1975, Barber *et al.* 1978). Moderately heavy reaction product was also seen in the deeper dorsal horn laminae IV–VI, the medial aspect to the intermediate gray (lamina VII), and the region around the central canal (lamina X). A moderately light concentration of GAD-positive reaction product was observed in the ventral horn, and punctate deposits of reaction product also were seen on motoneuron cell bodies. The visually observed punctate distribution of GAD-positive reaction product described above corresponded to GAD-positive synaptic terminals visualized by electron microscopy in comparable regions. Many more GAD-positive terminals were observed in dorsal horn laminae I–III than in deeper laminae IV–VI. GAD-containing terminals in the dorsal horn were presynaptic to dendrites, cell bodies, and other axon terminals. The latter were more numerous in laminae II and III. GAD-positive synaptic terminals were presynaptic to large and small dendrites and motoneuron somata in the motor nuclei. In addition, small GAD-containing terminals also were presynaptic to larger axonal terminals which were in turn preynaptic to motoneuron somata. The observation of GAD-positive terminals presynaptic to dendrites and cell bodies in both dorsal and ventral horns was compatible with the evidence suggesting that GABA terminals may mediate postsynaptic inhibition of spinal interneurons and motoneurons.

Multiple dorsal rhizotomies were performed unilaterally at lumbar levels L1–L4 in adult rats, and the spinal cords were examined 24 hours later (Barber *et al.* 1978). Large numbers of degenerating terminals, probably entirely from cutaneous afferents, were observed in the ipsilateral substantia gelatinosa, but not contralaterally. However, the distribution of GAD-positive reaction product, most intense within laminae II and III, appeared to be normal on both sides of the cord. Electron microscopically, primary afferent terminals were found in various stages of degeneration on the side of the rhizotomies, and GAD-positive axon terminals were found to be presynaptic to degenerating primary afferent terminals in the substantia gelatinosa. The data furnish a chemomorphological basis for the conclusion that the presynaptic inhibition of primary afferents is mediated by axoaxonal synapses formed between GABA-releasing interneurons and primary sensory neurons. A detailed analysis of the various synaptic relationships of GAD-positive terminals in the dorsal horn of the rat spinal cord has led to reasonable hypotheses about how release of GABA from such terminals could participate in such presynaptically modulated phenomena as primary afferent depolarization, the dorsal root reflex. and primary afferent hyperpolarization. A schematization of some of the relations of GABA-ergic neurons in the substantia gelatinosa is shown in Fig. 2.

Olfactory bulb

light microscopic studies demonstrated GAD-positive puncta throughout all layers of the olfactory bulb with the greatest concentration in the external plexiform layer in the glomeruli of the glomerular layer (Ribak *et al.* 1977). The cytoplasm of many neuronal somata in the granule and glomerular cell layers was GAD-positive, but not the cytoplasm of mitral and tufted cell somata. The GAD-positive staining of presumed granule and periglomerular neuronal somata also extended into their dendrites for many microns.

Electron microscopic observations confirmed the presence of GAD-positive reaction product within the cytoplasm of granule and periglomerular neurons. Also, in the external plexiform layer, reaction product filled many of the granule cell gemmules which form reciprocal dendrodendritic synapses with mitral cell dendrites. The presence of GAD within granule and periglomerular cells lends support to suggestions based on previous physiologic and pharmacologic studies that these inhibitory interneurons use GABA as their neurotransmitter.

Basal ganglia

Large amounts of GAD-positive reaction product, seen throughout the substantia nigra in the light microscopic preparations, appeared to be localized in punctate structures that were apposed to dendrites and somata (Ribak *et al.* 1976). Electron microscopic studies revealed that most of the axon terminals in the substantia nigra were filled with GAD-positive reaction product and formed both axodendritic and axosomatic synapses. Many dendrites were extensively surrounded by GAD-positive terminals, which most commonly formed symmetric synaptic junctions. The results were consistent with biochemical, pharmacologic, and physiologic data which previously had indicated that neurons of the neostriatum and globus pallidus could exert a GABA-mediated, postsynaptic inhibition upon the neurons of the substantia nigra. The GAD-positive somata in the globus pallidus were medium-sized neurons. In the striatum the medium-sized spiny neurons, with round or fusiform shapes, appeared to be GABA-ergic (Ribak 1978). The pattern of GAD-positive terminals associated with dendrites of pallidal neurons resembled that observed in the substantia nigra.

Cortex

GAD was observed in somata, proximal dendrites and axon terminals of nonpyramidal neurons in the rat visual cortex in all cortical layers, including the

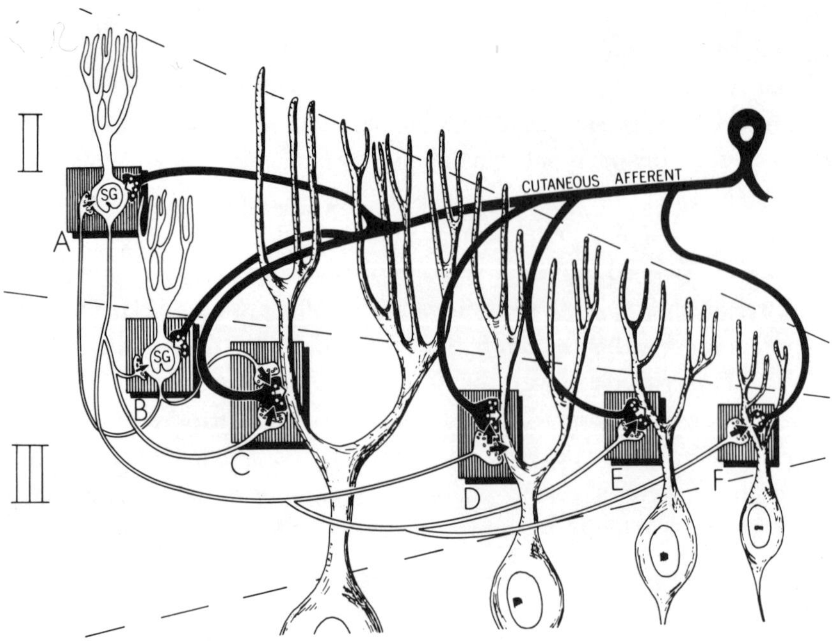

Fig. 2. Schematic representation of possible synaptic pathways within the substantia gelatinosa (Rexed's laminae II and III) which involve both GABA-ergic and primary afferent axon terminals. GABA-ergic, substantia gelatinosa neurons (SG) are white, and a primary afferent neuron is black. The single primary afferent neuron represents all of the different neurons of this class whose axons terminate in the substantia gelatinosa. Black arrows indicate the direction of GABA-ergic synaptic transmission, and white arrows indicate the direction of primary afferent synaptic transmission.

In a number of the synaptic complexes observed, a GAD-positive terminal was presynaptic to a primary afferent terminal, and in addition both kinds of terminals (i.e., GAD-positive and primary afferent terminals) were presynaptic to the same dendritic profile (Fig. 2D). In these cases, the same GABA-ergic axon terminal could mediate both presynaptic and postsynaptic inhibition. Depolarization of a primary afferent axon terminal by GABA could mean that a subsequent primary afferent volley would result in less transmitter being released. This reduced amount of released primary afferent transmitter would also have to exert its effect upon a postsynaptic dendrite that has been hyperpolarized by the action of a GABA-ergic axodendritic synapse. Consequently, there would be a further reduction of the effectiveness of the primary afferent transmitter substance in producing an excitatory postsynaptic potential in the second order neuron. It is plausible to assume that inhibitory synaptic complexes such as those established by the GABA-ergic terminals which make synaptic contacts with both pre- and postsynaptic elements (Fig. 2D) and those established by several GABA-ergic presynaptic terminals with the same primary afferent terminal (Fig. 2C) could form the center of the inhibitory gradient which has been described surrounding primary afferent fibers immediately following an afferent volley. The scheme illustrating possible synaptic pathways involved in a GABA-ergic modification of primary afferent activity (Fig. 2) is largely based upon data accrued from investigation of rat lumbar spinal cord. However, primary afferent depolarization has been shown to occur at several spinal levels as well as in the cuneate

immediate subjacent white matter (Ribak 1978). GAD-positive terminals formed symmetric synaptic junctions most commonly with dendritic shafts and somata of pyramidal and stellate neurons and less frequently with initial axon segments of pyramidal neurons and dendritic spines. Extensively pericellular plexus were formed by these terminals with the somata of pyramidal neurons in layers III and V. Detailed morphological study of the GAD-positive neurons indicate that they are aspinous and sparsely-spinous stellate interneurons with extensive intracortical axonal arborizations. At the light level GAD-positive somata were seen to have GAD-positive terminals upon their surfaces. The localization of GAD within these neurons in combination with physiologic and pharmacologic data indicate that these local circuit neurons mediate GABA-ergic inhibition and disinhibition in the neocortex and probably play a key rôle in information processing.

Virtually from the beginning of physiologic and pharmacologic observations of the GABA system it has been conjectured that decreases in the efficacy of this system could result in convulsive seizures (Roberts *et al.* 1960). The availability of the immunocytochemical techniques for visualization of GABA-ergic neurons and of sections from sensorimotor cortex obtained from five epileptic monkeys treated with alumina cream has made it possible to determine whether or not a correlation exists between epileptic activity and effects on GABA neurons (Ribak *et al.* 1978). Mean numbers of GAD-positive terminals determined in contiguous area from the bottom of layer VI to the middle of layer V showed in each instance a highly significant reduction in numbers of GAD-positive terminals at the site of alumina gel application (A) by comparison with the contralateral homotopic cortex (C). Ipsilateral sections further away from the alumina gel (B) showed significantly higher numbers of GABA-ergic endings than A and significantly lower ones than C. These results support the idea that a selective loss of inhibitory GABA-ergic neurons, aspinous and sparsely-spinous

---

nucleus, and it appears to be mediated by GABA in several species. Therefore, primary afferent depolarization that is mediated by the synaptic transmitter GABA would appear to be a rather general mechanism for the regulation of transmitter release from primary afferent terminals. On this basis, it is reasonable to suggest that synaptic pathways similar to those illustrated in Fig. 2 may be generally distributed throughout the substantia gelatinosa. Thus such pathways may provide repetitive units in which GABA-ergic interneurons presynaptically modulate the various exteroceptive impulses carried to the substantia gelatinosa by primary afferent fibers. (Fig. 2 taken from Barber *et al.* 1978)

stellate cells, could be responsible for the epileptic activity observed at seizure foci. Further work along this line is in progress.

Retina

Dense aggregations of GAD-positive puncta appear to form four separate sublayers within the inner plexiform layer of rat retina, a broad sublayer being adjacent to both the inner nuclear and ganglion cell layers, and two thin sublayers lying in the middle portion of the inner nuclear layer (Vaughn *et al.* 1978). GAD-positive staining was not observed in any of the other retinal layers. Electron microscopy showed GABA-ergic terminals from amacrine cells ending on bipolar and amacrine cell processes and on ganglion cell dendrites and somata. GAD-positive terminals were also postsynaptic to bipolar cells and occasionally were observed to form reciprocal synapses with bipolar terminals. It appears from the results that some classes of amacrine cells are the only GABA-ergic neurons in rat retina. It will be important to determine whether other transmitters, which are believed by some to be dopamine, glycine, and taurine, are found in some amacrine cells and what their relations are to the GABA-ergic amacrines.

Hippocampus

Some of the GAD-positive puncta appeared in light microscopy as pericellular baskets around pyramidal and granule cell somata and these puncta corresponded to the known distribution of basket cell axon terminals (Barber & Saito 1976, Ribak *et al.* 1978). Also GAD-positive reaction product was observed in somata and dendrites. GAD-positive reaction product filled the somata and bipolar dendrites of many horizontal neurons located near the boundary between stratum oriens and the alveus. The majority of the GAD-positive somata in stratum radiatum and stratum lacunosum corresponded to those of horizontal and other short-axon neurons. Granule and pyramidal cells did not appear to contain GAD-positive reaction product either in light or electron microscopic preparations. Some of the GAD-positive axon terminals formed symmetrical synaptic junctions with pyramidal and granule cell somata and their dendritic shafts. The GAD-positive terminals forming axosomatic synapses corresponded in location to the endings of basket cells, known indigenous inhibitory interneurons.

GABA NEURONS AND PROBLEMS OF FUNCTIONAL COORDINATION IN THE NERVOUS SYSTEM

The successful or adaptive operation of a nervous system requires a coordination of neuronal activity which can determine the ability of an individual to prevent the too-frequent firing of preprogrammed circuits of behavioral options spontaneously or maladaptively; and, under a variety of environmental circumstances, internal and external, it must maintain within physiologic limits the rates of operation of continuously needed neuronal circuits, such as those required for cardiac function, respiration, and maintenance of blood pressure. When gross malfunctions of the coordination of inhibitory and disinhibitiory neuronal system occur, there may result lethal effects either through generalized seizures or cessation of operation of some vital function; alternatively, some obviously severe neurological and psychological dysfunctions may occur.

When there is incoordination between the GABA system and other neurotransmitter systems, for whatever reason, the defect might be restricted to a local brain region, might include several regions, or might be global throughout the CNS. Under relatively simple environmental conditions, the nervous system in such individuals could function in an apparently adequate adaptive manner, which might appear to be in the normal range. As the complexity and intensity of environmental inputs is increased, there would be a correlated increased degree of incoordination. Then, those systems in the nervous system that are most poorly controlled will tend to break down under the stress and produce symptoms that are consequent to such a breakdown.

Let us suppose that for some reason in the entire brain or in specific regions, the inhibitory GABA neurons have a considerably lower-than-normal effectiveness on their recipient neurons, which, themselves, are normally effective. As the complexity and intensity of environmental inputs is increased, there would be an increase of excitatory influences on pacesetter neurons. More-than-normal numbers of behavioral options or inappropriate ones would be released (behavior disorders, mania, schizophrenia, etc.); choreic movements, seizures, or spasticity might occur; there might be hypersensitivity to pain,etc.; and abnormal fluctuations would be observed in autonomic functions. Recent experimental results suggest that GABA neurons may play an important role in control mechanisms in several hypothalamic centers. Thus, if specific hypothalamic regions were affected, greater-than-normal degrees of changes in responses might be observed in emotional reactivity, cardiac and respiratory functions, blood pressure, food and water intake, sweating, galvanic skin response, insulin secretion, liberation of gastric acid, motility of the colon, etc.

Application to Human Studies

It certainly seems likely that in epilepsy (Roberts *et al.* 1960, Ribak *et al.* 1978), schizophrenia (Roberts 1972, 1977, Bird *et al.* 1977), and Huntington's and Parkinson's diseases (Iversen *et al.* 1978, McGeer & McGeer 1978) deficiencies might exist in the relative numbers of GABA neurons in specific brain areas, or that there might be defects in the structural or functional relationships of GABA neurons to other neurons, which either might inhibit or excite them, or which they, themselves, presumably might inhibit. This would necessitate being able to locate the GABA neurons and/or their processes at both the histological and ultrastructural levels.

Application of the currently available immunocytochemical tools to human material is difficult, and at the present time probably would have to be restricted to studies at the light microscopic level. The immunocytochemical technique for GAD requires fixation for ultrastructural analysis by rapid and adequate perfusion, a procedure that normally would not be feasible in human material, which usually is obtained only at autopsy several hours after death. Furthermore, the techniques could only be applied to small, specific regions, since they do not lend themselves to broad screening approaches. It would seem to me that it would be minimally informative to study tissue with extensive pathological changes such as the striatum in Huntington's disease or the substantia nigra in advanced Parkinsonism. On the other hand, it might be most interesting to examine regions of the ventrobasal complex of the thalamus in Huntington's chorea, since, in the absence of grossly observable pathological changes in this region, quantitative cytometric measurements showed there to be a loss of more than 50% of small Golgi type II neurons (presumably GABA interneurons) in the ventrolateral thalamus by comparison with controls and a decrease in size of those cells remaining (Dom 1976, Dom *et al.* 1976). The latter type of neuron appeared unaffected in other thalamic sites. A loss of coordinative neural elements in the ventrolateral thalamus, a key relay station for processing information involved in motor control and muscle tone could be importantly related to the choreic symptoms of the disease. Detailed immunocytochemical study of GABA neurons in this region might give important leads about the primary degenerative changes that occur in Huntington's disease.

The largest and best controlled series of measurements on autopsy tissue obtained from schizophrenic and non-schizophrenic individuals has shown there to be a statistically significant reduction in the GAD level in the nucleus accumbens of the schizophrenic patients (Bird *et al.* 1977). The latter region could be profitably studied with the immunocytochemical technique for clues about possible neuropathologic correlates. Results of a much smaller series than the latter showed that of six brain regions measured, not including the nucleus accumbens or other limbic structures, only in the case of the thalamus were the values in the schizophrenic brains lower than those of the normal controls at the 5% level of significance (Roberts 1977). In this connection, it is of considerable interest that, of the various thalamic regions studied, only the pulvinar showed a significant decrement (40%) in the number of Golgi type II neurons in the brains of catatonic schizophrenic patients in comparison with controls (Dom 1976). Since the pulvinar plays an important rôle in coordinating visual and auditory inputs, the cellular defect observed might be associated with the well-known hallucinatory phenomena observed in the above state.

Many studies of the neuropathology of neurologic and psychiatric disorders will be helped greatly when the materials and techniques become more generally available not only for the visualization of GABA neurons and their processes, but also for the neurons specializing in the release of the other neurotransmitters or neuromodulators.

REFERENCES

Barber, R. & Saito, K. (1976) Light microscopic visualization of GAD and GABA-T in immunocytochemical preparations of rodent CNS. In: *GABA in Nervous System Function,* ed. Roberts, E. Chase, T. N. & Tower, D. B., pp. 113-132. Raven Press, N.Y.

Barber, R., Vaughn, J. E., Saito, K., McLaughlin, B. J. & Roberts, E. (1978) GABA-ergic terminals are presynaptic to primary afferent terminals in the substantia gelatinosa of the rat spinal cord. *Brain Res.* 141, 35–55.

Bird, E D., Spokes, E. G., Barnes, J., Mackay, A. V. P., Iversen, L. L. & Shepherd, M. (1977) Increased brain dopamine and reduced glutamic acid decarboxylase and choline acetyl transferase activity in schizophrenia and related psychoses. *Lancet* ii, 1157–1159.

Dom, R. (1976) *Neostriatal and Thalamic Interneurons: Their Role in the Pathophysiology of Huntington's Chorea, Parkinson's Disease and Catatonic Schizophrenia,* Catholic University of Leuven, Belgium.

Dom, R., Malfroid, M. & Baro, F. (1976) Neuropathology of Huntington's chorea: Studies of the ventrobasal complex of the thalamus. *Neurology* 26, 64–68.

Iversen, L. L., Spokes, E. & Bird, E. (1978) Agonist specificity of GABA binding sites in human brain and GABA in Huntington's disease and schizophrenia. This Symposium.

Matsuda, T., Wu, J.-Y. & Roberts, E. (1973) Immunocytochemical studies on glutamic decarboxylase from mouse brain. *J. Neurochem.* 21, 159–166.

Matsuda, T., Wu, J.-Y. & Roberts, E. (1973) Electrophoresis of glutamic acid decarboxylase from mouse brain in sodium dodecyl sulfate polyacrylamide gels. *J. Neurochem.* 21, 167–172.

McGeer, E. G. & McGeer, P. L. (1978) GABA-containing neurons in schizophrenia, Huntington's chorea and normal aging. This Symposium.

McLaughlin, B. J., Barber, R., Saito, K., Roberts, E. & Wu, J.-Y. (1975) Immunocytochemical localization of glutamate decarboxylase in rat spinal cord. *J. Comp. Neurol.* 164, 305–321.

McLaughlin, B. J., Wood, J., Saito, K., Barber, R., Vaughn, J. E., Roberts, E. & Wu, J.-Y. (1974) The fine structural localization of glutamate decarboxylase in synaptic terminals of rodent cerebellum. *Brain Res.* 76, 377–391.

McLaughlin, B. J., Wood, J. G., Saito, K., Roberts, E. & Wu, J.-Y. (1975) The fine structural localization of glutamate decarboxylase in developing axonal processes and presynaptic terminals of rodent cerebellum. *Brain Res.* 85, 355–371.

Ribak, C. E. (1977) The immunocytochemical localization of GAD within stellate neurons of rat visual cortex. *Anat. Rec.* 187, 692–693.

Ribak, C. E. (1978) Immunocytochemical localization of glutamic acid decarboxylase (GAD) in the rat corpus striatum. *Anat. Rec.* 190, 521.

Ribak, C. E. (1978) Aspinous and sparsely-spinous stellate neurons contain in the visual cortex of rats: glutamic acid decarboxylase. *J. Neurocytol.* 7, 461.

Ribak, C. E., Harris, A. B., Anderson, L., Vaughn, J. E. & Roberts, E. (1978) GABAergic axon terminals decrease at experimental seizure foci in monkey cerebral cortex. *Neurosci. Abst.* 4. In press.

Ribak, C. E. & Vaughn, J. E. (1976) Immunocytochemical localization of GAD in somata and dendrites of GABAergic neurons following colchicine treatment. *Neurosci. Abst.* 2, 796.

Ribak, C. E., Vaughn, J. E. & Saito, K. (1976) Immunocytochemical localization of glutamate decarboxylase (GAD) in the olfactory bulb. *Anat. Rec.* 184, 512–513.

Ribak, C. E., Vaughn, J. E. & Saito, K. (1978) Immunocytochemical localization of glutamic acid decarboxylase in neuronal somata following colchicine inhibition of axonal transport. *Brain Res.* 140, 315–332.

Ribak, C. E., Vaughn, J. E., Saito, K. & Barber, R. (1976) Immunocytochemical localization of glutamate decarboxylase in the substantia nigra of the rat. In: *The Basal Ganglia,* ed. Yahr, M. D., pp. 205–211. Raven Press, N.Y.

Ribak, C. E., Vaughn, J. E., Saito, K., Barber, R. & Roberts, E. (1976) Immunocytochemical localization of glutamate decarboxylase in rat substantia nigra. *Brain Res.* 116, 287–298.

Ribak, C. E., Vaughn, J. E., Saito, K., Barber, R. & Roberts, E. (1977) Glutamate decarboxylase (GAD) localization in neurons of the olfactory bulb. *Brain Res.* 126, 1–18.

Roberts, E. (1972) An hypothesis suggesting that there is a defect in the GABA system in schizophrenia. *Neurosci. Res. Program Bull.* 10, 468–482.

Roberts, E. (1976) Immunochemistry of the GABA system – a novel approach to an old transmitter. In: *Neurotransmitters, Hormones, and Receptors: Novel Approaches,* ed. Ferrendelli, J. A., McEwen, B. S. & Snyder, S. H., pp. 123–138. Society for Neuroscience, Bethesda, Md.

Roberts, E. (1977) The γ-aminobutyric acid system in schizophrenia. In: *Neuroregulators and Psychiatric Disorders,* ed. Usdin, E., Hamburg, D. A. & Barchas, J. D., pp. 347–357. Oxford University Press, N.Y.

Roberts, E. (1978) Rôles of GABA neurons in information processing in the vertebrate CNS. In: *Neuronal Information Transfer,* ed. Karlin, A., Tennyson, V. M & Vogel, H. J., pp, 213–239. Academic Press, N.Y.

Roberts, E., Baxter, C. F., Van Harreveld, A., Wiersma, C. A. G., Adey, W, R. & Killam, K. F. (1960) *Inhibition in the Nervous System and γ-Aminobutyric Acid,* Pergamon Press, Oxford.

Saito, K. (1976) Immunochemical studies of glutamate decarboxylase and GABA-α-ketoglutarate transaminase. In: *GABA in Nervous System Function*, ed. Roberts, E., Chase, T. N. & Tower, D. B., pp. 103–111. Raven Press, N.Y.

Saito, K., Barber, R., Wu, J.-Y., Matsuda, T., Roberts, E. & Vaughn, J. E. (1974) Immunohistochemical localization of glutamate decarboxylase in rat cerebellum. *Proc. Natl. Acad. Sci. (USA)* 71, 269–273.

Saito, K., Roberts, E. & Barber, R. (1977) Immunocytochemical identification of GABAergic neurons. In: *Structure and Function of Synapses*, ed. Kuriyama, K., pp. 143–157. Ishiyaku Shuppan Publ. Co., Tokyo, Japan.

Saito, K., Schousboe, A., Wu, J.-Y. & Roberts, E. (1974) Some immunochemical properties and species specificity of GABA-α-ketoglutarate. *Brain Res.* 65, 287–296.

Saito, K., Wu. J.-Y., Matsuda, T. & Roberts, E. (1974) Immunochemical comparisons of vertebrate glutamic acid decarboxylase. *Brain Res.* 65, 277–285.

Schousboe, A., Wu, J.-Y. & Roberts, E. (1973) Purification and characterization of the 4-aminobutyrate-2-ketoglutarate transaminase from mouse brain. *Biochemistry* 12, 2868–2873.

Schousboe, A., Wu, J.-Y. & Roberts, E. (1974) Subunit structure and kinetic properties of 4-aminobutyrate-2-ketoglutarate transaminase purified from mouse brain. *J. Neurochem.* 23, 1189–1195.

Vaughn, J. E., Barber, R., Saito, K., Roberts, E. & Famiglietti, Jr., E. V. (1978) Immunocytochemical identification of GABAergic neurons in rat retina. *Anat. Rec.* 190, 571–572.

Wong, E., Schousboe, A., Saito, K., Wu, J.-Y. & Roberts, E. (1974) Immunochemical studies of brain glutamate decarboxylase and GABA-transaminase of six inbred strains of mice. *Brain Res.* 68, 133–142.

Wood, J. G., McLaughlin, B. J. & Vaughn, J. E. (1976) Immunocytochemical localization of GAD in electron microscopic preprations of rodent CNS. In: *GABA in Nervous System Function*, ed. Roberts, E., Chase, T. N. & Tower, D. B., pp. 133–148. Raven Press, N.Y.

Wu, J.-Y. (1976) Purification, characterization, and kinetic studies of GAD and GABA-T from mouse brain. In: *GABA in Nervous System Function*, ed. Roberts, E., Chase, T. N. & Tower, D. B., pp. 7–55. Raven Press, N.Y.

Wu, J.-Y., Matsuda, T. & Roberts, E. (1973) Purification and characterization of glutamate decarboxylase from mouse brain. *J. Biol. Chem.* 248, 3029–3034.

Wu, J.-Y. & Roberts, E. (1974) Properties of brain L-glutamate decarboxylase: inhibition studies. *J. Neurochem.* 23, 759–767.

New Directions in GABA Research II: Some Observations Relevant to GABA Action and Inactivation

Eugene Roberts, Esther Wong, Diana N. Krause, Kazuo Ikeda & Phyllis Degener

Another area of major concern to us is the study of the detailed mechanisms of control of GABA synthesis, sequestration, and release and of the mechanisms of action of the released GABA on postsynaptic membranes and its subsequent synaptic inactivation. Recently we have begun to turn our attention to a few of the interesting unanswered problems. Both GABA and glutamate are present in GABA-ergic terminals, yet there is no evidence that glutamate is ever liberated from such terminals. Since glutamate is a potent depolarizing agent and probably is a major excitatory transmitter, liberation of glutamate from endings of nerves performing inhibitory functions certainly could have chaotic effects on information processing. The sequestration of the glutamate precursor pool from the GABA transmitter pool must be achieved in such a manner that only GABA is liberated by GABA-ergic neurons. Based in part on experiments performed during our purification of GAD (Wu *et al.* 1973), and in part on my interpretation of a large physiologic and morphologic literature, I would like to speculate that the increase in free Ca^{++} that occurs in nerve terminals during depolarization may result in the association of GAD with the outer surfaces of synaptic vesicles in the interior of the terminal. Glutamate in the cytoplasm may attach to active enzymatic sites of the GAD and be converted to GABA, which

* Division of Neurosciences, City of Hope National Medical Center, Duarte, CA., USA.

This work was supported in part by USPHS Grants NS01615 and NS12116 from the National Institute of Neurological and Communicative Disorders and Stroke, and Grant MH22438 awarded by the National Institute of Mental Health, DHEW. This paper was written while the author was a Fellow at the Center for Advanced Study in the Behavioral Sciences, Stanford, and supported in part by grant BNS-76-22943 from the National Science Foundation.

"GABA-NEUROTRANSMITTERS", Alfred Benzon Symposium 12, Munksgaard 1978

as a consequence of cooperative interaction of the enzyme and vesicular membrane during the enzymatic reaction, could be transported or pumped directly into the internal volume of the vesicles. The vesicles near the membrane surface are filled with transmitter to a capacity determined by the maximal extent to which their membranes can be stretched by the transmitter molecules and their associated water and binding materials. They then enter collimators that serve to select vesicles of the appropriate dimensions and guide them to the ultimate sites of transmitter release facing the synaptic cleft. The transmitter then is liberated by processes consequent to the depolarization of the presynaptic membrane by the invading action potential and the resulting influx of Ca^{++} ions. One key question with regard to the above scheme is whether or not GAD and the vesicular membrane can associate under suitable conditions to form the proposed coordinated enzymatic "pump and storage tank".

Techniques now are available to test the above hypothesis. Of course, such a mechanism could be proposed to exist for all transmitters believed to be formed from precursors within nerve terminals and subsequently liberated from vesicles contained in them.

Much evidence suggests that GABA-anionophore complexes exist in some excitable membranes which function in such a manner that, when GABA or a suitable agonist attaches to the GABA recognition site, anion channels are opened for the period during which GABA is attached to such sites. Recent work, summarized in several papers in this symposium, suggests that convulsants such as picrotoxin, bicuculline, penicillin and pentylenetetrazole and the anticonvulsants such as diphenylhydantoin, diazepam, and phenobarbital somehow decrease or increase, respectively, the efficacy of GABA synapses. It also is clear that the above substances do not compete effectively with GABA at the GABA recognition sites on the receptor and that probably several steps may be involved between the attachment of GABA to such a specific recognition site and the consequent increase in chloride conductance (Enna & Snyder 1975, Olsen *et al.* 1978a, b, Krogsgaard-Larsen 1978, DeFeudis 1977). The nature, number, and sequential activities of the entities involved must be elucidated. A search now is on for suitable high affinity ligands for the different steps in the processes intervening between GABA recognition and channel opening. Because of the probable cooperative interaction between a number of protein and lipid components in GABA-anionophore complexes, it is likely that the details of this interaction will differ at least in some discernible respects from species to species and probably from site to site in the same organism. Experimental results seem to bear this out in a number of instances (see literature citations in references given above).

GABA probably is inactivated at synapses by a mechanism that involves

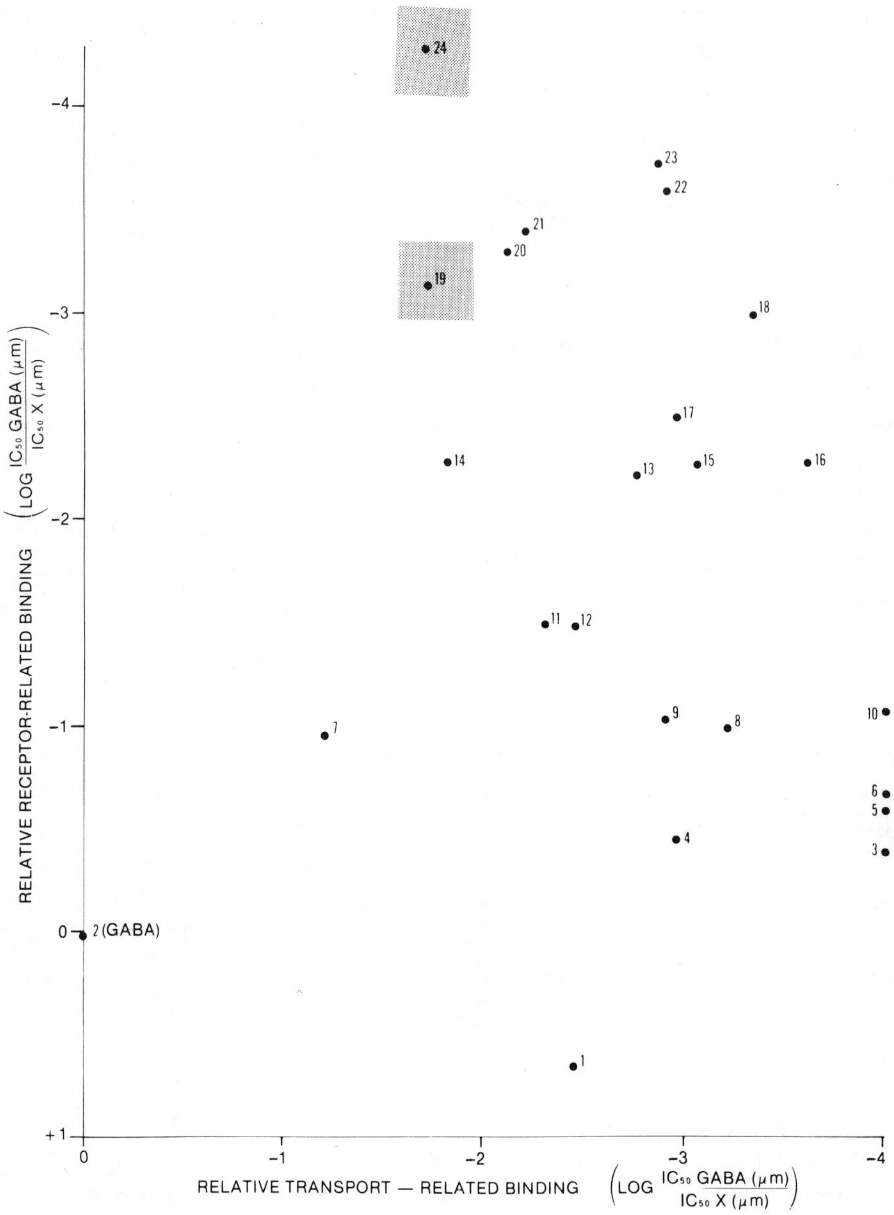

binding to unique membrane sites and the subsequent transport out of the synaptic junction by a process that is similar to that for many substances. Substances that potently and specifically block the binding of GABA to the GABA recognition site of the inactivation system, while not affecting the transport part of the process and possessing no mimetic or antagonistic properties at GABA receptor sites, and not eventually acting as false transmitters might be effective amplifiers of GABA action at synapses at which GABA normally is liberated.

STRUCTURE-ACTIVITY RELATIONS ON MEMBRANE RECEPTOR AND TRANSPORT GABA RECOGNITION SITES AND ON A CRUSTACEAN NEURON

We have studied a variety of chemical substances, many used similarly by others before, employing quantitative conductance measurements in the GABA-responding crayfish stretch receptor neuron (Swagel *et al.* 1973a, b, Hori *et al.* 1978, Krause *et al.* 1978). The same substances also were examined using adaptations of previously published procedures with membrane preparations from mouse brain to measure GABA binding to presumed GABA recognition sites of the receptor-anionophore complex (Enna & Snyder 1975) and to the GABA binding sites of the GABA transport system (Roberts *et al.* 1978).

In Fig. 1 are plotted the log potencies of GABA relative to those of a number of substances in displacing ^{3}H-GABA in receptor-related and transport-related GABA binding assay systems to mouse brain membrane preparations. The individual substances tested are listed in order of their potency in the receptor binding system in the legend to Fig. 1. Of the 24 substances studied, only

Fig. 1. The log potencies of GABA relative to those of a number of structurally related substances in displacing ^{3}H-GABA in receptor-related mouse brain membrane binding assays (log IC_{50} GABA) plotted *vs* the values found in the transport-related assay system.

The substances numbered in the order of their potency in the receptor-related assay are as follows: muscimol, 1; GABA, 2; isoguvacine, 3; 3-aminopropane sulfonate, 4; 3-aminopropane sulfinate 5; isonipecotate, 6; β-guanidinopropionate, 7; imidazole-4-acetate, 8; guanidoacetate, 9; THIP (4, 5, 6, 7-tetrahydroisoxazole-[5,4-c pyridine-3-ol] zwitterion), 10; DL-δ-hydroxy GABA, 11; δ-aminovalerate, 12; bicuculline, 13; β-alanine, 14; 1-methylimidazole-4-acetate, 15; imidazole-4-acetate, isopropyl ester, 16; GABA-L-histidine (homocarnosine), 17; taurine, 18; (±)nipecotate, 19; γguanidinobutyrate, 20; L-α,γ-diaminobutyrate, 21; imidazole-4-propionate, 22; δ-aminolevulinate, 23; L-α,β-diaminopropionate, 24. (Isoguvacine and THIP were gifts from Dr. P. Krogsgaard-Larsen, samples of 3-aminopropane sulfonate from Drs. R. Olsen and A. Mori, 3aminopropane sulfinate from Dr. A. Mori, and muscimol from Dr. E. Costa and Ciba-Geigy Corp. The rest of the chemicals were obtained commercially.)

muscimol (#1) was more potent than GABA in the receptor-related system. Compounds 3–12 all are related in structure to GABA. A detailed examination was made of CPK models of GABA and of all of the other substances tested. In Fig. 2a are shown projections of the faces of the fully extended GABA molecule, the side, top, and bottom views being depicted. A good deal of previous work has suggested that GABA acts on its receptor in the extended form, as

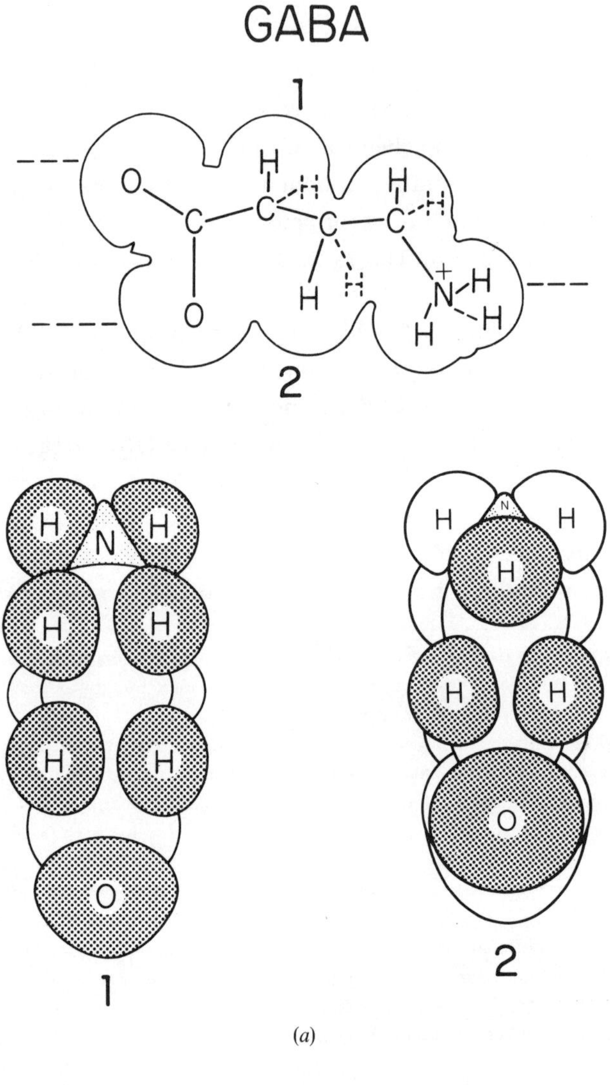

(*a*)

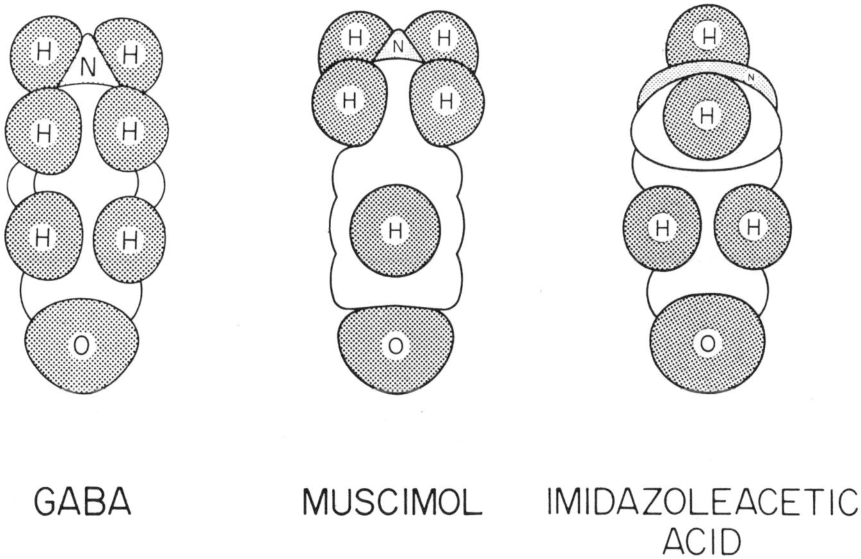

(*b*)

Fig. 2. (a) The faces of GABA as seen on projections of CPK space-filling models.
(b) Comparisons of "GABA-binding site" faces of projections of space-filling models of GABA (left), muscimol (center), and imidazoleacetic acid (right).

represented in Fig. 2a (Olsen *et al.* 1978a, Krogsgaard-Larsen 1978). Atoms that are shaded are those that protrude from the surface and might be the first ones to hit a membrane surface that would be approached by the faces of the molecules. Face 1 of the GABA molecule, as shown in Fig. 2a, resembles the surface of GABA that would be recognized by a receptor. Indeed, every one of compounds 3–12 can be shown from the models to have at least one possible configuration that presents a surface similar to face 1 of the GABA molecule, with closely similar distances between N and O atoms (see Fig. 2b for examples). Detailed structural considerations will be reported elsewhere. Strikingly, not a single one of the substances tested was nearly as potent as GABA, itself, in the transport-related binding system, 16 times the concentration of the next most potent compound, *β*-quanidinopropionate (no. 7), being required to achieve the same effect (IC_{50}) as GABA. (±) Nipecotate (no. 19) and L–*a*,*β*-diaminopropionate (no. 24) are emphasized on Fig. 1 because they were the most potent blockers of GABA binding to the recognition site of the transport-related system among the substances tested that also possessed very low affinities for the receptor-related sites. The two latter substances were chosen for subsequent study in the crayfish stretch receptor system. A careful study of CPK models of the most potent transport site inhibitors, compounds 7, 11, 14, 19, 20, 21, and 24, showed that each of the substances had at least one permissible configuration that closely resembled face 2 of GABA (Fig. 2a), the distances between the nitrogen and oxygen atoms and the shapes of the projecting surfaces being quite similar. Face 2 of the GABA model (Fig. 2a) may be the one that attaches to the binding site or sites involved in the transport of GABA.

From a number of previous studies in other laboratories, similar in principle to those above, it has been proposed that GABA may bind to its neuronal receptors in an extended conformation and to its transport sites in a folded conformation. Our data suggest another possibility. When the GABA molecule attaches to the receptor site in the extended form, *the other side of the GABA molecule* already is in the configuration that is recognized by the transport binding site. If the two sites are in close juxtaposition at the receptor complex, the removal of GABA from the receptor site by the transport binding site could occur automatically and immediately following the conformational changes that accompany membrane activation by the transmitter and anion channel opening. This would eliminate the physiological uncertainties that might attend processes involving the passive equilibrium dissociation of the transmitter from the active site and diffusion to removal sites and would ensure immediate removal of the transmitter from its recognition site and the closing of the associated ion channel. It would be compatible with the quantal and temporal requirements for precise synaptic function.

The data in Fig. 3 are the first, to our knowledge, in which in the same laboratory quantitative receptor-related binding data on mouse brain membranes have been correlated with quantitative conductance measurements of the effects of GABA and related substances in a physiologically responding system. With the method employed for plotting the data, there appears to be a curvilinear relationship between the relative efficacies of GABA and the other test substances in the two systems. In both the *in vitro* and *in vivo* test systems muscimol (no. 1) and GABA (no. 2) were the most potent substances examined by us. Further work is in progress to determine the structural and physicochemical parameters pertinent to determining relative efficacy in the two test systems. Meanwhile, we now have assurance that there is a *quantitative* correspondence between our measurements on mouse brain membranes and the crayfish stretch receptor neuron.

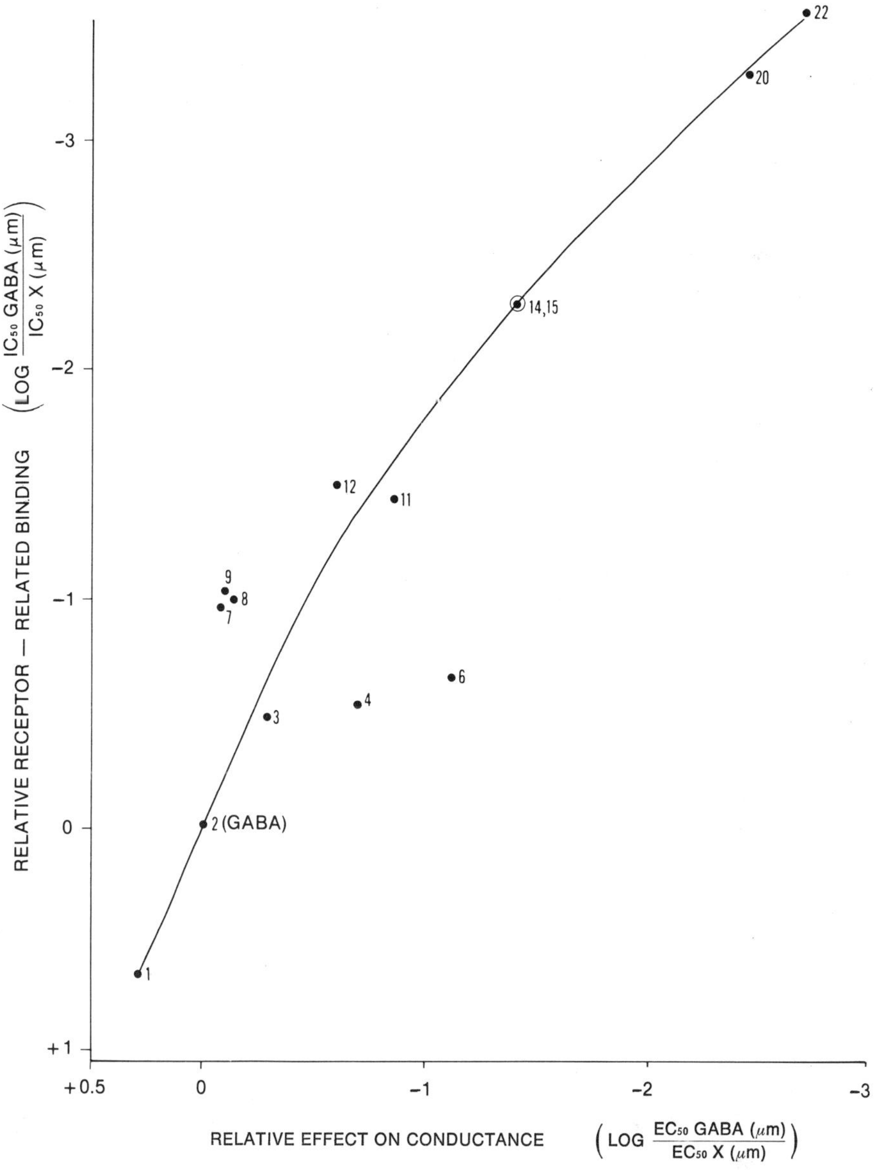

Fig. 3. The log potencies of GABA relative to those of several structurally related substances in displacing ^{3}H-GABA in receptor-related mouse brain membrane binding assays (log IC_{50} GABA) plotted *vs* the values found on conductance fond in the crayfish stretch receptor system. The numbers of the compounds tested are the same as those assigned in the legend to Fig. 1.

COMMENTS AND EXPERIMENTAL OBSERVATIONS RELEVANT TO THE PROPOSED COUPLED ACTION-INACTIVATION MECHANISM OF GABA FUNCTION

The hypothesis proposed above is that the attachment of GABA to its receptor recognition site ordinarily would be followed automatically by an extremely rapid removal by the coupled binding process, the inactivation step, consequent to which there would be closure of the anion channel opened by the action of GABA and uptake of the bound GABA into the cytoplasm of the postsynaptic site. The above processes would be operative regardless of the mechanisms (bath application or nerve stimulation) by which GABA reaches the recognition sites of the receptor complex. The termination of the action of GABA at receptor and diffusion only if the removal process coupled to receptor activation were and diffusion only in the removal process coupled to receptor activation were somehow blocked or inactivated or if the two processes were uncoupled. It would follow that GABA, itself, might be a potent enhancer of its own action, providing a concentration of GABA were attained that would keep at least some of the transport binding sites saturated, since GABA has by far the highest affinity for the transport related binding sites of the substances tested (Fig. 1). The IC_{50} values of GABA for the mouse brain membrane receptor and transport-related systems were found by us to be closely similar, 0.13 μm and 0.25 μm, respectively. Attaching with approximately the same affinity to both receptor and transport sites, GABA could, in a concentration dependent manner, enhance its own efficacy at the receptor site by decreasing the ratio of channels closed by the coupled mechanism to those whose inactivation would take place by the slower processes of dissociation and diffusion. The hypothesis suggests that with increasing GABA concentrations individual ion channels would tend to stay open longer, because GABA would remain attached longer to the GABA-recognition sites of the receptor-ionophore complex. At low ambient GABA concentrations, then, a given amount of GABA would be less effective in causing a conductance increase in a receptive membrane in the presence of a fully active inactivation mechanism, as described above, than would be the case if GABA were removed from the active sites solely by a dissociation-diffusion mechanism. At high ambient GABA concentrations, with the coupled transport sites already covered by GABA to a considerable extent, the efficacy of GABA in increasing membrane conductance should be greater. The log-dose conductance curve would be expected to increase more slowly at low GABA levels and then more rapidly at higher GABA levels than would be expected if the only processes taking place were the original attachment of GABA to receptor sites and its subsequent equilibrium dissociation. This situation could lead to erroneously high values for the slopes of Hill plots calculated in the usual manner, and a misconception of the number of transmitter molecules of GABA required to activate individual receptor sites.

In a current series of experiments in our laboratories with the crayfish stretch receptor neuron (Krause *et al.* 1978), an average value of the Hill coefficient for GABA of 3.41 was obtained from 11 preparations at 18° C, while values of approximately 2 were obtained for a series of GABA-mimetic substances tested: muscimol (no. 1), 1.8; isoguvacine (no. 3), 2.1; 3-aminopropane sulfonate (no. 4), 2.1; isonipecotate (no. 6), 2.2; and THIP (no. 10), 2.0. The effects of the latter substances might be considered to be "pure" in the sense that they all have extremely low affinities for the transport-related membrane system (Fig. 1), and their action, in contrast to that of GABA, would be expected to be terminated almost entirely by dissociation and diffusion away from receptor recognition sites.

If the above hypothesis were correct, antagonists of GABA binding to the recognition site of the transport system should be effective in enhancing the efficacy of GABA action on membranes by prolonging the time of association of GABA with the receptor complex and, therefore, the length of time of opening of anion channels for each association of transmitter with receptor recognition site. The results in Fig. 4 show, indeed, that addition of 10^{-3}M nipecotate (no. 19), which, by itself, is without any effect on membrane conductance at this concentration (see Fig. 5), markedly enhanced the conductance increase produced by a submaximally effective concentration of GABA (4×10^{-5}M). The results in Fig. 5 show that the above concentration of nipecotate shifted the GABA dose-conductance curve to the left, with the relative enhancement produced by nipecotate being greatest at the lower GABA concentrations. On the other hand, the curve for muscimol (no. 1), a substance with the very low affinity for the GABA transport recognition site (approximately one three-thousandths of that of GABA (Fig. 1), was not affected by addition of nipecotate (Fig. 5). Similar results to those above, not shown here, were obtained with L-α, β-diaminopropionate (no. 24, Fig. 1), another effective blocker of GABA attachment to the transport recognition site.

In studies with the crayfish stretch receptor neuron, the log-dose conductance curve for muscimol always began to rise at lower concentrations than did that for GABA (Hori *et al.* 1978, Krause *et al.* 1978), as illustrated in Fig. 5.

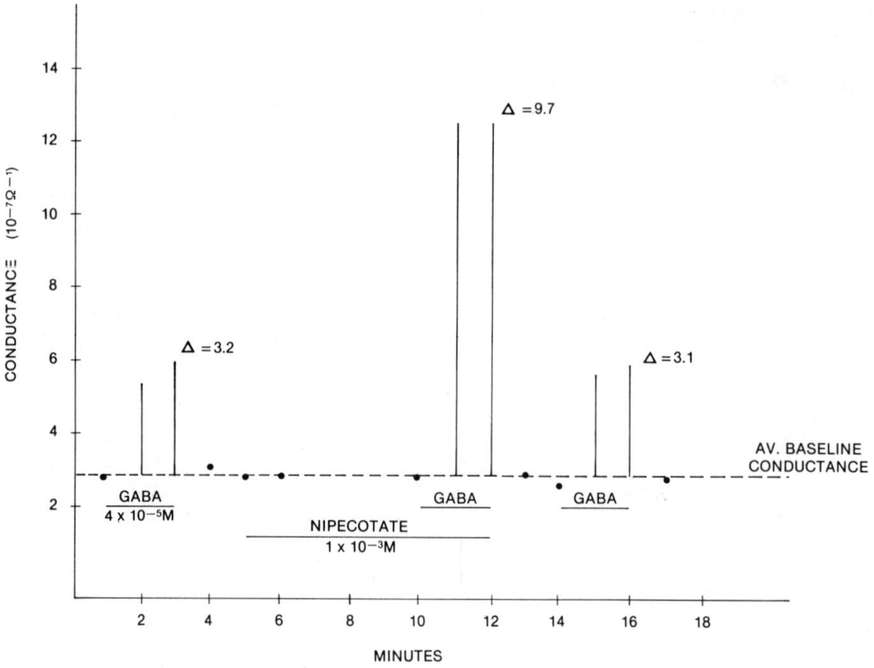

Fig. 4. The enhancing effect of nipecotate on the conductance change produced in the crayfish stretch by a submaximally effective concentration of GABA.

Invariably, however, at higher GABA concentrations the two curves crossed prior to attainment of the maximal conductance increase. Thus, at the lower concentrations muscimol appeared to be far more potent than GABA in producing conductance changes, while at higher concentrations GABA appeared to be more effective. This suggests that, when the problem of differential removal from active sites by the transport system is eliminated, GABA actually may have a greater affinity for the GABA recognition site than muscimol. From the point of view of practical pharmacology, muscimol is active at lower doses than GABA and the above observation may not be of great significance. It is unlikely that high extracellular levels of GABA would exist normally because most synaptic and nonsynaptic neural membranes (Sano & Roberts 1961, Sano & Roberts 1963, Weinstein *et al.* 1965, Varon *et al.* 1965) and glia (Iversen & Kelly 1975, Schousboe *et al.* 1977) possess high affinity binding-transport sites for GABA that probably remove any excess GABA that is not inactivated immediately by the coupled mechanism proposed here. However, the above observations do raise serious questions as to whether or not the greater efficacy of muscimol in the test systems employed to date allows one to conclude that the muscimol molecule has a structurally better fit to the transmitter-recognition site of the GABA receptor than does side 1 (Fig. 2) of the extended form of the GABA molecule, itself. Because several possible configurations of the flexible GABA molecule can exist in solution, the concentrations of the "active" form always will be lower than the total concentration of GABA employed; while there is a much better conformity between the two in the case of muscimol, which has a restricted conformation. New data in our laboratory (Wang *et al.* 1978) show that there is a slower rate of dissociation of muscimol than of GABA from the GABA-recognition sites of the receptor complexes in membranes from mouse brain. It still has not been ruled out that some of the effects of nipecotate and L-α, β-diaminopropionate described above could have occurred because of inhibition of uptake processes in presynaptic terminal, and sheath cells in the crayfish stretch receptor. A more definitive test of the above hypothesis might be obtained in study of the effects of GABA uptake blockers on single channel characteristics (noise analysis).

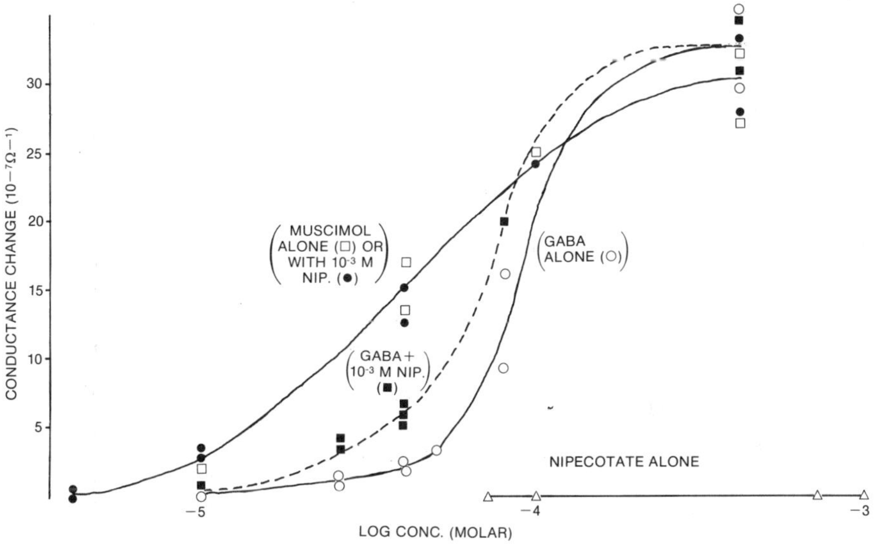

Fig. 5. Data showing that a concentration of nipecotate (10^{-3}M) which produces no effect on conductance alone, shifts the GABA log-dose conductance curve to the left while not exerting any effect on the muscimol curve.

CONCLUDING COMMENTS

It is obvious that the above studies, and others like them, are just beginning to scratch the surface of a meaningful pharmacology of the GABA system. A recent study of GABA-induced membrane current noise in crayfish muscle fibers showed the presence of "fast", synaptic channels, and "slow" extra-synaptic channels (Dudel *et al.* 1977), as has been shown to be the case for acetylcholine and glutamate synapses (Dreyer *et al.* 1976, Katz & Miledi 1973, Neher & Sakmann 1976). The effects of bath application af substances to preparations with reactive membranes may take place at both subsynaptic and extrasynaptic membranes. Iontophoretic studies have shown there to be a high degree of sensitivity to GABA localized to the rostral dendrites of the crayfish stretch receptor neuron, where inhibitory synapses are most numerous (Graelius 1976). However, GABA can affect non-synaptic sites as well in the latter preparation. It would seem that an improved way of getting information about the effects of bath applied substances would be to examine their influence on neurally evoked inhibitory responses at postsynaptic sites. Such measurements are feasible and currently are being set up in our laboratories. Maximally useful types of information would be obtained employing voltage clamp techniques in noise analysis (Gage 1976). The application of the latter technique to the crayfish stretch receptor neuron presents some formidable technical difficulties at present.

We chemists and pharmacologists must be modest in the claims we make for our measurements and most careful about making any dogmatic mechanistic interpretations of them. A great deal remains to be learned even about the biophysical and molecular events that take place at excitatory neuromuscular junctions, by far the best known synaptic connections. There still is almost everything to learn about the details of inhibitory synapses. Those of us who wish to work toward the understanding of their function at a molecular level probably have a long and exciting journey ahead of us.

REFERENCES

DeFeudis, F. V. (1977) GABA-receptors in the vertebrate nervous system. *Progress in Neurobiol.* 9, 123–145.

Dreyer, K., Müller, K.-D., Peper, K. & Sterz, R. (1976) The *M. omohyoideus* of the mouse as a convenient mammalian muscle preparation. A study of functional and extrajunctional acetylcholine receptors by noise analysis and cooperativity. *Pflügers Arch.* 367, 115–122.

Dudel, J., Finger, W. & Stettmeier, H. (1977) GABA-induced membrane current noise and the time course of the inhibitory synaptic current in crayfish muscle. *Neurosci. Letters* 6, 203–208.

Enna, S. J. & Snyder, S. (1975) Properties of γ-aminobutyric acid (GABA) receptor binding in rat brain synaptic membrane fractions. *Brain Res.* 100, 81–97.

Gage, P. W. (1976) Generation of end-plate potentials. *Physiol. Rev.* 56, 177–247.

Graelius, W. (1976) The distribution of GABA sensitivity on crayfish muscle receptor organs. *J. Physiol.* (Lond.) 263, 405–415.

Hori, N., Ikeda, K. & Roberts, E. (1978) Muscimol, GABA and picrotoxin: effects on membrane conductance of a crustacean neuron. *Brain Res.* 141, 364–370.

Iversen, L. L & Kelly, J. S. (1975) Uptake and metabolism of γ-aminobutyric acid by neurons and glial cells. *Biochem. Pharmacol.* 24, 933–938.

Katz, B. & Miledi, R. (1973) The characteristics of "end-plate noise" produced by different depolarizing drugs. *J. Physiol.* (Lond.) 230, 707–717.

Krause, D., Ikeda, K. & Roberts, E. (1978) Dose-conductance relationships of GABA and structurally-related compounds. *Neurosci. Abstr.* 4. In Press.

Krogsgaard Larsen, P. (1978) GABA agonists and uptake inhibitors of restricted conformations: structure-activity relations. In: *Amino Acids as Neurotransmitters,* ed. Fonnum, F., pp. Plenum Press, N. Y.

Neher, E. & Sakmann, B. (1976) Noise analysis of drug-induced voltage clamp currents in denervated frog muscle fibres. *J. Physiol.* (Lond.) 258, 705–729.

Olsen, R. W., Greenlee, D., Van Ness, P. & Ticku, M. K. (1978a) Studies on the gamma-aminobutyric acid receptor/ionophore proteins in mammalian brain. In: *Amino Acids as Neurotransmitters,* ed. Fonnum, F., pp. Plenum Press, N. Y.

Olsen, R. W., Ticku, M. K., Van Ness, P. C. & Greenlee, D. (1978) Effects of drugs on γ-aminobutyric acid receptors, uptake, release and synthesis in vitro. *Brain Res.* 139, 277–294.

Roberts, E., Wong, E., Svenneby, G. & Degener, P. (1978) Sodium-dependent binding of GABA to mouse brain particles. *Brain Res.* In Press.

Sano, K. & Roberts, E. (1961) Binding of γ-aminobutyric acid by brain preparations. *Biochem. Biophys. Res. Commun.* 4, 358–361.

Sano, K. & Roberts, E. (1963) Binding of γ-aminobutyric acid by mouse brain preparations. *Biochem. Pharmacol.* 12, 489–502.

Schousboe, A., Hertz, L. & Svenneby, G. (1977) Uptake and metabolism of GABA in astrocytes cultured from dissociated mouse brain hemispheres. *Neurochem. Res.* 2, 217–229.

Swagel, M. W., Ikeda, K. & Roberts, E. (1973a) Effects of GABA and bicuculline on conductance of crayfish abdominal stretch receptor. *Nature New Biol.* 244, 180–181.

Swagel, M. W., Ikeda, K. & Roberts, E. (1973b) Effects of GABA, imidazoleacetic acid, and related substances on conductance of crayfish abdominal stretch receptor. *Nature New Biol.* 246, 91–92.

Varon, S., Weinstein, H., Kakefuda, T. & Roberts, E. (1965) Sodium-dependent binding of γ-aminobutyric acid by morphologically characterized subcellular brain particles. *Biochem. Pharmacol.* 14, 1213–1224.

Wang, Y.-J., Roberts, E. & Salvaterra, P. (1979) Characterization of the binding of ^{3}H-muscimol to mouse brain membrane. *Molecular Pharmacol.* In Press.

Weinstein, H., Varon, S., Muhleman, D. R. & Roberts, E. (1965) A carrier-mediated transfer model for the accumulation of ^{14}C-γ-aminobutyric acid by subcellular brain particles. *Biochem. Pharmacol.* 14, 273–288.

Wu, J.-Y., Matsuda, T. & Roberts, E. (1973) Purification and characterization of glutamate decarboxylase from mouse brain. *J. Biol. Chem.* 248, 3029–3034.

The Distribution of Putative Monoamine, GABA, Acetylcholine and Glutamate Fibers in the Mesolimbic System

I. Walaas & F. Fonnum

It is generally acknowledged that the dopamine (DA) fibers from substantia nigra to neostriatum are involved in "extra-pyramidal" motor control, and that the hypothalamic tubero-infundibular DA fibers are involved in neuro-endocrine regulation. In contrast, the function(s) of the third major DA system in mammalian brain, the so-called "mesolimbic" system, is less clear. An involvement in psychotic phenomena has been proposed, and important interactions between these DA fibers and GABA neurons have been inferred (Stevens *et al.* 1974, Roberts 1976). The lack of information on the anatomical organization of the transmitter candidates present in the "mesolimbic" regions has, however, been an obstacle to more definite functional and pharmacological studies on this system.

The term "mesolimbic system" was originally coined by Ungerstedt (1971) as a description of the ascending DA fibers from the mesencephalic ventral tegmental area (VTA) to the so-called "limbic" region's nucleus accumbens, olfactory tubercle, bed nucleus of the stria terminalis and central amygdaloid nucleus. Later, corresponding DA fibers to the septum have been found (Lindvall 1975). The more recently discovered DA fibers to cortical areas (Thierry *et al.* 1973), whether "limbic" or not, are usually not included in the concept. Of the subcortical regions, three subdivisions can be made, e.g. the amygdala-related regions (the bed nucleus and the central amygdala), the "limbic striatal" or "ventral striatal" regions (the olfactory tubercle and the nucleus accumbens, see Heimer & Wilson 1975), and the septum. In the present

Norwegian Defence Research Establishment, Division for Toxicology, N-2007 Kjeller, Norway.

"GABA-NEUROTRANSMITTERS", Alfred Benzon Symposium 12, Munksgaard 1978

communication, we will present some results recently achieved in our laboratory on the organization of the monoamine, (in these regions mostly DA), acetylcholine (ACh), GABA and glutamate (GLU) fibers present in the septum, the ventral striatal regions and in the neostriatum, with special emphasis on possible GABA fibers. Neurochemical similarities between the dorsal and ventral striatum will also be discussed.

METHODS

In these experiments, we have studied the localization of transmitter candidates by means of topographical distribution studies of transmitter "markers", and by analysis of such markers after different lesions. The studies have been performed on rats, and we have employed electrocoagulations and knife or suction lesions, which are described in detail in the original papers. In addition, the recently reported technique of local application of kainic acid, which destroys local neurons but leaves afferents and fibers passing through intact (Schwarcz & Coyle 1977, Hattori & McGeer 1977), has been used (Fonnum & Walaas 1978, Walaas & Fonnum 1978). As the monoamine fibers have been mapped in detail by other techniques (Ungerstedt 1971, Fuxe & Jonsson 1974, Hökfeldt *et al.* 1977), we have restricted ourselves to aromatic amino acid decarboxylase (AAD) as a general marker for these fibers (Broch & Fonnum 1972, Fonnum 1975a). For ACh and GABA fibers, however, the specific markers choline acetyltransferase (ChAT) and glutamate decarboxylase (GAD) have been employed (Fonnum 1975a, b, Fonnum *et al.* 1977). In addition, possible glutamate or aspartate (ASP) fibers have been studied by means of the so-called high affinity uptake of GLU, which seems to be a suitable marker for such neurons (Young *et al.* 1974, Storm-Mathisen 1977, Fonnum & Walaas 1978). Autoradiographic studies on the high affinity uptake of D-aspartate (ASP) which travels by the GLU-uptake mechanism (Davies & Johnston 1976) have been performed by Dr. T. Taxt and Dr. J. Storm-Mathisen as previously described (Storm-Mathisen 1977).

RESULTS

Distribution of aminergic fibers

The distribution of AAD activity (Table I) as a measure of the density of catecholamine and indolamine fibers indicates the same degree of aminergic

Table I

Aromatic amino acid decarboxylase in "mesolimbic" and "extrapyramidal" regions of rat brain

Region	Unoperated brain μmol/h/g dry wt.	Lesioned brain % of unlesioned	Type of lesions
Medial accumbens	16.6±1.2	21±7*	Hemitran-
Lateral accumbens	10.4±0.8	25±3*	section
Olfactory tubercle	10.2±2.2	18±6*	"
Septum	6.2±0.6	33±3*	"
Neostriatum	14.2±2.6	14±3*	"
Ventral tegmental area	20.2±1.2	95±18	"
Substantia nigra compacta	15.0±2.6	99±11	"
Substantia nigra reticulata	4.0±0.6	75±15	"

Results presented as mean±S.E.M. Data from Fonnum *et al.* 1977, and unpublished.
* $P<0.01$.

innervation of the olfactory tubercle and nucleus accumbens as that of neostriatum. The innervation of septum is considerably less dense. A hemitransection through the globus pallidus decreases AAD in the telencephalic regions by 70–90%, demonstrating the ascending nature of all these fibers. The mesencephalic origins of the "mesolimbic" and nigrostriatal DA fibers also have very high AAD activities, probably mostly because of enzyme synthesis in local DA cells, but partly also because of serotonin and noradrenaline terminals in these regions (Saavedra *et al.* 1974, Versteeg *et al.* 1976).

Distribution of ACh fibers

The distribution of ChAT (Table II) indicates a dense cholinergic innervation comparable to that in neostriatum in both medial nucleus accumbens, olfactory tubercle and medial septum, with less density in lateral nucleus accumbens and lateral septum. The ChAT activity in all these regions is insensitive to a caudal hemitransection, but decreases by 60–90% after destruction of intrinsic neurons with kainic acid (Table II, Schwarcz & Coyle 1977, Walaas & Fonnum 1978, Malthe-Sørenssen, unpublished data). All ACh fibers in these regions therefore probably belong to local neurons. It is known that some of the ACh-cells in medial septum project to the hippocampus (Lewis *et al.* 1967, Fonnum & Walaas 1978). In agreement with this, we find that ChAT also decreases in hippocampus after kainic acid injection into the septum (Malthe-Sørenssen, unpublished). Whether some of the local ACh neurons in nucleus accumbens or olfactory tubercle could be part of the system of the "magnocellular nuclei of the forebrain" and thus be origin for probable cholinergic projections to cortex is at present unknown (Jones *et al.* 1976).

In comparison with the telencephalic regions, the ACh innervation of the mesencephalic DA-cells seems quite insignificant.

Table II

Choline acetyltransferase in "mesolimbic" and "extrapyramidal" regions of rat brain

Region	Unoperated brain μmol/h/g dry wt.	Lesioned brain % of unlesioned	Type of lesion
Medical accumbens	84±17	24±4*	Kainic acid
Lateral accumbens	41±8	28±4*	Kainic acid
Olfactory tubercle	96±6	114±8	Hemitransection
Medial septum	66±8	(decrease)	Kainic acid
Lateral septum	28±4	(decrease)	Kainic acid
Neostriatum	83±6	30±5*	Kainic acid
Ventral tegmental area	10±2	112±20	Hemitransection
Substantia nigra reticulata+compacta	3±1	120±28	Hemitransection

Results presented as mean±S.E.M. Data from Fonnum *et al.* 1977, Fonnum & Walaas 1978, Schwarcz & Coyle 1977, Walaas & Fonnum 1978, Malthe-Sørenssen, unpublished.
* $P<0.01$.

Table III

High affinity GLU uptake in "mesolimbic" and "extrapyramidal" regions of rat brain

Region	Unoperated brain μmol/h/g protein	Lesioned brain % of unlesioned	Type of lesion
N. accumbens	2.67±0.16	53±9*	Kainic acid
		55±6*	Fornic lesion
		17±5*	Kainic acid and fornix lesion
Olfactory tubercle	1.42±0.12	—	
Lateral septum	2.61±0.13	30±4*	Bilateral fornix lesion
Medial septum	0.95±0.14	91±9	Bilateral fornix lesion
Neostriatum	4.14±0.18	30± *	Frontal decortication
Globus pallidus	0.46±0.07	—	—

Results presented as mean±S.E.M. Data from Fonnum 1978, Fonnum & Walaas 1978, Walaas & Fonnum 1978.
* $P<0.01$.

Distribution of GLU fibers

The distribution of the high affinity uptake of GLU demonstrates (Table III) that the neostriatum has the highest density of GLU/ASP fibers, followed by lateral septum and nucleus accumbens. The olfactory tubercle is less densely innervated by such fibers, and the medial septum and globus pallidus has a very low GLU uptake. Different lesions (Table III) demonstrate that neocortex, particularly the frontal parts, gives rise to a GLU/ASP projection to neostriatum (Divac *et al.* 1977, Fonnum 1978), while allocortex sends such fibers to lateral septum (probably from the pyramidal cells in the hippocampus proper (Fonnum & Walaas 1978) and to nucleus accumbens (probably from the subiculum (Walaas & Fonnum 1978)). For both these GLU-projections, an anatomical substrate has been found (Swanson & Cowan 1977). Amino acid analysis indicates that all these fibers probably use GLU and not ASP as transmitter (Fonnum 1978, Fonnum & Walaas 1978, Walaas & Fonnum 1978). The olfactory tubercle has been suggested to receive GLU fibers from the olfactory bulb (Harvey *et al.* 1975, Yamamoto & Matsui 1976).

In nucleus accumbens, kainic acid lesion alone or in combination with fornix lesion results in a decrease in GLU uptake which indicates the existence of local GLU/ASP neurons. Whether such neurons are present in neostriatum or olfactory tubercle is unknown. The low activity in septum after lesions would seem to indicate that they are not numerous in this region.

Fig. 1 demonstrates by autoradiography the same distribution of GLU terminals as the biochemical results. Noteworthy is a region on the medial boundary of nucleus accumbens, which seems to be almost devoid of such terminals.

Distribution of GABA fibers

The distribution of GAD (Table IV) in the regions receiving ascending DA fibers indicates that the "mesolimbic" regions have a more dense GABA innervation than the neostriatum. The medial septum, which receives few, if any, DA fibers (Hökfelt *et al.* 1977), displays a definitely lower GAD activity than the other mesolimbic regions. Kainic acid lesions demonstrate that the GABA cells probably consist solely of local neurons (Table IV, Schwarcz & Coyle 1977, Walaas & Fonnum 1978, Malthe-Sørenssen, unpublished).

It is now well established that the neostriatum projects GABA fibers to substantia nigra (Fonnum *et al.* 1974, Fonnum *et al.* 1978) where the fibers terminate on the somata and dendrites of the local cells (Ribak *et al.* 1976). This

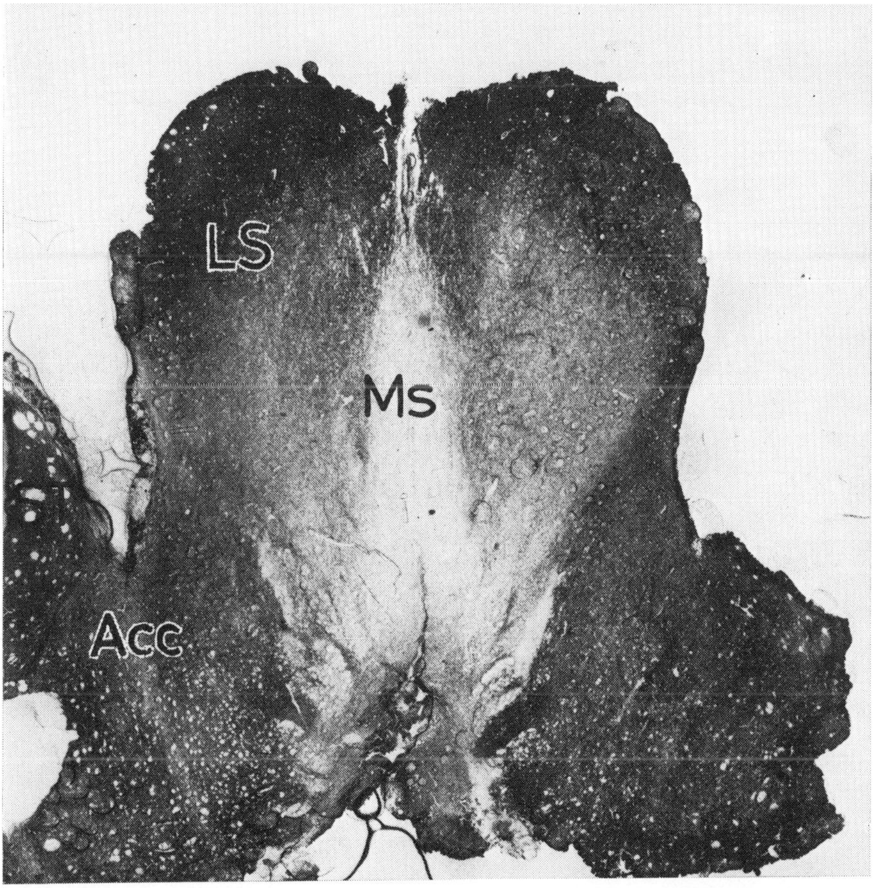

Fig. 1. Distribution of glutamate-accumulating terminals in the septum and nucleus accumbens. Autoradiographic study after uptake of D-aspartate (10^{-6}M) performed by T. Taxt & J. Storm-Mathisen (unpublished).

projection is both the most dense GABA tract yet reported in rat brain (Tappaz *et al.* 1976), and also an example of negative feedback of the nigrostriatal DA neurons. The possibility of comparable GABA projections from the "meso-limbic" regions has been suggested by many investigators. Both septum, nucleus accumbens and the olfactory tubercle have been found to project fibers to VTA, (Conrad & Pfaff 1976, Swanson 1976, Meibach & Siegel 1977), and an anatomical substrate for comparable feedback regulation of the mesolimbic DA cells is thus present. In addition, other major efferents pathways from these areas consist of septal fibers to hippocampus and to hypothalamus (Meibach &

Table IV
Glutamate decarboxylase in "mesolimbic" and "extrapyramidal" regions of rat brain

Region	Unoperated brain μmol/h/g dry wt.	Lesioned brain % of unlesioned	Type of lesion
Medial accumbens	220±11	29±9*	Kainic acid
Lateral accumbens	163±48	25±10*	Kainic acid
Olfactory tubercle	220±21	120±11	Hemitransection
Medial septum	62±9	(decrease)	Kainic acid
Lateral septum	160±12	(decrease)	Kainic acid
Neostriatum	90±11	32±6*	Kainic acid

Results presented as mean±S.E.M. Data from Fonnum *et al.* 1977, Schwarcz & Coyle 1977, Walaas & Fonnum 1978, Malthe-Sørenssen, unpublished.
* $P<0.01$.

Siegel 1977), fibers from nucleus accumbens and olfactory tubercle to a region commonly regarded as a rostral part of the substantia innominata (Heimer & Wilson 1975, Heimer 1978, Williams *et al.* 1977), and accumbens fibers to the ventromedial part of the globus pallidus and to substantia nigra (Swanson & Cowan 1975, Conrad & Pfaff 1976, Williams *et al.* 1977).

The distribution of GAD in some of these terminal regions (Table V) indicates that the fibers from nucleus accumbens and olfactory tubercle to substantia innominata terminate in a region with extremely dense GABA innervation, displaying even higher GAD activity than the pars reticulata of the substantia nigra and approximately twice the activity in globus pallidus. This region, which is clearly separated from the neighboring bed nucleus of the stria terminalis and horizontal nucleus of the diagonal band, therefore seems to be under very heavy GABA control. Preliminary results from our laboratory indicate that the GAD activity in this region decreases dramatically after an electrolytic lesion of the nucleus accumbens, without any decrease found in the adjoining bed nucleus, neostriatum or rostral globus pallidus (Walaas & Fonnum, unpublished). Also the GAD activity in substantia nigra is not significantly reduced by this lesion. This indicates that the nucleus accumbens, and, by inference, possibly the olfactory tubercle, projects GABA fibers to the rostral substantia innominata, while the alleged GABA nature of the projections to globus pallidus (Pycock & Horton 1976) and to substantia nigra remains unproven. However, due to insufficient knowledge on the termination of these projections in the rat (compare for example Conrad & Pfaff 1976, Williams *et al.* 1977), the necessary precision in dissection is difficult to achieve, and the results are therefore not definite. Hemitransections between globus pallidus and neostriatum, on the other hand, dramatically decrease GAD in globus pallidus, nucleus entopeduncularis (the homologue of the internal segment of globus pallidus in primates) and substantia nigra (Fonnum *et al.* 1978), without affecting the rather low GAD activity in VTA (Table V, Fonnum *et al.* 1977). Thus the striopallidal, strioentopeduncular and strionigral projections contain GABA fibers, while the septal-VTA, accumbens-VTA and olfactory tubercle-VTA fibers do not. Septal lesions also do not decrease GAD in hippocampus (Storm-Mathisen 1972, Fonnum & Walaas 1978) or hypothalamus (Tappaz & Brownstein 1978). These prominent septal projections are therefore also non-GABAergic.

DISCUSSION

The GABA system in the basal ganglia has been the subject of intense interest, and several aspects of this will be discussed by other workers in this symposium. Results reviewed in this communication demonstrate (Fig. 2) that these GABA fibers partly concist of intrinsic neostriatal neurons. A heavy neocortical excitatory GLU projection, ascending inhibitory DA and serotonin fibers, and local ACh cells may interact with these GABA neurons.

Further, GABA is a major transmitter in the communication of information

Table V

Glutamate decarboxylase in regions receiving fibers from "mesolimbic" and "extrapyramidal" regions

Region	Unoperated brain μmol/h/g dry wt.	Lesioned brain % of unlesioned	Type of lesion
Substantia innominata	1042±76	(decrease)	accumbens lesion
Globus pallidus	376±10	20−50	anterior hemitransection
Nucleus entopeduncularis	195±8	30−50	anterior hemitransection
Ventral tegmental area	95±8	98±12	hemitransection
Substantia nigra compacta	234±41	57±5*	hemitransection
Substantia nigra reticulata	615±43	19±4*	hemitransection

Results presented as mean±S.E.M., except for globus pallidus and n. entopeduncularis, where range is given. Data from Fonnum *et al.* 1977, 1978, Walaas & Fonnum, unpublished.
* $P<0.01$.

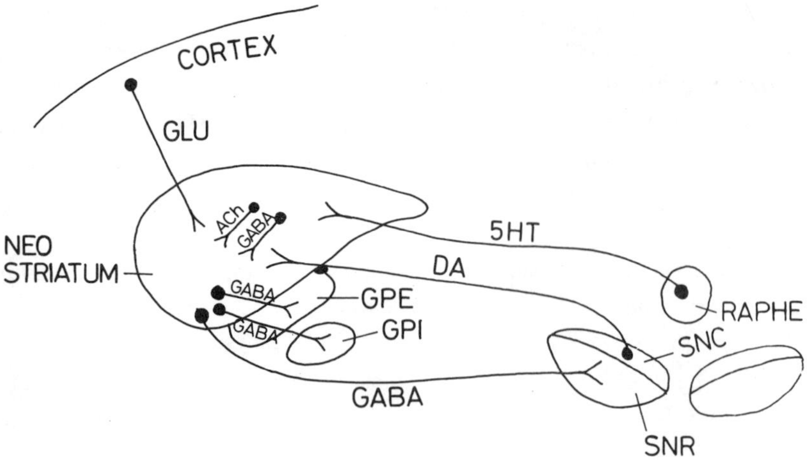

Fig. 2. Organization of putative aminergic, cholinergic, GABAergic and glutamergic fibers in the basal ganglia and related regions.

from neostriatum towards globus pallidus and nucleus entopeduncularis, from where the basal ganglia-output reaches thalamus. It therefore seems clear that these GABA systems will be prominent in the control of motor function.

Lastly, the GABA fibers to substantia nigra establish a direct "feedback loop" with the ascending DA system.

In comparison, the GABA systems in the "mesolimbic" regions seem to be organized differently.

In the *septum*, (Fig. 3) GABA is probably present only in local neurons which are concentrated in the lateral septum, where also most DA fibers are reported to end (Hökfelt *et al.* 1977). The dorsolateral septum receives most of an allocortical (hippocampal) excitatory GLU projection, while the medial septum contains most of the septal ACh system. The efferent projections which could represent possible feedback systems from the septum, e.g. those to hippocampus, to preoptic/hypothalamic regions and to VTA, do not seem to contain GABA fibers. The GABA system in septum is therefore probably exclusively involved in the internal processing of information arriving from different parts of the "limbic brain".

In the *nucleus accumbens*, (Fig. 4) GABA also seems to be present in local neurons, some of which probably are interneurons. No afferent GABA fibers have been found. The high density of GABA terminals in the medial accumbens seems to coincide with the most dense ACh and DA innervation. This medial

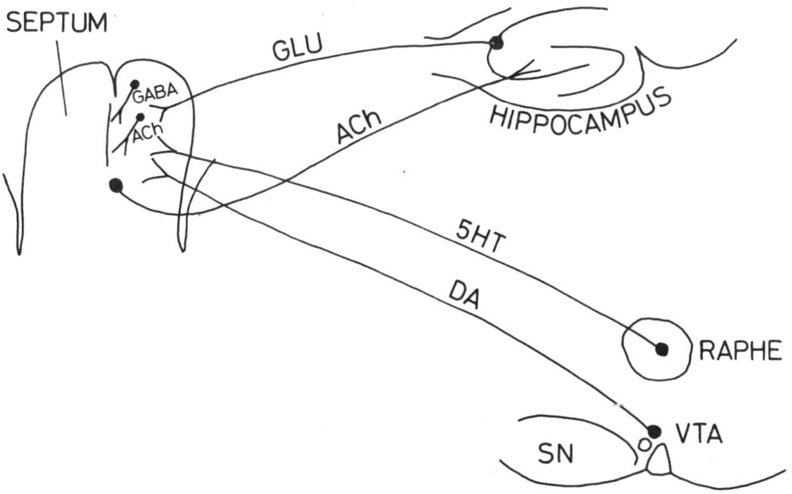

Fig. 3. Organization of putative aminergic, cholinergic, GABAergic and glutamergic fibers in the septum and related regions.

region is therefore probably a "center" for possible GABA/ACh/DA interactions in the nucleus accumbens.

In addition to these interneurons, the dominating efferent projection from nucleus accumbens, which terminate in the rostral so-called substantia innominata, probably contains a very heavy contingent of GABA fibers. Based on

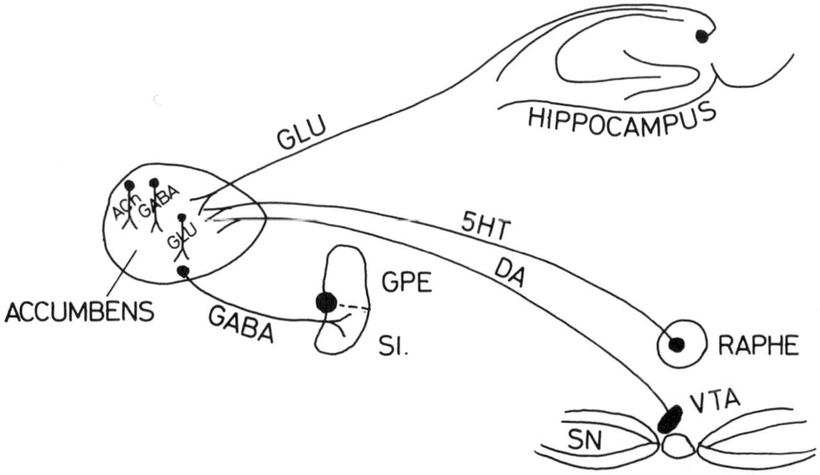

Fig. 4. Organization of putative aminergic, cholinergic, GABAergic and glutamergic fibers in the nucleus accumbens and related regions.

the GAD activity in the terminal region, this GABA projection, which to our knowledge has not been previously reported, seems to be one of the major GABA tracts in mammalian brain.

The substantia innominata is a rather enigmatic region, consisting of different cell groups which have different fiber connections (Jones *et al.* 1976, Heimer 1978). Our results indicate, in agreement with Heimer (1978), that the rostral part of this region were this GABA tract terminates (Fig. 5), probably should be regarded as a ventral part of globus pallidus, and that the fibers from nucleus accumbens thus constitute a ventral striatal-pallidal projection, comparable to the neostriatal-pallidal fibers both in anatomy and in transmitter chemistry. In contrast to this projection, our work indicates no feedback GABA systems to VTA, and the projections to globus pallidus and substantia nigra do not seem to contain important contingents of GABA fibers either.

In summary, the neurochemical defined circuitry of the nucleus accumbens therefore seems to be composed of ascending inhibitory DA and serotonin fibers from VTA and the mesencephalic raphe, respectively, allocortical excitatory

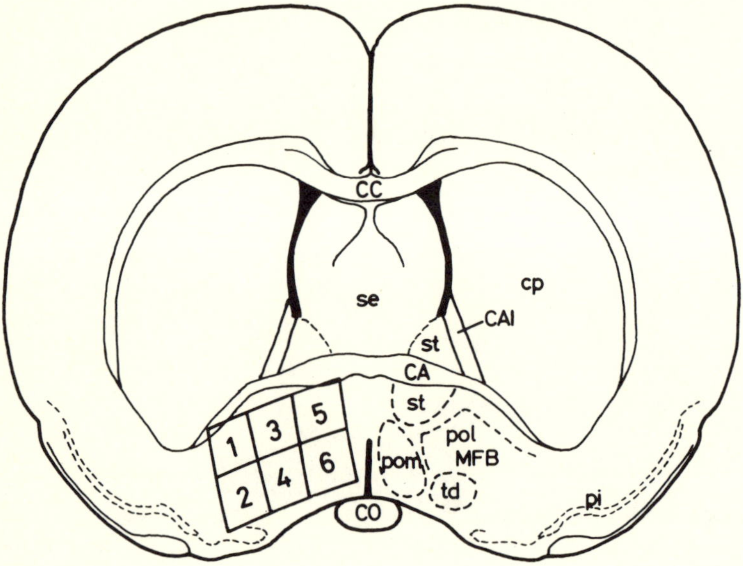

Fig. 5. Schematic drawing of a frontal section of rat brain through the rostral part of substantia innominata. Sample 3 denotes the region with highest GAD activity and also where the fibers from n. accumbens are reported to terminate. Abbrev.: CC – corpus callosum, CAI – internal capsule, cp – caudate putamen, CA – anterior commissure, MFB – medial forebrain bundle, pom – medial preoptic area, pol – lateral preoptic area, pi – pyriform cortex, st – bed nucleus of stria terminalis, td – nucleus of the horizontal limb of the diagonal band. From Fonnum *et al.* (1977).

GLU fibers from the subiculum, intrinsic GABA, ACh and GLU or ASP neurons, and a heavy GABA output to "ventral pallidum".

The olfactory tubercle, parts of which probably belong to the same neural mechanism as nucleus accumbens (Heimer 1978), has not been studied in the same detail. However, based on the similarities with nucleus accumbens in fiber connections, it may be proposed that allocortical GLU fibers from the piriform cortex might be present, in addition to the GLU fibers from the olfactory bulb, that the very dense ACh and GABA innervation is in the form of local neurons, some of them interneurons, and that the heavy projection to the ventrolateral part of the "ventral pallidum" could consist of GABA fibers, as do the corresponding fibers from accumbens. This scheme requires experimental verification, however. The "feedback" fibers from the olfactory tubercle to VTA are probably not GABA fibers.

These results thus demonstrate both similarities in the afferent transmitter systems, but also clear differences in the intrinsic and efferent transmitter systems in the septal and "striatal" parts of the "mesolimbic system". We therefore think it reasonable to assume that the transmitter interactions and functional roles of these regions will be different. The concept of *one* functionally unitary "mesolimbic system" is therefore an oversimplification, and studies on the neurobiology of these regions should preferably be interpreted with this fact in mind.

ACKNOWLEDGMENTS

We thank Dr. J. Storm-Mathisen and Dr. T. Taxt for the autoradiography picture in Fig. 1.

I. Walaas is a fellow of the Norwegian Council for Science and the Humanities.

REFERENCES

Broch, O. J. Jr. & Fonnum, F. (1972) The regional and subcellular distribution of catechol-O-methyl transferase in the rat brain. *J. Neurochem.* 19, 2049–2055.

Conrad, L. C. A. & Pfaff, D. W. (1976) Autoradiographic tracing of nucleus accumbens efferents in the rat. *Brain Research* 113, 589–596.

Davies, L. P. & Johnston, G. A. R. (1976) Uptake and release of D- and L-asparate by rat brain slices. *J. Neurochem.* 26, 1007–1014.

Divac, I., Fonnum, F. & Storm-Mathisen, J. (1977) High affinity uptake of glutamate in terminals of corticostriatal axons. *Nature* (Lond.) 266, 377–378.

Fonnum, F. (1975a) The localization of glutamate decarboxylase, choline acetyltransferase, and aromatic amino acid decarboxylase in mammalian and invertebrate nervous tissue. In: *Metabolic Compartmentation and Neurotransmission,* ed. Berl, S., Clarke, D. D. & Schneider, D. pp. 99–122. Plenum Press, New York.

Fonnum, F. (1975b) A rapid radiochemical method for the determination of cholineacetyltransferase. *J. Neurochem.* 24, 407–409.

Fonnum, F. (1978) Comments on neurotransmitters in striatum. In: *Amino Acids as Chemical Transmitters,* ed. Fonnum, F. NASI Life Science Series, Plenum Press. (In press).

Fonnum, F., Gottesfeld, Z. & Grofova, I. (1978) Distribution of glutamate decarboxylase, choline acetyltransferase and aromatic amino acid decarboxylase in the basal ganglia of normal and operated rats. Evidence for striatopallidal, striatoentopeduncular and striatonigral GABA-ergic fibers. *Brain Research* 143, 125–138.

Fonnum, F., Grofova, I., Rinvik, E., Storm-Mathisen, J. & Walberg, F. (1974) Origin and distribution of glutamate decarboxylase in substantia nigra of the cat. *Brain Research* 71, 77–92.

Fonnum, F., Walaas, I. & Iversen, E. (1977) Localization of GABAergic, cholinergic and aminergic structures in the mesolimbic system. *J. Neurochem.* 29, 221–230.

Fonnum, F. & Walaas, I. (1978) The effect of intrahippocampal kainic acid injections and surgical lesions on neurotransmitters in hippocampus and septum. *J. Neurochem.* (In press).

Fuxe, K. & Jonsson, G. (1974) Further mapping of central 5-hydroxytryptamine neurons: studies with the neurotoxic dihydroxytryptamines. *Adv. Biochem. Psychopharmacol.* 10, 1–12.

Harvey, J. A., Scholfield, C. N., Graham, L. T. jr. & Aprison, M. H. (1975) Putative transmitters in denervated olfactory cortex. *J. Neurochem.* 24, 445–449.

Hattori, T. & McGeer, E. G. (1977) Fine structural changes in the rat striatum after local injections of kainic acid. *Brain Research* 129, 174–180.

Heimer, L. (1978) The olfactory cortex and the ventral striatum. In: *The Continuing Evolution of the Limbic System Concept,* ed. Livingston, K. & Hornykiewicz, O., Plenum Press, New York. (In Press).

Heimer, L. & Wilson, R. D. (1975) The subcortical projections of the allocortex: similarities in the neural associations of the hippocampus, the pyriform cortex and the neocortex. In: *Perspectives in Neurobiology,* Golgi Centennial Symposium, ed. Santini, M., pp. 177–193, Raven Press, New York.

Hökfelt, T., Johansson, O., Fuxe, K., Goldstein, M. & Park, D. (1977) Immunohistochemical studies on the localization and distribution of monoamine neuron systems in the rat brain. In: *Rhinencéphale, Neurotransmetteurs et Psychoses,* ed. de Ajuriaguerra, J. & Tissot, R. pp. 79–113. Masson, Paris.

Jones, E. G., Burton, H., Saper, C. B. & Swanson, L. W. (1976) Midbrain, diencephalic and cortical relationships of the basal nucleus of Meynert and associated structures in primates. *J. Comp. Neurol.* 167, 385–419.

Lewis, P. R., Shute, C. C. D. & Silver, A. (1967) Confirmation from choline acetylase analyses of a massive cholinergic innervation to the rat hippocampus. *J. Physiol.* (Lond.) 191, 215–224.

Lindvall, O. (1975) Mesencephalic dopaminergic afferents to the lateral septal nucleus of the rat. *Brain Research* 87, 95–98.

Meibach, R. C. & Siegel, A. (1977) Efferent connections of the septal area in the rat: an analysis utilizing retrograde and anterograde transport methods. *Brain Research* 119, 1–20.

Pycock, C. & Horton, R. (1976) Evidence for an accumbens-pallidal pathway in the rat and its possible gabaminergic control. *Brain Research* 110, 629–634.

Ribak, C. E., Vaughn, J. E., Saito, K., Barber, R. & Roberts, E. (1976) Immunocytochemical localization of glutamate decarboxylase in rat substantia nigra. *Brain Research* 116, 287–298.

Roberts, E. (1976) Disinhibition as an organizing principle in the nervous system – the role of the GABA system. Application to neurologic and psychiatric disorders. In: *GABA in Nervous System Function,* ed. Roberts, E., Chase, T. N. & Tower, D. B. pp. 515–539. Raven Press, New York.

Saavedra, J. M., Brownstein, M. & Palkovits, M. (1974) Serotonin distribution in the limbic system of the rat. *Brain Research* 79, 437–441.

Schwarcz, R. & Coyle, J. T. (1977) Striatal lesions with kainic acid: neurochemical characteristics. *Brain Research* 127, 235–249.

Stevens, J., Wilson, K. & Foote, W. (1974) GABA blockade, dopamine and schizophrenia: experimental studies in the cat. *Psychopharmacologia* (Berl.) 39, 105–119.

Storm-Mathisen, J. (1977) Glutamic acid and excitatory nerve endings: reduction of glutamic acid uptake after axotomy. *Brain Research* 120, 379–386.

Swanson, L. W. (1976) An autoradiographic study of the efferent connections of the preoptic region in the rat. *J. Comp. Neurol.* 167, 227–256.

Swanson, L. W. & Cowan, W. M. (1975) A note on the connections and development of the nucleus accumbens. *Brain Research* 92, 324–330.

Swanson, L. W. & Cowan, W. M. (1977) An autoradiographic study of the organization of the efferent connections of the hippocampal formation in the rat. *J. Comp. Neurol.* 172, 49–84.

Tappaz, M., Brownstein, M. & Palkovits, M. (1976) Distribution of glutamate decarboxylase in discrete brain nuclei. *Brain Research* 108, 371–379.

Tappaz, M. & Brownstein, M. (1978) Origin of glutamate-decarboxylase (GAD) containing cells in discrete hypothalamic nuclei. *Brain Research.* (In press).

Thierry, A. M., Blanc, G., Sobel, A., Stinus, L. & Glowinski, J. (1973) Dopamine terminals in the rat cortex. *Science* 182, 499–501.

Ungerstedt, U. (1971) Stereotoxic mapping of the monoamine pathways in the rat brain. *Acta Physiol. Scand.,* Suppl. 367, 1–48.

Versteeg, D. H. G., van der Gugten, J., de Jong, W. & Palkovits, M. (1976) Regional concentrations of noradrenaline and dopamine in rat brain. *Brain Research* 113, 563–574.

Walaas, I. & Fonnum, F. (1978) The effects of surgical and chemical lesions on neurotransmitter candidates in nucleus accumbens. Submitted for publication.

Williams, D. J., Crossman, A. R. & Slater, P. (1977) The efferent projections of the nucleus accumbens in the rat. *Brain Research* 130, 217–227.

Yamamoto, C. & Matsui, S. (1976) Effect of stimulation of an excitatory nerve tract on release of glutamic acid from olfactory cortex slices *in vitro. J. Neurochem.* 26, 487–491.

Young, A., Oster-Granite, M. L., Herndon, R. M. & Snyder, S. H. (1974) Glutamic acid: selective depletion by viral induced granule cell loss in hamster cerebellum. *Brain Research* 73, 1–13.

GABA Neurons and Their Interaction with Monoamine Neurons. An Anatomical, Pharmacological and Functional Analysis.

K. Fuxe, K. Andersson, S.-O. Ögren, M. Perez De La Mora, R. Schwarcz, T. Hökfelt, P. Eneroth, J.-Å. Gustafsson & P. Skett.

In this laboratory we have for several years been concerned with the analysis of GABA-monoamine interactions in brain (Fuxe *et al.* 1975, 1977a,b). In this analysis it was found that putative GABA-ergic drugs such as Lioresal and aminooxyacetic acid preferentially reduced dopamine turnover within limbic areas especially after pimozide pretreatment (Fuxe *et al.* 1975, Andén and Wachtel 1978). Furthermore the dopamine receptor agonist apomorphine increased GABA turnover in dopamine-rich structures such as the neostriatum, the substantia nigra and subcortical limbic areas (Perez de la Mora & Fuxe 1977). Changes in GABA turnover were evaluated by measuring the accumulation of GABA after GABA transaminase inhibition which is nerve impulse-dependent (Perez de la Mora *et al.* 1977). These studies indicated the existence of important GABA-dopamine interactions in brain and *inter alia* suggested a strong inhibitory GABA-ergic control of the mesolimbic dopamine systems. In view of the dopamine hypothesis of schizophrenia claiming that blockade of limbic dopamine receptors is of importance for the therapeutic actions of antipsychotic drugs, it was speculated on the basis of the findings mentioned above that combined treatment of schizophrenia with neuroleptic drugs and

---

Departments of Histology and Chemistry, Karolinska Institute, Stockholm and the Hormone laboratory, Department of Obstetrics and Gynecology, Karolinska Hospital, Stockholm; Research laboratories, AB ASTRA, Södertälje and the Departemento de Biologia Experimental, Instituto de Biologia, UNAM Mexico D.F.

"GABA-NEUROTRANSMITTERS", Alfred Benzon Symposium 12, Munksgaard 1978

GABA-ergic drugs could improve treatment of schizophrenia (see also Roberts 1974). Thus, such treatment might allow a more preferential blockade of the limbic dopamine systems. Since then reports on reduced glutamic acid decarboxylase activity in certain brain nuclei of schizophrenic patients have appeared (Bird *et al.* 1977, Mc Geer & Mc Geer 1977). This work has now been continued along the following lines.

1. An anatomical analysis of the distribution of GABA nerve terminals in dopamine rich regions has been performed by producing specific antibodies against glutamate decarboxylase (GAD), using a GAD preparation obtained by affinity chromatography (Possani *et al.* 1977).

2. In order to understand if GABA mechanisms also exist beyond the dopamine receptors in the nucleus caudatus and nucleus accumbens and not only at the DA cell body and terminal level (Bartholini 1976, Fuxe *et al.* 1977), it has been evaluated whether the GABA receptor agonist muscimol or the GABA transaminase inhibitor gamma-acetylenic GABA (Schechter *et al.* 1977) can inhibit the apomorphine-induced stereotyped behavior and locomotor activity, respectively (see also Scheel-Krüger *et al.* 1978). Also it has been evaluated if the GABA-ergic drugs can increase the catalepsia produced by a neuroleptic drug such as haloperidol.

3. The effects of muscimol and gamma-acetylenic GABA have been evaluated on dopamine (DA) turnover within the neostriatum, within the subcortical limbic areas (tuberculum olfactorium and nucleus accumbens), and within the median eminence, since these two drugs are more specific than the previous putative GABA-ergic drugs we have used. Possible effects on noradrenaline (NA) turnover in the hypothalamic areas have also been studied.

4. The effects of the antipsychotic drugs chlorpromazine and sulpiride have been studied on GABA turnover, mainly in the cataleptic dose range. These drugs are DA receptor blocking agents.

5. The possible involvement of GABA mechanisms in the control of prolactin secretion has been studied in normal male rats by evaluating the effects of muscimol and gamma-acetylenic GABA on prolactin secretion. Possible involvement of catecholaminergic mechanisms in mediating the effects of increased GABA receptor activity on prolactin secretion were evaluated by simultaneous measurements of DA and NA turnover and levels within the median eminence and other parts of the hypothalamus and by pretreatment with CA receptor blocking agents. Previous studies indicate that GABA receptors may produce both decreases and increases of prolactin secretion (Makara &

Stark 1978, Mc Cann *et al.* 1978, Fuxe *et al.* 1977, see also Müller, this symposium).

Immunihistochemical studies on the distribution of GABA nerve terminals using antibodies against GAD

This work is made in collaboration with Drs. L. Possani, R. Tapia, L. Teran, and R. Palacios. The antibodies are prepared against the affinity sepharose bound GAD and cause a concentration-dependent inhibition of GAD activity. Furthermore, GAD antibodies give a single precipitation band in counter-immuno-electrophoresis when reacted against purified soluble GAD or crude extracts from mouse or rat brain. Large numbers of nigral GABA nerve terminals, probably making axo dendritic contacts with dopamine dendrites in the Substantia nigra, were demonstrated in agreement with the work of Roberts' group (see Roberts, this symposium). Furthermore, in the neuropile of the nucleus caudatus and nucleus accumbens diffuse networks of GABA nerve terminals were found. In the tuberculum olfactorium region networks of GABA nerve terminals were also found among the DA nerve terminals. However, a rich network of GABA terminals also appeared to establish axodendritic and axosomatic contacts with nerve cells present within the medial forebrain bundle area and with dendrites extending into the islands of Calleja and into parts of the cell body layer of the olfactory tubercule. Thus, at least within the tuberculum olfactorium it seems possible that GABA-ergic mechanisms may exist also in the pathways beyond the DA receptors since the outer layers of this structure at least partly project to the deeper structures, e.g. the islands of Calleja. The GABA receptors may here block or enhance the effects of postsynaptic dopamine receptor activation. Also it must be pointed out that there exists within the globus pallidus a dense GABA-ergic innervation which forms baskets around the large multipolar cells of this nucleus. Thus, by an action at the globus pallidus level GABA-ergic mechanisms could easily modify the influences of postsynaptic dopamine receptor activity on motor activity, since the efferent outflow of the neostriatum to large extent must pass via the globus pallidus and the thalamus to reach the motor cortex. Finally, mapping out of GABA neurons in the hypothalamus indicates existence of hypothalamo – infundibular GABA pathways.

Behavioral analysis of GABA-DA interactions

Muscimol significantly reduced apormorphine-induced stereotypies in the dose range 2–3 mg/kg (Figs. 1, 2). The effects of muscimol on the various stereotypic symptoms were highly dose-dependent and a steep dose-effect curve was observed. Muscimol in a dose of 0.5–1 mg/kg did not reduce the frequency of the stereotyped behavior. In a dose of 2 mg/kg, however, muscimol produced a very clearcut reduction of licking and biting but only slightly reduced sniffing and chewing (Figs. 1, 2). In a dose of 3 mg/kg muscimol produced a complete suppression of all stereotypic symptoms. Muscimol was more potent in blocking the increase in locomotion induced by apomorphine than the increase in apomorphine-induced stereotypies. Muscimol in a dose of 0.5 mg/kg caused a significant reduction in the apomorphine-induced increase in locomotion and a complete suppression was observed at 2 mg/kg (Fig. 2). The apomorphine-induced rearing activity was similarly affected by muscimol treatment. Bicuculline, a GABA receptor antagonist, in a dose of 1 mg/kg given 30 minutes prior to apomorphine, significantly antagonized the suppressive effects of muscimol on the apomorphine-induced stereotypies (Figs. 1, 2). Bicuculline also slightly but not significantly antagonized the reduction of apomorphine-induced locomotion produced by muscimol. Muscimol in a dose of 1 mg/kg did not cause any catalepsy and in a dose of 2 mg/kg it produced catalepsy in 50% of the animals. However, it should be noted that the catalepsy induced by muscimol was not identical to that produced by haloperidol. Muscimol in a dose of 3 mg/kg caused a pronounced sedation and a loss of the righting reflex in all the animals.

Gamma-acetylenic GABA in a dose of 100 mg/kg also produced a reduction of apomorphine-induced stereotypies when given 4 hours prior to apomorphine (Fig. 1). Gamma-acetylenic GABA caused a complete suppression of the apomorphine-induced increase in locomotion, rearing, licking and biting activity but had less pronounced effects on sniffing and chewing in line with the results obtained with muscimol. Gamma-acetylenic GABA produced clearcut sedation as well as catalepsy 4–8 hours after administration and a weak ptosis after 2–4 hours. This drug also produced a significant potentiation of haloperidol-induced catalepsy (Fig. 3). It should be pointed out that the catalepsy induced by gamma-acetylenic GABA appeared to be somewhat different from the type of catalepsy induced by haloperidol.

The inhibitory effects of muscimol and gamma-acetylenic GABA on apomorphine-induced locomotion and stereotypies and their partial counteraction by bicuculline give evidence that GABA receptor activity within the nesotriatum and nucleus accumbens located beyond the postsynaptic DA

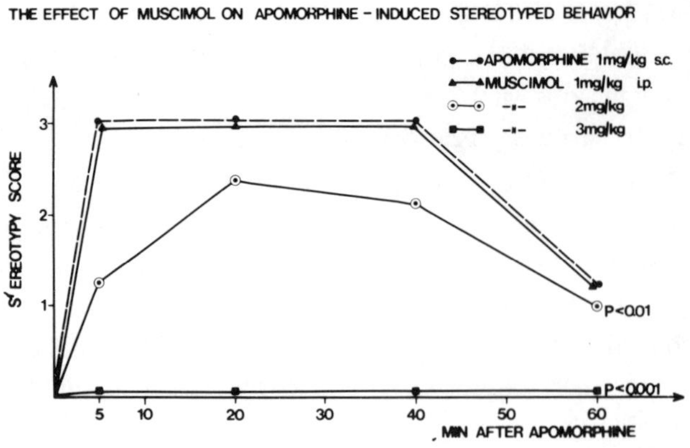

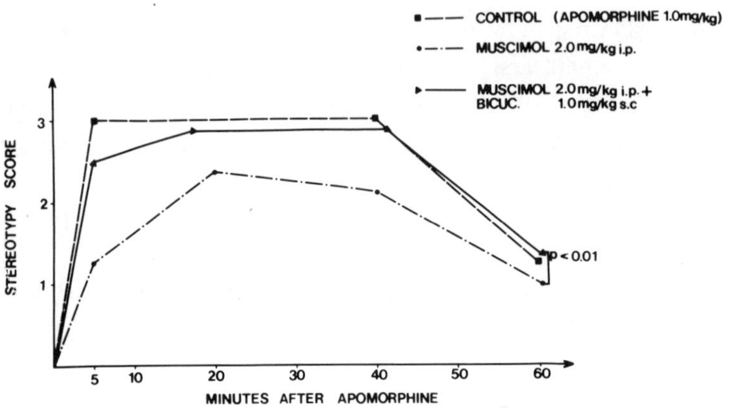

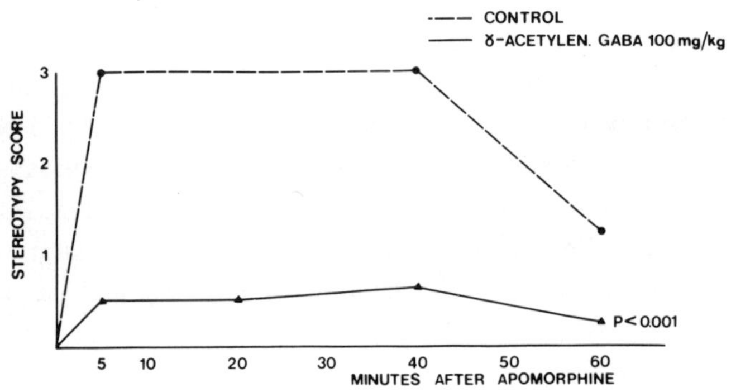

receptors can block the behavioral expression of DA receptor activity in these areas.

Fig. 1. The effects of muscimol, gamma-acetylenic GABA and combined treatment with muscimol and bicuculline on stereotyped behavior in rats induced by apomorphine. Muscimol was given 60 min before the apomorphine injection (1 mg/kg, s.c.) Gamma-acetylenic GABA was given 4 h before apomorphine and bicuculline was administered 30 min after muscimol. The stereotypies were assessed over an interval of 1 h. The intensity of the response was scored on a 1–3 scale. 0: No change in behavior, 1: Discontinuous sniffing, 2: Continuous sniffing, 3: Continuous sniffing chewing, biting and licking. Each value represents the mean score of eight animals. Statistical significance between the apomorphine control and the muscimol groups were evaluated by Mann-Whitney U-test. The same test was used when comparing the apomorphine group with the gamma-acetylenic GABA plus apomorphine group or the bicuculline plus muscimol plus apomorphine group.

Effects of muscimol and gamma-acetylenic GABA on DA turnover in the forebrain and on catecholamine turnover in the hypothalamus

Changes in DA and NA turnover have been evaluated by studying the disappearance of the catecholamine stores following the inhibition of tyrosine hydroxylase using the tyrosine hydroxylase inhibitor alphamethyltyrosine

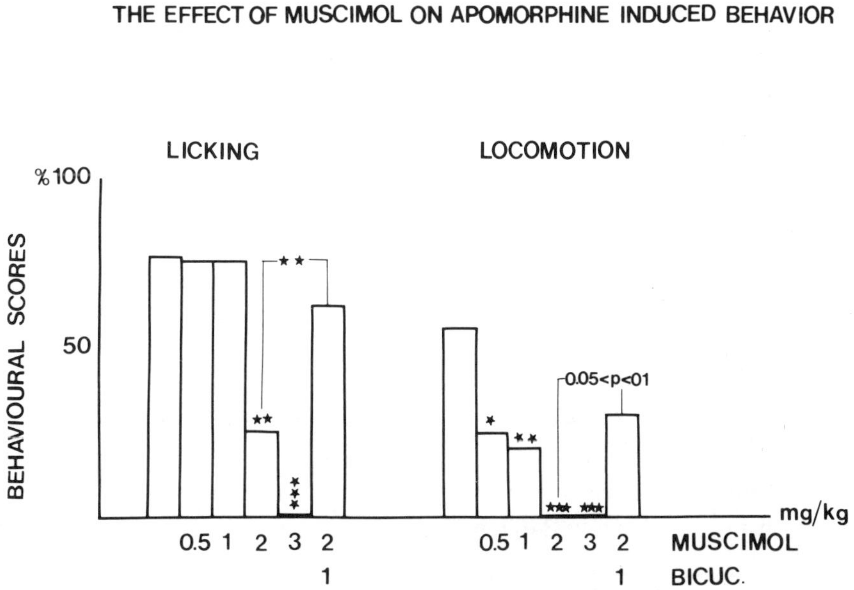

Fig. 2. The effect of muscimol on apomorphine induced stereotypies (licking) and increase in locomotion. Muscimol was given i.p. 60 min before the apomorphine injection (1 mg/kg, s.c.). Bicuculline in a dose of 1 mg/kg was given i.p. 30 min before the apomorphine injection. The results are the mean values of the total scores of an observation period of 60 min. Each value represents the mean scores of eight animals. Statistical significance was evaluated by Mann-Whitney U-test. x: $P<0.05$, xx: $P<0.01$ xxx: $P<0.001$.

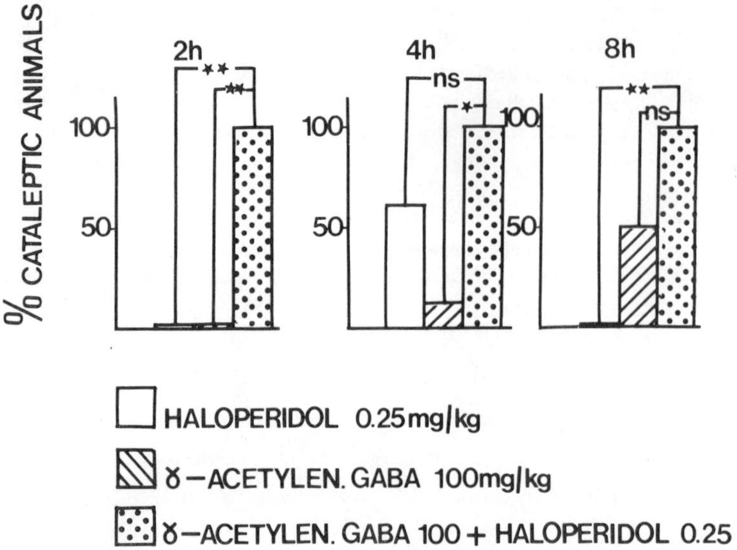

Fig. 3. The effect of gamma-acetylenic GABA in combination with haloperidol on cataleptic behavior in rats. The catalepsy was tested by placing the both front limbs over the horizontal bar and recording the time each animal stayed on the bar. The animal was defined as cataleptic if it stayed on the bar more than 60 sec. The percentage of animals with catalepsy were calculated from groups of 8–10 animals. The statistical analysis was performed by the Fisher exact probability test. x: $P<0.05$, xx: $P<0.01$, xxx: $P<0.001$. Haloperidol in a dose of 0.25 mg/kg was given i.p. together with gamma-acetylenic GABA (100 mg/kg, i.p.).

methyl ester (H44/68, 250 mg/kg/2 hours) before killing (see Fuxe *et al.* 1977b). As seen in Fig. 4, muscimol significantly increased DA turnover within the nucleus caudatus and produced a trend for an increase in nucleus accumbens (dotted type of DA terminal, posterior part) in doses of 0.3 mg/kg, while the DA turnover within the tuberculum olfactorium was not significantly affected. Furthermore, in the diffuse type of DA terminals of the nucleus accumbens (anterior part) a marked biphasic dose-effect curve was observed with a retarded DA depletion after H44/68 with the higher doses used (3 and 10 mg/kg), these groups being significantly different from the group treated with 1 mg/kg of muscimol.

The dopamine turnover within the lateral palisade zone (LPZ) of the median eminence was also significantly increased by muscimol in doses of 1–3 mg/kg (Fig. 5). The NA turnover within the subependymal layer (SEL) of the median eminence was significantly increased by muscimol in a dose of 3 mg/kg, while the increase of DA turnover in the medial palisade zone did not become

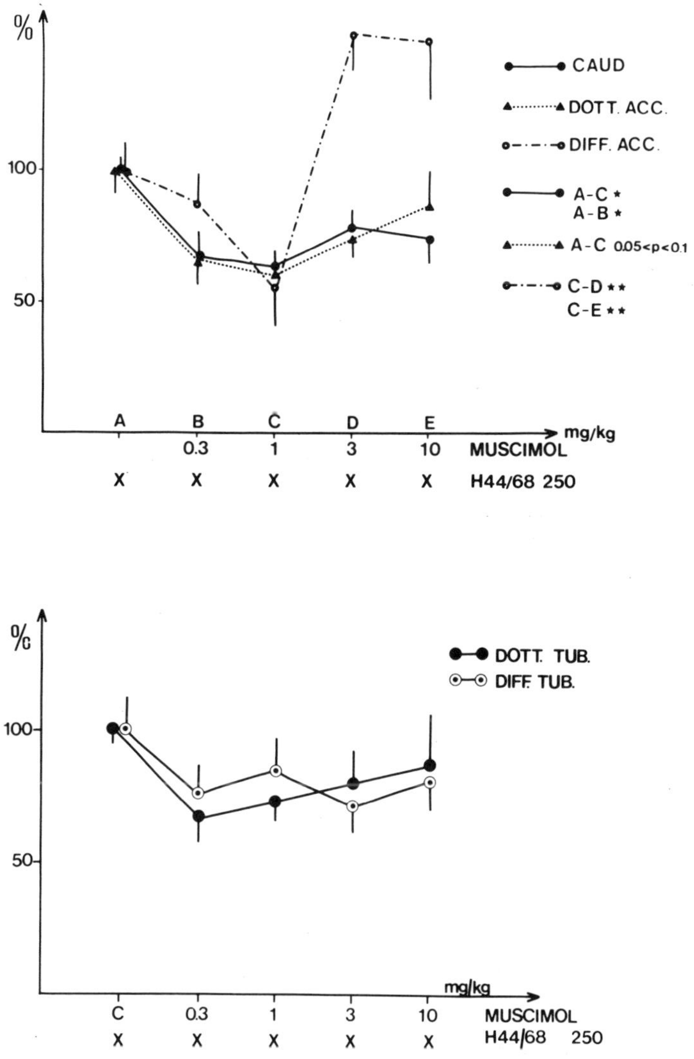

Fig. 4. The effects of muscimol on the H 44/68-induced DA fluorescence disappearance in various regions of the forebrain. H44/68 was given i.p. in a dose of 250 mg/kg 2 h before killing. Muscimol was administered at the same time i.p. On the x-axis the doses of muscimol are shown on a log scale. On the y axis the means ±S.E.M. of the DA fluorescence in each area is shown. The values are given in per cent of the respective H44/68 mean value. The Wilcoxon one-way classification: comparing all possible pairs of treatments was use. n = 5. x: $P<0.05$, xx: $P<0.01$. CAUD:anterior and medial part of nuc. caudatus, DOTT.ACC.: dotted type of DA terminal in posterior accumbens, DIFF.ACC.: diffuse type of DA terminal in the anterior accumbens, DOTT.TUB.: Dotted type of DA terminal in posterior tuberculum olfactorium, DIFF.TUB.: diffuse type of DA terminal in anterior tuberculum olfactorium.

significant (Fig. 5). In the anterior periventricular hypothalamic region (PUI), on the other hand, muscimol in a dose of 0.75 mg/kg produced a significant reduction of NA turnover. Thus, in contrast to previously studied GABA-ergic drugs, muscimol produced an increase of dopamine turnover in agreement with the work of Gessa's group, reporting increases of homovanillic acid levels in brain following muscimol treatment (Biggio *et al.* 1977). This increase is preferentially located in the motor centers (nucleus caudatus and nucleus

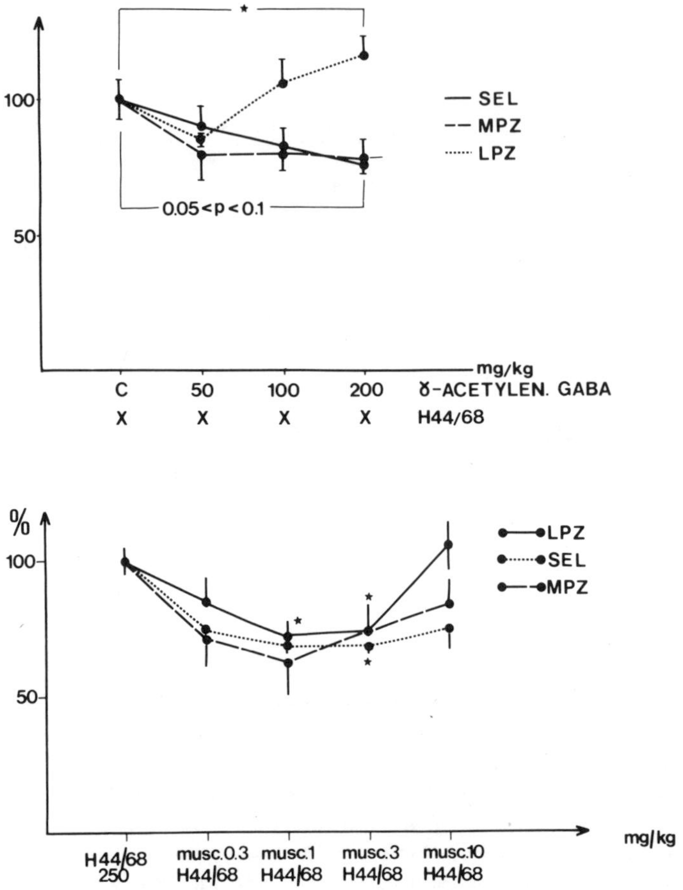

Fig. 5. The effects of gamma-acetylenic GABA and muscimol on the H44/68-induced CA fluorescence disappearance in the median eminence of rats. The GABA-ergic drugs were given i.p. at the same time as H44/68. The values are given in per cent of the H44/68 alone group mean value. Means ±S.E.M. are shown. For statistical analysis and significances see text to Fig. 4. SEL: subependymal layer, MPZ: medial palisade zone, LPZ: lateral palisade zone. The significances obtained are towards the H44/68 control group.

accumbens) and in the median eminence and disappears in the highest doses studied (3–10 mg/kg). After pretreatment with the DA receptor blocking agent pimozide, muscimol (0.75–3 mg/kg) could no longer produce signs of increases of DA turnover (Figs. 6, 7). Instead, even a significant reduction of DA turnover was observed in one region, i.e. in the dotted type of DA nerve terminal in the tuberculum olfactorium, using a dose of 3 mg/kg of muscimol.

Gamma-acetylenic GABA, on the other hand, decreased DA turnover in the LPZ but like muscimol increased NA turnover in the SEL (Fig. 5). Also, in contrast to muscimol, gamma-acetylenic GABA reduced DA turnover in the nucleus caudatus and left the nucleus accumbens (diffuse type of DA terminals) fairly unaffected (Fig. 8). The significant effects obtained with gammaacetylenic GABA were observed in a dose of 200 mg/kg, with this dose of gamma-acetylenic GABA also a significant increase of NA turnover was seen in the parvo cellular part of the hypothalamic region (Fig. 9). After pimozide pretreatment gamma-acetylenic GABA, like, e.g. lioresal preferentially and significantly reduced DA turnover in the nucleus accumbens (dotted type of DA terminal) and in the tuberculum olfactorium (diffuse type of DA terminals) (Figs. 6, 7).

The reason why muscimol increased dopamine turnover in the low dose range while the GABA transaminase inhibitor reduces dopamine turnover may be that muscimol in this dose range preferentially activates only *certain* types of GABA receptors. Muscimol-sensitive GABA receptors may be located perhaps mainly beyond the dopamine receptors and to a lesser degree on the DA dendrites in the substantia nigra and could in view of the behavioral data in this way elicit the compensatory increase of dopamine turnover observed. When the dose of muscimol is increased, however, the increase of DA turnover produced disappears and is in certain areas even reversed into a reduction. Thus, in high doses, muscimol may also activate other types of GABA receptors having an inhibitory influence on DA neurons. These GABA receptors are probably partly located within the substantia nigra and within the area of the A 10 group which sends DA fibers to the limbic regions (see Fuxe *et al.* 1976b). This interpretation would also be in line with the reductions of DA turnover obtained with gamma-acetylenic GABA, since in this case GABA may leak out from the GABA terminals to reach GABA receptors in all areas, and in this case the inhibitory influences on the dopamine pathways will predominate. In the case of the mesolimbic DA systems this is especially true when the DA receptors have been blocked, whereas the opposite seems to be true for the nigro-neostriatal DA system. Gamma-acetyletic GABA resembles lioresal and 5 ethyl, 5 phenyl-pyrrolidione in its ability to preferentially reduce DA turnover in the limbic areas (see Fuxe *et al.* 1977b). Thus, the latter two drugs may preferentially act on the GABA receptors having inhibitory influences on limbic DA pathways.

The fact that both muscimol and gamma-acetylenic GABA increase NA turnover within the SEL (Fig. 5) indicates the possible existence of a local GABA-ergic control of this NA nerve terminal system. A local GABA-ergic mechanism may also be involved in the control of NA release from the NA nerve terminal plexa of the parvocellular portion of the hypothalamic paraventricular

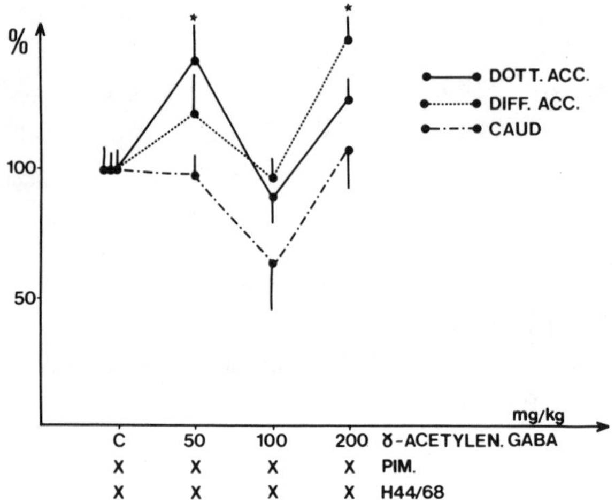

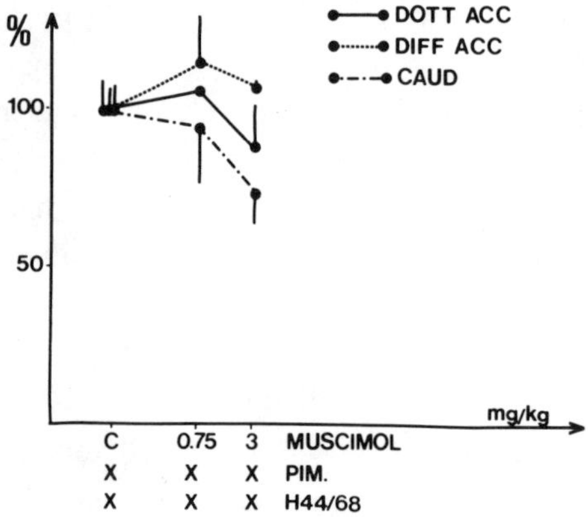

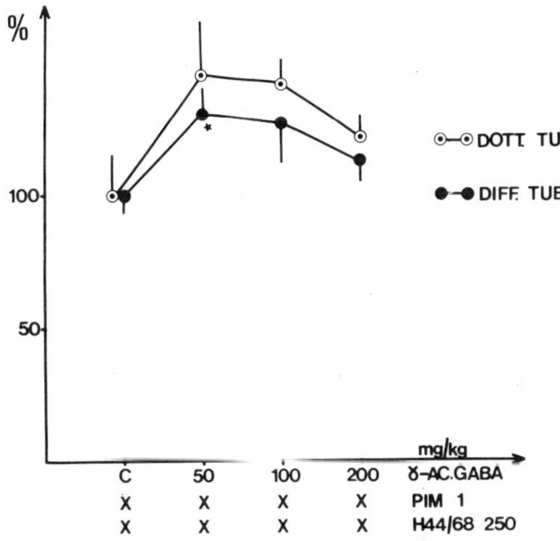

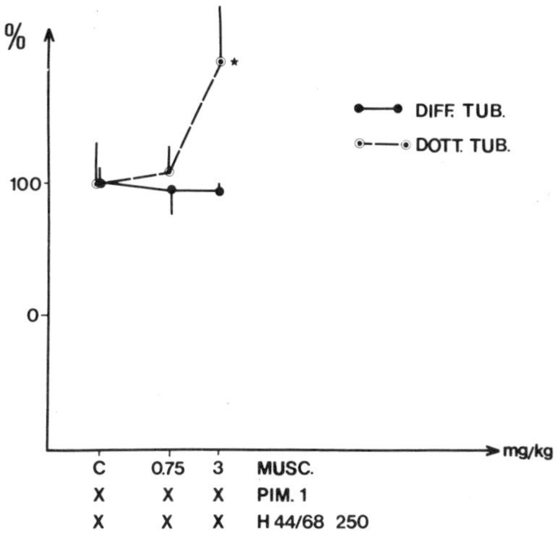

Figs. 6 and 7. The effects of gamma-acetylenic GABA and muscimol on the pimozide induced increase in the H44/68-induced DA fluorescence disappearance in the forebrain. Pimozide was given 2 h before the H44/68 injection in a dose of 1 mg/kg i.p. The GABA-ergic drugs were given at the same time as the H44/68. For further details see text to Fig. 4. The DA fluorescence values are given in per cent of the respective H44/68 group mean value. Means ±S.E.M. are shown. n = 5. For statistical analysis see text to Fig. 4. x: $P<0.05$. The significance obtained is always towards the H44/68 control group.

nucleus, in view of the dose-dependent increases of NA turnover observed after treatment with gamma-acetylenic GABA in a dose of 200 mg/kg.

The fact that muscimol (1–3 mg/kg) increased DA turnover in the LPZ of the

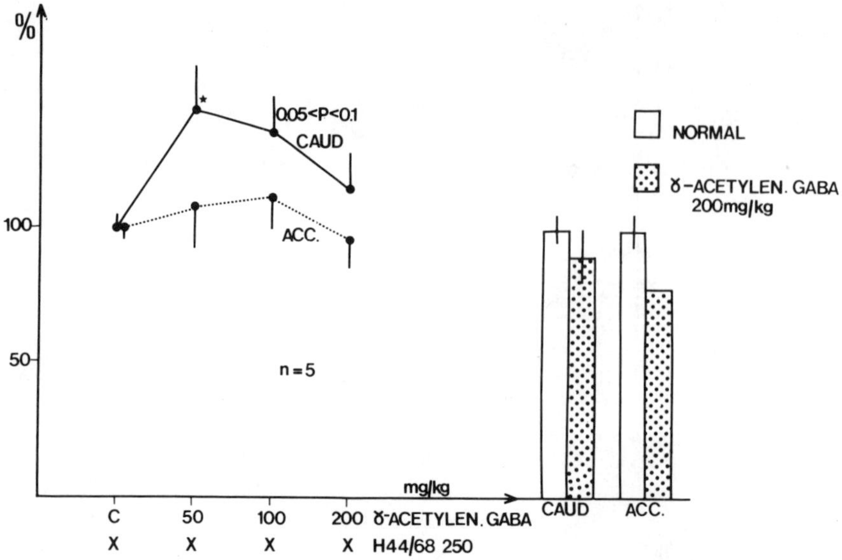

Fig. 8. The effects of gamma-acetylenic GABA on the H44/68-induced DA fluorescence disappearance in the nuc.caudatus and in the nuc.accumbens (diffuse type of DA terminal, anterior part). The GABA-ergic drug was given at the same time as the H44/68. For further details on treatment see text to Figs. 4 and 5. The fluorescence values are given in per cent of the H44/68 alone group mean value. Means ±S.E.M. ar shown. Statistical analysis as described in text to Fig. 4. Significances refer to the H44/68 control group. n = 5. x: $P<0.05$.

median eminence while gamma-acetylenic GABA (200 mg/kg) reduced DA turnover in this area could also be explained on the basis that muscimol in the lower dose range only activates certain types of GABA receptors which predominantly have an excitatory influence on the tubero-inferdibular DA systems. However, when the dose of muscimol is increased also other types of GABA receptors may be activated, including those having inhibitory influences on this DA system and the increase of DA turnover will disappear. After gamma-acetylenic GABA the inhibitory GABA-ergic influences obviously predominate and a reduction of DA turnover is observed. These results illustrate well the possible existence of both excitatory and inhibitory GABA-ergic influences on the tubero-inferdibular DA pathways. Thus, GABA-ergic mechanisms could in part mediate their neuroendocrine actions over this DA system. In agreement with this view is the fact that GABA and GABA-ergic drugs have been found to both decrease and increase, e.g. prolactin secretion (Makara & Stark 1978, Mc Cann *et al.* 1978).

Effects of DA receptor blocking agents on GABA turnover in DA rich regions
Changes in GABA turnover were evaluated by measuring the accumulation of GABA induced by gamma-acetylenic GABA. This accumulation is probably dependent on nerve impulses, since it is markedly reduced by interruption of the impulse flow. Changes in GABA accumulation may therefore reveal changes in the neuronal GABA pool. The results obtained with chlorpromazine and sulpiride are summarized in Tables I and II. Chlorpromazine (10 mg/kg) and sulpiride (100 mg/kg) both produced catalepsy. As seen in Tables I and II the drugs produced a trend for a selective reduction of the gamma-acetylenic GABA-induced accumulation of GABA in the substantia nigra. Furthermore, a non-cataleptogenic dose of sulpiride (15 mg/kg) produced a substantial depletion of the GABA stores within the substantia nigra and trends for depletion of GABA stores in the prefrontal cortex and in subcortical limbic regions (Table II). Lloyd & Hornykiewicz (1977) have previously observed that haloperidol acutely depletes GABA stores in the substantia nigra.

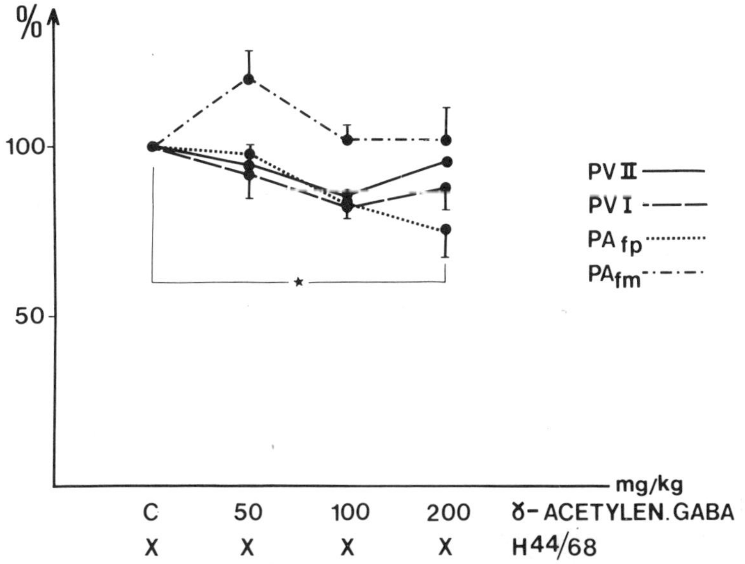

Fig. 9. The effects of gamma-acetylenic GABA on the H44/68-induced DA fluorescence disappearance in various NA nerve terminal plexa of the hypothalamus. Treatment as described in text to Fig. 8. The fluorescence values are given as per cent of the H44/68 alone group mean value. Means ±S.E.M. are shown. Statistical analysis as described in text to Fig. 4. x: $P<0.05$. PV I: Anterior periventricular hypothalamic region. PV II: Posterior periventricular hypothalamic region. PA_{fp}: the parvocellular part of the paraventricular hypothalamic nucleus. PA_{fm}: the magnocellular part of the paraventricular hypothalamic nucleus. n = 5.

The preferential effects found in the substantia nigra region might reflect an important dopaminergic control of GABA release in the nigral region. It may be that dendritic release of DA in the substantia nigra can control GABA synthesis and release in nigral GABA terminal, having an overall facilitory influence (Reubi *et al.* 1977). Therefore, blockade of DA receptors in the substantia nigra can lead to the reduction of GABA stores and turnover observed in the present experiments. These results are in line with our previous findings that apomorphine can increase GABA turnover within the substantia nigra region (Perez de la Mora & Fuxe 1977). The failure to see any effects on GABA turnover in the neostriatum after DA receptor blocking agents is in line with previous results obtained, e.g. with pimozide and haloperidol (Mao *et al.* 1978, Racagni *et al.* 1978). In view of these findings it should be considered that the apomorphine-induced increases of GABA turnover in the neostriatum and limbic structures (Perez de la Mora & Fuxe 1977) may reflect the existence of a dopaminergic mechanism, which only operates under special conditions to increase GABA nervous activity in these structures. Furthermore, we have recently observed

Table I

Effect of chlorpromazine on γ-acetylenic-GABA-induced GABA accumulation

Treatment	Region: *N. caudatus*	*Subcortical limbic region*	*Prefrontal cortex*	*Midbrain ventral tegmentum*	
Saline	100±12 (5)	100±11 (4)	100±7.4 (4)	100±5.1 (5)	
Chlorpromazine (10 mg/kg; 4h)	102± 6 (5)	89.7±9.1 (5)	94.4±13 (4)	85.9±5 (4)	
γ-acetylenic GABA (100 mg/kg; 4 h)	323±57 (4)	246±25 (4)	293±29 (4)	173±8 (4)	$P<0.1$
γ-acetylenic-GABA (100 mg/kg; 4 h) + Chlorpromazine (10 mg/kg; 4 h)	349±35 (5)	239±20 (5)	306±19 (5)	145±10 (4)	

Values are in per cent of the corresponding saline control group ±S.E.M. Absolute values (μmoles/g wet tissue) for the saline-treated group were: N. caudatus 1.3±0.16; subcortical limbic region, 2.7±0.31; prefrontal cortex, 1.1±0.08; midbrain ventral tegmentum 4.5±0.23. Double tailed Student's t-test was used for the statistical evaluation of the results. Chlorpromazine and γ-acetylenic-GABA treated groups were compared with the saline-treated group while γ-acetylenic-GABA + chloropromazine was compared with the corresponding γ-acetylenic-GABA-treated group. $P<0.001$ was found for the γ-acetylenic-GABA-group in all the regions. Number of animals in parenthesis.

Table II

Effects of sulpiride on γ-acetylenic-GABA-induced GABA accumulation

Treatment	Region N. caudatus	Subcortical limbic region	Prefrontal cortex	Midbrain ventral tegmentum
Saline	100±8.9 (7)	100±10.4 (7)	100±9.4 (5)	100±10.3 (7)
		$0.05<P<0.1$	$0.05<P<0.1$	$P<0.01$
Sulpiride (15 mg/kg; 4 h)	87.9±0.16 (7)	69.1±10.6 (7)	78.6±4.2 (5)	62±5.2 (6)
Sulpiride (100 mg/kg; 4 h)	92.9±7.1 (4)	87.7±5.3 (4)	-	73.9±9.8 (3)
γ-acetylenic-GABA (100 mg/kg; 4 h)	280±25 (7)	176±11 (7)	262±19 (5)	208±7.0 (6)
γ-acetylenic-GABA (100 mg/kg; 4 h) + Sulpiride (15 mg/kg; 4 h)	282±9.2 (6)	188±12 (6)	319±27 (4)	196±24 (6)
γ-acetylenic-GABA (100 mg/kg) + Sulpiride (100 mg/kg; 4 h)	277±22 (4)	232±30 (4)	-	175±17 (4)

Values are in per cent of the control saline-treated mean group ±S.E.M. Absolute values (μmoles/g wet tissue) for the control group were: N. caudatus, 1.83±0.16; subcortical limbic region, 4.5±0.47; prefrontal cortex, 1.17±0.11 and midbrain ventral tegmentum 4.95±0.5. Double tailed Student's t-test was used for the statistical evaluation of the results. Sulpiride alone and γ-acetylenic-GABA groups were compared with the saline-treated group while γ-acetylenic-GABA + sulpiride-treated group was compared with the corresponding γ-acetylenic-GABA-treated control group. $P<0.001$ was found for the γ-acetylenic-GABA in all the regions. Number of animals in parenthesis.

that another DA receptor agonist, bromocriptine, which only seems to activate DA receptors not related to adenylcyclase, preferentially *reduces* GABA turnover in subcortical limbic structures, indicating that different types of DA receptors can have opposite effects on GABA turnover. Such mechanisms could also contribute to the failure of DA receptor blocking agents to influence GABA turnover in the DA-rich areas of the forebrain.

Effects of muscimol and gamma-acetylenic GABA on prolactin secretion.
As seen in the Figs. 10 and 11 both muscimol and gamma-acetylenic GABA effectively reduce the hypersecretion of prolactin obtained after inhibition of the

catecholamine synthesis by maximal 90% and 50% respectively. The inhibitory effects on prolactin secretion by these drugs could also be obtained in the presence of the DA receptor blocking agent pimozide. However, after pimozide pretreatment the maximal inhibition by muscimol (Fig. 11) was only 50%. These findings indicate that GABA-ergic mechanisms can in part exert their inhibitory effects on prolactin secretion without involving an activation of the tubero-

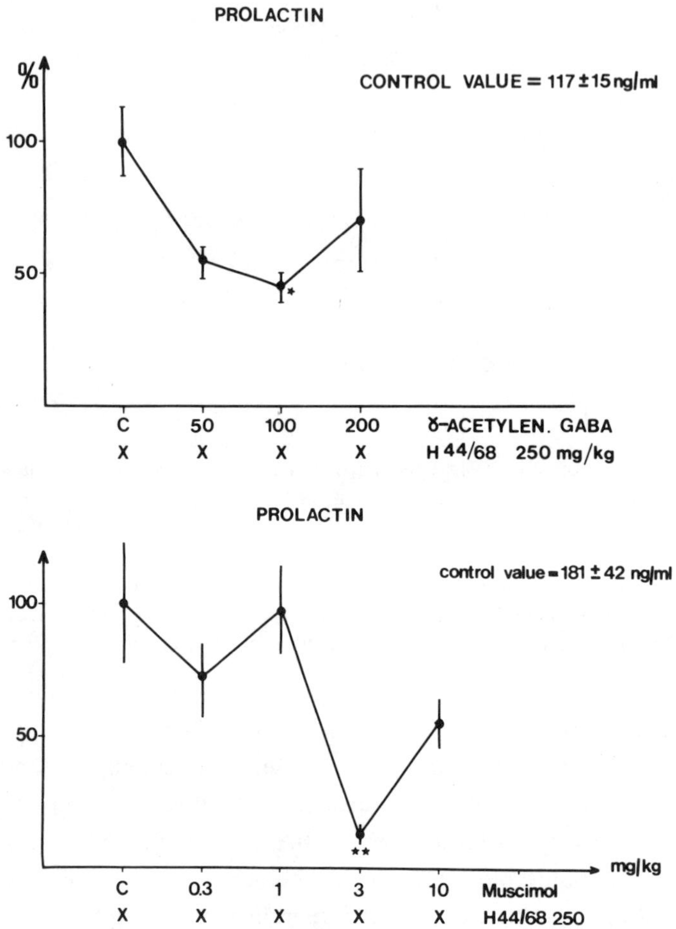

Fig. 10. The effects of gamma-acetylenic GABA and muscimol on the increase of prolactin secretion produced by H44/68 (250 mg/kg, i.p., 2 h before killing) in normal male Sprague-Dawley rats. The prolactin values are given in per cent of the H44/68 alone group mean value, which is given in the figure. Means ±S.E.M. are shown. Statistical analysis was made according to Wilcoxon one-way classification, treatment versus controls. x:$P<0.05$. xx:$P<0.01$.

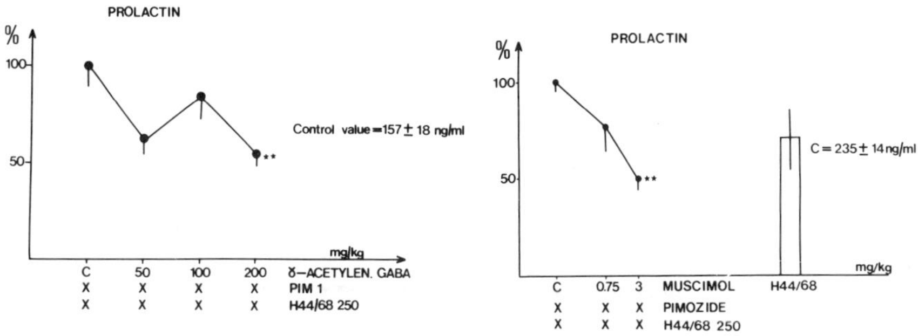

Fig. 11. Effects of gamma-acetylenic GABA and muscimol on the pimozide and H44/68-induced increase of prolactin secretion. Same treatment as described in text to Figs. 6 and 7. The values are given in per cent of the group treated with pimozide and H44/68 alone. Means ±S.E.M. are shown. The absolute values for the pimozide plus H44/68 group are shown in the figure. Statistical analysis as in text to Fig. 10. xx: $P<0.01$.

infundibular DA neurons, since the pituitary DA receptors in these experiments were blocked. Thus, GABA-ergic mechanisms could control also activity in the prolactin releasing factor containing systems and/or in thyroid hormone releasing hormone (THRH) – containing systems, since THRH also has the ability to release prolactin. It should be pointed out that muscimol may mainly inhibit prolactin secretion by a direct action on putative GABA receptors located on the prolactin gland cells (see Müller, this symposium, Guidotti, pers. comm.). In agreement with the idea that GABA terminals can control THRH – containing systems is the fact that gamma-acetylenic GABA increases NA turnover in the parvocellular part of the paraventricular nucleus which is rich in THRH cell bodies. This increase in NA turnover should lead to a facilitory influence on prolactin secretion, since NA mechanisms facilitates TSH secretion. A partial involvement of the inhibitory dopaminergic mechanisms in mediating the inhibitory effects of muscimol and gamma-acetylenic GABA on prolactin secretion is also likely in view of the fact that they both produce a trend for an increase of DA turnover in MPZ from which zone DA probably is released as a prolactin inhibitory factor.

SUMMARY

The present paper gives evidence for the existence of GABA-ergic mechanisms having both inhibitory and excitatory influences on ascending nigro-neostriatal and mesolimbic DA pathways as well as on the tubero-infundibular DA systems controlling, e.g. prolactin secretion. Certain selective hypothalamic NA terminal regions also show increases or decreases of NA turnover after treatment with GABA-ergic drugs, indicating the existence of local GABA-ergic mechanisms controlling certain hypothalamic NA terminal plexa.

The results obtained with various GABA-ergic drugs and especially with the GABA receptor agonist muscimol led to the hypothesis that muscimol preferentially stimulates GABA receptors with a facilitating influence on the DA systems. Thus, there may exist at least two types of GABA receptors in the brain. One type, which is inhibitory to the ascending DA systems, is *inter alia* located on the DA cell bodies, dendrites and terminals. The other type, which is excitatory to the ascending DA systems, is in view of the behavioral findings, showing blockade by GABA-ergic drugs of apomorphine-induced locomotion and stereotyped behavior, probably *inter alia* located beyond the DA receptors in the neostriatum, nuc accumbens and tuberculum olfactorium. The blockade of the behavioral expression of postsynaptic DA receptor activation by stimulation of this GABA receptor probably activates a compensatory mechanism to increase DA turnover.

After blockade of DA receptors it can be demonstrated that the limbic DA terminals are preferentially inhibited versus the neostriatal DA terminals by treatment with GABA-ergic drugs. Therefore, combined treatment with neuroleptics and GABA-ergic drugs may improve treatment of schizophrenia, since the antipsychotic activity of neuroleptic drugs may be related to blockade of limbic DA receptors. The preferential inhibitory effects by GABA-ergic drugs of locomotor activity versus stereotyped activity induced by apomorphine, the former being controlled by nuc. accumbens, gives further support to the idea that limbic DA mechanisms are preferentially inhibited by GABA-ergic drugs. Thus the findings suggest that muscimol and gamma-acetylenic GABA in the low dose range can preferentially inhibit the behavioral expression of DA receptor activation in limbic structures. In the high dose range, however, these two drugs could enhance haloperidol-induced catalepsia and by themselves produce catalepsia, suggesting blocking activity also of neostriatal DA mechanisms by GABA receptors.

Prolactin secretion seems to be under a predominantly inhibitory control by GABA pathways in view of the marked inhibitory effects observed on prolactin secretion in the pharmacological analysis. Inhibitory effects can be observed even in the presence of DA receptor blockade indicating that the main inhibitory action can involve another mechanism e.g. stimulation of putative GABA receptors in the anterior pituitary inhibiting prolactin recretion. Mapping out of GABA neurons indicates existence of hypothalamo-infundibular GABA neurons

ACKNOWLEDGMENTS

This work has been supported by a grant (MH 25504) from the National Institute of Health, by a grant (04X–715) from the Swedish Medical Research Council and by grants from M. Bergvalls Stiftelse and Karolinska Institutet. Muscimol was generously supplied by Professor P. Krogsgaard-Larsen.

"γ-acetylenic GABA was generously forwarded by the Centre de Recherche Merrell International, Strasbourg, France".

REFERENCES

Andén, N.-E. & Wachtel, H. (1978) Some effects of GABA and GABA-like drugs on central catecholamine mechanisms. In: *Interactions Between Putative Neurotransmitters in the Brain*, ed. Garttini, S., Pujol, J. F. & Samanin, R. pp. 161–174. Raven Press, New York.

Bartholini, G. (1976) Interactions of dopamine, acetyl-choline and γ-aminobutyric acid in limbic and striatal structures: relation to the therapy of schizophrenia. In: *Rhinencéphales Neurotransmetteurs et Psychoses*, ed. de Ajuriaguerra, J. & Tissot, R. pp. 241–251. Georg & S. A., Genève.

Biggio, G., Casu, M., Corda, M. G., Vernaleone, F. & Gessa, G. L. (1977) Effect of muscimol, a GABA-mimetic agent, on dopamine metabolism in the mouse brain. *Life Sci.* 21, 525–532.

Bird, E. D., Barnes, J., Iversen, L. L., Spokes, E. G., Mackay, A. V. P. & Shepherd, M. (1977) Increased brain dopamine and reduced glutamic acid decarboxylase and choline acetyl transferase activity in schizophrenia and related psychoses. *Lancet* 2 (8049), 1157–1159.

Fuxe, K., Hökfelt, T., Johansson, O., Ganten, D., Goldstein, M., Pérez de la Mora, M. Possani, L., Tapia, R., Terán, L., Palacios, R., Said & Mutt, V. (1976) Monoamine neurons system in the hypothalamus and their relation to the GABA and peptide-containing neurons, *INSERM, Colloque de Synthese 1976*, Action Thématique Rapport No. 7: Actions thématiques 22 et 35. Neuroendocrinologie, pp. 17–40.

Fuxe, K., Hökfelt, T., Ljungdahl, A., Agnati, L., Johansson, O., & Pérez de la Mora, M. (1975) Evidence for an inhibitory gabergic control of the mesolimbic dopamine neurons: Possibility of improving treatment of schizophrenia by combined treatment with neuroleptics and gabergic drugs. *Med. Biol.* 53, 177–183.

Fuxe, K., Pérez de la Mora, M., Agnati, L., Eneroth, P., Gustafsson, J.-Å. & Ögren, S.-O. (1977a) Possible involvement of central aminergic, histaminergic, cholinergic and gabaergic mechanisms in the central control of gonadotrophin secretion. A pharmacological analysis. *Acta Endocrinol.* Suppl. 212, 85, p. 15.

Fuxe, K., Pérez de la Mora, M., Hökfelt, T., Agnati, L., Ljungdahl, A. & Johansson, O. (1977b) GABA-DA interaction and their possible relation to schizophrenia. In: *Psychopathology and*

Brain Dysfunction, ed. Shagass, C., Gershon, S. & Friedhoff, A. J. pp. 97–111. Raven Press, New York.

Lloyd, K. G. & Hornykiewicz, O. (1977) Effect of chronic neuroleptic or L-Dopa administration on GABA levels in the rat substantia nigra. *Life Sci.* 21 (10), 1489–1496.

Makara, G. B. & Stark, E. (1978) Role of GABA in the hypothalamic control of the pituitary gland. In: *Interactions Between Putative Neurotransmitters in the Brain,* ed. Garttini, S., Pujol, J. F. & Samanin, R. pp. 263–284. Raven Press, New York.

Mao, C. C., Marco, E., Revuelta, A. & Costa, E. (1978) Antipsychotics and GABA turnover in mammalian brain nuclei. In: *Interactions Between Putative Neurotransmitters in the Brain,* ed. Garattini, S., Pujol, J. R. & Samanin, R. pp. 151–160. Raven Press, New York.

McCann, S. M., Krulich, L., Ojeda, S. R. & Vijayan, E. (1978) Control of prolactin release by putative synaptic transmitters. In: *Progress in Prolactin Physiology and Pathology,* ed. Robyn, C. & Harter, M. pp. 137–148. Elsevier/North Holland Biomedical Press.

McGeer, P. L. & McGeer, E. G. (1977) Possible changes in striatal and limbic cholinergic systems in schizophrenia. *Arch. Gen. Psychiatry* 34, 1319–1323.

Pérez de la Mora, M. & Fuxe, K. (1977) Brain GABA, dopamine and acetylcholine interactions. 1. Studies with oxotremorine. *Brain Res.* 135, 107–122.

Pérez de la Mora, M., Fuxe, K., Hökfelt, T. & Ljungdahl, A. (1977) Evidence for a nerve impulse-dependent GABA accumulation in the substantia nigra after treatment with γ-glutamylhydrazide. *Neurosci. Lett.* 5, 75–82.

Possani, L. D., Bayón, A. & Tapia, R. (1977) Synthesis of affinity chromatographic resins for the purification of brain glutamate decarboxylase. *Neurochem. Res.* 2, 51–57.

Racagni, G., Bruno, F., Cattabeni, F., Maggi, A., Di Guilio, A. M. & Groppetti, A. (1978) Interactions among dopamine, acetylcholine, and GABA in the nigrostriatal system. In: *Interactions Between Putative Neurotransmitters in the Brain,* ed. Garattini, S., Pujol, J. F. & Samanin, R. pp. 61–74, Raven Press, New York.

Reubi, J.-C., Iversen, L. L. & Jessel, T. M. (1977) Dopamine selectively increases ^{3}H-GABA release from slices of rat substantia nigra *in vitro. Nature* 268, 652–654.

Roberts, E. (1974) A hypothesis suggesting that there is a defect in the GABA system in schizophrenia. *Neurosci. Res. Program Bull.* 10, 468–482.

Schechter, P. J., Tranier, Y., Jung, M. J. & Böhlen, P. (1977) Audiogenic seizure protection by elevated brain GABA concentration in mice: Effects of γ-acetylenic GABA and γ-vinyl GABA, two irreversible GABA-T inhibitors. *Eur. J. Pharmacol.* 45, 319–328.

Scheel-Krüger, J., Christensen, A. V. & Arnt, J. (1978) Muscimol differentially facilitates stereotypy but antagonizes motility induced by dopaminergic drugs: a complex GABA-dopamine interaction. *Life Sci.* 22 (1), 75–84.

Turnover Rates of GABA in Striatal Structures: Regulation and Pharmacological Implications

F. Moroni, E. Peralta & E. Costa

Several lines of independent investigation have suggested that gamma-amino butyric acid (GABA) plays a fundamental role as a neurotransmitter in striatal structures (Costa *et al.* 1978). There are two types of GABA neurons in striatum: short axon GABA neurons which are intrinsic to the striatum (McGeer & McGeer 1975) and long axon GABA neurons which project from striatum to other nuclei such as the descending strio-nigra GABA-ergic pathway (Fonnum *et al.* 1974, Gale *et al.* 1977). Long axon GABA-ergic neurons have been postulated to play a role in the feedback regulation of dopaminergic nigro-striatal neurons (Ribak *et al.* 1976, Anden *et al.* 1964, Ungerstedt 1971, Lindvall & Bjorklund 1974). This background information and some reports on the inhibition by muscimol of the striatal tyrosine hydroxylase activation caused by haloperidol (Gale *et al.* 1977) suggest that GABA-ergic striatal-nigra neurons may play a role in determining the extrapyramidal side effects of classical antipsychotics (Carlsson & Lindqvist 1963). But, in fact, many attempts to produce convincing and more direct evidence that an inhibition of GABA-ergic mechanisms in substantia nigra is associated with the extrapyramidal side effects of classical antipsychotics turned out to be unsuccessful (Marco *et al.* 1978, Mao *et al.* 1977, Costa *et al.* 1978). The reasons for this lack of success can be explained by recent evidence on the role that striatal enkephalinergic (Hong *et al.* 1978) and substance P (Hong & Costa 1978) neurons play in the action of

---

Laboratory of Preclinical Pharmacology, National Institute of Mental Health, Saint Elizabeths Hospital, Washington, D.C. 20032 USA.

"GABA-NEUROTRANSMITTERS", Alfred Benzon Symposium 12, Munksgaard 1978

antipsychotics and in the regulation of feedback neuronal loops linking the N. caudatus to the substantia nigra.

Our knowledge of how putative neurotransmitters participate in the function of various neuronal loops strictly relates to the availability of appropriate electrophysiological, biochemical and histochemical methodology. Since further methodological developments are needed, our understanding of how drugs affect the function of various brain pathways is not complete. Among the biochemical methods available to assess the extent of neuronal participation into a given function, the procedure that still offers more advantages is the estimation of the turnover rate of neurotransmitters. This procedure acquires a greater impact when used in conjunction with anatomical and electrophysiological information. Recently it became possible to measure the turnover rate of GABA (Bertilsson *et al.* 1977); the present report will give an account of the information acquired using this approach to study the pharmacology of striatal GABA-ergic mechanisms.

MEASUREMENT OF GABA TURNOVER RATES

The development of a very sensitive method for the simultaneous quantitation by mass fragmentography of the glutamic acid and GABA content in brain tissue (Bertilsson & Costa 1976) has made it possible to measure the turnover rate of GABA in small brain structures. With this method, the carboxylic groups of glutamate and GABA are esterified with 1,1,1,3,3,3-hexafluoroisopropanol (HFIP) while the amino groups are acylated with pentafluoropropionic anhydride (PFPA). To obtain an estimation of the GABA utilization, the changes with time in the ^{13}C enrichment of GABA and glutamate during constant rate infusion of ^{13}C glucose are monitored (Bertilsson *et al.* 1977). Similar to the other methods to measure the turnover rate of catecholamines (Costa & Meek 1974) or acetylcholine (Cheney & Costa 1977), also this method is based on a certain number of assumptions and it involves a number of approximations. Therefore the measurement of GABA turnover is useful for comparative drug studies but fails to yield absolute values of turnover rates. As it was just proposed, the method tacitly implies that the glutamate pool present in a brain sample serves only as a precursor of GABA. Naturally, this is never completely true because glutamate functions not only as a GABA precursor but also as an intermediary metabolite and as a primary transmitter. The errors deriving from such a generalization can be minimized by collecting the samples very early during the infusion of ^{13}C glucose and by selecting those tissues where the pool size of glutamate functioning predominently as a GABA precursor prevails over that of the other two glutamate pools. In practice, with this method, the turnover rate of GABA can be estimated in the globus pallidus, substantia nigra, N. caudatus and N. accumbens, but it cannot be determined in the cerebellar cortex, deep cerebellar nuclei and various parts of the hippocampus where glutamate is an important transmitter.

Another problem that besets these measurements is the deviations from linearity caused by the recycling of the variant ^{13}C atom. GABA is metabolized to succinic semialdehyde which is a substrate for the tricarboxylic acid cycle. By this route the ^{13}C incorporated into GABA can return to glutamic acid. When the label is administered by pulse injection, the problems created by such a recycling are without a practical solution. Conversely, when the specific activity of label led glucose increases at a convenient rate, such as, for instance, during constant rate infusion, one can calculate the efflux rate of ^{13}C from the precursor-product relationship at a time when the deviations caused by ^{13}C recycling are minimal. Of course, even though the errors caused by recycling can be minimized, they cannot be excluded completely by using the constant rate infusion.

In the brain nuclei shown in Table 1, the value of the turnover rate of GABA is completely unrelated to the GABA content. GABA turnover is highest in N. caudatus and lowest in substantia nigra, but N. caudatus has the lowest and substantia nigra the highest GABA content.

SYNAPSES BETWEEN GABA-ERGIC NEURONS

In order to understand whether in striatum GABA-ergic neurons establish synaptic contacts with each other, two types of experiments were conducted. In one of them, muscimol (1,5 mg/kg), a potent and specific GABA receptor

Table I

GABA concentrations and turnover rate in regions of rat brain

Region	GABA (nmoles/mg prot)	k_{GABA}/hr	TR_{GABA} (nmoles/mg prot/hr)
Substantia nigra	95±4.4	3.1±0.5	290
Globus Pallidus	89±5.5	4.0±0.3	360
N. Caudatus	19±0.86	18±1.5	340
N. Accumbens	47±2.2	5.1±0.7	240

Each figure represents the average of at least six determinations.

agonist, (Curtis *et al.* 1971, Krossgard-Larsen *et al.* 1975) was administered intravenously to rats 40 min before beginning a constant rate infusion with ^{13}C glucose. Muscimol failed to change the GABA content but decreased the turnover rate of GABA in the N. caudatus and in substantia nigra (Table II). A change was not obtained in the globus pallidus and N. accumbens (Table II). The remarkable decrease in GABA turnover elicited by muscimol in N. caudatus indicates that in this nucleus, a major site for the metabolism of GABA is inhibited by the stimulation of GABA receptors. since a similar inhibition was not obtained in the N. accumbens nor in the globus pallidus, one can infer that in the N. caudatus but not in the N. accumbens, or the globus pallidus, the small GABA interneurons intrinsic to striatum are connected in a series. Since the injection of muscimol also reduces the turnover rate of GABA in the substantia nigra, we must conclude that also the cell bodies of the long axon GABA-ergic neurons of the caudate-nigra or of the caudate-pallidal pathways contain GABA receptors. However, there is also the possibility that GABA receptors regulate an excitatory pathway afferent to the long axon GABA-ergic neurons that connect caudatus to pallidus or caudatus to nigra.

It has been debated whether or not the GABA-ergic connection between the striatum and substantia nigra is a continuing pathway or is interupted by synapses. We have reasoned that if the pathway was interrupted by GABA-ergic synapses, the stimulation of N. caudatus should cause an inhibition of the turnover rate of GABA (TR_{GABA}) in substantia nigra. If it were continuous, the stimulation should cause an increase of TR_{GABA}.

A direct electrical current was applied unilaterally to the outer shell of the head of the nucleus caudatus while the rats were infused intravenously with ^{13}C-glucose (Mao *et al.* 1978). Stimulus intensities of 2 and 4 volts (20 Hz and 0.5 ms)

Table II

Action of muscimol (1.5 mg/kg) on the turnover rate of GABA in regions of rat brain

Region	TR_{GABA}(nmoles/mg prot/hr) Saline	Muscimol	% of Control
Substantia Nigra	290±32	110±15*	40
Globus Pallidus	360±45	400±41	111
N. Caudatus	340±30	66±12*	19
N. Accumbens	240±28	280±23	117

Each figure represents the average of at least six determinations.
*$P<0.05$

Table III

Striatal HVA content and GABA turnover rate following unilateral electrical stimulation of substantia nigra

Tissue Analyzed	HVA (pmol/mg prot)	TR_{GABA} (μmol/mg prot/hr)
Homolateral to stimulation	110±10*	280±40
Contralateral to stimulation	60±6	330±62

Stimulation at 15 Hz, 6 volts/ 2 ms for 20 min. Each value is the average of six animals.

failed to change the TR_{GABA}; however, both 8 and 10 volts doubled the TR_{GABA} in the substantia nigra ipsilateral to the stimulus without affecting the contralateral substantia nigra or the N. caudatus. These results give credence to the view that there is an uninterrupted neuronal link between the N. caudatus and the substantia nigra and that the TR_{GABA} stored in axon terminals may be a reliable biochemical index for the functional state of those terminals. That most of the GABA stored in substantia nigra is contained in nerve terminals is shown by lesion experiments of the strio-nigra pathway which causes a 75% decrease of the GABA content of substantia nigra (Gale *et al.* 1977).

Regulation of GABA metabolism by afferent dopaminergic neurons

This relationship was investigated by three different types of experiments: electrical stimulation of substantia nigra, injections of apomorphine, and acute or chronic treatment with dopamine receptor blockers endowed with anti-psychotic action. The substantia nigra was stimulated for various periods of time with bipolar electrodes at 15 Hz, 2 msec and various stimuli intensities. The bipolar electrode was inserted through a guide cannula previously positioned stereotaxically. Table III shows that a 20-min stimulation with an 6 volt intensity increases the N. caudatus content of HVA by about 100% but fails to modify the TR_{GABA} in this structure. Apomorphine was administered into the N. caudatus through a 22 – gauge guide cannula placed stereotaxically (8.2A; 2.8L; 4V) 3 days before the experiment. The dose administered was dissolved into 1 μl and delivered over a period of 30 to 40 sec. The rats were killed 30 min. after drug administration. The injection of apomorphine (25 nmoles) failed to change the GABA turnover rate in N. caudatus.

The GABA content and its rate of efflux were measured in the substantia nigra and in the N. caudatus of rats injected intraperitoneally with haloperidol, pimozide, chlorpromazine, clozapine and thioridazine at doses indicated in

Table IV

Change in the turnover rate of GABA elicited by antipsychotics in various regions of rat brain

		% of Control			
Drug	μmol/kg i.p.	Substantia nigra	Globus Pallidus	Nucleus Caudatus	Nucleus Accumbens
Haloperidol	1.3	–	240	–	225
Pimozide	3	–	330	–	250
Chlorpromazine	18	–	250	–	410
Clozapine	30	600	220	320	190
Thioridazine	50	150	260	170	280
d-Butaclamol	2.4	–	280	–	220
l-Butaclamol	2.4	–	–	–	–

Only those changes in the TR_{GABA} that are significant ($P\langle 0.05$) are reported. Dashes indicate that turnover was not changed from the values reported in Table I. Drugs at the doses indicated were injected 40 to 50 min. before measuring GABA turnover during ^{13}C glucose infusion at constant rate.

Table IV. All the drugs were tested at the minimal effective dose that causes maximal activation of striatal tyrosine hydroxylase (Zivkovic *et al.* 1975). None of the drugs changed the concentration of GABA in the brain regions listed in Table IV; only thioridazine and clozapine, two atypical antipsychotics that cause little or no extrapyramidal side effects, changed the TR_{GABA} in substantia nigra and N. caudatus. In order to exclude that this difference was due to specific dose effects, the dose of haloperidol was increased by threefold. It was found that even high doses of this cataleptogenic antipsychotic failed to change the GABA content or the TR_{GABA} in substantia nigra. However, the data reported in Table 4 shows that all the antipsychotics tested increase the TR_{GABA} in N. accumbens and globus pallidus. None of the drugs tested changed the GABA content of these two structures, significantly. In order to establish a relationship between the changes of TR_{GABA} and the antipsychotic action, the effect of d- and l-butaclamol was measured on the TR_{GABA} of various structures. As shown in Table IV only d-butaclamol, the pharmacological active form, changed the TR_{GABA} in N. accumbens and globus pallidus.

Several reports have shown that after chronic administration of antipsychotics, many of the affects that depend on the blockade of DA receptors develop tolerance. In contrast, the effects that depend on the blockade of the DA receptors in the limbic system show a greater resistance to the tolerance. The data reported in Table V show that such tolerance develops to the increase in TR_{GABA} caused by the antipsychotics in substantia nigra, globus pallidus and nucleus caudatus. In contrast, the increase in TR_{GABA} persists in the nucleus accumbens of rats given chronically antipsychotics (Table V). Hence, we believe that the increase of TR_{GABA} caused by the antipsychotics in the N. accumbens has to be considered of possible relevance for the interpretation of their therapeutic action.

These experiments have shown that:

1. There is no direct synaptic connection between dopaminergic terminals and GABA-ergic neurons in striatum; this direct connection probably exists in the N. accumbens.
2. The increased turnover rate of striatal DA caused by all the antipsychotics given in single doses is not caused by a decreased utilization rate of GABA in substantia nigra. Probably an increase in the activity of substance P neurons is operative (Hong *et al.* 1978).
3. The decreased ability of thioridazine and clozapine to cause extrapyramidal side effects may be related to an increase in GABA utilization elicited by both drugs in substantia nigra. Probably this increase could be operative in causing the lower incidence of tardive dyskinesia reported after both drugs. This consideration prompts one to study whether the association of GABA mimetics with classic antipsychotics may be a way to lower the incidence of tardive dyskinesia after chronic treatment with classic antipsychotics.

INTERACTIONS BETWEEN ENKEPHALINERGIC AND GABA-ERGIC NEURONS

The injection of various doses of morphine subcutaneously or of beta-endorphin intraventricularly decreases the TR_{GABA} in nucleus caudatus but increases the turnover rate of this putative neurotransmitter in the globus pallidus or

Table V

Change in the turnover rate of GABA elicited by chronic haloperidol or clozapine in various regions of rat brain

		% of Control			
Drug	μmol/kg i.p. twice daily for 7 days	Substantia nigra	Globus Pallidus	Nucleus Caudatus	Nucleus Accumbens
Haloperidol	4	–	–	–	310
Cozapine	30	–	–	–	240

Only those changes that are significant ($P\langle 0.05$) are reported. Dashes indicate that the TR_{GABA} was not changed from the values reported in Table I.

Table VI
GABA turnover rate in brain areas following subcutaneous morphine or intraventricular β-endorphin

	TR_{GABA} as % of Control		
Drug	N. Caudatus	Globus Pallidus	Substantia nigra
Morphine (70 μmol/kg s.c.)	34	130	220
β-Endorphin (2.9 nmol/intraventricular)	55	260	300

All the data are significantly different ($P < 0.05$) from saline-treated controls.

Table VII
Effects of unilateral intracaudatal morphine on the GABA turnover rate in various regions of rat striatum

Brain Area	Tissue Analyzed	μmol/mg prot/hr
N. Caudatus	Homolateral to injection	864±85
	Contralateral to injection	610±48*
Globus Pallidus	Homolateral to injection	1079±210
	Contralateral to injection	2750±150*
Substantia nigra	Homolateral to injection	474±78
	Contralateral to injection	400±32

Each value is the average of at least six experiments

substantia nigra (Table VI). These changes are dose related and are inhibited by naltrexone. The concentration of enkephalins and of opiate receptors is particularly elevated in the N. caudatus and globus pallidus (Hong *et al.* 1977, Yang *et al.* 1977), thus the action of morphine and beta – endorphin on the TR_{GABA} of striatum may reflect physiological mechanisms regulated by enkephalinergic transmission. In order to clarify whether or not the opiate receptors are located on the membrane of striatal GABA-ergic neurons, we have measured the TR_{GABA} in the N. caudatus, globus pallidus and substantia nigra, after intracaudatal injection of opiate receptor agonists and antagonists. The administration of morphine or beta – endorphin in the head of the N. caudatus decreases the TR_{GABA} in the N. caudatus, increases the TR_{GABA} in the globus pallidus but fails to change that of substantia nigra (Table VII). In other experiments we have shown that the intracaudatal injection of naltrexone can antagonize the increase in the TR_{GABA} elicited in the globus pallidus by subcutaneous injection of morphine. Thus, enkephalinergic neurons probably influence the GABA metabolism in interneurons of N. caudatus but not those of globus pallidus. Previous reports have shown that enkephalins inhibit neuronal activity when applied electrophoretically; thus we can surmise that morphine and beta-endorphin released extraneuronally decrease the release of GABA from caudatal interneurons. Since the TR_{GABA} in the globus pallidus increases after subcutaneous or intracaudatal injection of morphine, we can surmise that very probably the caudatal GABA-ergic interneurons exert transsynaptically an inhibitory influence on the pallidal GABA-ergic activity. However, these small GABA-ergic interneurons of N. caudatus fail to influence the activity of the long axon striatal GABA-ergic neurons that project to the substantia nigra. The increase in pallidal GABA metabolism is important for the cataleptogenic activity and for the extrapyramidal side effects of opioids and antipsychotics. In support of this view injections of muscimol into the globus pallidus also cause extrapyramidal rigidity. Thus it can be said that both opioids and neuroleptics cause an increase in GABA turnover of globus pallidus when they cause extrapyramidal rigidity. However, while the increase in the TR_{GABA} of globus pallidus caused by the opioids can be related to a decrease in the activity of

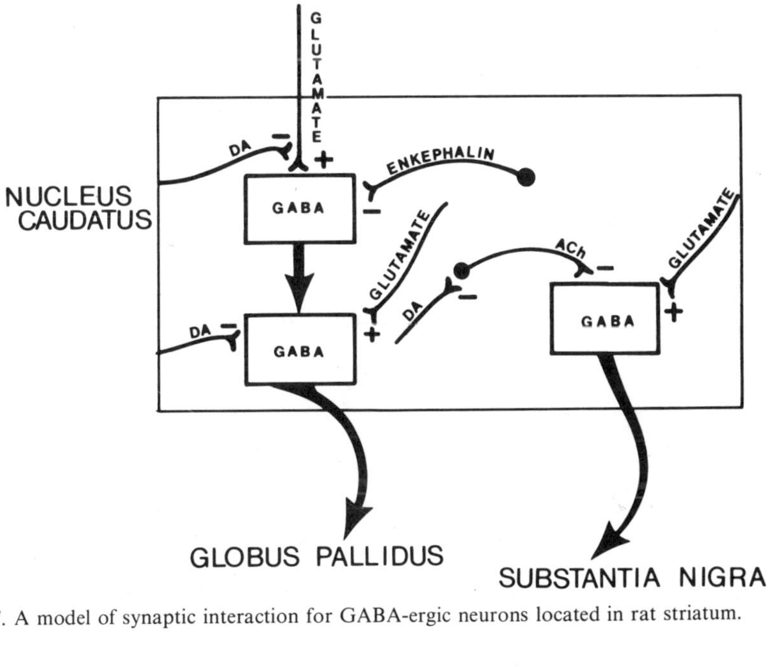

Fig. 1. A model of synaptic interaction for GABA-ergic neurons located in rat striatum.

GABA-ergic caudatal inhibitory interneurons (Fig. 1), that caused by the antipsychotics can be related to a direct increase in the activity of stimulatory afferents to the N. caudatus. This stimulation, for instance, may derive from the decreased efficiency of a presynaptic inhibition by dopaminergic neurons. Perhaps the cortical-striatal (glutamatergic?) pathway is normally inhibited presynaptically by the dopaminergic synapses (Fig. 1); in rats treated with haloperidol, this inhibition is nullified and as a result the pallidal GABA metabolism is stimulated. When a rat receives opiates, the effects of the cortical striatal excitatory pathway are enhanced because the inhibitory tone on caudatal cells by the GABA-ergic interneurons is reduced (Fig. 1). As a result, also in this case, the metabolism of GABA in pallidus is increased. Thus we can surmise that the cataleptogenic action of the antipsychotics and opioids is mediated by an increased release of GABA in the globus pallidus.

CONCLUSIONS

As shown in Fig. 1, there is evidence for three main populations of GABA-ergic neurons in striatum: caudatal interneurons, strio-pallidal (long axon) neurons, and strio-nigral (long axon) neurons. Of these three groups of GABA-ergic neurons, only the strio-pallidal may be directly inhibited by dopaminergic innervation. The strio-nigral pathway is not inhibited directly; probably a cholinergic interneuron which in turn is regulated by dopamine is operative in controlling the strio-nigra GABA-ergic neurons. This possibility is suggested by the increase in the turnover of nigral GABA caused by clozapine and thioridazine which block dopamine and acetylcholine receptors (see Zivkovic *et al.* 1975 for discussion). Opiate receptors regulate GABA-ergic interneurons located in N. caudatus and probably cause an inhibition. These interneurons are in contact with caudatal-pallidal but not with caudatal-nigral GABA-ergic neurons. When these interneurons are inhibited by morphine there is an increase of GABA metabolism in globus pallidus; this is associated with an extrapyramidal rigidity. The same rigidity can be caused by the antipsychotics which increase the GABA turnover of pallidus by relieving the DA inhibition of the cortical striatal (glutamatergic?) and the strio-pallidal (GABA-ergic) neurons (see Fig. 1). The increase in the GABA turnover in substantia nigra that is caused by opioids and atypical antipsychotics may be of value in limiting the occurrence of tardive dyskinesia which is associated with the extrapyramidal side effects caused by classic antipsychotics.

REFERENCES

Anden, N. E., Carlsson, A., Dahlstrom, A., Hillarp, N. A. & Larsson, L. (1964) Demonstration and mapping out of nigro-neostriatal dopamine neurons. *Life Sci.* 3, 523–530.

Bertilsson, L. & Costa, E. (1976) Mass fragmentographic quantitation of glutamic acid and gamma aminobutyric acid in cerebellar nuclei and sympathetic ganglia of rat. J. Chromatog. 118, 395–399.

Bertilsson, L., Mao, C. C. & Costa, E. (1977). Application of principles of steady state kinetics to the estimation of gamma-aminobutyric acid turnover rate in nuclei of rat brain. *J. Pharmacol. Exp. Ther.* 200, 277–284.

Carlsson, A. & Lindqvist, M. (1963) Effect of chlorpromazine or haloperidol on the formation of 3-methoxytyramine and normetanephrine in mouse brain. *Acta Pharmacol. Tox.* 20, 140–144.

Cheney, D. L. & Costa, E. (1977) Pharmacological implications of brain acetylcholine turnover measurements in the rat brain nuclei. *Ann. Rev. Pharmacol. Toxicol* 17, 369–386.

Costa, E. & Meek, J. L. (1974) Regulation of biosynthesis of catecholamines and serotonin in the C.N.S. *Ann. Rev. Pharmacol. Toxicol.* 14, 491–511.

Costa, E., Cheney, D. L., Mao, C. C. & Moroni, F. (1978) Action of antischizophrenic drugs on the metabolism of GABA and acetylcholine in neurons of striatum and N. accumbens. *Fed. Proc.*, 37, 2408–2414.

Curtis, D. R., Duggan, A. W., Fexix, D. & Johnston, C.A.R. (1971) Bicuculline, an antagonist of GABA and synaptic inhibition in the spinal cord of the cat. Brain Res. 32, 69–96.

Fonnun, F., Grofova, I., Rinvik, E., Storm-Mathisen, J. & Walberg, F. (1974) Origin and distribution of glutamate decarboxylase in substantia nigra of the cat. *Brain Res.* 71, 77–92.

Gale, K., Guidotti, A. & Costa, E. (1977) Dopamine-sensitive adenylatecyclase: location in substantia nigra. Sci. 195, 503–505.

Gale, K., Hong, J. S. & Guidotti, A. (1977). Presence of substance P in separate striatonigral neurons. *Brain Res.* 136, 371–375.

Hong, J. S., Yang, H. – Y.T. & Costa, E. (1978) Substance P content of substantia nigra after chronic treatment with antischizophrenic drugs. *Neuropharmacol.* 17, 83–85.

Hong, J. S., Yang, H. – Y.T. & Costa, E. (1977) On the location of methionine enkephalin neurons in rat striatum. *Neuropharmacol.* 16, 451–453.

Hong, J. S., Yang, H. – Y.T., Fratta, W. & Costa, E. (1978) Rat striatal methionine-enkephalin content after chronic treatment to cataleptogenic and noncataleptogenic antischizophrenic drugs. *J. Pharmacol. Exp. Ther.* 205, 141–147.

Krogsgaard-Larsen, P., Johnston, G.A.R., Curtis, D. R., Game, G.J.A. & McCulloch, R. M. (1975) Structure and biological activity of a series of conformationally restricted analogues of GABA. *J. Neurochem.* 25, 803–809.

Lindvall, O. & Bjorklund, A. (1974) The organization of the ascending catecholamine neuron systems in the rat brain as revealed by the glyoxylic acid fluorescence method. *Acta Physiol. Scand.* Suppl 412, 1–48.

Mao, C. C., Cheney, D. L., Marco, E., Revuelta, A. & Costa, E. (1977) Turnover times of gamma-aminobutyric acid and acetylcholine in nucleus caudatus, nucleus accumbens, globus pallidus and substantia nigra: effects of repeated administration of haloperidol. *Brain Res.* 132, 375–379.

Mao, C. C., Peralta, E., Moroni, F. & Costa, E. (1978). The turnover rate of gamma aminobutyric acid in the substantia nigra following electrical stimulation or lesioning of the descending strio-nigral pathway. *Brain Res.*, 155, in press.

Marco, E., Mao, C. C., Revuelta, A., Peralta, & Costa, E. (1978). Turnover rates of gamma-aminobutyric acid in substantia nigra, N. caudatus, globus pallidus and N. accumbens of rats injected with cataleptogenic and noncataleptogenic antipsychotics. *Neuropharmacol.*, 17, 589–596.

McGeer, P. L. & McGeer, E. G. (1975). Evidence for glutamic acid decarboxylase - containing interneurons in the neostriatum. *Brain Res.* 91, 331–335.

Ribak, C. E., Vaughn, V. E., Saito, K., Barber, R. & Roberts, E. (1976) Immunocytochemical localization of glutamate decarboxylase in rat substantia nigra. *Brain Res.* 116, 287–298.

Yang, H. - Y.T., Hong, J. S. & Costa, E. (1977) Regional distribution of leu- and met-enkephalin in rat brain. *Neuropharmacol.* 16, 303–307.

Zivkovic, B., Guidotti, A., Revuelta, A. & Costa, E. (1975). Effects of thioridazine, clozapine and other antipsychotics on the kinetic state of tyrosine hydroxylase and on the turnover rate of dopamine in striatum and N. accumbens. *J. Pharmacol. Exp. Ther.* 194, 37–46.

Gaba and Dopamine: Their Mutual Regulation in the Nigro-Striatal System

F. Cattabeni, A. Bugatti, A. Groppetti, A. Maggi, M. Parenti* & G. Racagni*

The many questions on the physiological role of GABA cannot be answered by considering only the effect of a given drug on this system as if it were an isolated entity, with its specific functions within the CNS.

It has become quite evident that physiological activities are regulated by several pre-programmed circuits and that the mutual regulation of this complex circuitry by different neurotransmitters is responsible for the so-called "activitas nervosa superior", typical of higher vertebrates, which reaches its maximal levels in man.

Although the final goal of understanding how the brain is put together is far from being even delineated, better understanding of the neuronal connections between dopamine, acetylcholine (Ach) and GABA in the nigro-striatal system is now available.

We describe here some of the results obtained along this line in our laboratories in the last few months.

The functional interaction between GABA, dopamine and Ach has been studied in the nigro-striatal system utilizing different approaches. GABA functional activity was assessed by measuring changes in the accumulation rate after inhibiting selectively its catabolism by ethanolamine-o-sulphate (EOS) (Fowler & Jhon 1972, Cattabeni *et al.* 1977). Activity of dopaminergic neurons was revealed by changes in concentrations of 3-methoxytyramine (3-MT), the dopamine metabolite which is thought to reflect almost exclusively neurotransmitter release (Kehr 1976, Di Giulio *et al.* in press). 3-MT was measured with a highly sensitive mass fragmentographic technique (Galli *et al.* 1976).

Institute of Pharmacology and Pharmacognosy, School of Pharmacy, and *Institute of Pharmacology, School of Medicine, University of Milan, 20129 Milan, Italy.

"GABA-NEUROTRANSMITTERS", Alfred Benzon Symposium 12, Munksgaard 1978

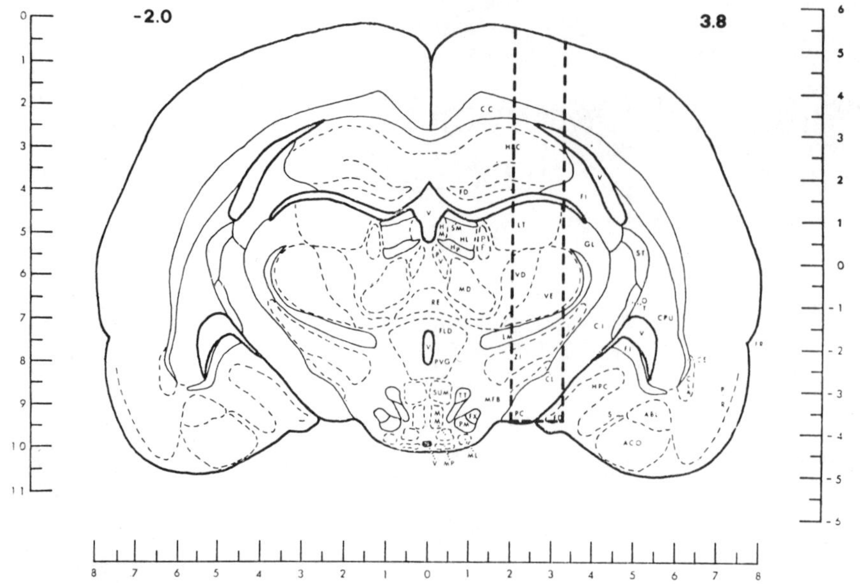

Fig. 1. Coronal section of the rat brain indicating at which level Crus Cerebri lesions were performed. The coordinates are those reported by Pellegrino & Cushman (1967).

Functional activities of GABA-ergic and dopaminergic neurons were studied in experimental conditions whereby one of these neurotransmitters was selectively decreased or increased by discrete mechanical lesions or by pharmacological treatments.

THE DESCENDING STRIO-NIGRAL GABA-ERGIC PATH AND ITS ACTIVITY ON ASCENDING DOPAMINERGIC FIBERS

Results obtained electrophysiologically (Precht & Yoshida 1971, Crossman *et al.* 1973) and pharmacologically (Andén & Stock 1973, Guidotti 1976) indicated that descending GABA-ergic nerve fibers inhibit dopamine cells in Substantia Nigra. However, more recent data have questioned this direct inhibition of GABA terminals on dopamine cell bodies. In fact, Chéramy *et al.* (1978) have recently reported that direct injections of GABA and GABA agonists into Substantia Nigra induced an increase of dopamine release in cat caudate.

These conflicting results prompted us to further investigate the role of GABA fibers originating in striatum and projecting to Substantia Nigra. It has been described that descending strio-nigral GABA-ergic fibers originate mainly in the caudal part of the striatum (Brownstein *et al.* 1977) and project to Substantia Nigra via Crus Cerebri. We have therefore performed a discrete lesion at the level of this brain area, close to the rostral end of Substantia Nigra (Fig. 1).

This lesion results in a decrease of GABA content in Substantia Nigra of the same extent as after extensive brain hemitransection (Table I), indicating that most of the discending GABA-ergic fibers have been interrupted.

The observation that in this experimental condition 3-MT is significantly increased in the striatum could therefore be interpreted as evidence that dopaminergic neurons have been disinhibited by the lack of GABA in Substantia Nigra. In this context we have also found that when GABA levels are elevated in Substantia Nigra, such as after intraventricular or intranigral administration of EOS, striatal 3-MT is consistently decreased (Table I).

These data seem therefore to indicate that GABA exerts an inhibitory role on dopaminergic cell bodies in Substantia Nigra. However, a more complex situation might be also operative in view of the data reported by Chéramy *et al.* (1978), who suggested that GABA can modulate dopamine cells either directly or indirectly through another inhibitory interneuron. Our data indicate that if this is the case, the summation of the effects on the electrical activity of dopamine cell bodies is inhibitory when GABA variations in Substantia Nigra are drastically changed.

Table I

Effects of GABA concentrations in Substantia Nigra on striatal 3-methoxytyramine levels

Treatment*	Substantia Nigra GABA nmoles/mg prot	Striatum 3-MT nmoles/g
Controls	78 ± 6.5	0.20 ± .03
Hemisection	35 ± 4.3	not determined
Crus Cer. Lesion	32 ± 1.9	0.38 ± .04
EOS (2 mg/kg i.vt.)	138 ± 14.0	0.08 ± .01
EOS (30 μg/in Sub. Nigra)	161 ± 13.0	0.10 ± .02

* The lesions were performed unilaterally and the intact sides served as controls. Animals were hemitransected according to Andén *et al.* (1972).

Crus Cerebri lesion was made using a stereotactically placed fine retractable knife-anterior 3.8, lateral 2.0 – according to Pellegrino & Cushman (1967). The animals were killed by high energy microwave irradiation 12 days after the lesions at 3.5 h after EOS treatment.

Each value represents the mean ± S.E.M. of at least six determinations.

All the figures are significantly different from controls ($P<0.05$).

Table II

Effect of hemisection and Crus Cerebri lesion on striatal dopamine and GABA and dopamine-sensitive adenylate cyclase (DA-AC) in Substantia Nigra

	Striatum	Substantia Nigra	
Treatment[a]	Dopamine (nmol/g)	GABA (nmoles/mg prot.)	DA-AC % Stimulation[b]
Controls	65±3.9	80±7.1	175
Hemisection	<0.5	34±2.1*	0
Crus Cerebri	66.5±3.5	32±1.9*	172

a The lesions were performed unilaterally and the intact sides served as controls.

b DA-AC values are given as percent of stimulation incubating the homogenates with $5 \cdot 10^{-5}$M dopamine.

Hemitransection and Crus Cerebri lesion were performed as described in Table I. The animals were killed by high energy microwave irradiation for dopamine and GABA measurements and by guillottine when measuring DA-AC.

Each value represents the mean±S.E.M. of at least six determinations.

* $P<0.05$.

Data taken in part from Racagni *et al.* 1978.

Recent evidence has been produced indicating that other mechanisms could participate in the regulation of dopaminergic nigro-striatal neurons. A dopamine-sensitive adenylate cyclase has been found in Substantia Nigra (Kebabian & Saavedra 1976). This enzyme has been suggested to be located on strio-nigral GABA-ergic fibers, since extensive lesions between striatum and Substantia Nigra decrease its activity (Gale *et al.* 1977, Spano *et al.* 1977). It is therefore conceivable that nigral GABA-ergic terminals could be directly modulated by the activation or the inhibition of this enzyme. The data reported in Table II seem to rule out this hypothesis, since a discrete lesion of the Crus Cerebri does not affect the enzymatic activity although it results in an extensive degeneration of GABA terminals.

DOPAMINE AND GABA IN STRIATUM: MEDIATION BY CHOLINERGIC INTERNEURONS OR DIRECT LINK?

Changes of the functional status of ascending dopaminergic fibers have been reported to affect striatal cell activity (Aghajanian & Bunney 1973). Pharmacological evidence has indicated that a major dopaminergic depressing action is on cholinergic interneurons (Racagni *et al.* 1976). Moreover, a large population of GABA neurons is also present in striatum. In the present study, we have investigated whether changes of the accumulation rate of GABA within this brain structure occur as a consequence of altered dopaminergic functional activity. In this context we have recently reported (Racagni *et al.* 1978) (Fig. 2) that interruption of the ascending dopaminergic fibers through hemitransection increases GABA accumulation rate. Moreover, Fig. 2 shows that the increase of striatal 3-MT after Crus Cerebri lesion is followed by a decrease of GABA accumulation rate in this nucleus. These findings indicate therefore that striatal dopamine not only modifies cholinergic cell activity, but is also able to induce changes in striatal GABA-ergic neurons.

However, the intimate connections between dopaminergic terminals, Ach and GABA intraneurons and GABA cell bodies projecting to Substantia Nigra still remain to be clarified. From previous findings it may be derived that if dopaminergic nerve terminals affect GABA neurons through Ach, cholinergic drugs should be able to induce similar changes. This does not seem to be the case in our experimental conditions. In fact, oxotremorine and psysostigmine do not alter GABA accumulation rate in striatum (Table III). However, the same

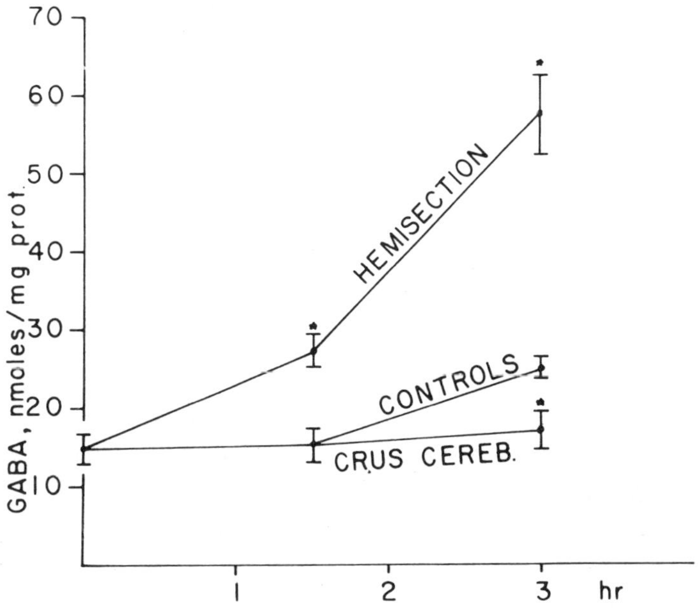

Fig. 2. Effect of brain hemisection and Crus Cerebri lesion (for details see Table I) on GABA accumulation rate in rat striatum, after blockade of its catabolism by i.vt. injections of EOS (2 mg/kg). $*P<0.01$.

Table III

Effect of cholinergic drugs on GABA accumulation rate in nigro-striatal system

Treatment (mg/kg i.p.)	GABA (nmoles/mg protein) Striatum	Subst. Nigra
Saline	10.0±0.4	81± 7
EOS (2 i.vt.)	24.0±2.0*	164±15*
EOS+Oxotremorine (1.5)	25.0±1.8*	333±34†
EOS+Physostigmine (2)	26.0±2.5*	250+24†

The animals were killed by high energy microwave irradiation 3.5 h after i.vt. injections of EOS. Oxotremorine and physostigmine were given 30 min before killing. The drugs themselves did not alter GABA levels.

Each value represents the mean±S.E.M. of at least five determinations.

* $P<0.01$ with respect to saline.

† $P<0.01$ with respect to EOS.

Table IV

Antagonism by artane of the oxotremorine-induced increase of GABA accumulation rate in Substantia Nigra

Treatment (mg/kg, i.p.)	GABA (nmoles/mg prot.)
Saline	81± 7
EOS (2, i.vt.)	164 ± 15[a]
EOS + Oxotremorine (1.5)	333 ± 34[b]
EOS + Oxotremorine (1.5) +Artane (10)	95 ± 5[c]

The animals were killed by high energy microwave irradiation 3.5 h after i.vt. injection of EOS. Oxotremorine was given 30 min before killing and artane was given 30 min before oxotremorine.

Each value represents the mean±S.E.M. of five determinations.

a $P<0.01$ with respect to saline.

b $P<0.01$ with respect to EOS.

c $P<0.01$ with respect to EOS+oxotremorine.

treatment induces an increase of GABA activity in Substantia Nigra (Table III). This effect is antagonized by trihexyphenidyl (artane), a muscarinic receptor blocker (Table IV). Hence, cholinergic receptors seem to be located on descending GABA-ergic fibers, whereas dopaminergic terminals in striatum may innervate directly GABA-ergic interneurons. The distribution of dopamine, Ach and GABA within the striatum seems to be in line with this hypothesis. In fact, while dopamine (Koslow *et al.* 1974) and dopamine-dependent adenylate cyclase (Fig. 3) have been reported to be concentrated mainly in the rostral and caudal part of the caudate, Ach has been found in high levels only in the anterior portion of this nucleus (Koslow *et al.* 1974). On the other hand, glutamic acid decarboxylase (GAD) (Fonnum *et al.* 1978, Scally *et al.* 1978) and GABA (Fig. 3) seem to be mainly distributed in the caudal part of the striatum.

These data, although preliminary, suggest that at least some dopaminergic nerve terminals are concentrated where a higher activity of dopamine-sensitive adenylate cyclase and a higher concentration of GABA are found.

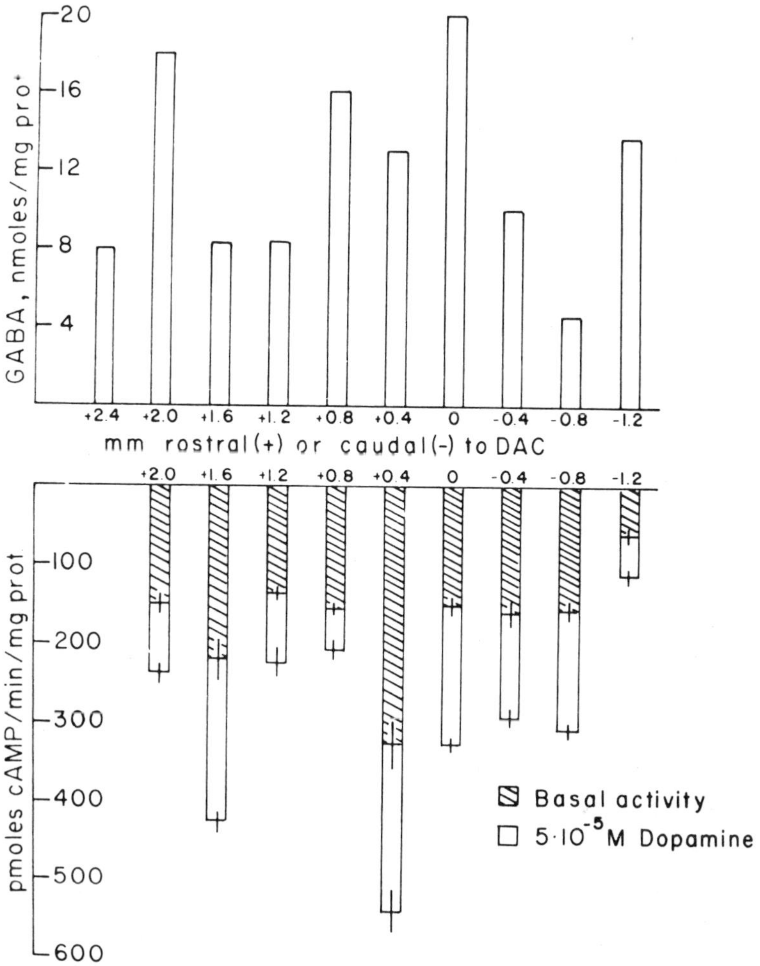

Fig. 3. Distribution of GABA and dopamine-sensitive adenylate cyclase in serial sections of the rat *N. Caudatus-putamen.* The reference point is the Decussation of Anterior Commissura (DAC).

DISCUSSION

It has become evident in these last few years that Substantia Nigra plays an important role in the regulation of striatal activity. Several neurotransmitters have been found to be present in this structure in concentrations which are the highest in the whole brain. However, the information about their mutual functional interplay is still controversial. For instance, conflicting data have been reported for the role of GABA on dopamine cell bodies in Substantia Nigra. In fact, despite substantial electrophysiological evidence suggesting that GABA terminals in Substantia Nigra exert an inhibitory effect on dopaminergic neurons, recent behavioral and biochemical findings have challenged this hypothesis: intranigral administration of muscimol has been found to produce controlateral circling behavior (Oberlander *et al.* 1977). However, this effect is not antagonized by haloperidol, suggesting therefore that this behavioral effect might be mediated by neuronal pathways other than dopaminergic ones, and hence the contradiction might be only apparent.

More difficult is the interpretation of the evidence produced by Chéramy *et al.* (1978), who showed that intranigral application of GABA in cat elicits a byphasic effect on striatal dopamine release, stimulatory at first and then inhibitory.

Our data support the electrophysiological studies, since we have found that a decrease of GABA in Substantia Nigra produces an enhancement of striatal dopamine release. The opposite occurs when GABA is increased.

The other results reported here concern the functional interplay of dopamine, Ach and GABA within the striatum. The data obtained indicate that GABA interneurons in this brain area may be modulated directly by dopamine nerve terminals. Vincent *et al.* (1978) have also suggested that a connection between dopamine and GABA might be operative in striatum, since 6-hydroxydopamine lesions in Substantia Nigra increase glutamate decarboxylase activity in striatum. On the other hand, the descending GABA-ergic fibers seem instead to be controlled by striatal cholinergic interneurons. In fact, after oxotremorine and physostigmine, GABA accumulation rate in Substantia Nigra is accelerated.

As expected striatal 3-MT concentrations are instead decreased by oxotremorine treatment (Fig. 4). This finding may be interpreted as further evidence to the hypothesis suggesting the existence of functional interactions in the nigrostriatal system operating as a regulatory feedback loop which involve striatal cholinergic interneurons, descending GABA-ergic fibers finally the ascending

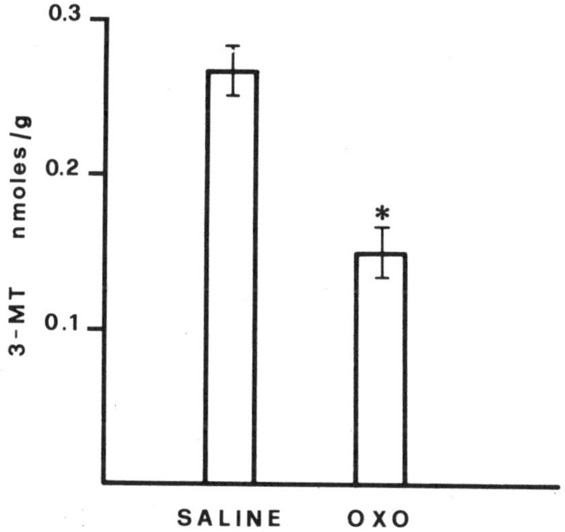

Fig. 4. 3-Methoxytyramine concentrations in rat striatum after i.p. injections of 1.5 mg/kg of oxotremorine, 30 min before killing the animals by high microwave irradiation. *$P<0.01$.

nigro-striatal dopamine tract. However, since cholinergic terminals have been reported to be present in Substantia Nigra, we cannot exclude that the effect of oxotremorine given systemically is due, at least in part, also to the activation of nigral cholinergic receptors. In this respect. Chéramy *et al.* (1978) have reported that benztropine, a cholinergic blocker, increases striatal dopamine release when injected in Substantia Nigra.

In conclusion, the body of evidence on the functional interaction of dopamine, Ach and GABA in the nigro-striatal system seems to indicate that these systems influence each other in both Substantia Nigra and striatum and that drugs acting on these systems may have several points of attack.

REFERENCES

Aghajanian, G. K. & Bunney, B. S. (1973) Central dopaminergic neurons: neurophysiological identification and responses to drugs. In: *Frontiers in Catecholamine Research,* ed. Usdin, E., pp. 643–648. Pergamon Press, New York.

Andén, N. E. & Stock, G. (1973) Inhibitory effect of gamma-hydroxybutyric acid and gamma-aminobutyric acid on dopamine cells of the Substantia Nigra. *Naunyn-Schmiedeberg's Arch. Pharmacol.* 279, 89–95.

Brownstein, M. J., Mroz, E. A., Tappaz, M. L. & Leeman, S. E. (1977) On the origin of substance P and glutamic acid decarboxylase (GAD) in the Substantia Nigra. *Brain Res.* 135, 315–323.

Cattabeni, F., Maggi, A., De Angelis, L., Bruno, F. & Racagni, G. (1977) A simple approach to study the effect of Haloperidol on GABA functional activity in the nigro-striatal system. *J. Neurochem.* 28, 1407–1408.

Chéramy, A., Nieoullion, A. & Glowinski, J. (1978) *In vivo* changes in dopamine release in cat caudate nucleus and Substantia Nigra induced by nigral application of various drugs including GABA-ergic agonists and antagonists. In: *Interactions Between Putative Neurotransmitters in the Brain,* ed. Garattini, S., Pujol, J. F. & Samanin, R., pp. 175–190. Raven Press, New York.

Crossman, A. R., Walker, R. J. & Woodruff, G. N. (1973) Picrotoxin antagonism of gamma-amino-butyric acid inhibitory responses and synaptic inhibition in the rat Substantia Nigra. *Brit. J. Pharmacol.* 49, 696–700.

Di Giulio, A. M., Groppetti, A., Cattabeni, F., Galli, C. L., Maggi, A., Algeri, S. & Ponzio, F. The significance of dopamine metabolites in evaluation of drugs acting on dopaminergic neurons. *Eur. J. Pharmacol.* In press.

Fonnum, F., Gottesfeld, Z. & Grofova, I. (1978) Distribution of glutamate decarboxylase, choline acetyltransferase and aromatic amino acid decarboxylase in the basal ganglia of normal and operated rats. Evidence for striato pallidal, striatoentopeduncular and striato-nigral GABA-ergic fibers. *Brain Res.* 143, 125–136.

Fowler, L. J. & Jhon, R. A. (1972) Active-site-directed irreversible inhibition of rat brain 4-aminobutyrate aminotransferase by ethanolamine-O-sulphate *in vitro* and *in vivo. Biochem. J.* 130, 569–573.

Gale, K., Guidotti, A. & Costa, E. (1977) Dopamine-sensitive adenylate cyclase: location in Substantia Nigra. *Science* 195, 503–505.

Galli, C. L., Cattabeni, F., Eros, T., Spano, P. F., Algeri, S., Di Giulio, A. M. & Groppetti, A. (1976) A mass fragmentographic assay of 3-methoxytyramine in rat brain. *J. Neurochem.* 27, 795–798.

Guidotti, A. (1976) Evaluation of GABA receptor agonists in the integrated function of mammalian CNS: a study of muscimol. In: *Abstracts of the Collegium Internationale Neuro-Psychopharmacologicum,* ed. Baronet-Lecroix, D., pp. 125, Abstract 176, Quebec.

Kebabian, J. W. & Saavedra, J. M. (1976) Dopamine-sensitive adenylate cyclase occurs in a region of Substantia Nigra containing dopaminergic dendrites. *Science* 193, 683–685.

Kehr. W. (1976) 3-Methoxytyramine as an indicator of impulse-induced Dopamine release in rat brain *in vivo. Naunyn-Schmiedeberg's Arch Pharmacol.* 293, 209–215.

Koslow, S. H., Racagni, G. & Costa, E. (1974) Mass fragmentographic measurement of norepinephrine, dopamine, serotonin and acetylcholine in seven discrete nuclei of the rat tel-diencephalon. *Neuropharmacol.* 13, 1123–1130.

Oberlander, C., Dumont, C. & Boissier, J. R. (1977) Rotational behavior after unilateral intranigral injection of muscimol in rats. *Eur. J. Pharmacol.* 43, 389–390.

Pellegrino, L. J. & Cushman, A. J. (1967) A stereotaxic atlas of the rat brain. In: *The Century Psychology Series,* ed. Elliott, R. M., Lindzey, G. & McCorgnodale K. Appleton-Century Crafts, New York.

Precht, W. & Yoshida, M. (1971) Blockade of caudate evoked inhibition in the Substantia Nigra by picrotoxin. *Brain Res.* 32, 229–233.

Racagni, G., Bruno, F., Cattabeni, F., Maggi, A., Di Giulio, A. M. & Groppetti, A. (1978) Interactions among dopamine, acetylcholine and GABA in the nigrostriatal system. In: *Interactions Between Putative Neurotransmitters in the Brain,* ed. S. Garattini, Pujol, J. F. & Samanin, R., pp. 61–72, Raven Press, New York.

Racagni, G., Cheney, D. L., Trabucchi, M. & Costa, E. (1976) *In vivo* actions of clozapine and haloperidol on the turnover rate of acetylcholine in rat striatum. *J. Pharmacol. Exp. Ther.* 196, 323–332.

Scally, M. C., Ulus, F. H., Wurtman, R. J. & Pettibone (1978) Regional distribution of neurotransmitter synthesizing enzymes and Substance P within the rat corpus striatum. *Brain Res.* 143, 556–560.

Spano, P. F., Trabucchi, M. & Di Chiara, G. (1977) Localization of nigral dopamine-sensitive adenylate cyclase on neurons originating from the corpus striatum. *Science,* 196, 1343–1345.

Vincent, R. S., Nagy, J. I. & Fibiger, H. C. (1978) Increased striatal glutamate decarboxylase after lesions of the nigro-striatal pathway. *Brain Res.* 143, 168–173.

Effect of Muscimol, AOAA and Na Valproate on the Activity of Dopamine Neurons and Dopamine Synthesis

J. R. Walters, J. M. Lakoski, N. Eng & B. L. Waszczak

Since Carlsson & Lindqvist (1963) first observed increases in striatal dopamine turnover following neuroleptic treatment, it has been thought that the striatonigral pathway may have an important influence on the activity of the nigrostriatal dopamine neurons. These workers postulated that the striatonigral part of this neuronal loop plays a compensatory role, increasing or decreasing the activity of the dopamine neurons to offset drug-induced alterations in stimulation delivered to the postsynaptic dopamine receptors. This hypothesis suggests that alterations in the activity in the striatonigral pathway are responsible for the increase in dopaminergic activity and dopamine metabolism observed after administration of dopamine receptor blocking drugs such as the neuroleptics. Similarly, drugs like amphetamine which release dopamine would cause an increased stimulation of postsynaptic dopamine receptors in the striatum and thereby produce a decrease in the activity of dopamine neurons by changing the activity of these nigral afferents.

Many studies have suggested that one of the transmitters utilized by this "feedback" pathway is γ-aminobutyric acid (GABA). These include the observations that striatal degeneration in Huntington's disease and interruption of the striatonigral pathway in animals both cause a decrease in nigral glutamic acid decarboxylase (GAD) (Kim *et al.* 1971, McGeer *et al.* 1971, Bird *et al.* 1973,

---

Presented at the Alfred Benzon Symposium 12: GABA-Neurotransmitters: Pharmacochemical, Biochemical and Pharmacological Aspects, Copenhagen, Denmark, May 21–25, 1978.

Experimental Therapeutics Branch, National Institute of Neurological and Communicative Disorders and Stroke, National Institutes of Health, 9000 Rockville Pike, Bethesda, Maryland 20014 U.S.A.

Perry *et al.* 1973, Fonnum *et al.* 1974, Kataoka *et al.* 1974), and the demonstration that a large proportion of the terminals synapsing on dendrites in the nigra contain GAD (Ribak *et al.* 1976). Such studies have made it seem very likely that nigrostriatal dopamine neurons are receiving a GABA-ergic striatonigral input which might be synonomous with the postulated striatonigral "feedback loop". The possibility that effects of dopamine receptor stimulating and blocking agents on the activity of dopamine neurons are mediated through a GABA-ergic striatonigral feedback loop has lead to the expectation that drugs which alter GABA-mediated function might also exert significant effects on dopaminergic activity. If this were so, pharmacologists would be provided with a new way to modify dopamine-mediated function and a new system for studying efficacy of GABA-active agents.

To explore these issues, we have examined the effects of three drugs which we thought might augment GABA-mediated neurotransmission on dopamine synthesis and unit activity. Two of these agents, aminooxyacetic acid (AOAA) and sodium valproate (valproate, n-dipropylacetate) produce an increase in brain GABA levels by preferentially inhibiting GABA catabolism (Baxter & Roberts 1961, Godin *et al.* 1969, Simler *et al.* 1973, Sawaya *et al.* 1975). Studies in the cortex and spinal cord have suggested that GABA-mediated neurotransmission can be augmented by increasing GABA levels with AOAA (Gottesfeld *et al.* 1972, Davidoff *et al.* 1973). The third drug, muscimol, has been reported to be an effective GABA agonist in both invertebrate and mammalian systems (Walker *et al.* 1971, Krogsgaard-Larsen *et al.* 1975, Johnson 1975, Wheal & Kerkut 1976). The results obtained in the present studies, however, do not suggest that tonic dopaminergic activity is readily inhibited by GABA-active drugs nor do they support the idea that changes in the activity of dopamine neurons provide a clear index of GABA-mimetic potential. They also raise questions about the role of the striatonigral GABA-ergic projection in regulation of dopaminergic activity.

EFFECTS OF GABA-T INHIBITORS ON DOPAMINERGIC ACTIVITY

Dopamine Synthesis

The accumulation of neostriatal DOPA in rats sacrificed 30 min after administration of a DOPA-decarboxylase inhibitor has been used as an indicator of the *in vivo* activity of tyrosine hydroxylase (Carlsson *et al.* 1972, Walters & Roth 1974). The ability of AOAA and valproate to alter the synthesis of dopamine was investigated by measuring the changes in striatal DOPA accumulation in animals treated with GABA-T (GABA: 2-oxoglutarate amino transferase) inhibitors before administration of the decarboxylase inhibitor (Fig. 1). Results obtained with valproate tended to support the idea that increasing GABA levels might attenuate dopamine synthesis. Valproate (400 mg/kg) administered 15 min before the decarboxylase inhibitor significantly lowered the apparent *in vivo* activity of tyrosine hydroxylase (Fig. 1) while it increased GABA levels by 46% in the striatum and 31% in the nigra (Table I).

However, when the effects of AOAA treatment were examined, the results cast doubt on the idea that valproate was altering dopamine synthesis by increasing GABA levels. AOAA, the more potent inhibitor of GABA catabolism, caused significantly greater increases in GABA levels but had less of an effect on dopamine synthesis. Fifty mg/kg AOAA caused a 132% increase in GABA levels in the striatum and a 73% increase in GABA in the substantia nigra within 45 min (Table I), but the rate of striatal DOPA accumulation during

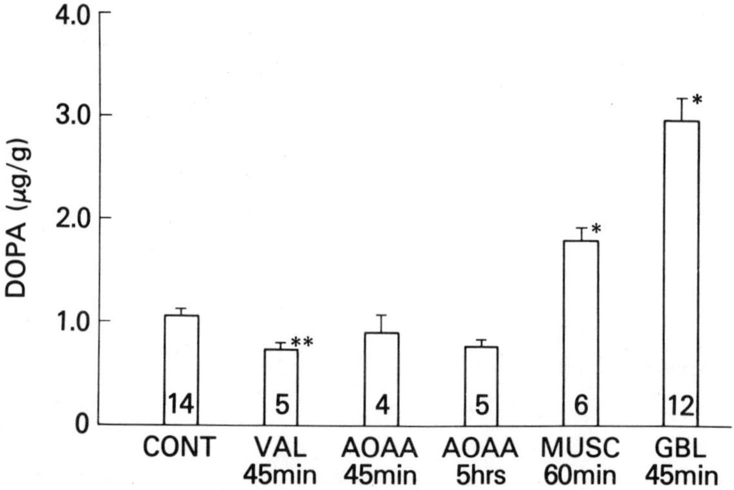

Fig. 1. Effect of GABA catabolism inhibitors and putative GABA agonists on neostritial DOPA accumulation. Rats were administered a DOPA decarboxylase inhibitor, R04–4602 (800 mg/kg, i.p.) 30 min before sacrifice. Valproate (VAL, 400 mg/kg), AOAA (50 mg/kg), muscimol (3.5 mg/kg) and GBL (600 mg/kg) were administered i.p. Times indicate the interval between drug administration and sacrifice. The bars represent the standard error of the mean and the numbers in the columns indicate the number of determinations. DOPA was assayed as described by Walters & Roth (1974).

* Significantly different from control, $P<0.001$.

** Significantly different from control, $P<0.025$.

Table I

Effect of valproate and AOAA on GABA levels in neostriatum and substantia nigra

Treatment	Neostriatum GABA (μg/mg protein)	N	Substantia Nigra GABA (μg/mg protein)	N
Control	1.25±.05	7	3.52±.29	7
Valproate (45 min)	1.83±.01*	4	4.60±.32†	4
AOAA (45 min)	2.90±.28*	7	6.08±.42*	7
AOAA (5 h)	6.02±.24*	3	11.65±.05*	3

Rats were administered either 400 mg/kg Na valproate or 50 mg/kg AOAA before death at the times indicated. Rats were killed by exposure to focussed microwave irradiation and brain regions were removed and assayed for GABA levels as described in Peričić *et al.* 1977. Values represent the mean+S.E.M., N=number of experiments.

* Significantly different from control, $P<.001$.

† Significantly different from control, $P<.05$.

the last half hour of the AOAA treatment was not significantly different from control. Even the 380% increase in striatal GABA and the 230% increase in nigral GABA observed 5 h after AOAA treatment did not significantly reduce the apparent *in vivo* synthesis of dopamine. Although valproate's effect remains to be explained, the results with AOAA suggest that substantial increases in GABA levels do not dramatically attenuate dopamine synthesis.

Single Unit Activity

The localization of dopamine-containing neurons by histofluorescence microscopy (Dählstrom & Fuxe 1964) made possible characterization of the neurophysiological properties of these cells by means of extracellular single-unit recording techniques (Bunney *et al.* 1973b, Guyenet & Aghajanian 1977, Walters *et al.*, in preparation). Such studies have shown that drugs thought to block the dopamine receptors, such as chlorpromazine and haloperidol, and those thought to activate dopamine receptors, such as amphetamine, L-dopa and apomorphine, do alter the firing rate of the 6-hydroxydopamine-sensitive cells in the pars compacta of the substantia nigra. These effects are consistent with the drugs' biochemical effects and proposed mechanisms of action. Moreover, these agents have no consistent, dose-dependent effects on the nondopaminergic neurons in the substantia nigra pars reticulata (Bunney *et al.* 1973a, b).

In the present study, the effects of AOAA and valproate on dopaminergic activity were examined in animals anesthetized with chloral hydrate, and in paralyzed rats, artificially respired and anesthetized locally with mepivacaine

HCl according to procedures described previously (Bunney *et al.* 1973b). Four dopamine cells monitored in anesthetized rats (one cell per rat) during and after the i.p. administration of 50 mg/kg AOAA showed no significant change in firing rate when baseline rates were compared with activities 25–30 min after drug administration (Fig. 2B). To determine whether chloral hydrate was in some way interferring with the effect of the GABA system on dopaminergic activity, similar experiments were performed with eight paralyzed, locally

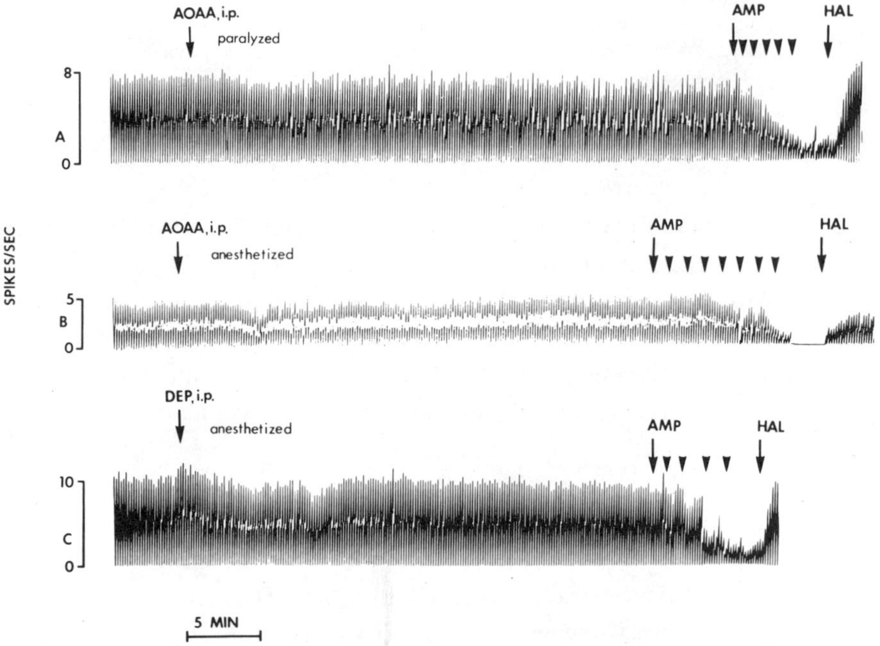

Fig. 2. Effect of GABA catabolism inhibitors on firing rates of dopamine cells located in the pars compacta of the substantia nigra. A. I.p. administration of 50 mg/kg AOAA to a gallamine-paralyzed, artificially respired rat treated with local anesthetic had no significant effect on the average firing rate of this cell. Amphetamine (AMP,0.2,0.2,0.4,1.6, and 3.2 mg/kg, i.v.) produced a decrease in activity which was reversed by administration of haloperidol (HAL, 1 mg/kg, i.v.). In both A and B, the sensitivity of the cells to amphetamine was less than that normally observed in animals not receiving AOAA pretreatment (Bunney *et al.* 1975). B. This response was typical of cells recorded in chloral hydrate-anesthetized rats. I.p. administration of 50 mg/kg AOAA had little effect on the single unit activity of this dopamine cell. Amphetamine (0.2, 0.2, 0.4, 0.8, 1.6, 3.2, 6.4 and 12.8 mg/kg, i.v.) caused a decrease in activity which was reversed by haloperidol (1 mg/kg, i.v.). C. Administration of valproate (DEP, depakine, n-dipropyl acetate, 400 mg/kg) also did not significantly change the firing rate of this cell recorded in an anesthetized rat. Haloperidol (1 mg/kg, i.v.) reversed the effect of amphetamine (0.1, 0.1, 0.2, 0.4, and 0.8 mg/kg, i.v.). Techniques as described by Bunney *et al.* (1973a).

anesthetized rats. Again, in these experiments, i.p. administration of 50 mg/kg AOAA had no significant effect on the activity of the monitored cells (Fig. 2A). To examine the effect of greater increases in GABA levels, six rats were pretreated with 50 mg/kg AOAA for 4 h. The firing rates of dopamine cells in several areas of the pars compacta of each rat were recorded and compared with activity of cells recorded in control animals, using the technique described by Nowycky *et al.* (1978). Of 33 cells with the neurophysiological characteristics of dopamine neurons which were recorded in the substantia nigra pars compacta of AOAA treated rats, the mean rate was 3.9±.3 (S.E.M.) spikes/sec, the median rate was 3.5, and the range was 0.2 to 8.4 spikes/sec. The mean of 41 cells recorded from five control animals was 3.6±.2 spikes/sec, the range was 0.7 to 6.7 spikes/sec, and the median was 3.5 spikes/sec. The distribution of firing rates in the two groups was not significantly different by the Mann–Whitney U-test.

In a separate group of experiments, chloral hydrate anesthetized rats were administered 400 mg/kg valproate, i.p., while the activity of a single pars compacta dopamine cell per rat was monitored (Fig. 2C). Although three cells showed slight decreases and one cell showed a slight increase in firing rate 25–30 min after the drug was administered, the average percent change from baseline rates at 30 min for nine cells was +0.5±2.6% (mean±S.E.M.).

These results support the biochemical studies with AOAA and indicate that simply increasing GABA levels in the striatum and nigra does not produce an obvious decrease in the tonic activity of the substantia nigra dopamine neurons. While it is possible that changes too subtle to be observed with the present technique might be occuring, or that changes might be observed if dopamine cells were monitored in awake, unrestrained rats, the lack of effect observed here is in marked contrast to the very obvious alterations in dopaminergic activity seen after administration of drugs like amphetamine and haloperidol (Figs. 2A, B, C).

Interaction with Amphetamine

Although significant changes in baseline activity of dopamine cells could not be seen with valproate or AOAA treatment, it seemed possible that release of the accumulated GABA might be facilitated and its effects made more evident if activity in the striatonigral pathway were stimulated. Amphetamine has been thought to inhibit the activity of dopamine neurons by increasing dopamine release and altering activity in the striatonigral "feedback loop" (Bunney & Aghajanian 1976). If this feedback loop corresponds to the striatonigral GABA-ergic neurons, then the amphetamine-induced inhibition of dopamine neurons should be associated with increased activity in GABA-ergic neurons. This train of thought led us to examine the effect of amphetamine on dopaminergic activity in rats pretreated for 1–2 h with 50 mg/kg AOAA or for 45 min with 400 mg/kg valproate. In each rat a single cell was recorded during i.v. administration of increasing doses of amphetamine, using procedures described previously (Bunney *et al.* 1975). Instead of seeing a facilitation of amphetamine's effects, we observed an attenuation of the effects of amphetamine in animals pretreated with AOAA (Fig. 3). Animals pretreated with valproate showed no change in their response to amphetamine. These results suggest that GABA-containing processes may affect dopaminergic activity at some levels but not in the manner the simplest model of the feedback loop would predict.

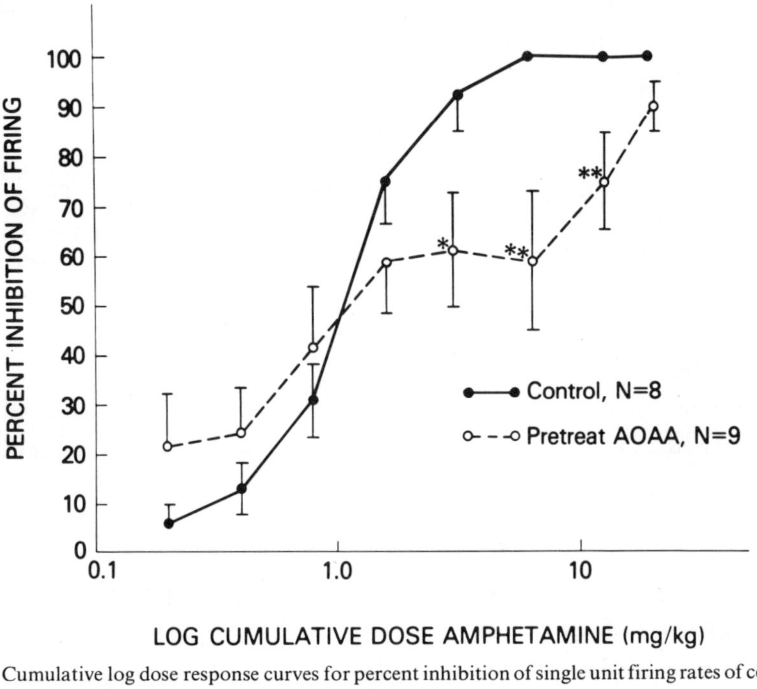

Fig. 3. Cumulative log dose response curves for percent inhibition of single unit firing rates of cells in the pars compacta substantia nigra induced by i.v. administration of increasing doses of *d*-amphetamine. Where indicated, rats were pretreated with AOAA (50 mg/kg, i.p.) for 3 h before being anesthetized with chloral hydrate and prepared for single unit recording.

* Significantly different from control, $P<0.05$.

** Significantly different from control, $P<0.25$.

EFFECT OF MUSCIMOL ON DOPAMINERGIC ACTIVITY

Dopamine Synthesis

In vivo dopamine synthesis was not altered by administration of 0.5 mg/kg or 2.0 mg/kg muscimol when given 5 min before inhibition of DOPA decarboxylase (Walters & Eng, unpublished observations). However, when 3.5 mg/kg muscimol was administered 30 min before the decarboxylase inhibitor, an 83% increase in dopamine synthesis was observed (Fig. 1). This effect is difficult to interpret. Although, the increase in dopamine synthesis suggests that muscimol might be increasing the activity of the dopamine neurons, dopamine synthesis is also known to increase when impulse flow in dopamine neurons is blocked by lesion of the nigrostriatal pathway or by administration of γ-butyrolactone (GBL), the precursor of γ-hydroxybutyric acid (GHB) (Fig. 1) (Carlsson *et al.* 1972, Walters *et al.* 1973). Thus, examination of dopamine synthesis suggested that this relatively high dose of muscimol could be causing either a gradual increase or an inhibition of dopaminergic activity.

Single Unit Activity

Dopamine cells recorded in rats anesthetized with chloral hydrate (N=8) were not inhibited by either i.p. administration of 3.5 mg/kg muscimol or by i.v. administration of up to lethal doses (Fig. 4A). This lack of effect was observed with doses which produced marked catalepsy in the awake animal. In paralyzed, locally anesthetized rats, dopamine cells were not inhibited by muscimol, and some increases in firing were observed with 64% of the cells recorded (Fig. 4B). The overall average change from baseline firing rates observed in the paralyzed rats was 28±9% (N=8) (Walters & Lakoski 1978). The time course of this effect after parenteral administration of muscimol was relatively slow and agreed with the observed effects on dopamine synthesis. These results also suggest that GABA can exert some effect on the activity of the dopamine neurons but do not support the idea that GABA agonists will preferentially attenuate activity in this pathway.

It is interesting to compare these results with those seen after administration of GBL or GHB (Roth *et al.* 1973, Walters & Roth 1976). Although GHB is inactive in *in vivo* and *in vitro* test systems used to screen for GABA-mimetic activity, it has sometimes been referred to as a GABA agonist because of its structural similarity to GABA and its ability to inhibit unit activity in the substantia nigra (for discussion see Peričić *et al.* 1978). If muscimol penetrates the CNS unaltered and acts there as a GABA agonist, the marked differences between the effects of GHB and muscimol on the dopamine system support the idea that GHB is not inhibiting nigral activity by stimulating GABA receptors at this site.

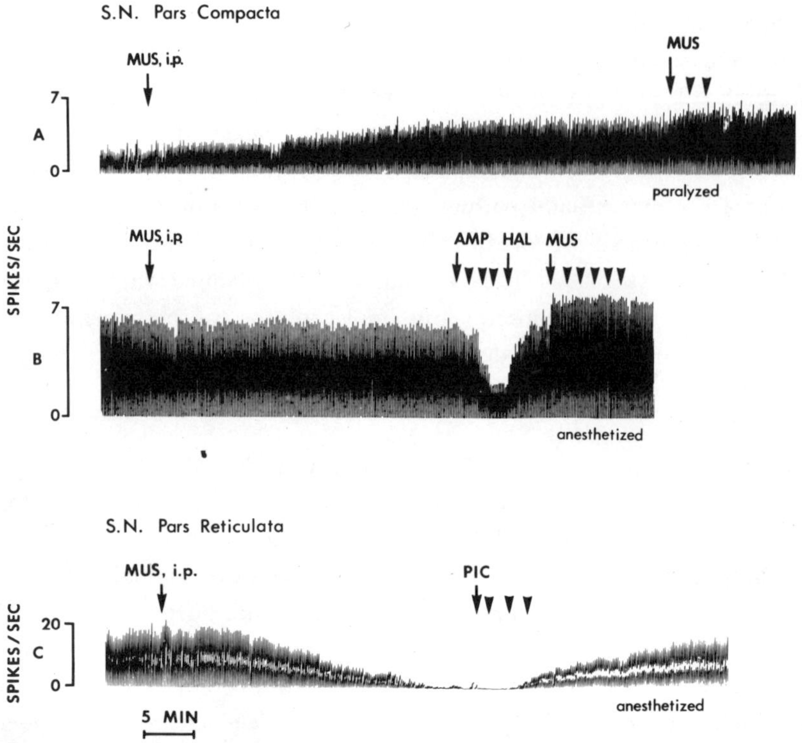

Fig. 4. Effect of muscimol administration on the firing rate of dopamine cells in the substantia nigra pars compacta and unidentified cells in the substantia nigra pars reticulata. A. I.p. administration of 3.5 mg/kg muscimol (MUS) caused a gradual increase in the firing rate of this dopamine cell recorded in a gallamine-paralyzed, artificially respired rat; additional administration of 0.4, 0.8, and 0.8 mg/kg i.v. had little further effect. Although the effect observed with this cell was greater than average, the majority of cells (64%) recorded under these conditions showed significant increases in rate. No cell showed a significant decrease. B. I.p. administration of 3.5 mg/kg muscimol caused no significant change in firing rate of this dopamine cell recorded in a chloral hydrate anesthetized rat, as was typically the case. Amphetamine (0.1, 0.1, 0.2, 0.4 mg/kg, i.v.) produced a typical decrease in activity which was reversed by administration of haloperidol (0.4 mg/kg, i.v.). Additional injections of muscimol (0.4, 0.4, 0.8, 0.8, and 0.8 mg/kg, i.v.) had no effect on unit activity. C. Effect of i.p. administration of 3.5 mg/kg muscimol upon firing rate of this unidentified cell recorded in the substantia nigra pars reticulata of a chloral hydrate anesthetized rat. The inhibition was reversed by i.v. administration of picrotoxin (0.4, 0.4, 0.8, and 1.6 mg/kg). Techniques as described by Bunney *et al.* (1973a). Data for A and B taken from Walters & Lakoski (1978).

EFFECT OF MUSCIMOL ON UNIT ACTIVITY IN THE SUBSTANTIA NIGRA PARS RETICULATA

Since the cells in the pars reticulata of the substantia nigra can also be considered possible sites of termination of the striatonigral GABA pathway, the effects of i.p. and i.v. administration of muscimol on the unit activity of these neurons were also examined (Waszczak *et al.* 1978). The results were quite different from those observed in the pars compacta. I.p. administration of 3.5 mg/kg muscimol completely inhibited the activity of reticulata cells in nine out of 10 animals (one cell per animal was monitored) (Fig. 4C). Activity declined gradually after the i.p. injection and the cells stopped firing after an average of 25 min. I.v. administration of muscimol caused a more rapid, dose-dependent inhibition of reticulata cell unit activity. After 1.6 mg/kg, i.v., alterations in firing rates could be seen within 20–30 sec. With this dose, significant decreases in unit activity were seen in 79% of cells recorded, increases in 14%, and no change in 7%. The average effect of muscimol upon the firing rate of these reticulata cells was inhibition to 70% of the baseline rate; activity remained depressed for more than 30 min. In some experiments, however, picrotoxin was administered, and unit activity returned to baseline levels. Although the response of the cells in the pars reticulata of the substantia nigra to changes in blood pressure and heart rate, etc., have not been well characterized, the activity of these cells is not altered in a consistent, dose-dependent way by drugs which do affect such functions, such as the dopamine receptor stimulating and blocking agents. Nevertheless, it cannot be ruled out that nonspecific or peripheral actions of muscimol at sites other than nigral GABA receptors could be responsible for the observed changes in reticulata cell activity. The results suggest, however, that a population of cells in the substantia nigra pars reticulata is sensitive to inhibition by muscimol at doses which do not inhibit the firing rates of pars compacta dopamine neurons. These findings are also consistent with the observations that the reticulata cells are more sensitive to iontophoresed GABA than the nigral dopamine cells (Aghajanian & Bunney 1974).

INTERACTION OF GABA-ACTIVE DRUGS WITH HALOPERIDOL

Several laboratories have reported that drugs which might be expected to potentiate GABA-mediated neurotransmission attenuate the increase in dopamine synthesis observed after haloperidol treatment (Andén 1974, Fuxe *et al.* 1975, Westerink *et al.* 1975, Kääriänen 1976, Keller *et al.* 1976). This is the effect

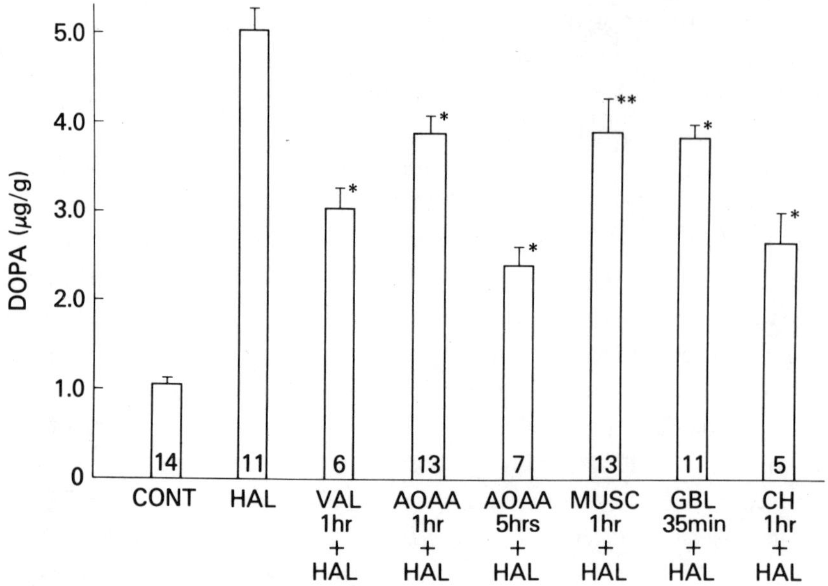

Fig. 5. Effect of GABA catabolism inhibitors and putative GABA agonists on the haloperidol-induced increase in *in vivo* neostriatal DOPA accumulation. Rats were administered R04–4602 (800 mg/kg, i.p.) 30 min before sacrifice. Haloperidol (HAL, 1 mg/kg) was administered, i.p., 45 min before sacrifice. Valproate (VAL, 400 mg/kg), AOAA (50mg/kg), muscimol (MUSC, 3.5 mg/kg), GBL (750 mg/kg) and chloral hydrate (CH, 400 mg/kg) were administered, i.p., before sacrifice at the times indicated. The bars represent the standard error of the mean and the numbers in the columns indicate the number of determinations. DOPA was assayed as described by Walters & Roth (1974). DOPA accumulation in all drug treated animals was significantly different from control ($P<.001$).

* Significantly different from haloperidol alone, $P<.001$.

** Significantly different from haloperidol alone, $P<.025$.

one might expect if the haloperidol-induced increase in dopaminergic activity were associated with decreased impulse flow in a GABA-ergic striatonigral pathway which tonically inhibits the dopamine neurons. Similarly, in the present study, all the drugs investigated were found to attenuate the effect of haloperidol on DOPA accumulation (Fig. 5). However, in most cases these effects were not correlated with the drug's apparent potency as a GABA-active agent, and with some drugs, the changes seen in the presence of haloperidol did not correlate with those observed in the absence of haloperidol (described above).

The results most consistent with the concept of a GABA-mediated decrease in dopaminergic activity after haloperidol treatment were observed with AOAA.

Both the attenuation of the haloperidol-induced increase in DOPA accumulation and the increase in GABA levels were greater after 5 h of AOAA pretreatment than after 1 h. In addition, AOAA pretreatment (4–5 h, 50 mg/kg) significantly reduced the single unit activity of dopamine neurons recorded in paralyzed, locally anesthetized rats treated with haloperidol (Walters, unpublished observations).

On the other hand, the changes caused by AOAA did not correlate well with those observed after administration of muscimol and valproate. Muscimol, which might have been expected to be the most potent GABA-mimetic agent, was one of the least effective at lowering DOPA accumulation after haloperidol. Conversely, valproate, which causes less of a change in GABA levels than does AOAA, was one of the most effective agents for reducing DOPA accumulation. Both this finding and the observation that valproate can also attenuate the increase in DOPA accumulation caused by GBL treatment (Walters & Eng, unpublished observations) support the view that valproate's effects on dopamine synthesis are not mediated by an increase in GABA levels or by GABA-mediated neurotransmission in the nigra. Since valproate does not prevent GBL from completely blocking dopaminergic activity (Walters, unpublished observations), its ability to alter DOPA accumulation when given with GBL indicates that valproate can affect dopamine synthesis in some way other than through altering dopaminergic firing rates. However, until single unit recordings are made, it is uncertain whether valproate and muscimol are more effective at reducing dopamine impulse activity to a greater extent after haloperidol treatment than in the absence of the neuroleptic.

In addition, results in Fig. 5 point out that reductions in the haloperidol-induced increase in DOPA accumulation can be caused by agents, such as GBL and chloral hydrate, which do not have well-established GABA-mimetic mechanisms of actions. Moreover, the attenuation can be greater with drugs which only slightly decrease firing after haloperidol than with drugs which completely inhibit dopamine unit activity. GBL, administered in conjunction with haloperidol, still completely inhibits dopamine activity (Walters & Roth 1977), and the resulting increase in DOPA accumulation is 24% less than that observed with haloperidol alone. Chloral hydrate, on the other hand, causes a 49% decrease in DOPA accumulation after haloperidol, yet only causes a relatively small decrease in dopaminergic unit activity (Walters, unpublished observations).

Finally, as with muscimol, the effect of chloral hydrate on the haloperidol-induced increase in dopamine activity is not consistent with the drug's action when it is administered in the absence of haloperidol: chloral hydrate slightly increases firing of dopamine neurons and synthesis of dopamine when administered to control rats (Bunney *et al.* 1973b, Bunney *et al.* 1975, Murrin *et al.* 1976).

While some of the changes observed here may in fact be induced through alterations in GABA-mediated neurotransmission, the lack of correlation between the demonstrated ability of these drugs to interact with GABA systems and their effects on dopaminergic activity makes it difficult to use this data as support for the idea that a GABA pathway is important in mediating haloperidol's effects. These results also caution against using attenuation of dopamine synthesis after haloperidol treatment as an index of GABA-mimetic potency or as an indication of how a drug might affect dopaminergic activity in the absence of a neuroleptic.

CONSIDERATIONS

In several respects, the results described here are not in obvious agreement with the hypothesis that dopaminergic activity is directly and tonically regulated by a GABA-ergic striatonigral feedback loop. Muscimol, a GABA receptor stimulating agent, inhibited neuronal activity more effectively in the pars reticulata of the substantia nigra than in the pars compacta. In fact, this drug increased dopamine synthesis and (under some conditions) firing rates of dopamine cells. Marked increases in GABA levels caused by AOAA treatment had little effect on tonic dopamine activity and attenuated rather than augmented the inhibitory action of amphetamine on dopaminergic single unit activity. Although a second inhibitor of GABA catabolism, valproate, had greater effects on dopamine synthesis, this drug did not appear to be acting through the GABA system because it caused smaller increases in GABA levels than did AOAA and altered dopamine synthesis in the absence of impulse flow. The GABA-mimetic drugs did attenuate effects of haloperidol, but not in a manner consistent with their assumed GABA-mimetic potencies.

One explanation for these inconsistencies may be that the drugs studied do not exert the predicted effect on GABA-mediated neurotransmission in the CNS, or that they have confounding interactions with other neurotransmitter systems. This seems especially possible with a drug like AOAA which interacts with pyridoxal-5'-phosphate, a cofactor required in many enzymatic reactions. It has also been argued that muscimol may not penetrate the CNS before it is metabolized (Enna *et al.* 1978). However, this seems unlikely, in view of the rapid changes in firing rates of pars reticulata cells observed upon i.v. administration of muscimol.

It is also possible that the striatonigral feedback loop affects dopamine neurons indirectly, through nigral interneurons or via local dendro-axonal and axo-dendritic interactions (Reubi *et al.* 1977). If several GABA synapses are involved in the feedback loop, it would be difficult to predict how GABA-mimetics would modify dopaminergic activity. GABA agonists might also produce a complex spectrum of effects if, besides interacting with postsynaptic GABA receptors, these drugs preferentially inhibit GABA neurons and/or interact with GABA receptors on dopamine terminals (Cheramy *et al.* 1977).

Another possibility is that the striatonigral GABA pathway does not even indirectly affect activity of the dopamine neurons (Garcia-Munoz *et al.* 1977). Other mechanisms may account for the changes in dopamine synthesis and neuronal firing rates induced by drugs which stimulate or block dopamine receptors (Di Chiara *et al.* 1977). Substance P containing neurons project from the striatum to the nigra (Hong *et al.* 1977, Kanazawa *et al.* 1977), and these could relay information from the postsynaptic dopamine receptors to the dopamine cell bodies. Dopamine may be released from dopamine dendrites in the nigra (Bjorklund & Lindvall 1975, Geffen *et al.* 1976, Korf *et al.* 1976), and it might directly modulate dopaminergic activity by interacting with auto-receptors on dopamine cell bodies (Aghajanian & Bunney 1977). Drugs could stimulate or inhibit the activity of dopamine neurons by interferring with the release or the action of dendritic dopamine (Korf *et al.* 1976, Paden *et al.* 1976, Nieoullon *et al.* 1977). Dopaminergic agents could also interact with presynaptic dopamine receptors on dopaminergic terminals to alter dopamine synthesis or release (Starke *et al.* 1977).

Whatever the reason for the difference between the results obtained here and those predicted by the striatonigral GABA "feedback loop" model, these studies do suggest that GABA-mimetic agents may not provide a useful way of decreasing the tonic activity of dopamine neurons. However, these issues will have to be reexplored as additional GABA-active agents become available, and as the pharmacology of the GABA system becomes better understood.

REFERENCES

Aghajanian, G. K. & Bunney, B. S. (1974) Dopaminergic and nondopaminergic neurons of the substantia nigra: Differential responses to putative transmitters. In: *Proceedings of the IXth Congress of the Collegium Internationale Neuropsychopharmacologicum,* pp. 444–452. Excerpta Medical Foundation, Paris.

Aghajanian, G. K. & Bunney, B. S. (1977) Dopamine "autoreceptors": Pharmacological characterization by microiontophoretic single cell recording studies. *Naunyn-Schmied. Arch. Pharmacol.* 297, 1–7.

Andén, N.-E. (1974) Inhibition of the turnover of the brain dopamine after treatment with the gamma-aminobutyrate: 2-oxyglutarate transaminase inhibitor aminooxyacetic acid. *Naunyn-Schmied. Arch. Exp. Path. Pharmak.* 283, 419–424.

Baxter, C. F. & Roberts, E. (1961) Elevation of γ-aminobutyric acid in brain: Selective inhibition of γ-aminobutyric-α-ketoglutaric acid transaminase. *J. Biol. Chem.* 236, 3287–3294.

Björklund, A. & Lindvall, O. (1975) Dopamine in dendrites of substantia nigra neurons: Suggestions for a role in dendritic terminals. *Brain Res.* 83, 531–537.

Bird, E. D., Mackay, A. V. P., Raynder, C. N. & Iversen, L. L. (1973) Reduced glutamic-acid-decarboxylase activity of post-mortem brain in Huntington's chorea. *Lancet* i, 1090–1092.

Bunney, B. S., Aghajanian, G. K. & Roth, R. H. (1973a) Comparison of effects of L-dopa, amphetamine and apomorphine on firing rate of rat dopaminegic neurons. *Nature* (New Biol.) 245, 123–125.

Bunney, B. S., Walters, J. R., Roth, R. H. & Aghajanian, G. K. (1973b) Dopaminergic neurons: Effect of antipsychotic drugs and amphetamine on single cell activity. *J. Pharmacol. Exp. Ther.* 185, 560–571.

Bunney, B. S., Walters, J. R., Kuhar, M. J., Roth, R. J. & Aghajanian, G. K. (1975) D- & L-amphetamine stereoisomers: Comparative potencies in affecting the firing of central dopaminergic and noradrenergic neurons. *Psychopharmacol. Comm.* 1, 177–190.

Bunney, B. S. & Aghajanian, G. K. (1976) d-Amphetamine-induced inhibition of central dopaminergic neurons: Mediation by a striato-nigral feedback pathway. *Science* 192, 391–393.

Carlsson, A. & Lindqvist, M. (1963) Effect of chlorpromazine or haloperidol on formation of 3-methoxytyramine and normetanephrine in mouse brain. *Acta Pharmacol. Toxicol.* 20, 140–144.

Carlsson, A., Kehr, W., Lindqvist, M., Magnusson, T. & Atack, C. V. (1972) Regulation of monoamine metabolism in the central nervous system. *Pharmacol. Rev.* 24, 371–384.

Cheramy, A., Nieoullon, A. & Glowinski, J. (1977) Effects of peripheral and local administration of picrotoxin on the release of newly synthesized ^{3}H-dopamine in the caudate nucleus of the cat. *Naunyn-Schmied. Arch. Pharmacol.* 297, 31–37.

Dahlström, A. & Fuxe, K. (1964) Evidence for the existence of monoamine-containing neurons in the central nervous system. *Acta Physiol. Scand.* 62, Suppl. 232, 1–55.

Davidoff, R. A., Grayson, V. & Adair, R. (1973) GABA-transaminase inhibitors and presynaptic inhibition in the amphibian spinal cord. *Am. J. Physiol.* 224, 1230–1234.

Di Chiara, G., Porceddu, M. L., Spano, P. F. & Gessa, G. L. (1977) Haloperidol increases and apomorphine decreases striatal dopamine metabolism after destruction of striatal dopamine-sensitive adenylate cyclase by kainic acid. *Brain Res.* 130, 374–381.

Fonnum, F., Grofova, I., Rinvik, E., Storm-Mathisen, J. & Walberg, F. (1974) Origin and distribution of glutamate decarboxylase in substantia nigra of the cat. *Brain Res.* 71, 77–92.

Fuxe, K., Hökfelt, T., Ljungdahl, A., Agnati, L., Johansson, O. & Perez de la Mora, M. (1975) Evidence for an inhibitory GABA-ergic control of the mesolimbic dopamine neurons: Possibility of improving treatment of schizophrenia by combined treatment with neuroleptics and GABA-ergic drugs. *Med. Biol.* 53, 177–183.

Garcia-Munoz, M., Nicolaou, N. M., Tulloch, I. F., Wright, A. K. & Arbuthnott, G. W. (1977) Feedback loop or output pathway in striato-nigral fibres? *Nature* 265, 363–365.

Geffen, L. B., Jessell, T. M., Cuello, A. C. & Iversen, L. L. (1976) Release of dopamine from dendrites in rat substantia nigra. *Nature* 260, 258–260.

Godin, Y., Heiner, L., Mark, J. & Mandel, P. (1969) Effects of di-n-propylacetate, an anti-convulsive compound, on GABA metabolism. *J. Neurochem.* 16, 869–873.

Gottesfeld, Z., Kelly, J. S. & Renaud, L. P. (1972) The *in vivo* neuropharmacology of amino-oxyacetic acid in the cerebral cortex of the cat. *Brain Res.* 42, 319–335.

Guyenet, P. G. & Aghajanian, G. K. (1977) Antidromic activation of dopaminergic and other neurons in the nigrostriatal pathway. *Soc. Neurosci. Abst.* 3, 38.

Hong, J. S., Yang, H.-Y. T., Racagni, G. & Costa, E. (1977) Projections of substance P-containing neurons from neostriatum to substantia nigra. *Brain Res.* 122, 541–544.

Johnston, G. A. R. (1975) Physiological pharmacology of GABA and its antagonists in the vertebrate nervous system. In: *GABA in Nervous System Function,* ed. Roberts, E., Chase, T. N. & Tower, D. B., pp. 395–412. Raven Press, New York.

Kanazawa, I., Emson, R. C. & Cuello, A. C. (1977) Evidence for the existence of substance P-containing fibres in striato-nigral and pallido-nigral pathways in rat brain. *Brain Res.* 119, 447–453.

Kataoka, K., Bak, I. J., Hassler, R., Kim, J. S. & Wagner, A. (1974) L-glutamate decarboxylase and choline acetyltransferase activity in the substantia nigra and the striatum after surgical interruption of the striatonigral fibers of the baboon. *Exp. Brain Res.* 19, 217–227.

Kääriänen, I. (1976) Effects of aminooxyacetic acid and baclofen on the catalepsy and on the increase of mesolimbic and striatal dopamine turnover induced by haloperidol in rats. *Acta Pharm. Toxicol.* 39, 393–400.

Keller, H. H., Schaffner, R. & Haefely, W. (1976) Interaction of benzodiazepines with neuroleptics at central dopamine neurons. *Naunyn-Schmied. Arch. Pharmacol.* 294, 1–7.

Kim, J. S., Bak, I. J., Hassler, R. & Okada, Y. (1971) Role of γ-aminobutyric acid (GABA) in the extrapyramidal motor system. 2. Some evidence for the existence of a type of GABA-rich strionigral neurons. *Exp. Brain Res.* 14, 95–104.

Korf, J., Zieleman, M. & Westerink, B. H. C. (1976) Dopamine release in substantia nigra? *Nature* 260, 257–258.

Krogsgaard-Larsen, P., Jonston, G. A. R., Curtis, D. R., Game, C. J. A. & McCulloch, G. M. (1975) Structure and biological activity of series of conformationally restricted analogues of GABA. *J. Neurochem.* 25, 803–810.

McGeer, P. L., McGeer, E. G., Wada, J. A. & Jung, E. (1971) Effects of globus pallidus lesions and Parkinson's disease on brain glutamic acid decarboxylase. *Brain Res.* 42, 425–431.

Murrin, L. C., Morgenroth, W. H. III, & Roth, R. H. (1976) Dopamine neurons: Effects of electrical stimulation on tyrosine hydroxylase. *Mol. Pharmacol.* 12, 1070–1081.

Nieoullon, A., Cheramy, A. & Glowinski, J. (1977) Release of dopamine *in vivo* from cat substantia nigra. *Nature* 266, 375–377.

Nowycky, M. C., Walters, J. R. & Roth, R. H. (1978) Dopaminergic neurons: Effect of acute and chronic morphine administration on single cell activity and transmitter metabolism. *J. Neural Trans.,* 42, 99–116.

Paden, C., Wilson, C. J. & Groves, P. M. (1976) Amphetamine-induced release of dopamine from the substantia nigra *in vivo. Life Sci.* 19, 1499–1506.

Peričić, D., Eng, N. & Walters, J. R. (1978) Post-mortem and aminooxyacetic acid-induced accumulation of GABA: Effect on gamma-butyrolactone and picrotoxin. *J. Neurochem.* 30, 767–773.

Perry, T. L., Hansen, S. & Kloster, M. (1973) Huntington's chorea: Deficiency of γ-aminobutyric acid in brain. *N. Eng. J. Med.* 288, 337–342.

Reubi, J.-C., Iversen, L. L. & Jessell, T. M. (1977) Dopamine selectively increases ^{3}H-GABA release from slices of rat substantia nigra *in vitro. Nature* 268, 652–654.

Ribak, E. C., Vaughn, J. E., Saito, K., Barber, R. & Roberts, E. (1976) Immunocytochemical localization of glutamate decarboxylase in rat substantia nigra. *Brain Res.* 116, 287–298.

Roth, R. H., Walters, J. R. & Aghajanian, G. K. (1973) Effects of impulse flow on the release and synthesis of dopamine in the rat striatum. In: *Frontiers in Catecholamine Research,* ed. Snyder, S. H. & Costa, E., pp. 567–574. Pergamon Press, New York.

Sawaya, M. C. B., Horton, R. W. & Meldrum, B. S. (1975) Effects of anticonvulsant drugs on the cerebral enzymes metabolizing GABA. *Epilepsia.* 16, 649–655.

Simler, S., Ciesielski, L., Maitre, M., Randrianarisoa, H. & Mandel, P. (1973) Effect of sodium n-dipropylacetate on audiogenic seizures and brain γ-aminobutyric acid level. *Biochem. Pharmacol.* 22, 1701–1708.

Starke, K., Taube, H. D. & Borowski, E. (1977) Presynaptic receptor systems in catecholaminergic transmission. *Biochem. Pharmacol.* 26, 259–268.

Walker, R. J., Woodruff, G. N. & Kerkut, G. A. (1971) The effect of ibotenic acid and muscimol on single neurons of the snail *Helix aspersa. Comp. Gen. Pharmacol.* 2, 168–174.

Walters, J. R. & Roth, R. H. (1974) Dopaminergic neurons: Drug-induced antagonism of the increase in tyrosine hydroxylase activity produced by cessation of impulse flow. *J. Pharmacol. Exp. Ther.* 191, 82–91.

Walters, J. R. & Roth, R. H. (1976) Dopamine neurons: An *in vivo* system for measuring drug interactions with presynaptic receptors. *Naunyn-Schmied. Arch. Pharmacol.* 296, 5–14.

Walters, J. R. & Lakoski, J. M. (1978) Effect of muscimol on single unit activity of substantia nigra dopamine neurons. *Eur. J. Pharmacol.* 47, 469–471.

Walters, J. R., Lakoski, J. M. & Eng, N. (1978) Dopamine neurons: Effect of lergotrile on unit activity and transmitter synthesis. In preparation.

Walters, J. R., Roth, R. H. & Aghajanian, G. K. (1973) Dopaminergic neurons: Similar biochemical and histochemical effects of gamma-hydroxybutyrate and acute lesions of the nigro-neostriatal pathway. *J. Pharmacol. Exp. Ther.* 186, 630–639.

Waszczak, B. L., Lakoski, J. M. & Walters, J. R. (1978) Effects of muscimol upon the activity of substantia nigra pars reticulata neurons. *Soc. Neurosci. Abst.* 4, 436.

Westerink, B. H. C. & Korf, J. (1975) Influence of drugs on striatal and limbic homovanillic acid concentration in the rat brain. *Eur. J. Pharmacol.* 33, 31–40.

Wheal, H. V. & Kerkut, G. A. (1976) The action of muscimol on the inhibitory postsynaptic membrane of the crustacean neuromuscular junction. *Brain Res.* 109, 179–183.

Effects of GABA and GABA-like Drugs on the Brain Dopamine and on the Motor Activity of Rats

N.-E. Andén, M. Grabowska-Andén & H. Wachtel

The brain GABA occurs at the highest concentrations in the substantia nigra and in the nucleus accumbens (Fahn & Côté 1968, Balcom *et al.* 1975). These two regions are also rich in dopamine (DA): the substantia nigra contains the cell bodies of the nigro-neostriatal DA neurons whereas the nucleus accumbens has a dense network of DA nerve terminals belonging to mesolimbic DA neurons. Changes in the activity of the DA cells in the substantia nigra can be revealed as alterations of the synthesis and the utilization of the DA of the nerve terminals in the corpus striatum. The nucleus accumbens is of great importance for the motor activity of rats as evidenced by the stimulatory effect of DA given locally into this area (Pijnenburg & van Rossum 1973, Jackson *et al.* 1975). In the present work we have studied the effects of GABA and the GABA-like agents gammahydroxybutyric acid (GHBA), baclofen (β-parachlorophenyl-GABA) and muscimol on the brain DA and on the motor activity of rats.

BIOCHEMICAL EFFECTS ON BRAIN DOPAMINE

Injections of GABA and GHBA into the substantia nigra of rats induced a rise in the concentration of DA in the forebrain (Andén & Stock 1973). The effect is probably specific since the analogues carnitine and betahydroxybutyric acid were ineffective. Intranigrally applied baclofen elevates the brain DA similarly (Kelly & Moore 1978). This effect of GABA and GHBA did not appear following application of even greater doses to the corpus striatum. Systemic

Department of Pharmacology, University of Göteborg, S-400 33 Göteborg, Sweden.

"GABA-NEUROTRANSMITTERS", Alfred Benzon Symposium 12, Munksgaard 1978

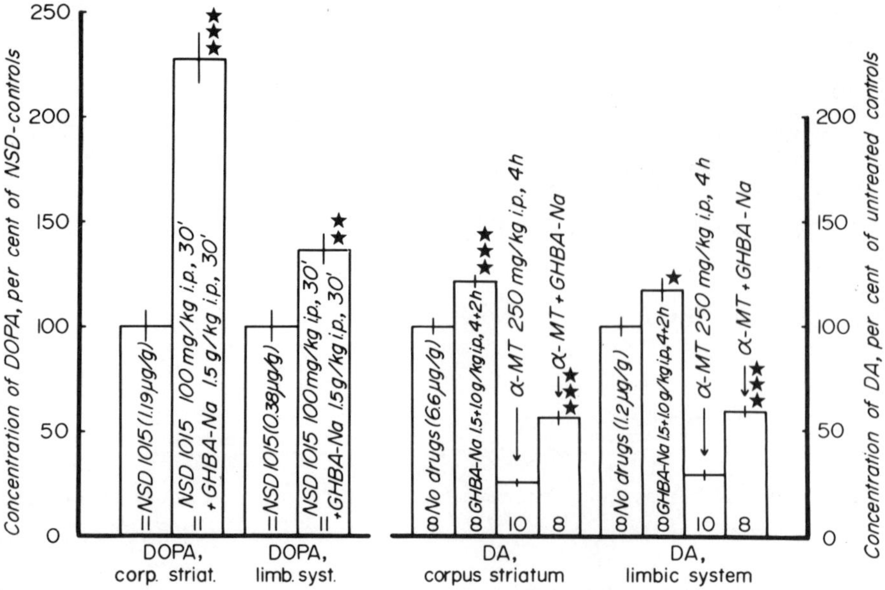

Fig. 1. Effects of gammahydroxybutyric acid (sodium form; GHBA-Na) on the accumulation of DOPA induced by NSD 1015 and on the disappearance of dopamine (DA) induced by α-methyltyrosine (α-MT) in the corpus striatum and in the limbic system of rats. The values are means ± S.E.M. with the number of experiments at the bottom of the columns. The statistical significances (Student's t-test) are indicated for the differences from the NSD-treated, the no drug or the α-MT-treated group, respectively (***: $P\langle 0.001$, **: $P\langle 0.01$, *: $P\langle 0.05$).

treatment with high doses of GHBA produces a similar or somewhat greater increase in the concentration of the brain DA than that following the injections of GHBA into the substantia nigra (Gessa *et al.* 1966). An axotomy of the ascending DA neurons to the forebrain leads to the same rapid elevation of the brain DA as treatment with GHBA. These data suggest that GABA and GHBA have an inhibitory influence on the DA cells in the substantia nigra (Stock *et al.* 1973, Walters *et al.* 1973). Actually, systemic treatment with GHBA blocks the firing rate of the nigro-neostriatal DA neurons (Roth *et al.* 1973). Locally given GABA can produce the same effect (Aghajanian & Bunney 1975).

In order to investigate how the GHBA-induced increase in the concentration of the brain DA is brought about, the synthesis and the utilization of the DA have been determined separately both in the corpus striatum and in the limbic system. The synthesis has been studied by the elevation of DOPA following inhibition of the aromatic amino acid decarboxylase by 3-hydroxybenzylhydrazine (NSD 1015, 100 mg/kg i.p., 30 min) (Carlsson *et al.* 1972). The utilization has been studied by the decrease in DA following inhibition of the tyrosine hydroxylase by *DL-a*-methyltyrosine methylester (*a*-MT, 250 mg/kg i.p., 4 or 2 h) (Spector *et al.* 1965, Corrodi & Hanson 1966, Andén *et al.* 1966a). The part designated the limbic system consisted of the DA-rich parts of the brain outside the corpus striatum such as the nucleus accumbens (medial part), the bed nucleus of the stria terminalis, the olfactory tubercles, the amygdala and the greater part of the limbic cortex (Andén *et al.* 1966b). It was obtained by sections through the rhinal fissures and the optic chiasm after removals of the corpus striatum. The corpus striatum had a high concentration of DA but not of noradrenaline (NA) (DA 6.6 μg/g, NA 0.23 μg/g) whereas the limbic system had high concentrations of both catecholamines (DA 1.2 μg/g, NA 0.75 μ/g). Therefore, the synthesis of DA in the limbic system has been calculated on the assumption that the synthesis of NA in the limbic system and that in the DA-poor parts of the brain such as the hemispheres and the brain stem are similar normally as well as after the various treatments.

GHBA increased the brain concentration of DA in a dose-related manner with a peak effect following 1.5 g/kg i.p. (Stock *et al.* 1973). This dose increased the synthesis and decreased the utilization of DA (Fig. 1). The synthesis of DA was increased by about 150% in the corpus striatum but only by about 80% in the limbic system. On the other hand, the *a*-MT-induced disappearance of DA was decelerated to about the same degree by GHBA in the corpus striatum and in the limbic system. Therefore, the rise in the concentration of DA following treatment with GHBA is in all likelihood the result of both an increase in the synthesis and a decrease in the utilization of DA. In Fig. 1, the maximal effect of GHBA on the concentration of DA had vanished since the last dose of GHBA was given 2h before sacrifice.

GHBA at a dose of 1.5 g/kg i.p. to rats produced a complete anesthesia with a slow respiration and a reduced muscle tone. The latter effect was even more pronounced than after equianesthetic doses of other agents such as barbiturates and diethylether. The presumed GABA agonist muscimol at a dose of 10 mg/kg i.p. also caused anesthesia, a slow respiration and a reduced muscle tone in rats but the effects were somewhat weaker than those of the high dose of GHBA. In contrast to GHBA, muscimol induced hypothermia and a general deterioration. Therefore, the treatment with this high dose of muscimol could not be studied for a longer time than 2 h.

Muscimol at a dose of 10 mg/kg i.p. to rats slightly accelerated the synthesis of

DA in the corpus striatum but it was almost ineffective in the limbic system (Fig. 2). The utilization of DA in the brain was clearly decelerated by 10 mg/kg of muscimol but it was only insignificantly reduced by lower doses. The concentration of DA was elevated, in all probability due to both the increased synthesis and the decreased utilization of DA. The α-MT-induced disappearance of NA was not changed by 10 mg/kg of muscimol but it was slightly accelerated following 5 and 2.5 mg/kg. In this connection, it is of interest that the turnover of NA in the brain is accelerated by GHBA, baclofen and the GABA transaminase inhibitor aminooxyacetic acid (AOAA) whereas the turnover of DA is decelerated by these drugs (Andén 1974, Andén & Wachtel 1977). The lack of effect on the NA utilization after 10 mg/kg of muscimol might be due to the above – mentioned deterioration and hypothermia.

The effects of GHBA, baclofen, AOAA and muscimol on the synthesis and the utilization of DA in the corpus striatum and in the limbic system are summarized in Table I. In the control rats, the fractional rate constants of the

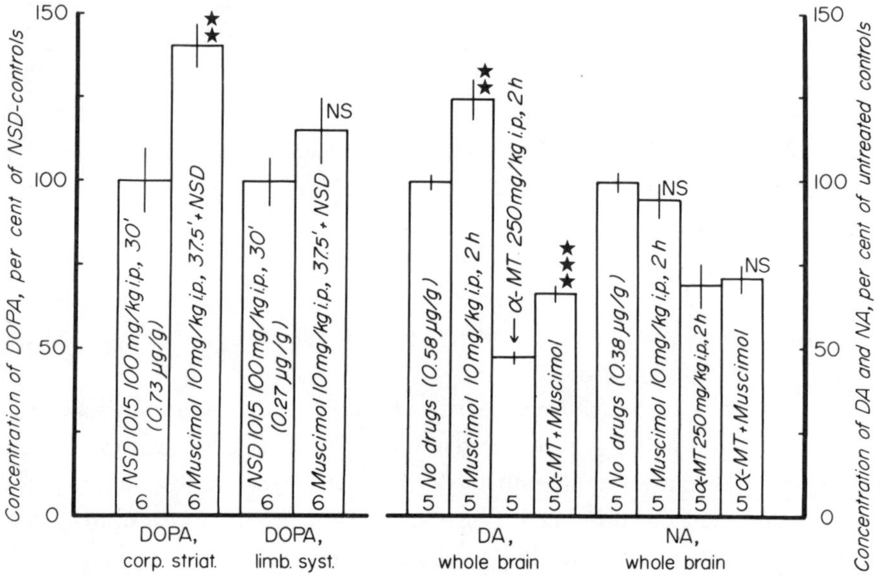

Fig. 2. Effects of muscimol on the accumulation of DOPA induced by NSD 1015 in the corpus striatum and in the limbic system of rats and on the disappearance of dopamine (DA) and noradrenaline (NA) in the whole brain of rats. The values are means ± S.E.M. with the number of experiments at the bottom of the columns. The statistical significances (Student's t-test) are indicated for the differences from the NSD-treated, the no drug or the α-MT-treated group, respectively (***: *P*⟨0.001, **: *P*⟨0.1, NS: no significance).

Table I

Rate constants (h^{-}) of the synthesis and the utilization of the dopamine in the rat brain. The synthesis was determined as the accumulation of DOPA following NSD 1015 (100 mg/kg i.p., 30 min before sacrifice). The utilization was determined as the disappearance of dopamine following a-methyltyrosine [a-MT, 250 mg/kg i.p., 4 or 2 (only muscimol) h before sacrifice]. The operation was performed and the drugs were given simultaneously with NSD 1015 and a-MT, apart from AOAA which was given 2 h before. In the a-MT experiments, GHBA was given at an additional dose of 1.0 g/kg i.p. 2 h after the first dose. The effect of muscimol on the utilization of dopamine was determined in the whole brain. The values are means of 5 – 12 experiments. Statistical significances (Student's t-test) of the differences from the control group are indicated

	SYNTHESIS (NSD 1015)		UTILIZATION (a-MT)	
TREATMENT	Corpus striatum	Limbic system	Corpus striatum	Limbic system
Controls	0.30	0.33	0.34	0.31
Axotomy	1.14***	0.72***	0.03***	0.06***
GHBA (1.5 g/kg i.p.)	0.77***	0.61**	0.14***	0.13***
Baclofen (75 mg/kg i.p.)	0.64***	0.47	0.08***	0.12***
Baclofen (12.5 mg/kg i.p.)	0.37	0.31	0.25*	0.21***
AOAA (50 mg/kg i.p.)	0.28	0.28	0.23***	0.22***
Muscimol (10 mg/kg i.p.)	0.42**	0.38	0.18***	

*** ($P<0.001$), ** ($P<0.01$), * ($P<0.05$) as compared to controls.

synthesis and of the utilization were approximately equal and they did not differ markedly between the corpus striatum and the limbic system. Axotomy of the DA neurons and treatments with high doses of GHBA and baclofen (Andén & Wachtel 1977) stimulated the synthesis of DA to a greater extent in the corpus striatum than in the limbic system. On the other hand, the utilization of DA was retarded similarly in the two regions. Baclofen at a dose six times lower than that described above did not significantly change the synthesis of DA and the same was true for the effect of a high dose of AOAA. The high dose of muscimol resembled the latter treatments in producing only a slight stimulation of the synthesis of DA in the corpus striatum. The treatments with muscimol, AOAA and the low dose of baclofen were effective, however, in decelerating the utilization of DA. Therefore, the increase in the synthesis of DA might occur only at a complete or an almost complete interruption of the nerve impulse flow in the DA neurons. On the other hand, a partial inhibition of the nerve impulse flow seems to be observed more easily as a deceleration of the utilization of DA.

Such a diminished firing of the DA neurons appears to be a common denominator of the four GABA-ergic drugs studied.

EFFECTS ON MOTOR ACTIVITY

The control rats injected with 0.9% NaCl bilaterally into the nucleus accumbens had a rather high activity during the first 10 min and it rapidly decreased later and reached stable and low levels after approximately 60 min (Fig. 3). Bilateral application of a high dose of GABA (2 × 250 μg) to the nucleus accumbens depressed the motor activity during the first 10 min. The GABA transaminase inhibitor AOAA at a dose not influencing the motor activity *per se* increased and prolonged the inhibitory effect of GABA on the motor activity. The hypoactivity was not followed by a hyperactivity after GABA alone and there was only a slight stimulation 60 min after the combined treatment with AOAA and GABA (Wachtel & Andén 1978).

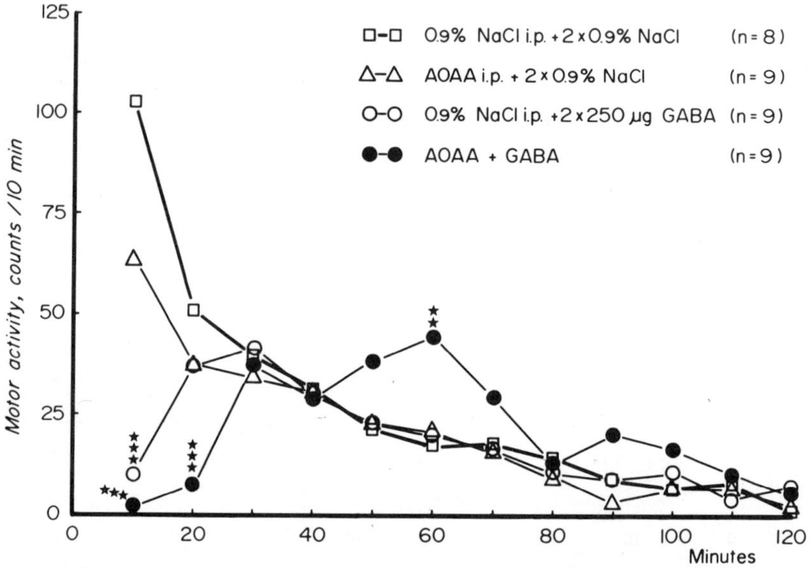

Fig. 3. Motor activity of rats at different time intervals following bilateral application of GABA or 0.9% NaCl (2 × 1 μl) to the nucleus accumbens. The rats were injected intraperitoneally with aminooxyacetic acid (AOAA, 15 mg/kg) or 0.9% NaCl 30 min before the start of the recordings. The counts were cumulated over each 10 min time interval. The values are means and the S.E.M. are usually between 10 and 30% of the mean (n=number of experiments). The statistical significances (Student's t-test) of the differences from the NaCl group are indicated (***: $P\langle 0.001$, **: $P\langle 0.01$). From Wachtel & Andén (1978).

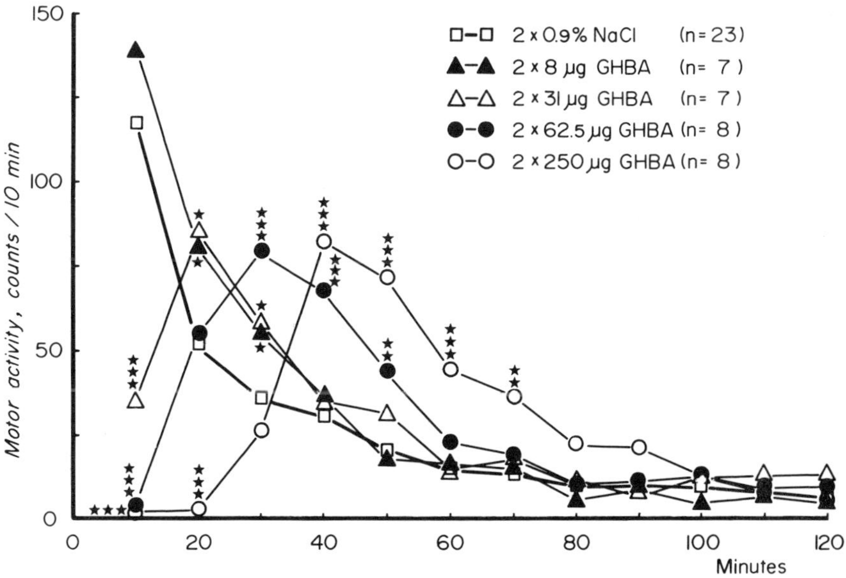

Fig. 4. Motor activity of rats at different time intervals following bilateral application of various doses of gammahydroxybutyric acid (sodium form; GHBA) or 0.9% NaCl (2 × 1 µl) to the nucleus accumbens. The values are means and the S.E.M. are usually between 10 and 30% of the mean (n=number of experiments). The statistical significances (Student's t-test) of the differences from the NaCl group are indicated (***: $P\langle 0.001$, **: $P\langle 0.01$, *: $P\langle 0.05$). From Wachtel & Andén (1978).

Injection of GHBA bilaterally into the nucleus accumbens led to a decrease followed by an increase in the motor activity (Fig. 4). The magnitude and the duration of the depression were dose-dependent and the same was true for the GABA-induced hypoactivity. The GHBA-induced stimulations of the motor activity subsequent to the suppressions had remarkably similar peak values after the various doses although they occurred later following the high doses. There was an increased activity only after 2 × 8 µg GHBA (Wachtel & Andén 1978).

The effects of GABA and GHBA in the nucleus accumbens on the motor activity appear to be specific since no or only small changes were observed following injections of the analogues carnitine and betahydroxybutyric acid (Wachtel & Andén 1978).

Injection of baclofen (2 × 0.025 µg) into the nucleus accumbens resulted in an initial suppression and a late stimulation of the motor activity. The peak activity was somewhat later than that following a dose of GHBA (2 × 31 – 62.5 µg) producing the same hypoactivity. Higher doses of baclofen induced a long lasting inhibition (Wachtel & Andén 1978).

As mentioned above, GABA, GHBA and baclofen can inhibit the firing rate of the DA neurons and the subsequent release of DA from the nerve terminals. Therefore it might be hypothesized that the depression of the motor activity observed following these drugs is caused by such an inhibition of the DA neurotransmission. In order to test this idea, GHBA and GABA were given into the nucleus accumbens of rats pretreated with reserpine and apomorphine. The apomorphine-induced hyperactivity of the reserpine-treated rats is in all probability due to stimulation of postsynaptic DA receptors. GABA and GHBA were able to inhibit this apomorphine-induced activity to about the same degree as they inhibited the normal motor activity. Therefore, it appears that GABA and GHBA did not evoke hypoactivity by inhibiting the release of DA but that they act mainly at sites in the nucleus accumbens beyond the DA synapses. It cannot be excluded that also other brain regions are involved in the depressions induced by GABA and GHBA since reductions of motor activity were observed following applications to the neostriatum and the paleostriatum. These hypoactivities were, however, smaller than those observed after applications of GABA and GHBA to the nucleus accumbens (Wachtel & Andén 1978).

The presumed GABA receptor blocking agent picrotoxin (Precht & Yoshida 1971, Crossman *et al.* 1973) induced a marked and long lasting increase in motor activity when applied bilaterally to the nucleus accumbens (Wachtel & Andén 1978). No hyperactivity was observed following treatment with other convulsive agents such as strychnine and pentylenetetrazole. The picrotoxin-induced stimulation was much smaller after injections into the neostriatum or the paleostriatum. Therefore, the increase in motor activity might be the result of a blockade of postsynaptic GABA receptors in the nucleus accumbens normally mediating a negative influence by neurally released GABA on motor activity. The inhibitory effects of GABA, GHBA and baclofen on motor activity might be caused by stimulations of such postsynaptic GABA receptors in the nucleus accumbens.

The stimulatory effect of low doses of GHBA on the motor activity might be hard to detect due to a high initial spontaneous activity of rats. Furthermore, the stimulations following high doses of GHBA might be compensatory to the previous suppressions. In order to exclude these possibilities, GHBA was given to rats habituated to the environment. Doses of GHBA up to $2 \times 16\,\mu g$ resulted in a rapid and clearcut activation of the habituated rats without any preceding hypoactivity. GABA was less potent than GHBA in this respect, in agreement with the less pronounced late stimulation by GABA following high doses (Wachtel & Andén 1978).

The effects of picrotoxin and GHBA indicate differences between the receptors mediating the increases and the decreases in the motor activity. The GHBA-induced changes in the motor activity are a mirror image of those produced by apomorphine. This DA receptor agonist has been reported to reduce the motor activity following low doses and to initially increase and subsequently decrease the motor activity following high doses (Maj *et al.* 1972, Puech *et al.* 1974, Thornburg & Moore 1974). The depression by apomorphine may be due to preferential stimulation of DA autoreceptors on the DA neurons, leading to impaired DA neurotransmission, whereas the stimulation should be due to a direct stimulation of postsynaptic DA receptors (Strömbom 1976). In an analogous way, the GHBA-induced increases and decreases in motor activity can be explained as stimulations of GABA autoreceptors and postsynaptic GABA receptors, respectively. It appears that GABA is relatively weaker than GHBA in activating the hypothetical GABA autoreceptors in comparison to the

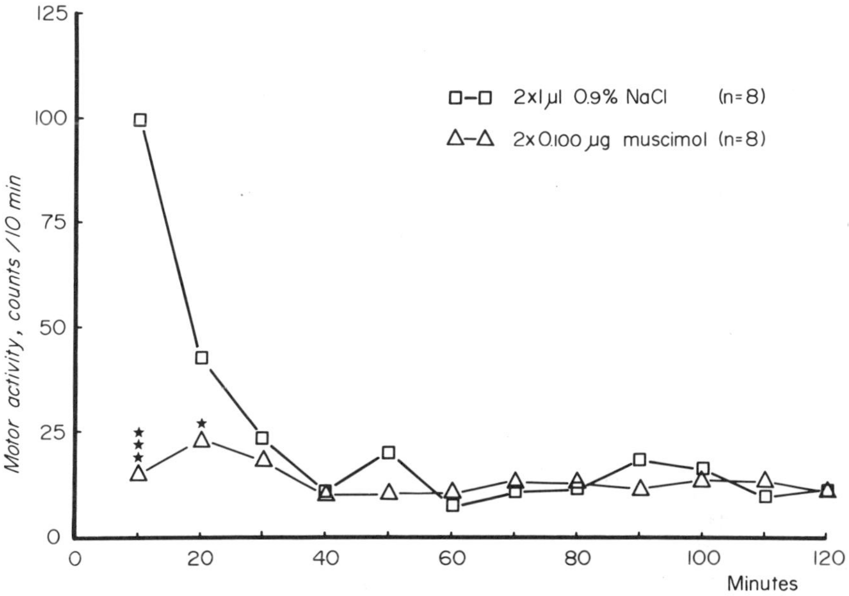

Fig. 5. Motor activity of rats at different time intervals following bilateral application of muscimol or 0.9% NaCl (2 × 1 µl) to the nucleus accumbens. The values are means and the S.E.M. are usually between 10 and 30% of the mean (n=number of experiments). The statistical significances (Student's t-test) of the differences from the NaCl group are indicated (***: $P<0.001$, *: $P<0.05$).

postsynaptic receptors. There are also other examples that exogenous agonists have a greater relative affinity for autoreceptors than the neurotransmitters, for instance, clonidine at the noradrenaline synapses and LSD at the 5-hydroxytryptamine synapses.

Application of muscimol (2 × 0.1 μg) to the nucleus accumbens induced a marked hypoactivity of a relatively short duration (Fig. 5). No subsequent hyperactivity was observed. Thus, muscimol resembles GABA rather than GHBA in affecting the motor activity following bilateral application to the nucleus accumbens.

SUMMARY

Local application of GABA, gammahydroxybutyric acid (GHBA) and baclofen to the substantia nigra elevated the brain dopamine similarly to systemic treatments with GHBA, baclofen and, to a smaller extent, muscimol. The effects were caused by increased synthesis in combination with decreased utilization of dopamine, probably due to inhibition of the firing of the dopamine neurons.

Local application of GABA, GHBA, baclofen and muscimol to the nucleus accumbens suppressed the motor activity whereas the GABA receptor antagonist picrotoxin stimulated it. GHBA and baclofen at low doses or at late intervals following high doses increased the motor activity. The hypokinesias are probably the result of postsynaptic GABA receptor stimulation whereas the hyperkinesias induced by GHBA and baclofen might be caused by activation of GABA autoreceptors.

ACKNOWLEDGMENTS

This work was supported by the Swedish Medical Research Council (04X–502) and Schering AG. Skillful technical assistance was provided by Inger Oscarsson and Maria Lindbäck.

REFERENCES

Aghajanian, G. K. & Bunney, B. S. (1975) Dopaminergic and non-dopaminergic neurons of the substantia nigra: differential responses to putative transmitters. In: *Neuropsychopharmacology*, ed. Boissier, J. R., Hippius, H. & Pichot, P., pp. 444–452. Excerpta Medica Foundation, Amsterdam.

Andén, N.-E. (1974) Inhibition of the turnover of the brain dopamine after treatment with the gammaaminobutyrate: 2-oxyglutarate transaminase inhibitor aminooxyacetic acid. *Naunyn-Schmiedeberg's Arch. Pharmacol.* 283, 419–424.

Andén, N.-E., Corrodi, H., Dahlström, A., Fuxe, K. & Hökfelt, T. (1966 a) Effects of tyrosine hydroxylase inhibition on the amine levels of central monoamine neurons. *Life Sci.* 5, 605–611.

Andén, N.-E., Fuxe, K., Hamberger, B. & Hökfelt, T. (1966 b) A quantitative study on the nigro-neostriatal dopamine neuron system in the rat. *Acta physiol. scand.* 67, 306–312.

Andén, N.-E. & Stock, G. (1973) Inhibitory effect of gammahydroxybutyric acid and gamma-aminobutyric acid on the dopamine cells in the substantia nigra. *Naunyn-Schmiedeberg's Arch. Pharmacol.* 279. 89–92.

Andén, N.-E. & Wachtel, H. (1977) Biochemical effects of baclofen (β-parachlorophenyl-GABA) on the dopamine and the noradrenaline in the rat brain. *Acta Pharmacol.* (Kbh.) 40, 310–320.

Balcom, G. J., Lenox, R. H. & Meyerhoff, J. L. (1975) Regional γ-aminobutyric acid levels in rat brain determined after microwave fixation. *J. Neurochem.* 24, 609–613.

Carlsson, A., Davis, J. N., Kehr, W., Lindqvist, M. & Atack, C. V. (1972) Simultaneous measurement of tyrosine and tryptophan hydroxylase activities in brain *in vivo* using an inhibitor of the aromatic amino acid decarboxylase. *Naunyn-Schmiedeberg's Arch. Pharmacol.* 275, 153–168.

Corrodi, H. & Hanson, L.C.F. (1966) Central effects of an inhibitor of tyrosine hydroxylation. *Psychopharmacologia (Berl.)* 10, 116–125.

Crossman, A. R., Walker, R. J. & Woodruff, G. N. (1973) Picrotoxin antagonism of γ-aminobutyric acid inhibitory responses and synaptic inhibition in the rat substantia nigra. *Brit. J. Pharmacol.* 49, 696–698.

Fahn, S. & Côté, L. J. (1968) Regional distribution of γ-aminobutyric acid (GABA) in brain of the rhesus monkey. *J. Neurochem.* 15, 209–213.

Gessa, G. L., Vargiu, L., Crabai, F., Boero, G. C., Caboni, F. & Camba, R. (1966) Selective increase of brain dopamine induced by γ-hydroxybutyrate. *Life Sci.* 5, 1921–1930.

Jackson, D. M., Andén, N.-E. & Dahlström, A. (1975) A functional effect of dopamine in the nucleus accumbens and in some other dopamine-rich parts of the rat brain. *Psychopharmacologia* (Berl.) 45, 139–149.

Kelly, P. H. & Moore, K. E. (1978) Dopamine concentrations in the rat brain following injections into the substantia nigra of baclofen, γ-aminobutyric acid, γ-hydroxybutyric acid, apomorphine and amphetamine. *Neuropharmacol.* 17, 169–174.

Maj, J., Grabowska, M., Gajda, L. & Michaluk, J. (1972) On the central action of apomorphine in mice. *Dissert. Pharm. Pharmacol.* 24, 351–364.

Pijnenburg, A. J. J. & van Rossum, J. M. (1973) Stimulation of locomotor activity following injection of dopamine into the nucleus accumbens. *J. Pharm. Pharmacol.* 25, 1003–1005.

Precht, W. & Yoshida, M. (1971) Blockage of caudate-evoked inhibition of neurons in the substantia nigra by picrotoxin. Brain Res. 32, 241–254.

Puech, A.-J., Simon, P., Chermat, R. & Boissier, J. R. (1974) Profil neuropsychopharmacologique de l'apomorphine. *J. Pharmacol. (Paris)* 5, 241–254.

Roth, R. H., Walters, J. R. & Aghajanian, G. K. (1973) Effect of impulse flow on the release and synthesis of dopamine in the rat striatum. In: *Frontiers in Catecholamine Research,* ed. Usdin, E. & Snyder, S. H., pp. 567–574. Pergamon Press, New York.

Spector, S., Sjoerdsma, A. & Udenfriend, S. (1965) Blockade of endogenous norepinephrine synthesis by α-methyltyrosine, an inhibitor of tyrosine hydroxylase. *J. Pharmacol. Exp. Ther.* 147, 86–95.

Stock, G., Magnusson, T. & Andén, N.-E. (1973) Increase in brain dopamine after axotomy or treatment with gammahydroxybutyric acid due to elimination of the nerve impulse flow. *Naunyn-Schmiedeberg's Arch. Pharmacol.* 278, 347–361.

Strömbom, U. (1976) Catecholamine receptor agonists. Effects on motor activity and rate of tyrosine hydroxylation in mouse brain. *Naunyn-Schmiedeberg's Arch. Pharmacol.* 292, 167–176.

Thornburg, J. E. & Moore, K. E. (1974) A comparison of effects of apomorphine and ET 495 on locomotor activity and circling behavior in mice. *Neuropharmacol.* 13, 189–197.

Wachtel, H. & Andén, N.-E. (1978) Motor activity of rats following intracerebral injections of drugs influencing GABA mechanisms. *Naunyn-Schmiedeberg's Arch. Pharmacol.* 302, 133–139.

Walters, J. R., Roth, R. H. & Aghajanian, G. K. (1973) Dopaminergic neurons: similar biochemical and histochemical effects of γ-hydroxybutyrate and acute lesions of the nigro-neostriatal pathway. *J. Pharmacol. Exp. Ther.* 186, 630–639.

Chapter II
GABA Receptors and Structure-Activity Studies on GABA Agonists and Inhibitors of GABA-T and GABA Uptake

Systematic Study of GABA Analogues of Restricted Conformation

Graham A. R. Johnston, Robin D. Allan, Sue M. E. Kennedy & Bruce Twitchin

The need to investigate GABA analogues of restricted conformation was recognized in the very early studies of the pharmacology of this inhibitory neurotransmitter. Purpura *et al.* (1959) commented that "Studies are underway with substances that have fewer degrees of rotational freedom such as unsaturated ω-amino acids", while Curtis & Watkins (1960) speculated on the two-charge character of the GABA receptor stating that "these charges are located upon molecular chains, the conformations of which are capable of variation. Changes in these conformations... may be induced by the amino acid". McGeer *et al.* (1961) studying the effects of GABA, imidazole-4-acetic acid and related compounds including dopamine on the crayfish stretch receptor, commented that all appreciably active compounds "had an acidic and basic function and could be oriented in such a way that these groups were approximately 4 Å apart and were sterically unhindered": these studies by McGeer *et al.* (1961) can be regarded as the first to use GABA analogues of restricted conformation to probe molecular aspects of GABA-receptor interactions. With respect to the CNS, there was little further progress in this field until the realization that glycine was an inhibitory synaptic transmitter (Aprison & Werman 1968) interacting with a different population of receptors to those for GABA, and the development of relatively selective antagonists for glycine and GABA receptors, strychnine and bicuculline respectively (Curtis *et al.* 1968, 1970). Inhibitory amino acids could then be classified as "glycine-like", i.e. strychnine-sensitive, bicuculline-insensitive, as "GABA-like", i.e. bicuculline-sensitive, strychnine-insensitive, or as having an action different to either glycine

Department of Pharmacology, John Curtin School of Medical Research, Australian National University, P.O. Box 334, Canberra City, A.C.T., 2601. Australia.

"GABA-NEUROTRANSMITTERS", Alfred Benzon Symposium 12, Munksgaard 1978

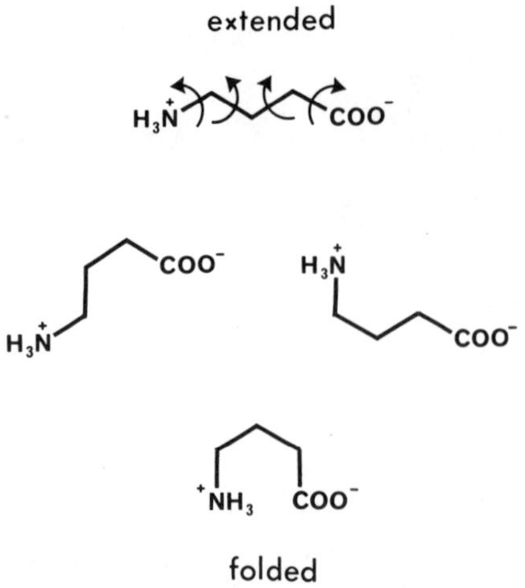

Fig. 1. Bond rotation in the GABA molecule producing different conformations.

or GABA, e.g. taurine was a strychnine-sensitive, bicuculline-sensitive inhibitor in the cat cerebral cortex (Curtis *et al.* 1971). Slowly, perhaps because the chemistry of these small water soluble compounds was difficult, new GABA analogues of restricted conformation began to be reported in the literature and tested for "GABA-like" activity on neurones, and also for effects on other GABA processes such as high affinity uptake (Beart *et al.* 1972a) and GABA transamination (Beart *et al.* 1972b). Recently ligand binding has been added to this list of GABA processes examined with these analogues (Enna & Snyder 1975). The new GABA analogues included muscimol (Johnston *et al.* 1968), 4-aminotetrolic acid (Beart *et al.* 1971), cis and trans-4-aminocrotonic acid, cis- and trans-3-aminocyclohexanecarboxylic acid (Beart *et al.* 1972a, Johnston *et al.* 1975), cis- and trans-3-aminocyclopentanecarboxylic acid (Segal *et al.* 1975). These studies were accompanied by structure-activity speculations particularly with respect to charge separation, and whether extended (Beart *et al.* 1971, Johnston *et al.* 1975) and/or folded (Steward *et al.* 1971, Van Gelder, 1971) conformations of GABA are important (Fig. 1). Chemists became increasingly interested in the field and provided information from x-ray crystallographic (Brehm *et al.* 1972) and proton magnetic resonance studies (Ham 1974) and from theoretical molecular orbital calculations (Andrews & Johnston 1973).

This article summarizes studies of GABA analogues of restricted conformation in a systematic manner based on the chemical means by which conformational restriction is achieved. This approach has proved useful with respect to other neurotransmitters such as acetylcholine and dopamine, providing information on the "active conformations" of these molecules (see e.g. Martin-Smith *et al.* 1967). The basic aim of these studies is a better understanding of the molecular processes involved in the interaction of transmitters and specific binding sites associated with metabolizing enzymes, transport carriers and neuronal receptors.

The GABA molecule has considerable flexibility as a result of free rotation around the single bonds as illustrated in Fig. 1. This conformational mobility can be reduced in analogues of GABA by the incorporation of unsaturation, ring structures or both into the basic transmitter molecule. Such conformational restriction usually results in compounds having more selective actions than that of the transmitter itself, or in having no action at all on GABA processes. Substituents can also produce restriction of otherwise relatively free rotation around single bonds as is discussed below for methyl-substituted muscimol derivatives.

There are ten possible ways (Fig. 2) of joining atom pairs of the three carbon atoms, the amino nitrogen and the carboxyl group of GABA in such a way as to restrict conformational mobility. Only strict GABA analogues are considered,

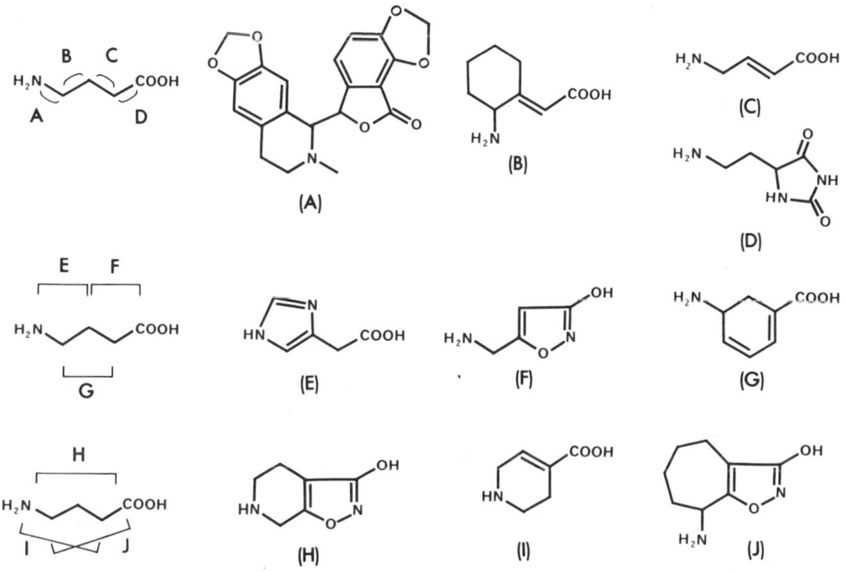

Fig. 2. Ten ways of restricting the conformation of GABA and examples of GABA analogues thus restricted.

Table I
GABA analogues of restricted conformation

GABA Analogue	IC50(μM) Binding	Uptake	GABA-T	GABA-T Substrate	Ref.
(GABA)	(0.34)	(20)	-	1.0	
(A) *Restriction of rotation around N-C4 bond*					
1. (+)-bicuculline methochloride	7	n.s.	n.s.	n.s.	c,h
2. (−)-bicuculline methochloride	500	?	?	?	h
(B) *Restriction of rotation around C4-C3 bond*					
3. (2-Aminocyclohexylidene)-acetic acid	n.s.	n.s.	?	?	u
4. (2-Aminocyclopentylidene)-acetic acid	n.s.	ca 500	?	?	u
(C) *Restriction of rotation around C3-C2 bond*					
5. Trans-4-aminocrotonic acid	0.14	24	-	1.79	d,e,u
6. Cis-4-aminocrotonic acid	25	n.s.	n.s.	-	i,u
7. 4-Aminotetrolic acid	?	450	580	n.s.	d,f
8. Trans-2-(aminomethyl)cyclopropane-carboxylic acid	0.26	>500	-	0.48	b
9. Cis-2-(aminomethyl)cyclopropane-carboxylic acid	19	n.s.	n.s.	-	b
10. Cis-2-(aminomethyl)cyclohexane-carboxylic acid	n.s.	n.s.	n.s.	-	u
11. o-Aminomethylbenzoic acid	n.s.	n.s.	n.s.	-	u
Derivatives of trans-4-aminocrotonic acid:					
12. N-Methyl	>100	500	8	8	u
13. 2-Fluoro	0.5	69	-	0.18	u
14. 2-Chloro	0.27	90	-	0.56	u
15. 2-Bromo	0.36	470	-	0.52	u
16. 2-Methyl	1.1	51	-	1.92	u
17. 3-Chloro	0.38	260	n.s.	-	u
18. 3-Bromo	n.s.	n.s.	94	n.s.	u
19. 3-Methyl	2.2	428	n.s.	-	u
20. 4-Methyl S(−)-isomer	1.8	n.s.	n.s.	-	u
21. 4-Methyl R(+)-isomer	81	34	n.s.	-	u
22. 4,4-Dimethyl	n.s.	n.s.	?	?	u
(D) *Restriction of rotation around C2-C1*					
23. 5-(2-Aminoethyl)hydantoin	n.s.	n.s.	>1000	-	u
(E) *Restriction of conformation by linking N and C3*					
24. Imidazole-4-acetic acid	0.24	>1000	?	-	g
25. Piperidine-3-acetic acid	n.s.	372	n.s.	n.s.	u

Table I

GABA Analogue	IC$_{50}$(μM) Binding	Uptake	GABA-T	GABA-T Substrate	Ref.
(F) *Restriction of conformation by linking C3 and C1*					
26. Muscimol	0.024	>1000	n.s.	-	j
27. Thiomuscimol	0.12	n.s.	n.s.	-	l
28. Isomuscimol	377	n.s.	n.s.	-	l
29. Azamuscimol	>100	n.s.	n.s.	-	l
30. 5-(1-Aminoethyl)-3-isoxazolol	7	n.s.	n.s.	-	k
31. 4-Methyl-5-aminomethyl-3-isoxazolol	48	n.s.	n.s.	-	k,u
(G) *Restriction of conformation by linking C4 and C3*					
(i) *6-membered ring:*					
32. Gabaculine	n.s.	69	3	n.s.	a
33. Cis-3-aminocyclohexanecarboxylic acid	n.s.	85	n.s.	-	e,u
34. Trans-3-aminocyclohexanecarboxylic acid	n.s.	1400	n.s.	-	e,u
35. Cis-5-aminocyclohex-3-enecarboxylic acid	n.s.	131	>1000	-	u
(ii) *5-membered ring:*					
36. Cis-3-aminocyclopentanecarboxylic acid	35	45	-	0.50	u
37. Trans-3-aminocyclopentanecarboxylic acid	0.8	63	n.s.	-	u
38. Cis-4-aminocyclopent-2-enecarboxylic acid	34	159	-	0.27	u
39. 4-Aminocyclopent-1-enecarboxylic acid	0.77	21	-	0.20	u
40 3-Aminocyclopent-1-enecarboxylic acid	31	15	-	0.26	u
(iii) *4-membered ring:*					
41. Cis-3-aminocyclobutanecarboxylic acid	3.1	>500	-	0.47	b
42. Trans-3-aminocyclobutanecarboxylic acid	20	n.s.	n.s.	n.s.	b
(H) *Restriction of conformation by linking N and C1*					
43. THIP	2.6	n.s.	n.s.	-	k
44. 2-Pyrrolidone	?	n.s.	n.s.	-	u
(I) *Restriction of conformation by linking N and C2*					
45. Isoguvacine	1.4	n.s	n.s	-	k
46. Piperidine-4-carboxylic acid	15	>500	n.s.	-	e,k
47. β-Proline	n.s.	453	?	-	u
48. Isoxazolidine-5-carboxylic acid	n.s.	n.s.	n.s.	-	u
49. Azetidine-2-carboxylic acid	?	n.s.	n.s.	-	u
(J) *Restriction of conformation by linking C4 and C1*					
50. 8-Aminocyclohepteno[1,2-*d*]-isoxazol-3-ol	n.s.	n.s.	n.s.	-	j

IC$_{50}$Values (concentrations giving 50% inhibition) were determined against sodium-independent binding of GABA to rat brain membranes (frozen-thawed-washed) (as described in ref. g), sodium-dependent high affinity uptake of GABA into rat brain sliced (ref. e) and transamination of GABA

Table I

by extracts of rat brain mitochondria (ref. f). Activity as a GABA-T substrate was determined as in ref. d and is expressed as relative to that of GABA. n.s. = not significant.

References:

a. Allan *et al.* (1977)
b. Allan *et al.* (1978)
c. Beart & Johnston (1972)
d. Beart & Johnston (1973)
e. Beart *et al.* (1972a)
f. Beart *et al.* (1972b)
g. Enna & Snyder (1975)
h. Enna *et al.* (1977)
i. Johnston *et al.* (1975)
j. Krogsgaard-Larsen & Johnston (1975)
k. Krogsgaard-Larsen & Johnston (1978)
l. Krogsgaard-Larsen *et al.* (1977b)

u. Unpublished observations of R. D. Allan, G. A. R. Johnston, S. M. E. Kennedy & B. Twitchin.

i.e. those in which there are three atoms in the chain separating the amino- and carboxyl-functions or their equivalents. Table I lists 50 of these GABA analogues of restricted conformation, together with their activities with respect to inhibition of sodium-independent binding of GABA to rat brain membranes (Enna & Snyder 1975), sodium-dependent high affinity uptake of GABA into rat brain slices (Beart *et al.* 1972a) and the transamination of GABA catalyzed by extracts of rat brain mitochondria (Beart *et al.* 1972b), and their activities as substrates for GABA-transaminase (GABA-T) activity in extracts of rat brain mitochondria (Beart & Johnston 1973).

(A) Restriction of rotation around N–C4 bond

The only formal analogue of this type tested so far appears to be the GABA antagonist, (+)-bicuculline (Fig. 2A) and related compounds. This alkaloid contains a type F conformational restriction which is likely to be more important than the type A since rotation around the N–C4 bond in GABA itself does not influence the conformation of GABA. Furthermore, molecular orbital calculations indicate that rotation around the single bond joining the two-ring structures in (+)-bicuculline (C1–C9) is also restricted (Andrews & Johnston 1973). Structural similarities between GABA and (+)-bicuculline (N–C–C–C–CO of GABA being equivalent to N–C–C–O–CO of bicuculline) were noted in the first paper describing the action of (+)-bicuculline as an antagonist of the inhibitory action of GABA on the firing of cat spinal neurones (Curtis *et al.* 1970). Subsequent studies on the antagonism *in vivo* by (+)-bicuculline of muscimol, 4-aminotetrolic acid, trans-4-aminocrotonic acid (but not the cis-isomer), cis- and trans-3-aminocyclopentanecarboxylic acid further emphasized these structural similarities (Johnston 1976). Ligand binding studies using GABA, (+)-bicuculline methiodide and muscimol provide evidence that these substances share some common binding sites (Enna *et al.* 1977, Möhler & Okada 1977, Beaumont *et al.* 1978). With respect to GABA antagonist action *in vivo* and to certain binding sites *in vitro*, bicuculline has a stereoselective action, the (−)-isomer being much less active. (+)-Bicuculline has other actions but as far as GABA processes are concerned appears to be selective for GABA receptors with no effect on GABA high affinity uptake or GABA transamination (Beart & Johnston 1972, Johnston 1976, 1978).

(B) Restriction of rotation around C4–C3 bond

(2-Aminocyclohexylidene)acetic acid (Fig. 2B), and the corresponding cyclopentylidene analogue were prepared recently (R. D. Allan, unpublished) following consideration of the structures of the new class of GABA agonists based on isoguvacine (Fig. 2I) (Krogsgaard-Larsen *et al.* 1977b). Isoguvacine showed surprisingly high activity as a GABA agonist in view of its nitrogen being a secondary amine and the relative inactivity of N-methyl-GABA and N-methyl-trans-4-aminocrotonic acid as GABA agonists. It was hoped that by using a type B restriction of rotation that the amino- and carboxyl functions of trans-4-amino-crotonic acid (Fig. 2C) could be held in a position equivalent to those in isoguvacine (Fig. 2I) while maintaining the primary amine function. Unfortunately these type B analogues proved to be inactive.

(C) Restriction of rotation around C3–C2 bond

Many GABA analogues of this type are known.

Trans-4-aminocrotonic acid (Fig. 2C) shows higher activity than GABA with respect to GABA binding sites and as a substrate for GABA transaminase, and shows activity comparable with that of GABA with respect to high affinity uptake. The cis-isomer is very weak with respect to GABA binding and inactive against GABA uptake and transamination. *In vivo*, the trans-isomer is a potent bicuculline-sensitive, strychnine-insensitive inhibitor of neuronal firing, while the cis-isomer is only a weak neuronal inhibitor insensitive to both bicuculline and strychnine (Johnston *et al.* 1975). These findings supported the concept that extended conformations of GABA were important with respect to bicuculline-sensitive postsynaptic receptors, high affinity uptake and transamination, and led to the proposal that folded conformations of GABA might interact with bicuculline-insensitive receptors (Johnston 1976, 1978). More recent studies with the cyclopropane analogues, trans- and cis-2-(aminomethyl)cyclopropane-carboxylic acid, have provided similar results with respect to receptors and binding sites although the trans-cyclopropane analogue is weaker than the trans-crotonic acid derivative in all its actions (Allan *et al.* 1978).

As a result of the development of a general synthesis of substituted crotonic acids (Allan & Twitchin 1978), a number of derivatives of trans-4-aminocrotonic acid have become available. Some of these derivatives show relatively selective actions at the price of some loss of activity compared to the parent trans-4-aminocrotonic acid. The 3-bromo derivative is a selective inhibitor of GABA-T without influence on GABA binding or uptake; the GABA-T inhibition is time-dependent and may be of the catalytic type. The 2-bromo derivative is a GABA-T substrate, and is 1000-fold more potent as an inhibitor of GABA binding than of GABA uptake. The 4-methyl derivative shows stereoselectivity with the S(−)-isomer being more active than the R(+)-isomer against GABA binding and less active against GABA uptake. The 2-methyl compound is a very active substrate for GABA-T; kinetic studies with this compound and with the parent trans-4-aminocrotonic acid indicate that they show similar affinity to GABA with the pyridoxal form of the enzyme but react with a higher V_{max}. It would appear that these derivatives of trans-4-aminocrotonic acid will provide valuable information as to the detailed mechanism of GABA transamination.

The triple bond analogue, 4-aminotetrolic acid, is a weak bicuculline-sensitive inhibitor of the firing of spinal neurones (Beart *et al.* 1971), a weak inhibitor of GABA uptake (Beart *et al.* 1972a) and a dead-end inhibitor of GABA transaminase with a similar affinity to that of GABA for the active site of the enzyme but failing to undergo transamination (Beart *et al.* 1972b).

(D) Restriction of rotation around C2–C1

5-(2-Aminoethyl)hydantoin (Fig. 2D) is an example of this type of GABA analogue in which the carboxyl group is incorporated into a heterocyclic ring structure which has some acidic properties. It is inactive with respect to GABA binding, uptake and transamination.

(E) Restriction of conformation by linking N and C3

Imidazole-4-acetic acid (Fig. 2E) has been long known as a GABA agonist (McGeer *et al.* 1961) and has a potent bicuculline-sensitive inhibitory action on

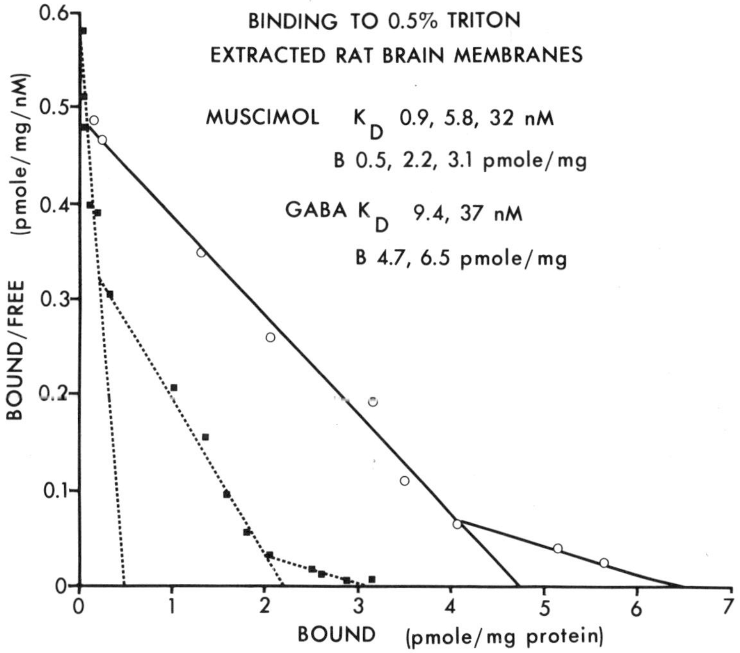

Fig. 3. Scatchard plots of the binding of radioactive muscimol and GABA to rat brain membranes extracted with 0.5% Triton X-100. Solid symbols and broken lines – muscimol. Open symbols and solid lines – GABA. (G. A. R. Johnston & S. M. E. Kennedy, unpublished).

the firing of spinal neurones (Curtis *et al.* 1971). It is a potent inhibitor of GABA binding (Enna & Snyder 1975) with little action on GABA uptake or transamination.

(F) Restriction of conformation by linking C3 and C1

Muscimol (Fig. 2F) is a potent and selective bicuculline-sensitive GABA agonist in which the 3-isoxazolol moiety acts as a masked carboxyl group and restricts conformation (Johnston *et al.* 1968, Curtis *et al.* 1971).

Ligand binding studies with radioactive muscimol have shown that muscimol binds to rat brain membranes with higher affinity than GABA, and inhibition data indicate that muscimol and GABA bind to some common sites (Beaumont *et al.* 1978). As illustrated by the Scatchard plots of Fig. 3, muscimol binds to about half the number of sites that bind GABA in 0.5% Triton X-100 extracted rat brain membrane preparations, and furthermore, muscimol shows three apparent binding components rather than the two shown for GABA,

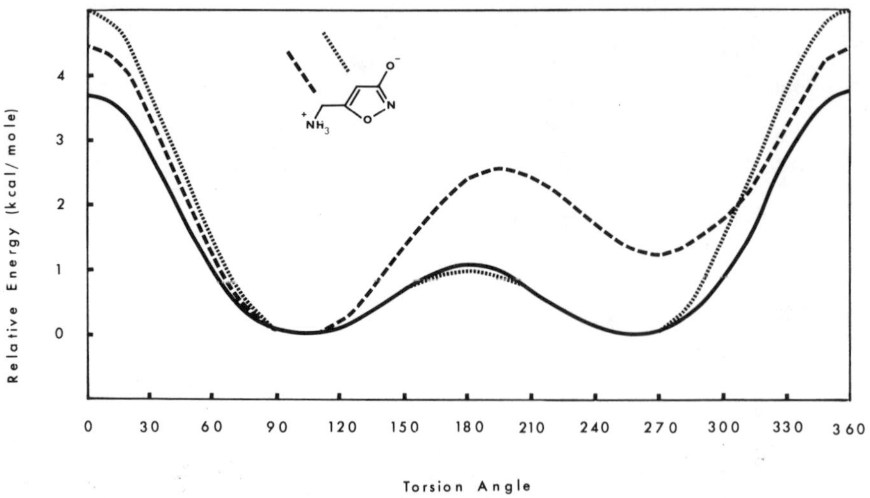

Fig. 4. Calculated potential energy barriers of rotation around the C5–C6 bond in muscimol and two related isoxazoles. Solid line – muscimol. Broken line – 5-(1-aminoethyl)-3-isoxazolol. Dotted line – 4-methyl-5-aminomethyl-3-isoxazolol.

suggesting that muscimol binds to some sites that do not bind GABA (G.A.R. Johnston & S. M. E. Kennedy, unpublished).

Muscimol has only a low affinity for the GABA high affinity uptake system (Johnston 1971) and is taken up relatively inefficiently (K_m 1 mM, V_{max} 0.1 μmol/g/min) into rat brain slices (G. A. R. Johnston *et al.* unpublished). It can be estimated that muscimol binds to some GABA receptors with approximately six orders of magnitude higher affinity than to GABA transport carriers. Muscimol is not a substrate for or an inhibitor of GABA transaminase.

Extensive structure-activity studies have been carried out on muscimol (Krogsgaard-Larsen & Johnston 1975, 1978; Krogsgaard-Larsen *et al.* 1975, 1977a, b). Of the heterocyclic analogues of muscimol tested thus far, only thiomuscimol shows appreciable activity as a GABA agonist. Structure-activity studies on substituted isoxazol-3-ols led to the development of the nipecotic acid series of GABA uptake inhibitor-substrates (Krogsgaard-Larsen & Johnston 1975), nipecotic acid having a higher affinity than GABA for transport carriers, and to the isoguvacine series of selective GABA agonists (Krogsgaard-Larsen *et al.* 1977b).

Calculations using the MINDO/3 molecular orbital method indicate that the aminomethyl side chain of muscimol has preferred conformations with respect to the isoxazole ring, the N7–C6–C5–C4 torsion angle in muscimol of lowest energy being near 100° and 260° (P. R. Andrews & G. A. R. Johnston, unpublished) which is close to that found in muscimol crystals (Brehm *et al.* 1972). Rotation of the aminomethyl side chain with respect to the isoxazole ring can be further restricted by methyl substitution on the side chain, as in 5-(1-aminoethyl)-3-isoxazolol, or on the ring, as in 4-methyl-5-aminomethyl-3-isoxazolol (Fig. 4). Consideration of the activities of these and related compounds as GABA agonists indicate that the "active conformations" might be those with torsion angles in the range 32–46° (P. R. Andrews & G. A. R. Johnston, unpublished). Fig. 5 illustrates muscimol in the conformation which affords maximum overlap with (+)-bicuculline in a low energy conformation

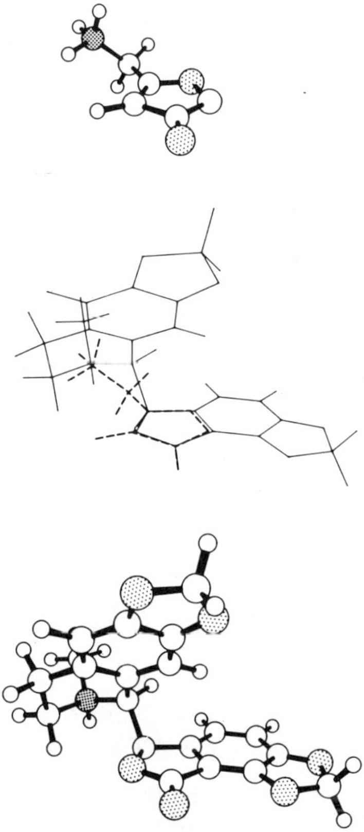

Fig. 5. Conformation of muscimol (torsion angle 39°) which affords maximum overlap with (+)-bicuculline (H–C1–C9–H angle 90°). Upper diagram: muscimol. Lower diagram: (+)-bicuculline. Middle diagram: overlay of muscimol (dotted lines) on (+)-bicuculline (solid lines). Light and dark shadings represent the oxygen and nitrogen atoms respectively.

consistent with molecular orbital and proton magnetic resonance data (Andrews & Johnston 1973 and unpublished).

(G) Restriction of conformation by linking C4 and C2

There is a large number of this class of GABA analogue in which C4 and C2 of GABA is part of a 6-, 5- or 4-membered ring.

Gabaculine (Fig. 2G) is a particularly potent catalytic site inhibitor of GABA-transaminase (Rando 1977), a moderately potent inhibitor of GABA uptake and has little or no action on GABA binding or on the firing of spinal neurones (Allan *et al.* 1977). Saturation of one (cis-5-aminocyclohex-3-enecarboxylic acid) or both (cis- and trans-3-aminocyclohexanecarboxylic acid) of the double bonds in gabaculine leads to substances that have little affinity for GABA transaminase and reduced affinity for the GABA uptake system. One of these derivatives, however, cis-3-amino-cyclohexanecarboxylic acid, appears to be a selective inhibitor of the uptake of GABA into nerve terminals with little activity in respect of the uptake of GABA into glial cells (Bowery *et al.* 1976).

The cyclopentane analogues, cis- and trans-3-aminocyclopentanecarboxylic acid are bicuculline-sensitive inhibitors of hippocampal and spinal neurones (Segal *et al.* 1975, Johnston 1976). Their effects on the binding of GABA and muscimol to rat brain membranes suggest differences between the binding sites for GABA and muscimol (Hitzemann & Loh 1978, Beaumont *et al.* 1978). Many of the cyclopentane analogues of GABA show activity as substrates for GABA transaminase.

The cyclobutane analogues are interesting in that the cis-isomer shows higher activity as an inhibitor of GABA binding than the trans-isomer, i.e. the opposite to that found for the isomers of aminocrotonic acid, 2-(aminomethyl)cyclopropanecarboxylic acid, and 3-aminocyclopentanecarboxylic acid where the trans is the more potent isomer.

(H) Restriction of conformation by linking N and C1

It has been known for a long time that the cyclized GABA analogue, 2-pyrrolidone, is inactive as a GABA agonist (McGeer *et al.* 1961, Curtis & Watkins 1960). While this lactam is inactive in most respects concerning GABA, higher lactams show convulsant activity, e.g. caprolactam, which may be associated with GABA antagonist properties (Kerr *et al.* 1976).

THIP (Fig. 2H) is a bicyclic isoxazole in which the N and C1 atoms of GABA are linked. This relatively rigid derivative is a selective GABA agonist (Krogsgaard-Larsen *et al.* 1977b).

(I) Restriction of conformation by linking N and C2

Isoguvacine (Fig. 2I) is the parent compound of a series of relatively rigid GABA agonists developed out of structure-activity studies on muscimol (Krogsgaard-Larsen *et al.* 1977b).

β-Proline is a weak inhibitor of GABA uptake in rat brain slices, but is more potent as an inhibitor of β-alanine uptake (IC_{50} 274 μM) which suggests that it shows some selectivity as an inhibitor of the glial uptake system for GABA (G. A. R. Johnston & B. Twitchin, unpublished).

(J) Restriction of conformation by linking C4 and C1

The only available derivative of this type is the bicyclic compound 8-aminocyclohepteno[1,2-*d*]isoxazol-3-ol (Fig. 2J). This was prepared as an analogue of muscimol in which rotation of the aminomethyl side chain was restricted by incorporation into a cycloheptene ring, but it showed no activity as an inhibitor of GABA binding (Krogsgaard-Larsen & Johnston 1978).

CONCLUSION

This survey of GABA analogues of restricted conformation has served to identify types of analogues that have been well studied and those that have been almost ignored. Clearly, some analogues have selective actions on particular GABA processes often acting with higher potency than GABA itself. There are examples of analogues of restricted conformation having selective actions on GABA postsynaptic receptors (muscimol, isoguvacine and THIP as agonists; derivatives of (+)-bicuculline as antagonists), GABA neuronal (cis-3-amino-cyclohexanecarboxylic acid) and glial (β-proline) uptake, and GABA transaminase (trans-2-methyl-4-aminocrotonic acid as a GABA-T substrate; gabaculine as a catalytic inhibitor; 4-aminotetrolic acid as a dead-end inhibitor). The actions of some of the analogues provide evidence for a multiplicity of GABA receptors, e.g. muscimol binding to some but not all GABA receptors and the possibility of (+)-bicuculline-insensitive receptors for folded analogues of GABA. These and further studies of GABA analogues should provide a basis for the rational design of selective, therapeutically useful drugs acting at GABA synapses.

ACKNOWLEDGMENTS

The authors are grateful to Drs. P. R. Andrews, P. M. Beart, and P. Krogsgaard-Larsen for helpful discussions.

REFERENCES

Allan, R. D., Johnston, G. A. R., Curtis, D. R., Lodge, D., Kennedy, S. M. E. & Twitchin B. (1978) The activity of cyclopropane and cyclobutane analogues of GABA on GABA processes.*Proc. Aust. Physiol. Pharmac. Soc.* 9, 93P.

Allan, R. D., Johnston, G. A. R. & Twitchin, B. (1977) Effects of gabaculine on the uptake, binding and metabolism of GABA. *Neurosci. Letters* 4, 51–54.

Allan, R. D. & Twitchin, B. (1978) Synthesis of some substituted 4-aminobut-2-enoic acids as analogues of the neurotransmitter GABA. *Aust. J. Chem.* In Press.

Andrews, P. R. & Johnston, G. A. R. (1973) Molecular orbital and proton magnetic resonance studies of bicuculline. *Nature New Biol.* 243, 29–30.

Aprison, M. H. & Werman, R. (1968) A combined neurochemical and neurophysiological approach to identification of central nervous system transmitters. *Neurosci. Res.* 1, 143–174.

Beart, P. M., Curtis, D. R. & Johnston, G. A. R. (1971) 4-Aminotetrolic acid: a new conformationally-restricted analogue of γ-aminobutyric acid. *Nature New Biol.* 234, 80–81.

Beart, P. M. & Johnston, G. A. R. (1972) Bicuculline and GABA-metabolising enzymes. *Brain Res.* 38, 226–227.

Beart, P. M. & Johnston, G. A. R. (1973) Transamination of analogues of γ-aminobutyric acid by extracts of rat brain mitochondria. *Brain Res.* 49, 459–462.

Beart, P. M. Johnston, G. A. R. & Uhr, M. L. (1972a) Competitive inhibition of GABA uptake in rat brain slices by some GABA analogues of restricted conformation. *J. Neurochem.* 19, 1855–1861.

Beart, P. M., Uhr, M. L. & Johnston, G. A. R. (1972b) Inhibition of GABA transaminase activity by 4-aminotetrolic acid. *J. Neurochem.* 19, 1849–1854.

Beaumont, K., Chilton, W. S., Yamamura, H. I. & Enna, S. J. (1978) Muscimol binding in rat brain: association with synaptic GABA receptors. *Brain Res.* 148, 153–162.

Bowery, N. G., Jones, G. P. & Neal, M. J. (1976) Selective inhibition of neuronal GABA uptake by cis-1,3-aminocyclohexane carboxylic acid. *Nature, Lond.* 264, 281–284.

Brehm, L., Hjeds, H. & Krogsgaard-Larsen, P. (1972) The structure of muscimol, a GABA analogue of restricted conformation. *Acta Chem. Scand.* 26, 1298–1299.

Curtis, D. R., Duggan, A. W., Felix, D. & Johnston, G. A. R. (1970) GABA, bicuculline and central inhibition. *Nature, Lond.* 226, 1222–1224.

Curtis, D. R., Duggan, A. W., Felix, D. & Johnston, G. A. R. (1971) Bicuculline, an antagonist of GABA and synaptic inhibition in the spinal cord. *Brain Res.* 32, 69–96.

Curtis, D. R., Hösli, L. & Johnston, G. A. R. (1968) A pharmacological study of the depression of spinal neurones by glycine and related amino acids. *Exp. Brain Res.* 6, 1–18.

Curtis, D. R. & Watkins, J. C. (1960) The excitation and depression of spinal neurones by structurally related amino acids. *J. Neurochem.* 6, 117–141.

Enna, S. J., Collins, J. F. & Snyder, S. H. (1977) Stereospecificity and structure-activity required of GABA receptor binding in rat brain. *Brain Res.* 124, 185–190.

Enna, S. J. & Snyder, S. H. (1975) Properties of γ-aminobutyric acid (GABA) receptor binding in rat brain synaptic membrane fractions. *Brain Res.* 100, 81–97.

Ham, N. S. (1974) NMR studies of solution conformations of physiologically active amino-acids. In: *Molecular and Quantum Pharmacology*, ed. Bergmann, E. D. & Pullman, B. pp. 261–268. Reidel Publ. Co., Dordrecht.

Hitzemann, R. J. & Loh, H. H. (1978) Effects of some conformationally restricted GABA analogues on GABA membrane binding and nerve ending transport. *Brain Res.* 144, 63–73.

Johnston, G. A. R. (1971) Muscimol and the uptake of γ-aminobutyric acid by rat brain slices. *Psychopharmacologia* 22, 230–233.

Johnston, G. A. R. (1976) Physiologic pharmacology of GABA and its antagonists in the vertebrate nervous system. In: *GABA in Nervous System Function*, ed. Roberts, E., Chase, T. N. & Tower, D. B. pp. 395–411. Raven Press, New York.

Johnston, G. A. R. (1978) Amino acid receptors. In: *Receptors in Pharmacology*, ed. Smythies, J. R. & Bradley, R. J. pp. 295–333. Dekker, New York.

Johnston, G. A. R., Curtis, D. R., Beart, P. M., Game, C. J. A., McCulloch, R. M. & Twitchin, B. (1975) *Cis*- And *trans*-4-amino-crotonic acid as GABA analogues of restricted conformation. *J. Neurochem.* 24, 157–160.

Johnston, G. A. R., Curtis, D. R., de Groat, W. C. & Duggan, A. W. (1968) Central actions of ibotenic acid and muscimol. *Biochem. Pharmacol.* 17, 2488–2489.

Kerr, D. I. B., Dennis, B. J., Breuker, E. L. M., Prager, R. H., Ward, A. D. & Duong, T. (1976) Antagonism of GABA-mediated inhibition in the central nervous system by caprolactam derivatives. *Brain Res.* 110, 413–416.

Krogsgaard-Larsen, P., Hjeds, H., Curtis, D. R., Lodge, D. & Johnston, G. A. R. (1977a) Thiomuscimol, isomuscimol, and related compounds as GABA agonists. *Proc. Int. Soc. Neurochem.* 6, 626.

Krogsgaard-Larsen, P. & Johnston, G. A. R. (1975) Inhibition of GABA uptake in rat brain slices by nipecotic acid, various isoxazoles and related compounds. *J. Neurochem.* 25, 797–802.

Krogsgaard-Larsen, P. & Johnston, G. A. R. (1978) Structure-activity studies on the inhibition of GABA binding to rat brain membranes by muscimol and related compounds. *J. Neurochem.* In Press.

Krogsgaard-Larsen, P., Johnston, G. A. R., Curtis, D. R., Game, C. J. A. & McCulloch, R. M. (1975) Structure and biological activity of a series of conformationally restricted analogues of GABA. *J. Neurochem.* 25, 803–809.

Krogsgaard-Larsen, P., Johnston, G. A. R., Lodge, D. & Curtis, D. R. (1977b) A new class of GABA agonist. *Nature,* Lond. 268, 53–55.

McGeer, E. G., McGeer, P. L. & McLennan, H. (1961) The inhibitory action of 3-hydroxytyramine, gamma-aminobutyric acid (GABA) and some other compounds towards the crayfish stretch receptor neuron. *J. Neurochem.* 7, 36–49.

Martin-Smith, M., Smail, G. A. & Stenlake, J. B. (1967) The possible role of conformational isomerism in the biological actions of acetylcholine. *J. Pharm. Pharmac.* 19, 561–589.

Möhler, H. & Okada, T. (1977) GABA receptor binding with $^{3}H(+)$ bicuculline methiodide in rat CNS. *Nature*, Lond. 267, 64–67.

Purpura, D. P., Girado, M., Smith, T. G., Callan, D. A. & Grundfest, H. (1959) Structure activity determinants of pharmacological effects of amino acids and related compounds on central synapses. *J. Neurochem.* 3, 238–268.

Rando, R. R. (1977) Mechanism of the irreversible inhibition of γ-aminobutyric acid-α-ketoglutaric acid transaminase by the neurotoxin gabaculine. *Biochemistry* 16, 4604–4610.

Segal, M., Sims, K. & Smissman, E. (1975) Characterization of an inhibitory receptor in rat hippocampus: a microiontophoretic study using conformationally restricted amino acid analogues. *Br. J. Pharmac.* 54, 181–188.

Steward, E. G., Player, R., Quilliam, J. P., Brown, D. A. & Pringle, M. J. (1971) Molecular conformation of GABA. *Nature New Biol.* 233, 87–88.

van Gelder, N. M. (1971) Molecular arrangement for physiological action of glutamic acid and γ-aminobutyric acid. *Can. J. Physiol. Pharmac.* 49, 513–519.

GABA Receptor and Ionophore Binding Sites: Interaction with Various Drugs

Richard W. Olsen, Maharaj K. Ticku, Donald Greenlee & Paul Van Ness

Postsynaptic membrane macromolecules involved in the action of neurotransmitters can be assayed *in vitro* by suitable radioactive ligand binding. Identification of binding sites as physiological receptors requires satisfaction of strict criteria regarding binding affinity, quantity, tissue and subcellular location, and chemical specificity. Receptor sites for the inhibitory neurotransmitter gamma-aminobutyric acid (GABA) have been identified by binding of radioactive GABA itself (Zukin *et al.* 1974, Enna & Snyder 1975, Olsen *et al.* 1978b), or of the potent and specific GABA agonist, muscimol (Beaumont *et al.* 1978). The convulsant plant substance picrotoxin inhibits the postsynaptic increase in chloride permeability which is the physiological result of GABA binding to its receptor (Ticku & Olsen 1977). Nevertheless, picrotoxin does not inhibit the GABA recognition site itself, but some other component of the receptor-ionophore system. Radioactive α-dihydropicrotoxinin is used to label these sites (Olsen *et al.* 1978b, Ticku *et al.* 1978a).

This report discusses the interaction of various drugs with GABA receptor-ionophore binding sites and some properties of the binding sites relevant to interpretation of these drug interactions.

GABA RECEPTOR BINDING SITES IN MAMMALIAN BRAIN

GABA binding sites in mammalian brain membrane fractions meet several criteria expected of receptor sites (Zukin *et al.* 1974, Enna & Snyder 1975, Enna *et al.* 1977, Olsen *et al.* 1978a,b, Greenlee *et al.* 1978a,b, Lester & Peck 1978, Krogsgaard-Larsen & Johnston 1978). The receptor-like sites are best measured

---

Department of Biochemistry, University of California, Riverside, CA USA

"GABA-NEUROTRANSMITTERS", Alfred Benzon Symposium 12, Munksgaard 1978

in sodium-free buffer (Enna & Snyder 1975) or with Triton X-100 washed membranes (Enna & Snyder 1977), to prevent GABA uptake-binding to nonreceptor sites, and with thoroughly washed, frozen and thawed, or detergent treated membranes, to remove endogenous inhibitors of GABA binding (Greenlee *et al.* 1978a, Johnston & Kennedy 1978). Under these

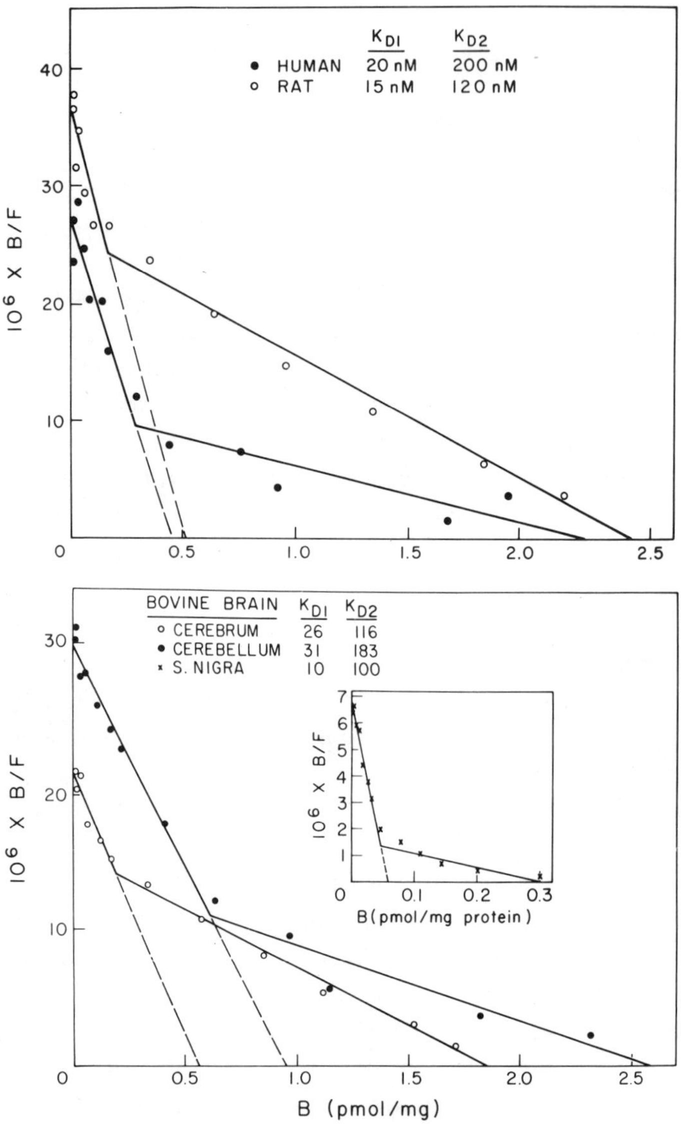

conditions, GABA binding curves for crude mitochondrial plus microsomal fractions from various species of mammalian brain suggest two classes of sites differing in affinity. The computer-drawn linear regressions of Scatchard plots (Fig. 1) suggest apparent K_D values of 20 ± 10 nM and 150 ± 50 nM (average of six). The same plot was obtained whether or not the membranes were pretreated with Triton X–100 (Greenlee *et al.* 1978a).

The Scatchard plots, best fit by two slopes, were very similar for GABA binding to rat brain, human brain (Fig. 1a) or bovine brain (Fig. 1b). Although the quantity of sites (B_{max} values) varied with brain region, the K_D values were remarkably similar in the three species and in the three regions of bovine brain shown. Furthermore there was no significant difference in the ratio of low affinity to high affinity sites in these different tissues; this ratio was always about 3:1. It should also be pointed out that more than two classes of binding sites may be present but not obvious in the graphs.

At this time the function of the two GABA binding sites is unknown. They may represent two types of receptor found on the same or different cells; they may represent interconvertible states of a single class of receptor, which might have interesting regulatory significance. This heterogeneity raises a problem in determining drug interactions with GABA receptors. Both (or all) of these sodium-independent GABA binding sites meet various criteria expected of receptors, and are inhibited by appropriate GABA structural analogues and drugs (Olsen *et al.* 1978a,b, Greenlee *et al.* 1978b, Enna *et al.* 1977, Krogsgaard-Larsen & Johnston 1978, Lester & Peck 1978).

Thus muscimol and related structures were found to inhibit these GABA

Fig. 1. Scatchard plots of sodium-independent GABA receptor binding to mammalian brain. Crude mitochondrial plus microsomal fratctions were osmotically disrupted, repeatedly frozen and thawed, and washed with 50 mM Tris buffered to pH 7.0 with citric acid at 0°. Binding was assayed in this buffer by centrigugation, specific binding being taken as pelleted radioactivity which could be displaced by 0.1 mM nonradioactive GABA. The concentration of [^{3}H]GABA (54 Ci/mmol, Amersham) was varied for the four lowest concentration points and the concentration of nonradioactive GABA was varied, with constant [^{3}H] GABA=4 nM, for the eight higher concentration points. Each point is the mean of triplicates; variation from the mean was $<5\%$. Each plot is typical of four or more experiments. Solid lines represent linear regressions of the data points without correction for additive functions. Protein concentrations in all assays were 1.3 ± 0.3 mg/ml. B refers to moles of GABA specifically bound per mg protein; F refers to the concentration of free GABA in the assay.

A. Total rat brain and human cerebellar cortex (post-mortem).

B. Bovine cerebral cortex, cerebellar cortex, and substantia nigra.

Table I.
Inhibitors of gamma-aminobutyric acid receptor binding sites in rat brain

Compound	IC_{50} (μM)
1. Muscimol	0.03±0.02
2. Homotaurine	0.07±0.02
3. Isoguvacine	0.16±0.07
4. GABA	0.20±0.10
5. *trans*-Aminocyclopentane-3-carboxylic acid	0.27±0.03
6. *trans*-Amino-4-crotonic acid	0.43±0.20
7. THIP	0.45±0.2
8. Homohypotaurine	0.6±0.1
9. β-Hydroxy GABA	0.7±0.3
10. Imidazole acetic acid	0.9±0.1
11. β-Guanidino-propionic acid	1.8±1.2
12. 3-Hydroxy-5-aminoethyl isoxazole	3±1
13. N-Lauroyl GABA	3±2
14. (+) Bicuculline	4±2
15. 4-Aminovaleric acid	5±1
16. *cis* 1-Aminocyclopentane 3-carboxylic acid	5.2±0.8
17. β-Alanine	42±14
18. Taurine	44±8
19. Homomuscimol	50±10
20. Benzyl pencillin	50±30
21. d-Tubocurarine	85±25
22. (+)β-p-(chlorophenyl) GABA (Lioresal)	100±50
23. (−) Lioresal	100±50
24. L-Glutamic acid	150±50
25. 3-Hydroxy,4-methyl,5-aminomethylisoxazole	>100
26. Azamuscimol	
27. 5-Aminolevulinic acid	
28. L-2,4-Diaminobutyric acid (DABA)	
29. (−) Nipecotic acid	
30. 2-Aminoethyl dithiocarbamic acid	
31. 1-Piperidine propane sulfonic acid	
32. 6-aminopenicillanic acid	
33. Chlorpromazine	
34. Diazepam	
35. Pentobarbital	
36. Diphenylhydantoin	
37. Pentylenetetrazole	
38. Picrotoxinin	
39. Caprolactam	
40. t-butyl Bicyclophosphate	
41. Isopropyl Bicyclophosphate	

binding sites with a potency correlating well with biological activity as GABA agonists on mammalian central neurons (Greenlee *et al.* 1978b, Olsen *et al.* 1978b, Krogsgaard-Larsen & Johnston 1978). Muscimol is an agonist more potent than GABA on all systems tested, and competitively (Greenlee *et al.* 1978b) inhibits sodium-independent GABA binding in the nanomolar concentration range (Olsen *et al.* 1978a,b, Enna *et al.* 1977, Krogsgaard-Larsen & Johnston, 1978). By contrast, muscimol inhibits GABA transport or enzymes only in the millimolar concentration range (Olsen *et al.* 1978a, Krogsgaard-Larsen & Johnston, 1978), thus providing the potent and *specific* drug needed to distinguish receptor binding from extraneous binding. Pharmacological effects of muscimol *in vivo* thus seem related to GABA synapses.

Inhibition studies of over 50 drugs revealed no exceptions to the conclusion that drugs highly active *in vivo* as GABA agonists or antagonists were the best inhibitors of sodium-independent GABA binding; compounds inactive on GABA synapses were poor inhibitors (Olsen *et al.* 1978a,b, Greenlee *et al.* 1978b). Analogues specific for GABA transport, such as nipecotic acid or L-2,4,diaminobutyrate (Krogsgaard-Larsen & Johnston 1978) did not inhibit sodium-independent GABA binding up to 100 μM (see Table I).

In contrast to the specific interaction of muscimol with GABA receptors, lioresal (baclofen, β-chlorophenyl GABA) did not potently or stereospecifically inhibit these presumed GABA receptor binding sites ($IC_{50}=100$ μM) (Olsen *et al.* 1978a), suggesting pharmacological effects of this drug involve primarily other sites of action.

The GABA binding sites were not inhibited by the synaptic antagonist picrotoxinin (50 μM), which we believe acts at another site in the GABA receptor-ionophore system (see below). Bicuculline, however, inhibited GABA binding in the micromolar concentration range (Olsen *et al.* 1978a b, Lester & Peck 1978) in a stereospecific manner (Enna *et al.* 1977). Nonlinear inhibition plots for bicuculline (Greenlee *et al.* 1978b) may be explained by heterogeneity of the GABA (and bicuculline) binding sites (Greenlee *et al.* 1978a), or by potentially interesting allosteric effects of bicuculline on the GABA receptor

← The following substances had no effect up to 200 μM; Tetramethylenedisulfotetramine, Haloperidol, Imipramine, 3-Hydroxy-5-(1-aminopropyl) isoxazole, 3-Hydroxy-4-(2-aminoethyl)5-methyl isoxazole, D-Glutamic acid, Glycine, *p*-Chlorophenyl silatrane, t-Butyl-bicyclo-orthocarboxylate, Barbital, Phenobarbital, Dimethyl butyl barbiturate, Cambendazole. GABA binding was determined in sodium-free buffer using frozen and thawed, thoroughly washed membranes as described in Fig. 1.

sites. Supporting this theory that the GABA and bicuculline binding sites may be distinct are observations of differential effects of chaotropic salts and mild detergents on the binding of GABA and bicuculline (Enna & Snyder 1977, Möhler & Okada 1978). This would not be the case if both drugs bound competitively to the same class of sites.

Which of the GABA receptor binding sites, if any, is affected by a given drug

Table II
Inhibitors of picrotoxinin binding in rat brain

Compound	IC50 (μM)
I. Picrotoxin analogues	
Picrotoxinin	0.4±0.2
Tutin	0.4±0.2
α-Dihydropicrotoxinin	1.1±0.2
Picrotin	70±15
Picrotoxinin acetate	>200
Alkali-hydrolyzed picrotoxinin	>200
II. Barbiturates	
(±) DMBB	0.05±0.02
CHEB	0.7±0.04
(±) MPPB	1.0±0.1
(±) Mephobarbital	5±2
(±) Metharbital	10±3 .
(±) Pentobarbital	50±12
Barbital	50±12
Primidone	170±30
Phenobarbital	400±80
III. Bicyclophosphates [R-C-($CH_2O)_3$-P=0]: R Substituent	
t-Butyl-	2±1
iso-Propyl-	8±3
n-Propyl-	8±4
Ethyl-	5±3
Methyl-	150±50
IV. *t*-Butyl Bicyclocarboxylates [*t*-Butyl-C-($CH_2O)_3$-C-R']: R' Substituent	
H-	1±1
Methyl-	1.5±1
Ethyl-	20+8
iso-Propyl-	20±6
n-Propyl-	10±4
n-Butyl-	25±10
Phenyl-	40±15

Table II

Compound		IC50 (μM)
V. Miscellaneous		
	TETS	4±2
	P-Chlorophenyl-silatrane	9±3
	Diphenylhydantoin	140±15
	Benzyl penicillin	150±20
	Bicuculline	100±35
	Strychnine	100±50
	Diazepam	>10
	Pentylenetetrazole	>10
	GABA	>1000

Fresh rat brain membranes (crude mitochondrial plus microsomal fraction) were incubated for 15 min at 0° with 63 nM [^{3}H]DHP (12Ci/mmol, Amersham), and centrifuged for 10 min at 50,000 x g. The assay buffer was 0.2 M NaCl, 5mM sodium phosphate buffer, pH 7.0. Specific binding was determined as pelleted radioactivity which could be displaced by 0.1 mM nonradioactive DHP. Quadruplicate samples included varying concentrations of displacing agent. DMBB=dimethyl-butyl barbiturate; CHEB=cyclohexylidene-ethyl barbiturate; MPPB=N-methyl, phenyl, propyl barbiturate; TETS=tetramethylene disulfotetramine. See Fig. 4 for the chemical structures of caged convulsant compounds.

in *vivo* will require determination of how many receptor binding proteins for GABA exist in the CNS, the effect of the drug on each of these individually, an identification of regional and cellular location of each receptor class, and comparison to neurophysiological-pharmacological observations made on those regions and cells. Only then will the effects of interesting drugs such as muscimol and benzodiazepines be really understood. Biochemical isolation of the GABA receptors should be useful in achieving these objectives.

In addition, there is at least one example involving GABA binding which shows drug interactions with fresh brain membranes which are less pronounced with frozen and washed membranes. Guidotti *et al.* (1978) observed an apparent allosteric activation of GABA rceptor binding in fresh brain membranes by diazepam. We found no significant effect of this drug up to 10 μM on GABA binding to frozen and thawed, thoroughly washed brain membranes (Olsen *et al.* 1978a,b). Thus even the simple preparation of very crude homogenates may have resulted in the loss of interesting regulatory or "native" properties, subject to drug interactions. For example, drugs could interact with the endogenous inhibitors of GABA binding (Guidotti *et al.*, this volume). Nevertheless, we use frozen-thawed and washed membranes because reproducible and quantitative

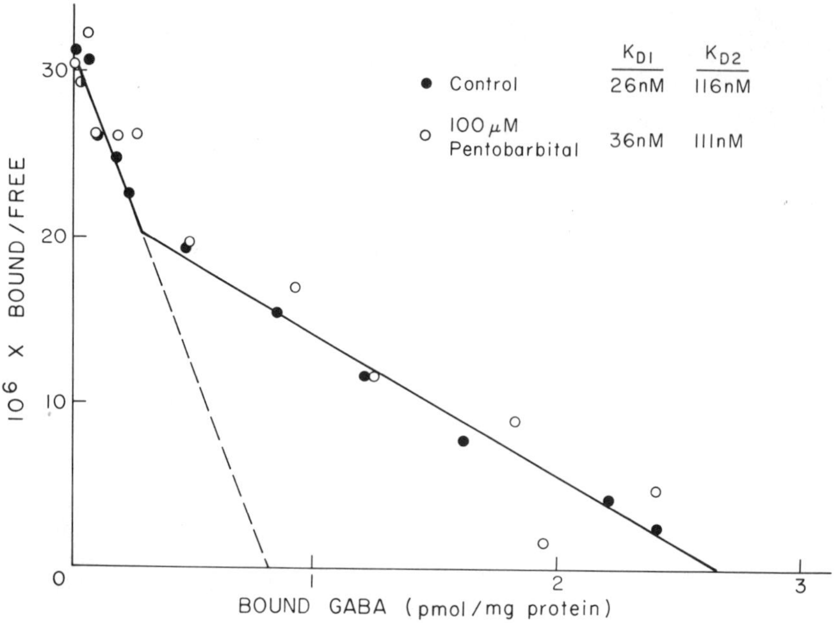

Fig. 2. Lack of effect of pentobarbital on GABA binding curve. Scatchard plot of GABA binding to bovine cerebral cortex as a function of [GABA], in the absence or presence (during assays and preincubation for 30 min at 0°) of 100 μM pentobarbital. Tissue preparation and assay as described in Fig. 1, with varying [^{3}H]GABA, 54 Ci/mmol, and protein=1.5 mg/ml.

binding data are difficult or impossible to obtain with fresh tissue (Greenlee *et al.* 1978a).

PICROTOXININ BINDING SITES IN MAMMALIAN BRAIN

Radioactive α-dihydropicrotoxinin (DHP) binds specifically to saturable sites (apparent K_D 1 μM) in crayfish muscle (Olsen *et al.* 1978c) and mammalian brain homogenates (Ticku *et al.* 1978a). DHP binding sites show a quantity, a regional and subcellular distribution, and an ontogenetic development similar to, but not identical to, sodium-independent GABA (receptor) binding sites (Ticku *et al.* 1978a,b,). DHP binding is inhibited by picrotoxin structural analogues (Table II) in a rank order and at drug concentrations which correlate with biological activity (Ticku *et al.* 1978a). GABA, however, does not affect DHP binding, and differential sensitivity to chemical treatments suggest that the DHP and GABA binding sites are distinct (Olsen *et al.* 1978b, Ticku *et al.* 1978b). DHP thus appears to label some postsynaptic macromolecule related to GABA ionophore function but not the GABA receptor.

The conclusion that DHP sites are related to the pharmacological action of the drug in blocking GABA ionophore activation is strengthened by studies demonstrating that DHP binding is also inhibited by a variety of other convulsant and depressant drugs which may act at the level of GABA-mediated inhibitory synaptic transmission, namely, the barbiturates and the so-called 'cage' convulsant compounds. We have found that barbiturates up to 0.1mM have no effect on GABA uptake or release from nerve endings (Olsen *et al.* 1978a) nor on GABA rceptor binding (Fig. 2). Table II lists the IC_{50} values for inhibition of DHP binding by numerous examples of these drugs.

Barbiturates, both depressant and excitant, inhibited DHP binding (Fig. 3), with depressants such as pentobarbital (IC_{50}=50 μM) and metharbital (IC_{50}= 10 μM) being more potent than the anticonvulsant phenobarbital (IC_{50}=400 μM). The inhibition by pentobarbital appeared competitive with DHP by double reciprocal plot (Ticku & Olsen 1978). ^{1}N-methylation appears to increase the potency of inhibition of DHP binding (compare metharbital to barbital and mephobarbital to phenobarbital). Convulsant barbiturates, such as 5-dimethylbutyl-5-ethyl barbiturate (DMBB, IC_{50}=50 nM), 5-cyclohexylidene-ethyl-5-ethyl-barbiturate (CHEB, IC_{50}=0.7 μM) or N-methyl-5-phenyl-5-pro-

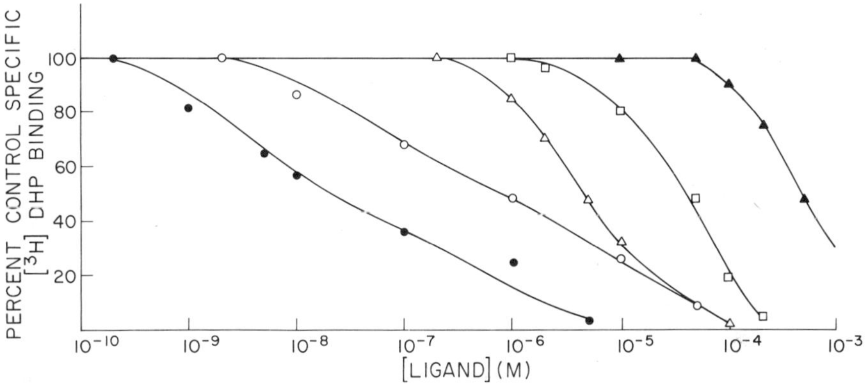

Fig. 3. Displacement of specific [^{3}H] DHP binding to rat brain membranes by barbiturates. Tissue preparation and assay are described in the Legend to Table I. Each point is the mean of quadruplicate samples and two or more experiments; variation from the mean was less than 20%. [Ligand] refers to varying concentrations of (●)DMBB; (○) CHEB: (△) mephobarbital: (□) pentobarbital; (▲) phenobarbital. (Taken from Ticku & Olsen 1978.)

pyl barbiturate (MPPB, $IC_{50}=1$ μM) were more potent inhibitors of DHP binding than were depressants.

The *in vivo* activity of hypnotic or anticonvulsant barbiturates is difficult to quantitate due to complex pharmacokinetic variables. Nevertheless, the effects of barbiturates on DHP binding indicate a relationship between barbiturate action and GABA synapses. For example, the concentrations of barbiturates which inhibit DHP binding (e.g. 50 μM for pentobarbital) are equivalent to or less than the concentrations required in the nervous system for anesthesia (e.g. Richards 1972). Furthermore, pentobarbital at similar concentrations has been found to mimic or potentiate GABA-mediated inhibitory synaptic transmission (Nicoll 1975, Nicoll *et al.* 1975, Ransom & Barker 1976), apparently at the postsynaptic level (Nicoll 1975, Ransom & Barker 1976); pentobarbital also reverses the convulsant and GABA antagonist activity (Bowery & Dray 1976, Casida *et al.* 1976, MacDonald & Barker 1978) of picrotoxin and related compounds. Pentobarbital was ten times more active than phenobarbital in these neurophysiological studies on GABA synapses (MacDonald & Barker 1978), as it is also in inhibiting DHP binding. More *in vitro* studies of this type would be useful in comparing structure-activity relationships for barbiturate effects at potentiating GABA action and in inhibition of DHP binding.

Diphenylhydantoin, at high but therapeutic concentrations ($IC_{50}=140$ μM), inhibited DHP binding. Diazepam (10 μM) had no effect on DHP binding (nor on GABA receptor binding) under our condition.

Numerous compounds with a caged structure (Fig. 4) such as tetramethylene disulfotetramine (TETS), silatranes, bicyclophosphate esters [R-$(CH_2O)_3P{=}0$], P=0], and bicyclocarboxylate ortho esters [R-$(CH_2O)_3$-C-R'], cause tonic-clonic convulsions and death in higher animals in a manner similar to picrotoxin (Casida *et al.* 1976). These substances have been shown to inhibit GABA postsynaptic responses (Bowery *et al.* 1977) and to have other actions resembling GABA antagonists, such as elevation of cerebellar cyclic GMP (Mattson *et al.* 1976). These actions of cage convulsants are reversed by barbiturates (Bowery & Dray 1976, Casida *et al.* 1976).

As shown in Table II, these substances inhibited DHP binding well, with IC_{50} values in the micromolar range. In the series of alkyl substituted bicyclophosphates, there was an excellent correlation between toxicity and inhibition of DHP binding, with t-$C_4H_9 > i$-$C_3H_7 = C_2H_5 \gg CH_3$. The same order of potency was observed for inhibition of GABA depolarization of superior cervical ganglion (Bowery *et al.* 1977). Although some bicyclophosphates of modest biological activity were reported to inhibit GABA receptor binding (Enna *et al.* 1977), in our hands none of these compounds up to 0.1 mM gave any inhibition of GABA binding.

Using the most active R substituent, *t*-butyl, studies on a series of R' substituted bicyclo-carboxylates revealed that the compounds with smaller substituents (such as -H,-CH_3) on the orthocarboxylate carbon were the best inhibitors of DHP binding. These derivatives are also highly toxic; however, whereas inhibition of DHP binding fell off gradually with larger substituents at that position, toxicity fell off dramatically with branched side chain groups, but returned with large alkyl or aromatic substituents (Milbrath *et al.* 1978). This lack of correlation between DHP binding inhibition and toxicity for the bicyclocarboxylates with large R' substituents may reflect a second and distinct mechanism of toxicity for these larger substances, which have not yet been tested on GABA synaptic preparations.

In light of these interactions of cage convulsant drugs with DHP binding, we propose that their convulsant properties, as well as those of the excitatory barbiturates, are likely to involve effects on the GABA receptor-ionophore system at the picrotoxinin site. Fig. 5 is a schematic model of the GABA postsynaptic system consisting of two functional parts, the GABA recognition

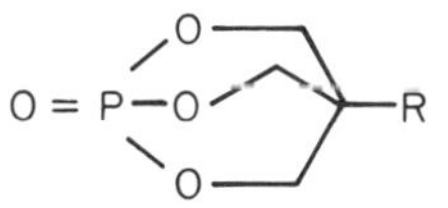

BICYCLOPHOSPHATES
(4-SUBSTITUTED-1-PHOSPHA-2,6,7-TRIOXABICYCLO [2.2.2] OCTANE-1-OXIDES)

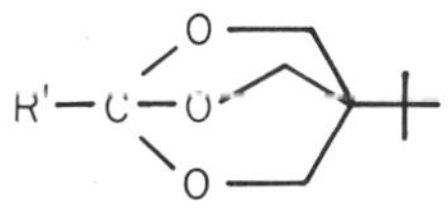

t-BUTYL BICYCLOCARBOXYLATES
(1-SUBSTITUTED-4-*t*-BUTYL-2,6,7-TRIOXABICYCLO [2.2.2] OCTANES)

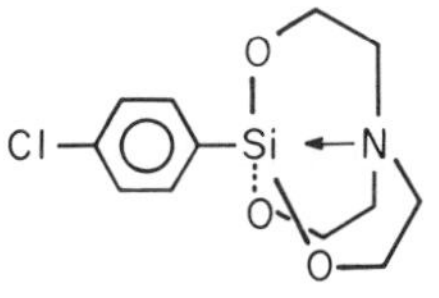

p-CHLOROPHENYL SILATRANE
(1-[*p*-CHLOROPHENYL]-2,8,9,-TRIOXA-5-AZA-1-SILABICYCLO [3.3.3] UNDECANE)

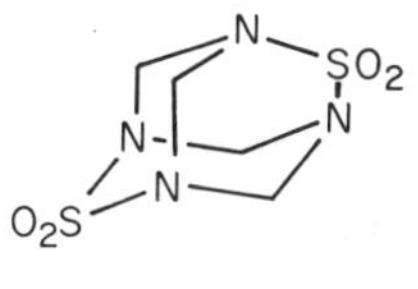

TETRAMETHYLENEDISULFOTETRAMINE
(2,6-DITHIA-1,3,5,7-TETRAZA-TRICYCLO [3.3.1.1^{3,7}] DECANE-2,2,6,6-TETRAOXIDE)

Fig. 4. Chemical structures and names of convulsant 'cage' compounds.

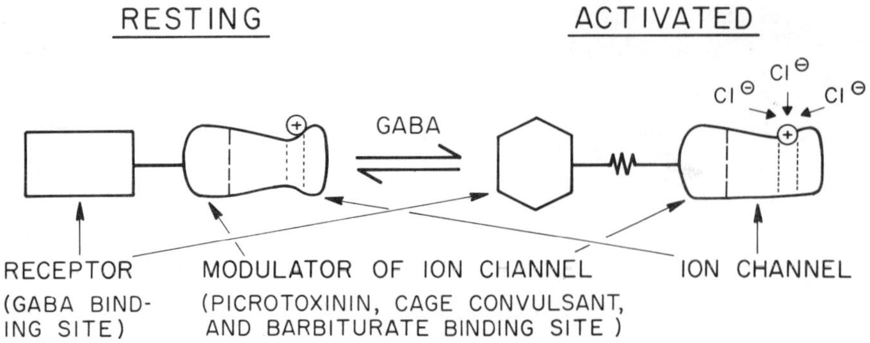

Fig. 5. Model of GABA receptor-ionophore indicating interaction of GABA, picrotoxinin, related cage convulsants, and barbiturates. The receptor (GABA binding site) and chloride ion channel (containing a 'modulator' section with the picrotoxinin, cage convusant, and barbiturate binding site) exist in two states: resting and activated. Binding of GABA or depressant barbiturates favors the activated state, whereas binding of picrotoxinin, convulsant barbiturates, and 'cage' compounds favors the inactive state.

or regulatory component (receptor) and the catalytic or functional component (ionophore). GABA binding to the receptor favors the activated state, and picrotoxin and convulsant binding to the ionophore favors the inactive state. We can further speculate that depressant barbiturates may potentiate and prolong GABA responses by binding to the ionophore and favoring the activated state. In this model, barbiturate action could cause positive or negative modulation of the GABA ionophore.

It should be stressed that the experimental testing of this model is by no means complete or simple to achieve. Ideally, comparisons should be made between neuro-chemical and -pharmacological-physiological studies of GABA, picrotoxinin, barbiturates, and cage convulsants, using tissue containing a homogeneous cell population and a single type of GABA synapse. Within the mammalian brain, it has not yet been conclusively demonstrated which binding proteins for GABA and DHP are associated with which physiological functions and therefore with which drug actions. It is possible that more than one class of pharmacological GABA receptors exists, and/or that all GABA receptors are not coupled to the same ionophores. This is supported by our observation of two affinities for GABA binding and by the lack of a strict 1:1 correspondence or coupling between GABA receptor binding sites and DHP binding sites. Furthermore, the displacement of DHP binding by convulsant barbiturates follows a different concentration dependence curve from that of depressants or

DHP itself (Fig. 3), and suggests either negative cooperativity or heterogeneity in DHP binding sites, with the latter possibility being more likely. Thus there may be more than one class of DHP binding site as well as more than one class of GABA receptor binding site. While current evidence supports the notion that these binding sites are involved in GABA receptor-ionophore function, and that drug interaction with the binding sites suggests a mechanism of action for at least some of the effects of the drugs discussed, the actual relationships between these drugs and GABA synapses *in vivo* will be shown only by further investigation.

ACKNOWLEDGMENTS

We thank Matt Ban for technical assistance, and Brad Meiners for helpful discussions. We thank Dr. James Collins for drawing our attention to the caged compounds, and Dr. John Casida for the kind gift of numerous caged compounds and for providing experimental results on the biological activity of these substances prior to publication. We thank H. Downes and Eli Lilly Corporation for providing barbiturates. We thank P. Krogsgaard-Larsen and G. A. R. Johnston for providing GABA analogues. Supported by NSF Grant BNS 77-24414, NIH Grants NS 12422 and RCDA NS 00224, and the Alfred P. Sloan Foundation.

REFERENCES

Beaumont, K., Chilton, W., Yamamura, H. I., & Enna, S. J. (1978) Muscimol binding in rat brain: association with synaptic GABA receptors. *Brain Res.* 148, 153–162.

Bowery, N. G. & Dray, A. (1976) Barbiturate reversal of amino acid antagonism produced by convulsant agents. *Nature* 264, 276–278.

Bowery, N. G., Collins, J. F. & Hill, R. G. (1976) Bicyclic phosphorus esters that are potent convulsants and GABA antagonists. *Nature* 261, 601–603.

Bowery, N. G, Collins, J. F., Hill, R. G., & Pearson, S. (1977) t-Butyl bicyclo phosphate: a convulsant and GABA antagonist more potent than bicuculline. *Br. J. Pharmac.* 60, 275P–276P.

Casida, J. E., Eto, M., Moscioni, A. D., Engel, J. L., Milbrath, D. S. & Verkade, J. G. (1976) Structure-toxicity relationships of 2,6,7-trioxabicyclo [2.2.2]-octanes and related compounds. *Tox. App. Pharmacol.* 36, 261–279.

Enna, S. J. & Snyder, S. H. (1975) Properties of gamma-aminobutyric acid binding to receptor sites in rat central nervous system. *Brain Res.* 100, 81–97.

Enna, S. J. & Snyder, S. H. (1977) Influences of ions, enzymes and detergents on GABA receptor binding in synaptic membranes of rat brain. *Mol. Pharmacol.* 13, 442–453.

Enna, S. J., Collins, J. F. & Snyder, S. H. (1977) Stereospecificity and structure-activity required of GABA receptor binding in rat brain. *Brain Res.* 124, 185–190.

Greenlee, D. V., Van Ness, P. C. & Olsen, R. W. (1978a) Endogenous inhibitor of GABA binding in mammalian brain. *Life Sciences.* 22, 1653–1662.

Greenlee, D. V., Van Ness, P. C. & Olsen, R. W. (1978b) Gamma-aminobutyric acid binding in mammalian brain: receptor-like specificity of sodium independent sites. *J. Neurochem.* In press.

Guidotti, A., Toffano, G., Grandison, L., & Costa, E. (1978) Second messenger responses and regulation of high affinity receptor binding to study pharmacological modifications of GABA-ergic transmission. In: *Amino Acids as Chemical Transmitters,* ed. Fonnum, F., Plenum Press, New York. In press.

Johnston, G. A. R. & Kennedy, S. M. E. (1978) GABA receptors and phospholipids. In: *Amino Acids as Chemical transmitters,* ed. Fonnum, F.,pp. 507–516. Plenum Press, New York.

Krogsgaard-Larsen, P. & Johnston, G. A. R. (1978) Structure-activity studies on the inhibition of GABA binding to rat brain membranes by muscimol and related compounds. *J. Neurochem.* 30, 1377–1382.

Lester, B. R. & Peck, E. J. (1978) Kinetic and pharmacological characterization of gamma-aminobutyric acid receptive sites from mammalian brain. *Brain Res.* In press.

MacDonald, R. L. & Barker, J. L. (1978) Different actions of anticonvulsant and anesthetic barbiturates revealed using cultured mammaliam neurons. *Science.* In press.

Mattson, H., Brandt, K. & Heilbronn, E. (1977) Bicyclic phosphorus esters increase the cyclic GMP level in rat cerebellum. *Nature* 268, 52–53.

Milbrath, D. S., Engel, J. L., Verkade, J. G. & Casida, J. E. (1978) Structure-toxicity relationships of 1-substituted-4-alkyl-2,6,7-trioxabicyclo [2.2.2.] octanes. *Tox. App. Pharmacol.* In press.

Möhler, H. & Okada, T. (1978) Properties of GABA receptor binding with $^{3}H(+)$ becuculline methiodide in rat cerebellum. *Mol. Pharmacol.* 14, 256–265.

Nicoll, R. A. (1975) Pentobarbital: action on frog motoneurons. *Brain Res.* 96, 119–123.

Nicoll, R. A., Eccles, J. C., Oshima, T. C. & Rubia, F. (1975) Prolongation of hippocampal inhibitory post-synaptic potentials by barbiturates. *Nature* 258, 625–627.

Olsen, R. W., Ticku, M. K., Van Ness, P. C. & Greenlee, D. (1978a) Effects of drugs on gamma-aminobutyric acid receptors, uptake, release and synthesis *in vitro. Brain Res.* 139, 277–294.

Olsen, R. W., Greenlee, D. Van Ness, P. & Ticku, M. K. (1978b) Studies on the gamma-aminobutyric acid receptor/ionophore proteins in mammalian brain. In: *Amino Acids as Chemical Transmitters,* ed. Fonnum, F., pp. 467–486. Plenum Press, New York.

Olsen, R. W., Ticku, M. K., & Miller, T. (1978c) Dihydropicrotoxinin binding to crayfish muscle sites possibly related to gamma-aminobutyric acid receptor/ ionophores. *Mol. Pharmacol.* 14, 381–390.

Ransom, B. R. & Barker, J. L. (1976) Pentobarbital selectively enhances GABA-mediated post-synaptic inhibition in tissue cultured mouse spinal neurons. *Brain Res.* 114, 530–535.

Richards, C. D. (1972) On the mechanism of barbiturate anesthesia. *J. Physiol.* 227, 749–767.

Ticku, M. K. & Olsen, R. W. (1977) Gamma-aminobutyric acid-stimulated chloride permeability in crayfish muscle. *Biochim. Biophys. Acta* 464, 519–529.

Ticku, M. K. Ban, M. & Olsen, R. W. (1978a) Binding of [^{3}H]α-dihydropicrotoxinin, a γ-aminobutyric acid synaptic antagonist, to rat brain membranes. *Mol. Pharmacol.* 14, 391–402.

Ticku, M. K., Van Ness, P. C., Haycock, J. W., Levy, W. B. & Olsen, R. W. (1978b) Dihydropicrotoxinin binding sites in rat brain: comparison to GABA receptors. *Brain Res.* 150, 642–647.

Ticku, M. K. & Olsen, R. W. (1978) Interaction of barbiturates with dihydropicrotoxinin binding sites related to the GABA receptor-ionophore system. *Life Sciences.* 22, 1643–1652.

Zukin, S. R., Young, A. B., & Snyder, S. H. (1974) Gamma-aminobutyric acid binding to receptor sites in rat central nervous system. *Proc. Natl. Acad. Sci.* (Wash.) 71, 4802–4807.

Agonist Specificity of GABA Binding Sites in Human Brain and GABA in Huntington's Disease and Schizophrenia

L. L. Iversen, E. Bird, E. Spokes, S. H. Nicholson & C. J. Suckling**

The finding that the degenerative changes which occur in human brain in Huntington's disease are accompanied by a selective loss of GABA and its biosynthetic enzyme (Bird & Iversen 1974, 1977) has encouraged further biochemical studies of the GABA system in human brain. In addition to measurements of GABA and related enzymes, Enna *et al.* (1976a,b, 1977a) and Lloyd *et al.* (1977a) found that high affinity sodium-independent binding of ^{3}H-GABA to receptor sites could also be measured in human postmortem tissue. The present paper will describe studies of the agonist specificity of such binding sites and their presence in normal and pathological material. In addition recent postmortem findings on the marker enzyme GAD in Huntington's disease and in schizophrenia will be discussed, emphasizing some of the pitfalls that may be encountered in interpreting such data.

AGONIST SPECIFICITY OF GABA BINDING IN HUMAN CEREBELLUM

We have used the method of Enna & Snyder (1975, 1977) to study the binding of ^{3}H-GABA to synaptic membranes prepared from human cerebellum. A crude synaptic membrane preparation is obtained by the method of Enna & Snyder (1975) from whole cerebellum, obtained at autopsy and not stored frozen. The membrane preparation is stable for several months when stored at −20 °C, and is used at a dilution of approximately 0.5 mg protein/ml after resuspension and

MRC Neurochemical Pharmacology Unit, University of Cambridge, England.
* Department of Pure & Applied Chemistry, University of Strathclyde, Scotland.

Table I

Inhibition of ^{3}H-GABA binding in human cerebellar membranes by GABA analogues

Compound	IC 50 – μM
GABA	0.07
Muscimol	0.02
β-HydroxyGABA	0.10
Imidazoleacetic acid	0.50
Guanidinoacetic acid	2.10
γ-MethylGABA	3.50
5-Aminopentanoic acid	4.10
N-amino-piperidine-3-sulphonic acid	13.50
β-MethylGABA	14.50
α-MethylGABA	22.00
β-Guanidinopropionic acid	26.00
Piperidine-3-sulphonic acid	30.00
β-ParachlorophenylGABA (Baclofen)	80.00
γ-DimethylGABA	100.00
β-PhenylGABA	360.00
α-γ-DimethylGABA	740.00
2-Aminomethylbenzoic acid	>1000.00
3-Aminomethylbenzoic acid	>1000.00
Pyridine-3-sulphonic acid	>1000.00
3-Aminobenzoic acid	inactive at 1mM
2-Aminophenylacetic acid	inactive at 1mM

Compounds were tested in triplicate at three to six concentrations for their ability to inhibit specific binding of ^{3}H-GABA; IC50=concentration required for 50% inhibition, determined by log/probit analysis. ^{3}H-GABA concentration=15 nM.

washing with incubation buffer prior to use. Since human cerebellum, as in the rat, contains a relatively high density of GABA binding sites, very favorable ratios of "specific" to "non-specific" binding (defined with 1mM nonradioactive GABA) are obtained. When incubations were performed with 15 nM ^{3}H-GABA for 10 min at 0°C, specific binding represented 70–80% of total binding. Various structural analogues of GABA have been tested in this assay in the hope that such results might provide information on the structure-activity requirements for agonist binding at human brain GABA receptors. The results (Table I) show that the structural specificity of the GABA binding sites in human brain is remarkably similar to that described in previous studies in animals. The potent GABA agonists, muscimol, imidazoleacetic acid and β-hydroxy GABA are effective inhibitors of GABA binding at submicromolar concentrations.

The results with a series of newly synthesized substituted 4-aminobutanoic acids, and with other possible GABA-mimetic substances, provide useful information on the probable conformation in which GABA binds to its postsynaptic receptors (Nicholson *et al.* 1978). The observation that muscimol and β-hydroxy GABA bind strongly to the receptor suggests that there is a preference for a polar substituent at the β-position, and that hydrogen bonding may take place between this group and the receptor. Methyl groups α- to the negatively charged end of GABA cause the greatest decrease in affinity, and methyl groups α- to the amino group the least decrease in affinity. Similar observations have been made in a series of isoxazoles by Krogsgaard-Larsen & Johnston (1978). Our results support the conclusion that GABA binds to its receptor in a conformation that is close to planar, eclipsed and partially folded.

GABA RECEPTOR BINDING IN HUNTINGTON'S DISEASE

The finding that ^{3}H-GABA binding sites are detectable in postmortem brain, and are stable under postmortem conditions (Enna *et al.* 1976a, b, 1977a) implies that it is possible from such measurements to determine whether the densities of GABA receptors are normal in pathological states. The first studies of this type, by Enna *et al.* (1976a, b), suggested that GABA binding sites were present in normal densities in basal ganglia tissue from patients dying with Huntington's disease. There was a significant increase in the number of GABA sites in substantia nigra, presumably reflecting their location on the dopaminergic neurons in this area which survive in Huntington's disease (Enna *et al.* 1976b). Lloyd *et al.* (1977a) also reported normal amounts of GABA binding in basal ganglia tissue from patients dying with Parkinson's disease, but in this case there was a significant loss of these sites from substantia nigra, paralleling the degeneration of the dopaminergic elements. The evidence presented by Enna *et al.* (1976a, b) for persistence of GABA receptors in Huntington's disease has important implications for the possible therapeutic benefits that might be obtained by treating such patients with GABA-mimetic drugs. However, a subsequent study by Lloyd *et al.* (1977b) reported quite different findings. They observed a large (75–80%) and highly significant decrease in the densities of GABA binding sites in caudate nucleus and putamen from patients dying with Huntington's disease, and an unexpected twofold increase in the density of GABA sites in cerebellar tissue from such patients. Because of this discrepancy, we have recently carried out measurements of ^{3}H-GABA binding in control and

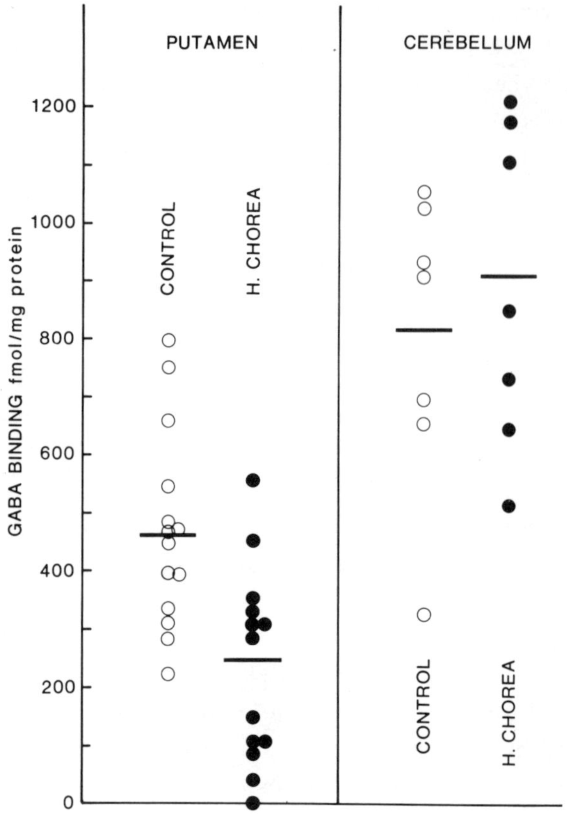

Fig. 1. GABA receptor binding in human postmortem brain. Each value represents the sodium-independent binding of ^{3}H-GABA (displacable by 1 mM non radioactive GABA) measured in an individual control or Huntington's disease brain (mean of triplicate measurements). The results are expressed per mg protein in the detergent-treated membrane preparations used for binding measurements; ^{3}H-GABA concentration = 15 nM. Horizontal bars indicate mean values.

Huntington's disease brains (Fig. 1). Unlike Lloyd *et al.* (1977b) we did not find any difference in the density of GABA binding sites in cerebellar tissue, but we did confirm that there was a substantial decrease in the average density of GABA binding sites in putamen samples from 14 Huntington's disease patients. The results obtained were very variable, with some samples showing essentially normal densities of GABA sites, and others very low values. The variability between patients perhaps explains why no difference in GABA binding was observed in our previous study (Enna *et al.* 1976a, b), and suggests that "GABA therapy" may be applicable only to some Huntington's disease patients.

RADIORECEPTOR ASSAY OF GABA IN HUMAN CSF

Enna *et al.* (1977b) and Wood *et al.* (1978) reported the use of the GABA receptor binding assay as a method to measure the very small amounts of GABA normally present in human cerebrospinal fluid (csf). The radioreceptor assay method involves measurements of the displacement of ^{3}H-GABA binding from brain membranes by nonradioactive GABA present in csf samples. We have confirmed the usefulness of this simple experimental method, using human cerebellar membrane preparations for the ^{3}H-GABA binding measurements. Using the standard 1 ml incubation volume, as little as 2 pmol GABA can be detected in 125 μl samples of csf, and 20 pmol GABA causes a 50% displacement of ^{3}H-GABA binding. Measurements of GABA in a collection of csf samples from 37 patients suffering from various neurological illnesses (other than Huntington's disease) showed a wide range of values ranging from less than 50 pmol GABA/ml csf to more than 1000 pmol/ml. The mean value for these 37 samples was 224 pmol/ml ($\pm$215 s.d.). This approach seems likely to be valuable in the clinical assessment of GABA function in various disease states.

GAD IN HUMAN POSTMORTEM BRAIN IN HUNTINGTON's DISEASE AND SCHIZOPHRENIA

Our initial experience in measurements of glutamate decarboxylase (GAD) activity in human postmortem brain (Bird *et al.* 1973, Bird & Iversen 1974) was encouraging. The enzyme appeared to be relatively stable in postmortem brain tissue, and a severe decrease in GAD activity was detected in basal ganglia tissue from patients dying with Huntington's disease, confirming the existence of a GABA deficit first observed by Perry *et al.* (1973). Although this finding has been confirmed by several other laboratories (McGeer *et al.* 1973, Stahl & Swanson 1974, McGeer & McGeer 1976), the value of postmortem brain measurements of GAD has been questioned because of the finding that GAD activity is lowered in many brain regions in Parkinson's disease (Lloyd *et al.* 1975, McGeer & McGeer 1976), senile dementia (Bowen *et al.* 1974, 1976, Perry *et al.* 1977) and chronic depression (Perry *et al.* 1977, 1978). We also found a highly significant reduction in GAD activity in various brain regions from

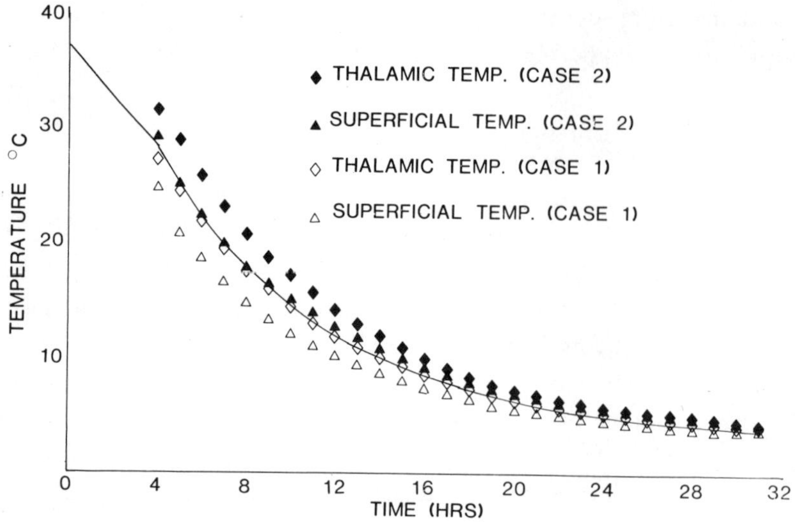

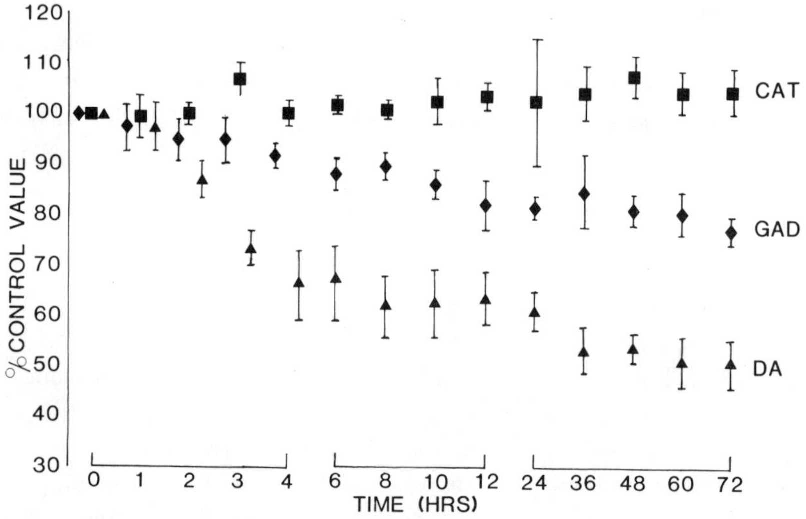

Fig. 2. Calculated mean cooling curve for human brain postmortem (A), measured with thermoprobes inserted in parietal cortex and thalamus in two cadavers. Transfer to mortuary refrigerator at 4°C took place 3–4 h after death.

Biochemical results (B), for choline acetyltransferase (CAT), glutamate decarboxylase (GAD) and dopamine (DA) in mouse brain were obtained from animals in which the brains were subjected to programmed cooling to simulate human postmortem data. Values are means ± S.E.M. for at least four cerebral hemispheres. Control values (time zero) were as follows: – DA = 7.1 ± 0.16 μg/g protein; GAD = 191 ± 5.5 μmol/h/g protein; CAT = 155.8 ± 1.3 μmol/h/g protein.

schizophrenic patients (Bird *et al.* 1977), although others failed to detect any difference in postmortem GAD values in such patients (Perry *et al.* 1978, Crow *et al.* 1978). It appears that some of these findings may be spurious, since postmortem GAD values can be markedly influenced by various factors not related to these illnesses.

POSTMORTEM STABILITY OF GAD

Knowledge of the postmortem stability of GAD is essential for the interpretation of postmortem measurements of enzyme activity, since the interval between death and autopsy is variable and not easily standardized. Previous studies on GAD activity in human and animal brain postmortem suggest, however, that this enzyme is relatively stable after a rapid initial decline (Bird & Iversen 1974, McGeer *et al.* 1973, Perry *et al.* 1977), although Crow *et al.* (1978) reported that GAD activity was significantly lower in brain samples stored for more than 48 h at 4°C than in those stored for shorter periods.

We have re-examined this question in both animal and human brain. An animal model was established by Spokes & Koch (1978) on the basis of direct measurements of the rate of cooling of human postmortem brain by insertion of microprobe thermometers in the brains of two cadavers. Brain tissue cools only slowly towards ambient temperature, and removal of the cadaver to a mortuary refrigerator within 2–4 h after death only slightly accelerates this cooling. During storage at 4°C the brain temperature takes 24 h to cool to this temperature (Fig. 2). Mice were killed and kept in an incubator subject to a programmed cooling to mimic in the mouse brain the normal rate of cooling observed in human material. Under these conditions there was a rapid initial decline in GAD activity within the first few hours to approximately 80% of initial values, and thereafter GAD remained at a stable plateau (Fig. 2). These results thus confirm earlier suggestions that GAD declines rapidly during the initial postmortem period but is then remarkably stable. This conclusion is also strongly supported by comparisons of postmortem GAD values obtained from patients in which the interval between death and autopsy was more than or less than 48 h (Table II). Measurements from a large series of cases show no significant reduction in GAD activity in those cases in which autopsy was delayed. It thus seems unlikely that postmortem delays and storage conditions play an important role in determining differences in GAD activity between groups.

Table II

Influence of the interval between death and necropsy on measured GAD values in control brain

Region	GAD activity – μmol/h/g protein <48 h	>48 h
Caudate	47.9±3.9(31)	45.2± 6.2(14)
Putamen	58.9±5.3(33)	56.9± 7.0(16)
Nucleus Accumbens	82.8±9.1(22)	80.0±11.4(10)

Values are means±S.E.M. for number of brains in brackets.

Table III

Comparison of GAD values in control, choreic and psychotic patients dying suddenly (SD) and from broncho-pneumonia (BP)

Region		GAD activity – μmol/h/g protein Control	Choreic	Psychotic
Caudate	SD	45.4± 3.3(48)	19.1± 3.6(14)	53.5± 8.4(8)
	BP	31.0± 9.0(7)	10.6± 1.6(32)	22.6± 2.9(13)
Putamen	SD	58.0± 4.1(51)	21.5± 4.1(16)	56.6±10.3(7)
	BP	40.4± 8.4(9)	11.6± 2.1(33)	26.3± 4.9(10)
Nucleus	SD	78.5± 6.6(40)	56.6±17.8(10)	70.5± 7.6(12)
Accumbens	BP	52.0±11.9(4)	27.1± 3.6(16)	38.9± 6.0(14)

Values are means±S.E.M. for number of brains in brackets.

EFFECT OF PREMORTEM STATE ON GAD

Although postmortem factors do not present insurmountable problems in the postmortem analysis of GAD, another uncontrollable factor, the immediate postmortem conditions appears to be of crucial importance in determining postmortem GAD activity. Bowen *et al.* (1976) were the first to emphasize that low postmortem GAD values were obtained from patients dying with conditions likely to lead to cerebral hypoxia. Perry *et al.* (1977) also pointed out the influence of premortem status, and found that GAD activity was significantly lower in several brain regions from a group of chronically hospitalized patients than in a group of normal people who had suffered sudden deaths. This suggests that spuriously low GAD activities may easily be recorded in various pathological conditions in which postmortem brain samples are obtained from elderly patients dying after chronic hospitalization, in whom the immediate cause of death is often broncho-pneumonia or a related condition likely to lead to terminal hypoxia. The results obtained in our own laboratory (Table III) strongly support this conclusion, and show that death from broncho-pneumonia in control, Huntington's disease or schizophrenia patients does lead to drastically lower GAD activities in various brain regions. Because of the preponderance of broncho-pneumonia deaths in the Huntington's disease and schizophrenia groups, this means that GAD values may be seriously underestimated in these conditions.

GAD IN HUNTINGTON'S DISEASE

In view of these findings, we have re-examined the postmortem GAD values measured in various regions of brains from Huntington's disease patients who died suddenly, and compared these values with those from a group of controls

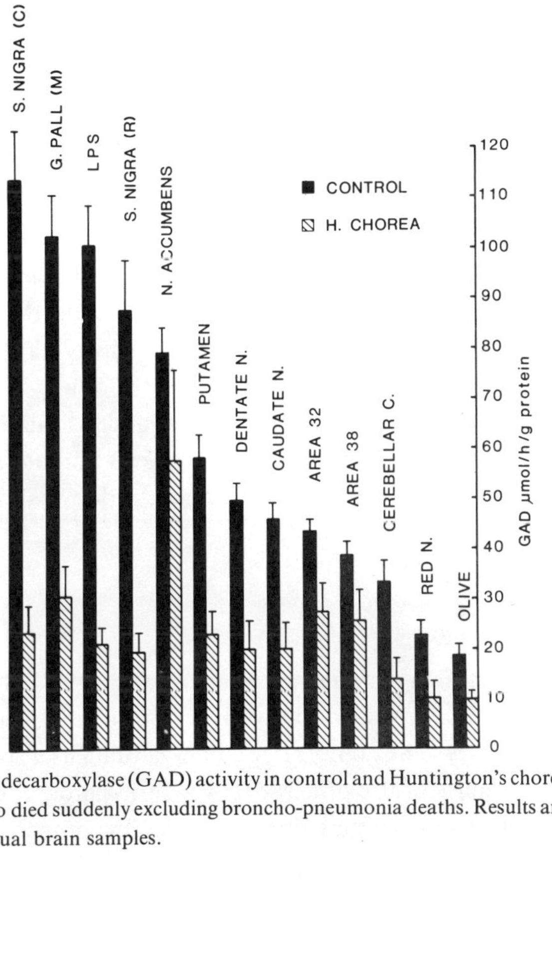

Fig. 3. Glutamate decarboxylase (GAD) activity in control and Huntington's chorea brains obtained from patients who died suddenly excluding broncho-pneumonia deaths. Results are means ± S.E.M. for 10–50 individual brain samples.

Table IV
Influence of mode of death on GAD values in psychotic patients

Region	GAD activity – μmol/h/g protein Sudden death	Broncho-pneumonia	Suicide	Others
Caudate	53.5± 8.4(8)	22.6±2.9(13)	44.3± 9.5(6)	26.6± 1.8(5)
Putamen	56.6±10.3(7)	26.3±4.9(10)	64.5±17.0(6)	41.2±14.9(6)
Nucleus accumbens	70.5± 7.6(12)	38.9±6.0(14)	63.7±16.6(6)	46.4±10.2(10)

Values are means±S.E.M. for number of brains in brackets.

who also died suddenly. The results (Table III and Fig. 3) confirm that there is a marked depletion of GAD, especially from basal ganglia regions in Huntington's disease, while some brain areas (Area 38 of cerebral cortex and nucleus accumbens) do not show any significant loss of GAD. However, the depletion of GAD from basal ganglia areas is not as severe as originally estimated, and certain other regions of brain – notably cerebellum and dentate nucleus – also show significant decreases in GAD activity.

GAD IN SCHIZOPHRENIA

The elimination of GAD values obtained from patients dying with bronchopneumonia and other conditions in which there is a slow death (Table IV) leads us to reinterpret our original finding that GAD activity is markedly reduced in various brain regions in schizophrenia. The absence of any significant differences when GAD values from patients suffering sudden deaths or suicides are compared with control values (Table III, IV) suggests that our earlier findings can be explained in terms of the cause of death, rather than the psychiatric illness.

CONCLUSIONS

The results of biochemical studies on human postmortem brain have to be interpreted with caution because of the many uncontrollable factors which may influence such findings. The ability to use human brain as a source of *in vitro* preparations for studies of drug interactions with receptors for GABA and a variety of other neurotransmitters offers considerable promise as a means of directly comparing the specificity of such receptors in man and experimental animals.

Interpretation of postmortem results on GABA receptor densities and the marker enzyme GAD in Huntington's disease and in schizophrenia is fraught with difficulties because of the marked individual variations in these measurements, and the influence of extraneous factors such as the premortem status. The present results emphasize the importance of the latter factor, and suggest that schizophrenia is not associated with any deficit in cerebral GAD. In Huntington's disease there are marked reductions in GAD in many brain regions, including some outside the basal ganglia. The variable reduction in GABA receptor binding sites in basal ganglia tissue in Huntington's disease suggests that the benefits of therapy with a future generation of GABA-mimetic drugs may be unpredictable.

REFERENCES

Bird, E. D. & Iversen, L. L. (1974) Huntington's chorea: postmortem measurement of glutamic acid decarboxylase, choline acetyltransferase and dopamine in basal ganglia. *Brain* 97, 457–472.

Bird, E. D. & Iversen, L. L. (1977) Neurochemical findings in Huntington's chorea. In: *Essays in Neurochemistry and Neuropharmacology,* vol. 1, eds. Youdim, M. B. H., Lovenberg, W., Sharman, D. F. & Lagnado, J. R., pp. 177–195. John Wiley & Sons, London.

Bird, E. D., Mackay, A. V. P., Rayner, A. N. & Iversen, L. L. (1973) Reduced glutamic acid decarboxylase activity of postmortem brain in Huntington's chorea. *Lancet* i, 1090–1092.

Bird, E. D., Spokes, E. G., Barnes, J., Mackay, A. V. P., Iversen, L. L. & Shepherd, M. (1977) Increased brain dopamine and reduced glutamic acid decarboxylase and choline acetyltransferase activity in schizophrenia and related psychoses. *Lancet* ii, 1157–1159.

Bowen, D. M., White, P., Flack, R. H. A., Smith, C. D. & Davison, A. N. (1974) Brain decarboxylase activities as indices of pathological changes in senile dementia. *Lancet* i, 1247–1249.

Bowen, D. M., Smith, C. B., White, P. & Davison, A. N. (1976) Neurotransmitter-related enzymes and indices of hypoxia in senile dementia and other abiotrophies. *Brain* 99, 459–496.

Crow, T. J., Owen, F., Cross, A. J., Lofthouse, R. & Longden, A. (1978) Brain biochemistry in schizophrenia. *Lancet* i, 36–37.

Enna, S. J. & Snyder, S. H. (1975) properties of gamma-aminobutyric acid (GABA) receptor binding in rat brain synaptic membrane fractions. *Brain Res.* 100, 81–98.

Enna, S. J. & Snyder, S. H. (1977) Influences of ions, enzymes and detergents on γ-aminobutyric acid receptor binding in synaptic membranes of rat brain. *Mol. Pharmacol.* 13, 442–453.

Enna, S. J., Bird, E. D., Bennett, J. P., Bylund, D. B., Yamamura, H. I., Iversen, L. L. & Snyder, S. H. (1976a) Huntington's chorea: changes in neurotransmitter receptors in the brain. *New Engl. J. Med.* 294, 1305–1309.

Enna, S. J., Bennett, J. P., Bylund, D. B., Snyder, S. H., Bird, E. D. & Iversen, L. L. (1976b) Alterations of brain neurotransmitter receptor binding in Huntington's chorea. *Brain Research* 116, 531–537.

Enna, S. J., Bennett, J. P., Bylund, D. B., Creese, I., Burt, D. R., Charness, M. E., Yamamura, H. I., Simantov, R. & Snyder, S. H. (1977a) Neurotransmitter receptor binding: regional distribution in human brain. *J. Neurochem.* 28, 233–236.

Enna, S. J., Wood, J. H. & Snyder, S. H. (1977b) γ-Aminobutyric acid (GABA) in human cerebrospinal fluid: radioreceptor assay. *J. Neurochem.* 28, 1121–1124.

Krogsgaard-Larsen, P. & Johnston, G. A. R. (1978) Structure-activity studies on the inhibition of GABA binding to rat brain membranes by muscimol and related compounds. *J. Neurochem.* 30, 1377–1382.

Lloyd, K. G., Möhler, H., Heitz, P. & Bartholini, G. (1975) Distribution of choline acetyltransferase and glutamate decarboxylase within the substantia nigra and in other brain regions from control and Parkinsonian patients. *J. Neurochem.* 25, 789–795.

Lloyd, K. G., Shemen, L. & Hornykiewicz, O. (1977a) Distribution of high affinity sodium-independent ^{3}H-gamma-aminobutyric acid (^{3}H-GABA) binding in the human brain: alterations in Parkinson's disease. *Brain Res.* 127, 269–278.

Lloyd, K. G., Dreksler, S. & Bird, E. D. (1977b) Alterations in ^{3}H-GABA binding in Huntington's chorea. *Life Sci.* 21, 747–754.

McGeer, P. L., McGeer, E. G. & Fibiger, H. C. (1973) Choline acetylase and glutamic acid decarboxylase in Huntington's chorea. *Neurol.* (Minneap.) 23, 912–917,

McGeer, P. L. & McGeer, E. G. (1976) Enzymes associated with the metabolism of catecholamines, acetylcholine and GABA in human cortex and patients with Parkinson's disease and Huntington's chorea. *J. Neurochem.* 26, 65–76.

Nicholson, S. H., Suckling, C. J. & Iversen, L. L. (1978) GABA analogues: conformational analysis of effects on ^{3}H-GABA binding to postsynaptic receptors in human cerebellum. *J. Neurochem.*, in press.

Perry, T. L., Hansen, S. & Kloster, M. (1973) Huntington's chorea, deficiency of gamma-aminobutyric acid in brain. *New Engl. J. Med.* 288, 337–342.

Perry, E. K., Gibson, P. H., Blessed, G., Perry, R. H. & Tomlinson, B. E. (1977) Neurotransmitter enzyme abnormalities in senile dementia. Choline acetyltransferase and glutamic acid decarboxylase activities in necropsy brain tissue. *J. Neurol. Sci.* 34, 247–265.

Perry, E. K., Blessed, G., Perry, R. H. & Tomlinson, B. E. (1978) Brain biochemistry in schizophrenia. *Lancet* i, 35–36.

Spokes, E. G. & Koch, D. J. (1978) Postmortem stability of dopamine, glutamate decarboxylase and choline acetyltransferase in mouse brain under conditions simulating the handling of human autopsy material. *J. Neurochem.*, in press.

Stahl, W. L. & Swanson, P. D. (1974) Biochemical abnormalities in Huntington's chorea brains. *Neurol.* (Minneap.) 24, 813–819.

Wood, J. H., Glaeser, B. S., Enna, S. J. & Hare, T. A. (1978) Verification and quantification of GABA in human cerebrospinal fluid. *J. Neurochem.* 30, 291–293.

Pharmacological Characteristics of GABA Receptors in Different Brain Regions

S. J. Enna, J. W. Ferkany & P. Krogsgaard-Larsen

Regional distribution studies of the synaptic receptor site for GABA in mammalian brain have revealed the ubiquity of this system (Enna & Snyder 1975, Enna *et al.* 1975, Enna *et al.* 1977, Lloyd *et al.* 1977). If all synaptic GABA receptors are identical, attempts to pharmacologically manipulate this system in specific brain areas may be unsuccessful, since side effects resulting from an action of the drug on other brain GABA receptors may override the desired behavioral or biochemical action.

In the past, the limited number of GABA receptor agonists and antagonists precluded a thorough and systematic investigation of the pharmacological characteristics of GABA receptors in various brain areas (Enna *et al.* 1976b). Recently, Krogsgaard-Larsen (1978) has synthesized and studied a number of rigid GABA analogues. The results of this and other studies (Krogsgaard-Larsen *et al.* 1975, Krogsgaard-Larsen *et al.* 1977) have revealed important information about the preferred structural conformation of the GABA receptor and have yielded a number of interesting compounds having a wide range of potency as GABA receptor agonists.

In the present study, using *in vitro* receptor binding techniques, some biochemical and pharmacological characteristics of GABA receptors in various regions of the human and rat brain are investigated and compared by exploring the relative potencies of numerous GABA receptor agonists to inhibit the

Departments of Pharmacology and of Neurobiology and Anatomy, The University of Texas Medical School at Houston, P. O. Box 20708, Houston, Texas, U.S.A. 77025. Department of Chemistry, The Royal Danish School of Pharmacy DK-2100 Copenhagen, Denmark.

"GABA-NEUROTRANSMITTERS", Alfred Benzon Symposium 12, Munksgaard 1978

receptor binding of this neurotransmitter agent. In addition, detailed kinetic studies using ^{3}H-GABA and ^{3}H-muscimol as ligands for the GABA receptor were undertaken. The results suggest that while all brain GABA receptors appear to be pharmacologically identical in terms of the relative potencies of agonists and antagonists, the affinity of the receptor for agonists may vary significantly among different brain areas.

MATERIAL AND METHODS

Human brains were obtained at autopsy and placed immediately into ice-cold 0.32M sucrose. All brains were dissected within 1 h post-mortem, and the brain regions were stored at -20°C until assayed. Though the causes of death varied widely, brains of individuals who had infections or neoplasia of the central nervous system were not used, nor were samples used when there was a delay of more than 20 h between death and freezing of the brain tissue.

For assay, the tissue was prepared and GABA receptor binding studied as previously described (Enna *et al.* 1976a, Enna *et al.* 1976b). Briefly, the frozen tissue was homogenized with a Polytron in 20 vol of distilled water, centrifuged at 48,000 x g for 10 min and the tissue washed two times by resuspending and centrifuging as above. Following the final centrifugation, the tissue was resuspended in 100 vol of 0.05M Tris-citrate buffer (pH7.1 at 4°C) for assay. In some cases the tissue was incubated in buffer containing 0.05% (v/v) Triton X-100 for 30 min at 37°C prior to washing with distilled water. The sodium-independent binding of ^{3}H-GABA (54 Ci/mmole) was employed to identify apparent synaptic GABA receptors (Enna & Snyder 1975, Enna & Snyder 1977). To study the ability of unlabeled compounds to displace receptor-bound ^{3}H-GABA, various concentrations of each drug were placed into the incubation tubes containing the ^{3}H-GABA and brain membranes and the amount of specifically bound ^{3}H-GABA calculated in the presence and absence of drug. The concentration of drug which displaced 50% of the receptor bound GABA (IC_{50}) was estimated using log-probit analysis. The IC_{50} value is a rough estimate of the receptor affinity for the drug (Hollenberg 1978).

To study rceptor binding in rat brain, membranes obtained from rat brain P_2 fractions were prepared, frozen, thawed, and treated with Triton X-100 as previously described (Enna & Snyder 1977). Using membrane fragments obtained from the same brains, GABA receptor binding was studied using both ^{3}H-GABA and ^{3}H-muscimol as ligands (Enna & Snyder 1977, Beaumont *et al.*

Table I

Binding site concentration and ligand affinity for ^{3}H-muscimol and ^{3}H-GABA binding in rat brain regions

	^{3}H-GABA		^{3}H-Muscimol	
Brain Region	B_{max} (pmoles/mg protein)	K_d (nM)	B_{max} (pmoles/mg protein)	K_d (nM)
Cerebral Cortex	2.5	10	2.6	2
Hippocampus	2.4	12	2.6	2
Striatum	1.3	15	0.8	2
Midbrain	1.3	10	1.4	2
Medulla-pons	0.8	11	0.7	2
Cerebellum	4.8	14	4.3	3

Binding was conducted on membranes from P_2 fractions prepared from each brain area. All membranes were treated with 0.05% Triton X-100 as described in Methods. Saturation studies were conducted by incubating the membranes with increasing concentrations of ^{3}H-muscimol or ^{3}H-GABA in the presence of either 10^{-5}M unlabeled muscimol or 10^{-3}M unlabeled GABA respectively. Specific binding at each concentration was determined by subtracting the amount of tritium remaining in the tissue in the presence of unlabeled ligand from the amount bound in the absence of unlabeled substance. Scatchard analysis of the amount of specifically bound ligand at each concentration revealed binding site concentration (B_{max}) and receptor affinity (K_d).

Each value is the mean of five to eight experiments, each performed in triplicate.

1978). For this study, the kinetic characteristics of GABA receptor binding were investigated by determining the amount of ligand specifically bound to the tissue with increasing concentrations of isotope. From these data, receptor affinity (K_d) and number of binding sites (B_{max}) were calculated by Scatchard analysis.

RESULTS

Kinetic analysis of ^{3}H-GABA and ^{3}H-muscimol binding sites in various regions of rat brain

Saturation studies of ^{3}H-GABA and ^{3}H-muscimol binding in six different regions of rat brain indicated that the total number of binding sites (B_{max}) for the two different ligands was virtually identical in all areas (Table I). In addition, though the receptor affinity (K_d) for GABA was five times less than that observed for muscimol, no significant differences were noted in receptor affinity of each ligand in the different areas, with the K_d being approximately 12 nM for GABA and 2 nM for muscimol.

Compound	Formula
GABA	
Muscimol	
Thiomuscimol	
Isoxazole 2	
Isoxazole 6	
Isoxazole 9	
Isoxazole 14	
Isoxazole 16	
Isoxazole 20	
Piperidine-4-Carboxylic Acid (P-4-CA)	
Isoguvacine	

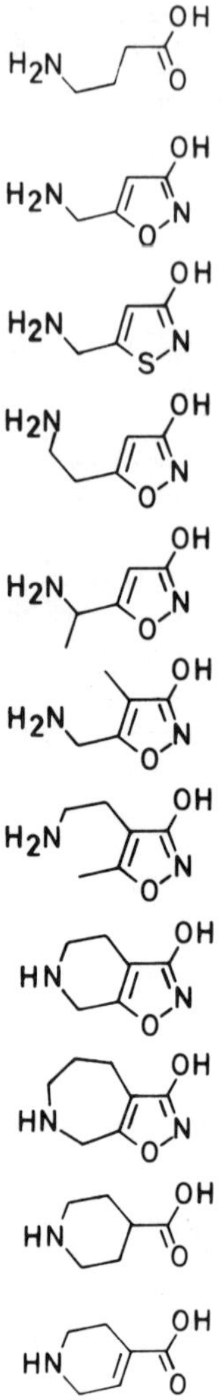

Fig. 1. Chemical formulas of some GABA analogues used in this study.

Relative potencies of drugs on GABA receptor binding in various areas of the human brain

To study the pharmacological characteristics of GABA receptors in human brain, the potency of a series of GABA analogues (Fig. 1) in displacing specifically bound GABA was determined. Most of the compounds studied were isoxazole derivatives or monocyclic amino acids related to isoxazole 16 (isoguvacine and piperidine-4-carboxylic acid). In addition, the GABA agonists 3-aminopropanesulfonic acid (APSA) and imidazoleacetic acid (IAA) and the antagonist bicuculline were also investigated. Preliminary experiments with selected compounds using membranes obtained from human caudate nucleus and treated with Triton X-100 revealed that dose-response curves for these compounds are parallel suggesting competitive inhibition (Fig. 2).

The IC_{50} value for the displacement of specifically bound ^{3}H-GABA in seven different regions of the human brain was determined for each compound (Table II). In this series of experiments the tissue was treated with Triton. In all areas, the order of drug potency was virtually identical, with muscimol being substantially more active than GABA in displacing receptor – bound ^{3}H-GABA and with thiomuscimol and APSA being approximately equipotent to GABA. In decreasing order of potency these compounds are followed by isoguvacine, isoxazole 16, IAA, P-4-CA and isoxazoles 2 and 6 which all have some activity in displacing bound ^{3}H-GABA but are from 2 to 100 times less potent than GABA itself. Isoxazoles 9, 14 and 20 are without any appreciable activity and

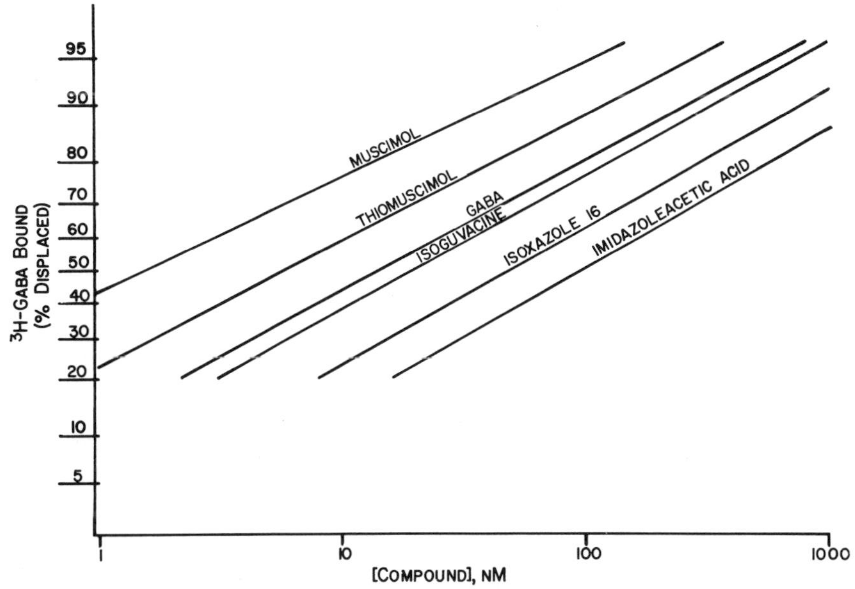

Fig. 2. Displacement of specifically bound ^{3}H-GABA from Triton treated membranes obtained from human caudate nucleus. Each point is the mean of three to six experiments, each performed in triplicate. Data are plotted on a log-probit (logit) scale.

Table II

Potencies of various compounds in displacing receptor-bound ^{3}H-GABA from different regions of the human brain

	IC50 (nM) Brain Region						
Compound	Caudate Nucleus	Frontal Cortex	Hippo-campus	Cere-bellar Cortex	Mid brain	Sub-stantia Nigra	Dentate Nucleus
Muscimol	3	3	1	1	5	6	7
Thiomuscimol	13	11	22	10	20	10	52
GABA	17	14	13	16	20	31	21
3-Aminopropanesulfonic acid	14	40	25	20	35	20	57
Isoguvacine	22	35	50	18	53	143	80
Isoxazole 16	96	80	90	52	64	170	135
Imidazoleacetic acid	80	90	120	90	321	300	120
P-4-CA	500	900	270	320	800	900	650
Isoxazole 2	1700	1200	1600	900	785	1500	1000
Isoxazole 6	2300	2000	1200	720	3000	3300	950
Isoxazole 9	N.S.*	N.S.	N.S.	N.S.	N.S.	N.S.	N.S.
Isoxazole 14	N.S.	N.S.	N.S.	N.S.	N.S.	N.S.	N.S.
Isoxazole 20	N.S.	N.S.	N.S.	N.S.	N.S.	N.S.	N.S.
Bicuculline	5000	4000	4000	8000	9000	5000	7000

Membranes were prepared from post-mortem human brain samples and were treated with 0.05% Triton X-100 as described in Methods. The ability of each compound to displace membrane-bound ^{3}H-GABA was determined by incubating samples with six different concentrations of each test substance. The concentration of drug which inhibited ^{3}H-GABA binding 50% (IC_{50}) was determined by log-probit analysis. Each value is the mean of three to six experiments, each performed in triplicate.

* $IC_{50} > 10{,}000$ nM

bicuculline, though active, is much weaker than GABA. The IC_{50} values for any given compound remain approximately the same in the different brain regions.

Effect of Triton X-100 treatment on IC_{50} values in various regions of the human brain

Since treating membranes with Triton enhances the apparent affinity of GABA for the receptor site (Enna & Snyder 1977), it was of interest to determine the relative potency of the various compounds in tissue which had not been treated with this detergent. Using five agonists, it was found that the relative potencies of these agents in the seven brain regions was the same as that seen using tissue treated with Triton (Table III). However, it is noteworthy that while Triton treatment substantially decreased the IC_{50} of the compounds in most of the brain areas, it appears to have significantly less effect in the dentate nucleus. This is better illustrated by calculating the ratio of the IC_{50} values in the absence and presence of Triton for these five compounds (Table IV). Thus, Triton has virtually no effect in decreasing the IC_{50} for muscimol, thiomuscimol and GABA in the dentate, where the Triton ratio for these compounds is close to 1, whereas the ratio in the caudate nucleus and midbrain for these compounds varies from 4–15. Furthermore, Triton treatment decreases the IC_{50} for isoguvacine and isoxazole 16 about five fold, which is substantially less than the 25-to 50-fold decreases observed in the midbrain and caudate for these two compounds.

Table III

Effect of Triton X-100 treatment on the potencies of various compounds to displace receptor-bound ^{3}H-GABA from different regions of the human brain

		IC_{50} (nM) Brain Region						
Compound	Triton*	Caudate Nucleus	Frontal Cortex	Hippo-campus	Cere-bellar Cortex	Mid-brain	Sub-stantia Nigra	Dentate Nucleus
Muscimol	−	39	45	16	27	22	47	14
	+	3	3	1	1	5	12	7
Thiomuscimol	−	200	280	510	450	127	170	60
	+	13	11	22	10	20	101	52
GABA	−	210	94	107	70	200	145	19
	+	17	14	13	16	20	31	21
Isoguvacine	−	725	650	900	460	1315	2000	200
	+	22	35	50	18	35	143	80
Isoxazole 16	−	5000	1300	2500	950	2400	2500	700
	+	96	80	90	52	64	170	135

Experiments were conducted and analyzed as described in Table II, except that tissue was not preincubated with Triton X-100. The values for tissue treated with Triton are taken from Table II. Each value is the mean of three to six experiments, each performed in triplicate.

* −, no Triton treatment; +, Triton treatment.

Table IV

Ratios of IC_{50} values obtained in non-Triton vs. Triton treated tissue

Compound	IC_{50} Ratio (Non-Triton/Triton) Brain Region		
	Caudate	Midbrain	Dentate
Muscimol	13	4	2
Thiomuscimol	15	6	1
GABA	12	10	1
Isoguvacine	33	25	3
Isoxazole 16	52	40	5

Each figure represents the ratio of the IC_{50} values obtained without and with Triton treatment as shown in Table III.

DISCUSSION

The finding that the total number of binding sites (B_{max}) for ^{3}H-GABA and ^{3}H-muscimol is identical in six regions of the rat brain suggests that, at least in these brain areas, there are no muscimol-insensitive GABA receptor sites. These results suggest that, pharmacologically, the GABA receptor is homogeneous throughout the brain. Further evidence for this belief is provided by the fact that the relative potencies of 13 GABA agonists and one antagonist are identical in seven different human brain regions. The significance of this correlation is established by the fact that the potencies of the compounds studied varied over a 1000-fold range. Thus, as reported earlier for rat brain (Krogsgaard-Larsen 1978), of the new GABA analogues studied, muscimol, thiomuscimol, isoguvacine, isoxazole 16 and P-4-CA appear to be useful GABA receptor agonists. However, the recent discovery that muscimol may not penetrate the brain and that the behavioral effects observed after systemic administration may be due to some derivative (A. Maggi & S. J. Enna, submitted) suggests that isoxazole derivatives may not be clinically useful agents for activating GABA receptors.

Though the present results indicate that the relative sensitivity of GABA receptors to various agonists appears to be the same throughout the brain, they also reveal that certain brain regions, such as the dentate nucleus, may have an inherently greater affinity for GABA agonists than other brain areas. The basis for this apparently higher affinity may be related to the results obtained by comparing IC_{50} values obtained using tissue before and after treatment with

Triton. Thus, Triton has very little or no effect on increasing GABA receptor affinity in the dentate nucleus whereas GABA receptor affinity in other brain areas is substantially increased by treatment with this detergent.

Recently it has been proposed that there is an endogenous competitive inhibitor of the GABA receptor in brain and that treatment with Triton rids the brain of this substance (Johnston & Kennedy 1978). Thus, the extent to which Triton enhances the potency of agonists would be a crude measure of the amount of endogenous inhibitor present in any brain region. Accordingly, the present results suggest that the dentate nucleus contains much less of this inhibitor than do areas such as the caudate nucleus, cerebral cortex, and hippocampus, meaning that for a given amount of GABA agonist present in brain, the dentate would respond to a much greater extent than cortical or striatal areas.

Previous studies using a single concentration of radioactive GABA have shown that the dentate nucleus is one of the lowest areas in the brain in terms of GABA receptor binding (Enna *et al.* 1977, Lloyd *et al.* 1977). This finding was surprising in light of the fact that the primary input to the dentate nucleus is from cerebellar Purkinje cells which utilize GABA as their transmitter agent. The present results demonstrating a high affinity GABA receptor site in the dentate may provide a plausible explanation as to why this nucleus does not require a large number of receptor sites to manage the extensive GABA input to this region.

The present results do not completely rule out the possibility of pharmacologically distinct GABA receptors such as exist for the adrenergic and cholinergic systems. Rather they demonstrate that the GABA receptors labeled using this binding technique have uniform pharmacological characteristics. However, the discovery that the affinity of these GABA receptors may vary significantly among different brain regions, possibly due to the amount of endogenous inhibitor present, may be of therapeutic importance since regions possessing a higher affinity for this neurotransmitter will be more greatly affected by a given dose of a GABA agonist. It is conceivable that many areas of the brain have, like the dentate nucleus, a relatively higher affinity for GABA. If these areas were known, the behavioral, biochemical and perhaps side effects of GABA therapy may be more predictable.

ACKNOWLEDGMENTS

Supported in part by grants from the Pharmaceutical Manufacturers Association, the Huntington's Chorea Foundation, Merck Sharp and Dohme and USPHS RCDA NS-00335 (S.J.E.). We thank Ms. Elaina Mann for her excellent technical assistance.

REFERENCES

Beaumont, K., Chilton, W. S., Yamamura, H. I. & Enna, S. J. (1978) Muscimol binding in rat brain: association with synaptic GABA receptors. *Brain Res.* 148, 153–162.

Enna, S. J., Bennett, J. P., Bylund, D. B., Creese, I., Burt, D. R., Charness, M. E., Yamamura, H. I., Simantov, R. & Snyder, S. H. (1977) Neurotransmitter receptor binding: regional distribution in human brain. *J. Neurochem.* 28, 233–236.

Enna, S. J., Bennett, J. P., Bylund, D. B., Snyder, S. H., Bird, E. D. & Iversen, L. L. (1976a) Alterations of brain neurotransmitter receptor binding in Huntington's disease. *Brain Res.* 116, 531–537.

Enna, S. J., Bird, E. D., Bennett, J. P., Bylund, D. B., Yamamura, H. I., Iversen, L. L. & Snyder, S. H. (1976b) Huntington's chorea: change in neurotransmitter receptors in the brain. *N. Eng. J. Med.* 294, 1305–1309.

Enna, S. J., Kuhar, M. J. & Snyder, S. H. (1975) Regional distribution of postsynaptic receptor binding for gamma-aminobutyric acid (GABA) in monkey brain. *Brain Res.* 93, 168–174.

Enna, S. J. & Snyder, S. H. (1975) Properties of γ-aminobutyric acid (GABA) receptor binding in rat brain synaptic membrane fractions. *Brain Res.* 100, 81–97.

Enna, S. J. & Snyder, S. H. (1977) Influences of ions, enzymes, and detergents on γ-aminobutyric acid receptor binding in synaptic membranes of rat brain. *Mol. Pharmacol.* 13, 442–453.

Hollenberg, M. D. (1978) Receptor models and the action of neurotransmitters and hormones. In: *Neurotransmitter Receptor Binding,* eds. Yamamura, H. I., Enna, S. J. & Kuhar, M. J., Raven Press, New York. pp. 13–39.

Johnston, G. A. R. & Kennedy, S. M. (1978) GABA receptors and phospholipids. In: *Amino Acids as Chemical Transmitters,* ed. Fonnum, F., Plenum Press, New York. In press.

Krogsgaard-Larsen, P. (1978) GABA agonists and uptake inhibitors of restricted conformations: structure-activity relations. In: *Amino Acids as Chemical Transmitters,* ed. Fonnum, F., Plenum Press, New York. In press.

Krogsgaard-Larsen, P., Johnston, G. A. R., Curtis, D. R., Game, C. J. A. & McCulloch, R. M. (1975) Structure and biological activity of a series of conformationally restricted analogues of GABA. *J. Neurochem.* 25, 803–809.

Krogsgaard-Larsen, P., Johnston, G. A. R., Lodge, D. & Curtis, D. R. (1977) A new class of GABA agonists. *Nature* 268, 53–55.

Lloyd, K. G., Shemen, K. & Hornykiewicz, O. (1977) Distribution of high affinity sodium-independent ^{3}H-gamma-aminobutyric acid (^{3}H-GABA) binding in the human brain: alterations in Parkinson's disease. *Brain Res.* 127, 269–278.

GABA Receptor Agonists: Design and Structure-Activity Studies

Povl Krogsgaard-Larsen, Tage Honoré & Karen Thyssen

Based on extensive physiological and biochemical studies, γ-aminobutyric acid (GABA) is generally considered to be the major inhibitory transmitter in the brain. However, many functional aspects of GABA neurones including their interactions with other central transmitter systems are far from being completely understood. Elucidation of these complex problems have become essential in the light of the recent findings that the GABA system is involved in the development of certain neurological and psychiatric disorders. Compounds with potent and specific actions on different functions of GABA neurones are vital tools for studies of the GABA system at the cellular and molecular level. Furthermore these model compounds represent important steps in our attempts to develop therapeutically useful GABA-ergic drugs.

SPECIFIC GABA RECEPTOR AGONISTS: DESIGN AND DEVELOPMENT

The mechanism of activation of GABA receptors (deFeudis 1977) and the termination of this process (Martin 1976) are key problems in the physiology of the GABA system. A considerable degree of conformational flexibility is a trait of the molecule of GABA. This molecular characteristic apparently is essential for the synaptic activity of GABA, but it inherently makes GABA itself inapplicable for studies of its "active conformations". GABA can adopt a variety of almost equi-energetic conformations (Ham 1974, Pullman 1976, Pullman & Berthod 1975), but attempts to deduce the "active conformations" of GABA at different synaptic sites based on these studies only are meaningless.

Department of Chemistry BC, Royal Danish School of Pharmacy, 2, Universitetsparken, DK-2100 Copenhagen, Denmark.

"GABA-NEUROTRANSMITTERS", Alfred Benzon Symposium 12, Munksgaard 1978

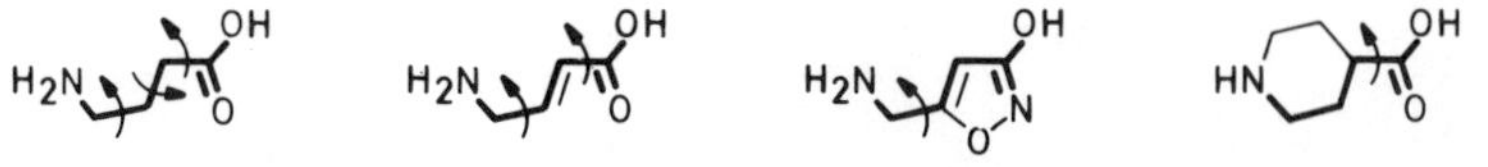

Fig. 1. The conformational mobility of the molecules of GABA, *trans*-ACA, muscimol, and isonipecotic acid as illustrated by the rotational freedom round carbon-carbon single bonds.

An approach to these problems involves design and investigation of the GABA-ergic activities of analogues of GABA of more rigid structure. In Fig. 1 the structures of some model compounds are depicted, in which various parts of the molecule of GABA are conformationally immobilized. *Trans*-4-Aminocrotonic acid (*trans*-ACA) is still relatively flexible, and it is able to interact with the GABA receptors (Johnston *et al.* 1975a), the GABA transport carrier (Beart *et al.* 1972), and GABA: 2-oxoglutarate aminotransferase (GABA-T) (Beart & Johnston 1973). Muscimol and isonipecotic acid, however, are relatively rigid compounds, in which the structure of GABA is incorporated into different ring structures. Based on structure-activity studies on model compounds related to muscimol and isonipecotic acid, it has been concluded that the "receptor-active conformation" of GABA is different from the conformation in which GABA is transported by the uptake system (Krogsgaard-Larsen *et al.* 1975, 1977a, Krogsgaard-Larsen 1978, Krogsgaard-Larsen & Johnston 1978). These conformations in turn seem to be different from that adopted by GABA at the active site of GABA-T (Allan *et al.* 1977).

Muscimol and muscimol analogues

Muscimol is a psychoactive natural product of unique structure (Brehm *et al.* 1972) produced by *Amanita muscaria* (Eugster 1969). The 3-isoxazolol moiety of muscimol can be regarded as a masked carboxyl group of frozen conformation. Muscimol is a very potent and selective GABA receptor agonist (Johnston *et al.* 1968, Curtis *et al.* 1971), being also a weak inhibitor of the uptake of GABA into rat brain slices (Johnston 1971) and cultured astrocyte cells (Schousboe *et al.* 1978). There is relatively free rotation of the aliphatic side chain of muscimol. Consequently the "receptor-active conformation" of muscimol can not be unequivocally deduced from studies of low energy conformations of this compound. Using muscimol as a model compound a variety of related monocyclic (Krogsgaard-Larsen & Christensen 1974, Brehm *et al.* 1974, Hjeds & Krogsgaard-Larsen 1976, Krogsgaard-Larsen *et al.* 1978) and bicyclic compounds

(Krogsgaard-Larsen & Hjeds 1974, Krogsgaard-Larsen 1977, Krogsgaard-Larsen *et al.* 1977b) have been developed, and the relationship between structure and activity of some of these compounds is illustrated in Table I. As emphasized in the formulas, all of the compounds are structural analogues of GABA.

Table I

Muscimol analogues as inhibitors of GABA receptor binding and as depressants of neuronal firing as determined by microelectrophoretic techniques

Compound	Structure	pK$_A$ Values	% Inhibition at 10^{-4}M	IC$_{50}$ (μM)	Rel. Potency in vivo	Antagonism by BMC
GABA	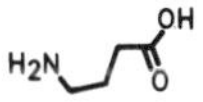	4.0; 10.7		0.033±0.004	– – –	+
Muscimol	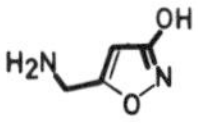	4.8; 8.4	103	0.024±0.003	– – – –	+
RS-5-(1-Aminoethyl)-3-isoxazolol	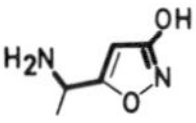	4.7; 8.5	98	2.2±0.1	– – –	+
S-(–)- —"—	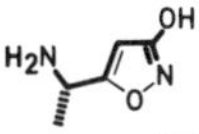	4.7; 8.5	97	0.64±0.08	n.t.	
R-(+)- —"—	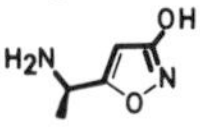	4.7; 8.5	92	19±1	n.t.	
1	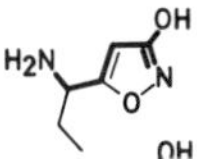	4.7; 8.4	n.s.		– –	0
2	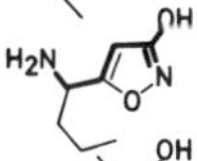	4.7; 8.5	n.s.		– –	0
3	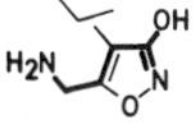	4.8; 8.8	13		–	0
4	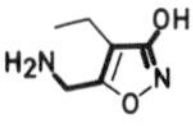	–	n.s.		0	
5	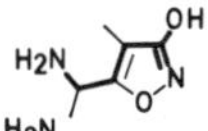	4.6; 8.6	n.s.		n.t.	
6	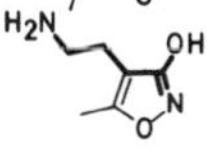	5.1; 10.4	n.s.		0	
THIP	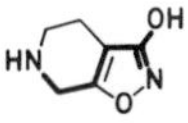	4.4; 8.5	98	0.13±0.01	– – –(–)	+
7	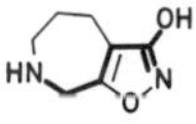	4.6; 8.6	21		n.t.	
8	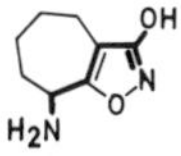	4.5; 8.3	n.s.		n.t.	

All GABA receptor binding experiments described in this chapter were performed according to the method of Enna & Snyder (1975).

However, an immediate structural similarity with GABA is evidently not a sufficient condition for interaction with the GABA receptors. Structure-activity studies on THIP (4,5,6,7-tetrahydroisoxazolo[5,4-*c*]pyridin-3-ol), an almost rigid muscimol analogue led to the conclusion that the depicted conformation of the muscimol molecule represents the conformation capable of activating GABA receptors. The ability of a compound to adopt this conformation may be a prerequisite for interaction with GABA receptors. The alkylated analogues of muscimol are relatively weak or inactive as GABA receptor agonists, and they may find it difficult to adopt the required conformations. Direct steric effects may further impede contact between the compounds concerned and the receptor sites.

Stereostructure-activity studies

The optical antipodes of 5-(1-aminoethyl)-3-isoxazolol have different affinities for the GABA receptors, indicating that the chiral carbon atom has a close

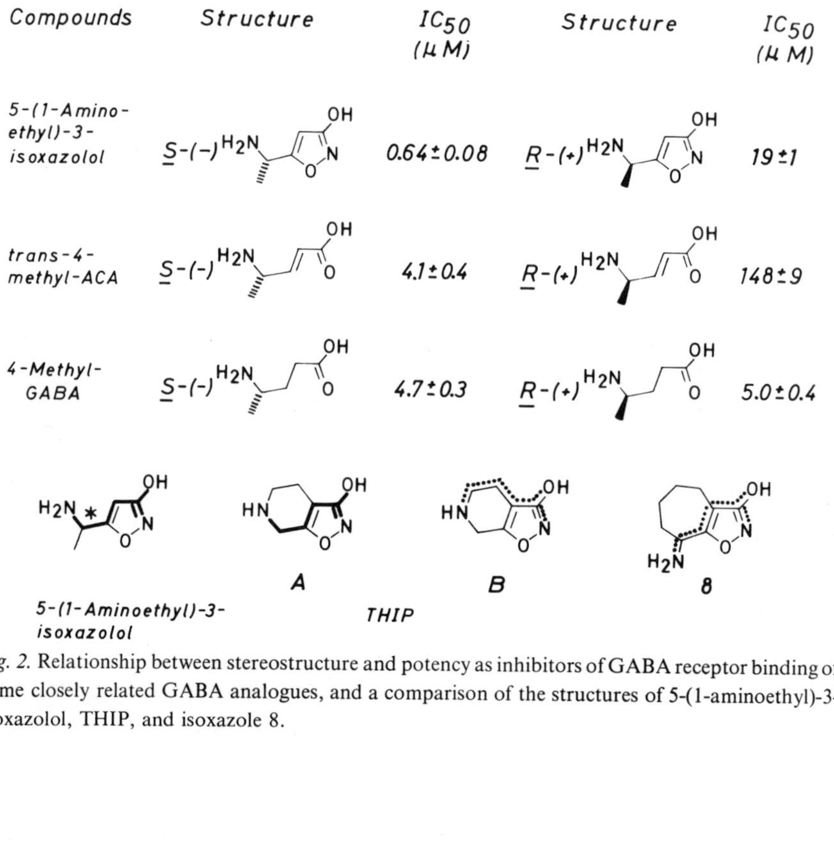

Fig. 2. Relationship between stereostructure and potency as inhibitors of GABA receptor binding of some closely related GABA analogues, and a comparison of the structures of 5-(1-aminoethyl)-3-isoxazolol, THIP, and isoxazole 8.

contact with the receptor macromolecule. This finding supports the theory that the corresponding carbon atom of THIP (Fig. 2) is involved in the binding of THIP to the receptor and that the structural element accentuated in formula A rather than that in B (dotted line) reflects the active conformation of muscimol. The elaborated part of the inactive isoxazole 8 reflects the low energy conformation of muscimol in the crystalline state (cf. Fig. 4), suggesting that the "receptor-active conformation" of muscimol is different from the observed low energy conformation.

In a striking contrast to the optical antipodes of 4-methyl-GABA, those of 5-(1-aminoethyl)-3-isoxazolol and *trans*-4-methyl-ACA exhibit a pronounced and similar degree of stereoselectivity with respect to interaction with the GABA receptor sites. Consequently the mode of interaction of the flexible GABA analogue 4-methyl-GABA with the receptor must be different from that of the conformationally restricted analogues concerned. These differences may be attributed to different degrees of intimacy of binding of the respective compounds to the receptor sites. An alternative interpretation of these stereostructure-activity studies is that 4-methyl-GABA interacts with a binding site of the GABA receptor different from that activated by the methylated derivatives of muscimol and *trans*-ACA. Two binding sites for GABA showing different binding characteristics have been detected on synaptic membranes treated with detergent (Enna & Snyder 1977, Wong & Horng 1977), and the possibility that different conformational modes of GABA interact with different GABA receptor sites must be considered. The inhibition of the binding of ^{3}H-muscimol to GABA receptor sites on rat brain membranes by the optical antipodes of 5-(1-aminoethyl)-3-isoxazolol, *trans*-4-methyl-ACA,and 4-methyl-GABA is being studied.

The structure-activity studies on muscimol and related compounds have shed light on the "receptor-active conformations" of muscimol and probably GABA. However, the ability of GABA analogues for adopting this particular conformation is not necessarily a sufficient condition for activation of the GABA receptors. From these studies it might be concluded that muscimol easily adopts an almost optimum "receptor-active conformation" close to that represented by THIP. Its partially flattened structure, however, is quite different from the structure of GABA, and it might be possible to design a GABA receptor agonist which fits the receptor even better than muscimol. These aspects have been elucidated by structure-activity studies on pertinent heterocyclic GABA analogues related to muscimol and THIP.

Table II

Heterocyclic muscimol analogues as inhibitors of GABA receptor binding and as depressants of neuronal firing as determined by microelectrophoretic techniques

Compound	Structure	pK_A Values	% Inhibition at $10^{-4}M$	IC_{50} (μM)	Rel. Potency in vivo	Antagonism by BMC
RS-4,5-Dihydromuscimol	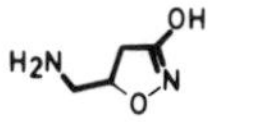	5.8; 9.3	101	0.009 ± 0.001	----	+
Muscimol	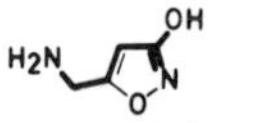	4.8; 8.4	103	0.024 ± 0.003	----	+
Thiomuscimol	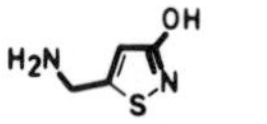	6.1; 8.9	114	0.12 ± 0.01	----	+
Isomuscimol	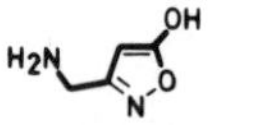	2.6; 9.0	42	377 ± 55	-	0
9	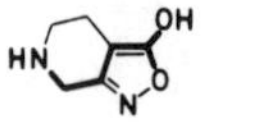	3.0; 9.1	54	83 ± 12	n.t.	
Azamuscimol	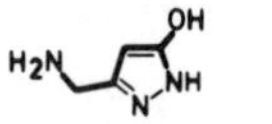	6.2; 9.8	16		--	0
10	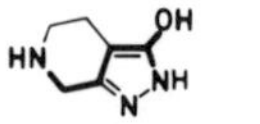	6.3; 9.9	n.s.		n.t.	
1-Methylazamuscimol	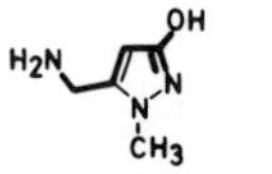	8.0; 10	26		n.t.	
11	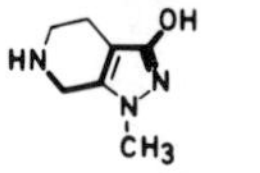	-	n.s.		n.t.	
2-Methylazamuscimol	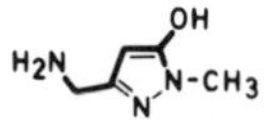	5.5; 9.8	17		n.t.	
12	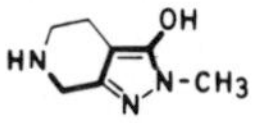	-	n.s.		n.t.	

Other heterocyclic GABA analogues

In the muscimol analogue 4,5-dihydromuscimol, the non-aromatic heterocyclic ring is devoid of the planar structure characteristic of the 3-isoxazolol ring in muscimol. 4,5-Dihydromuscimol has an affinity for the GABA receptors comparable with that of muscimol and it may be able to adopt a conformation which almost perfectly reflects a "receptor-active conformation" of GABA (Table II). The potency of 4,5-dihydromuscimol as a GABA-like depressant of neuronal firing has been compared with that of muscimol by using microelectrophoretic techniques (Fig. 3) (Curtis *et al.*, unpublished).

The degree of delocalization of the negative charge of GABA analogues may be important for their affinity for the GABA receptors. Like muscimol, 4,5-dihydromuscimol has a zwitterionic structure. Contrary to muscimol, in which the negative charge of the 3-isoxazolol ring apparently is slightly delocalized over the whole ring, the charge distribution of 4,5-dihydromuscimol may be similar to that of GABA (Fig. 5). Isomuscimol is a very weak GABA receptor agonist (Table II), and the negative charge of the 5-isoxazolol ring of

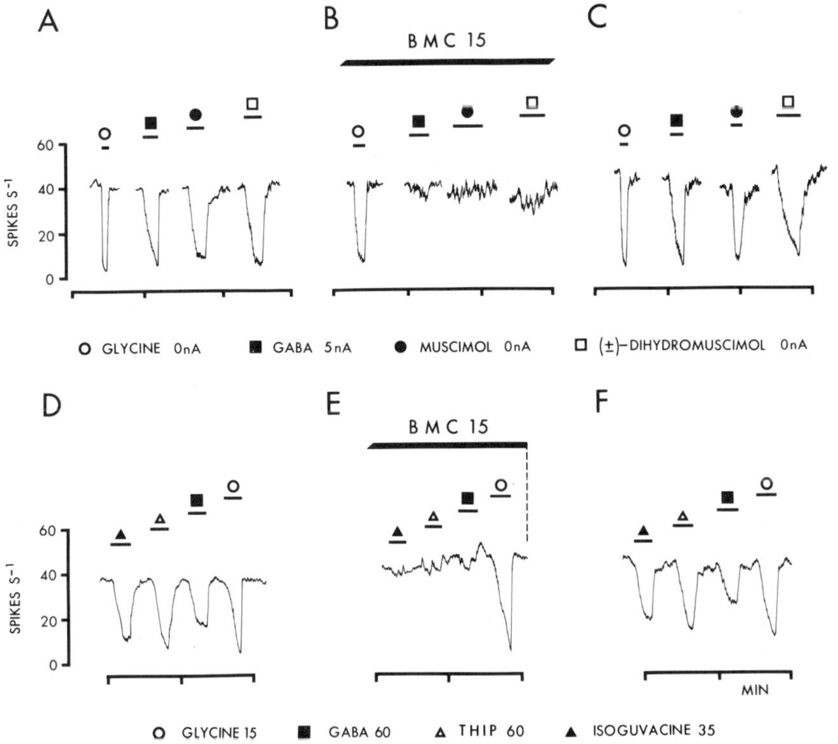

Fig. 3. A,B,C. The effect of bicuculline methochloride (BMC) on the inhibition of the firing of a spinal interneurone by glycine (○, 0 nA, 0.5 M); GABA (■, 5 nA, 0.2 M); muscimol (●, 0 nA, 0.1 M) and (±)-dihydromuscimol (□, 0 nA, 0.2 M), all ejected microelectrophoretically for the times indicated by the symbols and horizontal bars. The neurone was fired by the continuous ejection of DL-homocysteate (10 nA, 0.2 M). A, before; B, during BMC; C, 4 min after the BMC ejection was terminated.

D,E,F. The effect of bicuculline methochloride (BMC) on the inhibition of the firing of another spinal interneurone by glycine (○, 15 nA, 0.5 M); GABA (■, 60 nA, 0.2 M); THIP (△, 60 nA, 0.1 M) and isoguvacine (▲, 35 nA, 0.1 M) ejected as above. The current used to eject DL-homocysteate was 10 nA. D, before; E, during BMC, terminated at the vertical broken line; F, 3 min after E. Ordinates: firing frequency in spikes s^{-1}. Abscissae: time in min.

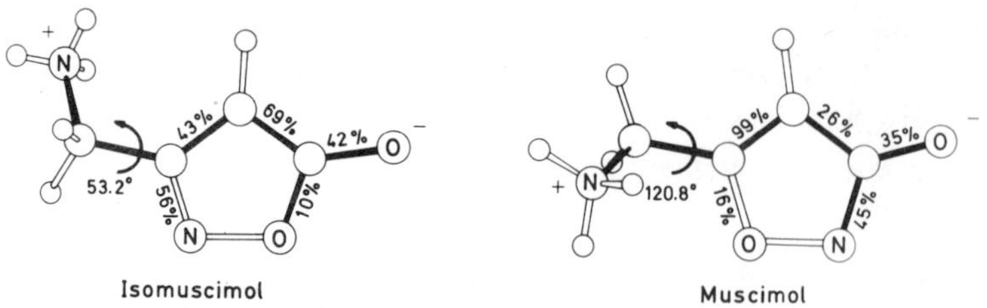

Fig. 4. The conformations of isomuscimol and muscimol in the crystalline states as established by x-ray analyses. The approximate double bond character per cent of the bonds of the heterocyclic rings is calculated by the method of Pauling (1944).

isomuscimol is highly delocalized as depicted in Fig. 5. This charge delocalization of isomuscimol is supported by x-ray crystallography (Honoré & Brehm, in preparation). In Fig. 4 the structures of isomuscimol and muscimol as determined by x-ray crystallographic methods are compared. The approximate double bound character per cent calculated by the method of Pauling (1944) from the bond distances of the heterocyclic rings reflects a pronounced resonance effect in isomuscimol. This charge delocalization of isomuscimol is also evident from the fact that its pK_A value is significantly lower than that of muscimol. The low energy conformation of isomuscimol in the crystalline state is very similar to that proposed to be a "receptor-active conformation" of muscimol and GABA. This finding supports the critical importance of charge distributions in GABA analogues for GABA agonist activity. The bicyclic isomuscimol analogue 9, which is closely related to THIP, is slightly more potent that isomuscimol (Table II). The very low affinity for GABA receptors of azamuscimol and related 3-pyrazolol derivatives may be explained by similar arguments, but so far little is known about the charge distribution of negatively charged 3-pyrazolols.

It must be emphasized that it is difficult to study the exact electronic structure of charged molecules under physiologically relevant conditions. Useful information can be obtained from x-ray crystallographic structure determinations and molecular orbital calculations and from studies of protolytic properties (pK_A values) of pertinent model compounds. As already mentioned, low pK_A values of acidic functions normally indicate a high degree of delocalization of the negative charge of the corresponding anion. The compounds depicted in Fig. 5 are all GABA analogues of zwitterionic structure. However, the distributions of the negative charges of, e.g. GABA, FAP (2-fluoro-5-aminomethylphenol), and DFAP (2,4-difluoro-5-aminomethylphenol) (Honoré *et al.*, unpublished) must be different. A comparison of the protolytic properties of the compounds depicted in Fig. 5 with their affinity for the GABA receptors supports the theories about the importance of electronic distributions in GABA analogues for affinity for GABA receptors.

Compounds which interact specifically and irreversibly with GABA receptors may be useful biochemical and pharmacological tools. Like isomuscimol, isoxazole 9 has a 5-isoxazolol nucleus (Table II). 5-Isoxazolol (isoxazolin-5-one) derivatives are highly reactive compounds (Quilico 1962). Consequently

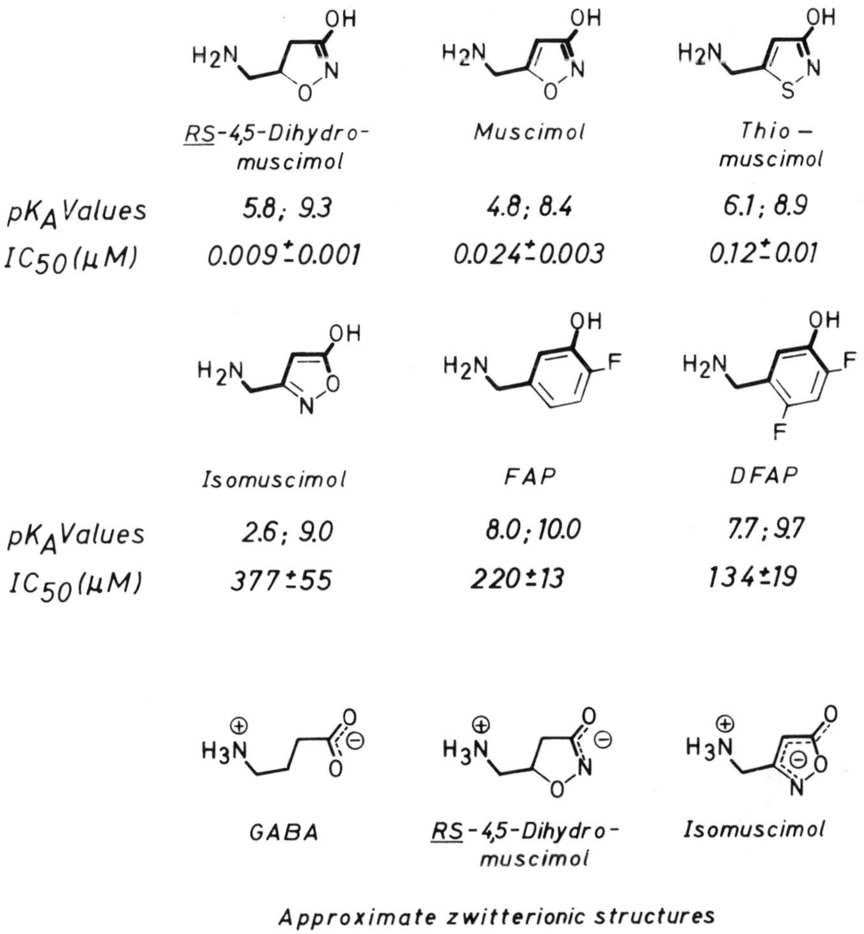

Fig. 5. Relationship between structure, protolytic properties, and potency as inhibitors of GABA receptor binding of some GABA analogues, and the approximate zwitterionic structures of GABA, (*RS*)-4,5-dihydromuscimol, and isomuscimol.

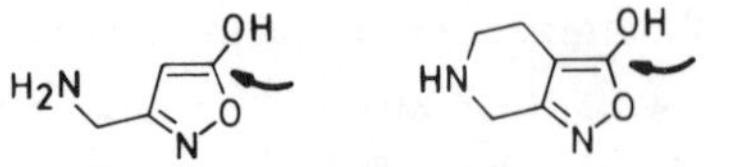

	Isomuscimol	9
IC_{50} (μM)	377±55	83±12

Fig. 6. The structures of isomuscimol and isoxazole 9. The acylating sites of these compounds are indicated by arrows.

isomuscimol and isoxazole 9, which is a moderately potent inhibitor of binding of ^{3}H-GABA to receptor sites, may interact irreversibly with the GABA receptor macromolecules. The acylating sites of isomuscimol and isoxazole 9 are indicated in Fig. 6. The mechanism of interaction of isoxazole 9 with the GABA receptor sites is being studied.

Isoguvacine, isonipecotic acid, and related GABA analogues

THIP is a key model compound for studies of the "receptor-active conformations" of muscimol and probably GABA. Structure-activity considerations of THIP prompted investigations of the structurally related compounds isoguvacine, isonipecotic acid, and (±)-cis-3-hydroxyisonipecotic acid as potential GABA receptor agonists (Fig. 7).Isonipecotic and isoguvacine acid in

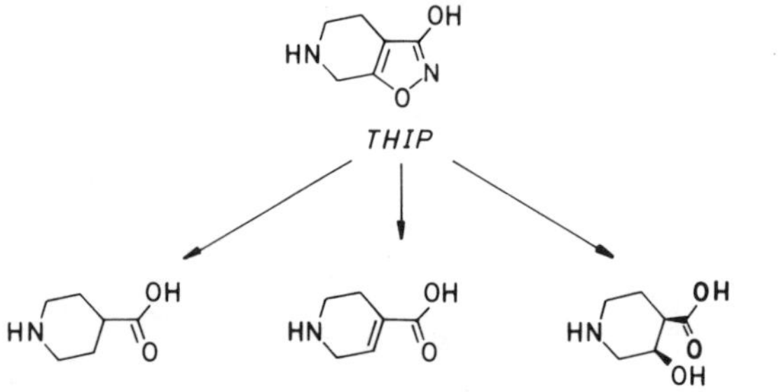

	Isonipecotic acid	Isoguvacine	(±)-cis-3-OH-Isonipecotic acid
pK_A Values	3.8;10.5	3.6;9.8	3.7; 10.0
IC_{50} (μM)	0.33±0.02	0.015±0.001	12±1
Rel. Potency in Vivo	---	----	-
Antagonism by BMC	+	+	

Fig. 7. Isonipecotic acid, isoguvacine, and (±)-*cis*-3-hydroxyisonipecotic acid as inhibitors of GABA receptor binding and as depressants of neuronal firing as determined by microelectrophoretic techniques, and the structural relationship between these cyclic amino acids and THIP.

Table III

Isoguvacine, isonipecotic acid, and related compounds as inhibitors of GABA receptor binding

	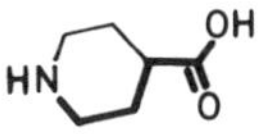 *Isonipecotic acid*	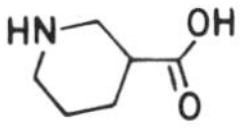 *Nipecotic acid*	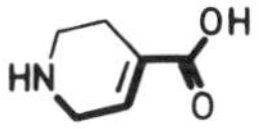 *Isoguvacine*	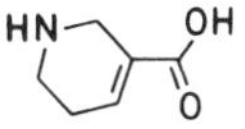 *Guvacine*
IC_{50} (μM)	0.33±0.02	> 1000	0.015±0.001	> 1000
	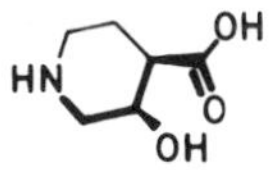 (±)-*cis*-3-OH-Isonipecotic acid	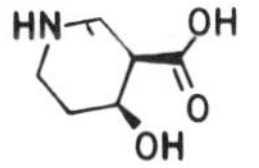 (±)-*cis*-4-OH-Nipecotic acid	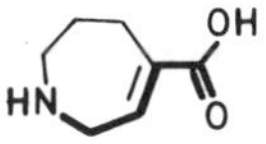 13	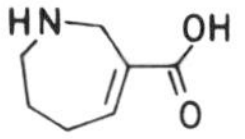 14
IC_{50} (μM)	12±1	> 1000	23±2	> 1000
	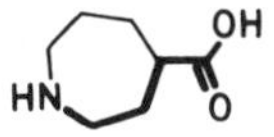 15	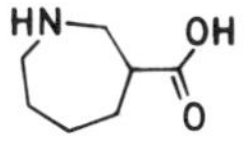 16	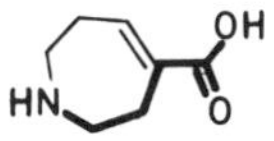 17	
IC_{50} (μM)	212±9	> 1000	15±1	

particular are potent and specific GABA agonists (Krogsgaard-Larsen *et al.* 1977a, Krogsgaard-Larsen & Johnston 1978). Among cyclic amino carboxylic acids the structure of isoguvacine seems to be almost optimum for activation of the GABA receptors.

A variety of related compounds has been developed (Krogsgaard-Larsen *et al.* unpuplished) and tested as inhibitors of binding of ^{3}H-GABA to GABA receptor sites (Table III). It is evident from these studies that the presence of a "GABA structure element" in the molecules is a prerequisite for interaction of this type of zwitterions with the GABA receptors. The conformation of these structural elements in the semirigid compounds is different, which may explain their different affinity for the GABA receptor sites.

(*R*)-(−)-Nipecotic acid (Krogsgaard-Larsen & Johnston 1975, Johnston *et al.* 1976a, b), guvacine (Johnston *et al.* 1975b), and (±)-cis-4-hydroxynipecotic acid (Krogsgaard-Larsen 1978), on the other hand, are potent inhibitors of GABA uptake into rat brain slices and of the uptake of GABA into cultured astrocyte cells (Schousboe *et al.* 1978). These compounds have very little or no affinity for the GABA receptors (Krogsgaard-Larsen & Johnston 1978).

GABA RECEPTOR AGONISTS IN NEUROPHARMACOLOGY

Impaired function of the central GABA system is involved in the development of neurological and psychiatric disorders like Huntington's chorea (McGeer & McGeer 1976a, b, Enna *et al.* 1977, Lloyd *et al.* 1977a), Parkinson's disease (Hornykiewicz *et al.* 1976, Lloyd *et al.* 1975, Lloyd *et al.* 1977b, McGeer & McGeer 1976b), and possibly schizophrenia (Roberts 1974, Van Kammen 1977). Consequently GABA replacement therapies based on specific GABA receptor agonists may be relevant for the treatment of these diseases. However, the full consequences of this type of therapy are unpredictable. GABA neurons are ubiquitous in the mammalian central nervous system, whereas the degeneration of GABA neurons in at least Huntington's chorea and Parkinson's disease seems to be restricted to discrete brain areas. GABA receptor agonists may be able to relieve the problems in the impaired parts of the brain, but activation of the entire GABA system may result in uncontrollable situations. However, GABA receptors in brain areas with impaired GABA systems may exhibit supersensitivity to GABA agonists (Champochiaro *et al.* 1977). Furthermore GABA receptors in different brain areas may exhibit different substrate specificity (see Enna *et al.*, this volume). Consequently, controlled and selective pharmacological manipulations of the GABA system using GABA receptor agonists may be a realistic possibility.

Being a very potent GABA receptor agonist at the cellular level in the spinal cord of cats (Johnston *et al.* 1968, Curtis *et al.* 1971, Krogsgaard-Larsen *et al.* 1975) muscimol has in recent years been extensively used as a pharmacological tool. However, the central actions of muscimol are not necessarily purely GABA-mimetic. The previously discussed stereostructure-activity studies may suggest that the mechanism of interaction of muscimol with GABA receptors is partially different from that of GABA. Alternatively muscimol may activate a limited population of GABA receptors. The depressant action of muscimol on single neurons is enhanced by simultaneous microelectrophoretic application of inhibitors of GABA uptake (Curtis *et al.* 1977) in agreement with the recent findings that muscimol is taken up by the neuronal GABA uptake system (Johnston *et al.*, unpublished). Furthermore, muscimol apparently is metabolized in mice (Ott *et al.* 1975) and metabolites of muscimol may contribute to the effects observed after systemic administration of muscimol (Naik *et al.* 1976). These aspects of the mode of action of muscimol must be considered in the interpretation of its pharmacological effects.

Beside muscimol the compounds depicted in Fig. 8 have pharmacological interest. Muscimol is a rather toxic compound when administered to mice (Theobald *et al.* 1968, Biggio *et al.* 1977). Whether the toxicity can be ascribed to

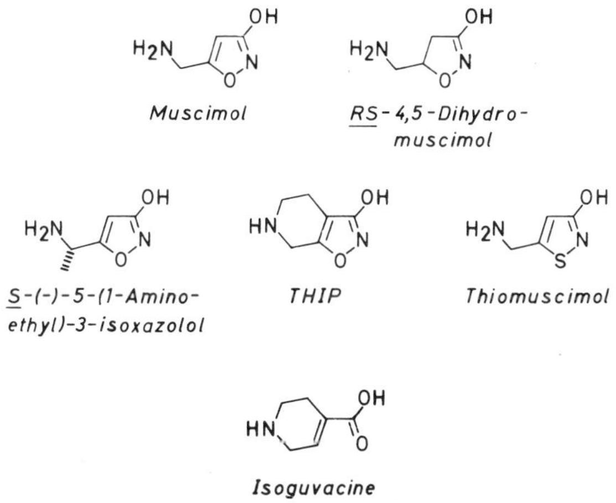

Fig. 8. Some GABA receptor agonists of pharmacological interest.

muscimol itself or to its metabolites is unknown. Since the side chain of muscimol may be susceptible to metabolism, compounds like (*S*)-(−)-5-(1-aminoethyl)-3-isoxazolol and in particular THIP may be more stable *in vivo.* In fact THIP has been shown to be a relatively non-toxic compound in rats and dogs and furthermore THIP seems to penetrate very easily into the brain after systemic administration. The pharmacology of THIP has been extensively studied in a variety of animal models (see Scheel-Krüger *et al.,* this volume), and in general the effects of THIP are slightly weaker than, but qualitatively similar to, those observed for muscimol.

A variety of muscimol analogues have been injected into substantia nigra in rats (Arnt *et al.,* in preparation). The doses required for initiation of contralateral turning behavior are in reasonable agreement with the potencies of the compounds as determined in GABA receptor affinity binding and micro-electrophoretic experiments. The duration of this effect of thiomuscimol is very short whereas isoguvacine has a prolonged effect.

Isoguvacine apparently does not easily penetrate the blood-brain barrier after systemic administration. However, pertinent derivatives of isoguvacine, which may be able to penetrate into the brain and subsequently be hydrolyzed to give isoguvacine, may be therapeutically useful "pro-drugs" of isoguvacine.

The availability of potent GABA receptor agonists combined with pharmaco-chemical insight may lead to the design and development of drugs for the treatment of diseases characterized in impaired functions of the GABA system.

ACKNOWLEDGMENTS

This project has been supported by grants from The Danish Medical Research Council. The microelectrophoretic experiments were performed by Professor D. R. Curtis; Professor D. R. Curtis and Dr. G. A. R. Johnston, The Australian National University, Canberra, Australia are gratefully acknowledged for collaboration and for stimulating advice and discussions. The authors wish to thank our colleagues Drs. L. Brehm, H. Hjeds, and E. Falch for fruitful collaboration and Mrs. B. Hare and Mrs. S. Stilling for skillful secretarial and technical assistance.

REFERENCES

Allan, R. D., Johnston, G. A. R. & Twitchin, B. (1977) Effects of gabaculine on the uptake, binding and metabolism of GABA. *Neuroscience Letters* 4, 51–54.

Beart, P. M. & Johnston, G. A. R. (1973) Transamination of analogues of γ-aminobutyric acid by extracts of rat brain mitochondria. *Brain Res.* 49, 459–462.

Beart, P. M., Johnston, G. A. R. & Uhr, M. L. (1972) Competitive inhibition of GABA uptake in rat brain slices by some GABA analogues of restricted conformation. *J. Neurochem.* 19, 1855–1861.

Biggio, G., Casu, M., Corda, M. G., Vernaleone, F. & Gessa, G. L. (1977) Effect of muscimol, a GABA-mimetic agent, on dopamine metabolism in the mouse brain. *Life Sci.* 21, 525–531.

Brehm, L., Hjeds, H. & Krogsgaard-Larsen, P. (1972) The structure of muscimol, a GABA analogue of restricted conformation. *Acta Chem. Scand.* 26, 1298–1299.

Campochiaro, P., Schwarcz, R. & Coyle, J. T. (1977) GABA receptor binding in rat striatum: localization and effects of denervation. *Brain Res.* 136, 501–511.

Curtis, D. R., Duggan, A. W., Felix, D. & Johnston, G. A. R. (1971) Bicuculline, an antagonist of GABA and synaptic inhibition in the spinal cord of the cat. *Brain Res.* 32, 69–96.

Curtis, D. R., Johnston, G. A. R. & Lodge, D. (1977) *In vivo* effects of GABA uptake inhibitors on the response of cat spinal neurons to GABA analogues. *Br. J. Pharmacol.* 61, 148P.

DeFeudis, F. V. (1977) GABA-receptors in the vertebrate nervous system. In: *Progress in Neurobiology*, eds. Kerkut, G. A. & Phillis, J. W. 9, 123–145. Pergamon Press, Oxford.

Enna, S. J. & Snyder, S. H. (1975) Properties of γ-aminobutyric acid (GABA) receptor binding in rat brain synaptic membrane fractions. *Brain Res.* 100, 81–97.

Enna, S. J. & Snyder, S. H. (1977) Influences of ions, enzymes, and detergents on γ-aminobutyric acid-receptor binding in synaptic membranes of rat brain. *Molec. Pharmacol.* 13, 442–453.

Enna, S. J., Stern, L. Z., Wastek, G. J. & Yamamura, H. I. (1977) Neurobiology and pharmacology of Huntington's disease, *Life Sci.* 20, 205–211.

Eugster, C. H. (1969) Chemie der Wirkstoffe aus dem Fliegenpilz. *Fortschr. Chem. Org. Naturst.* 27, 261–321.

Ham, N. S. (1974) NMR studies of solution conformations of physiologically active amino acids. In: *Molecular and Quantum Pharmacology*, eds. Bergmann, E. & Pullman, B., pp. 256–263, D. Reidel Publ. Comp., Dordrecht–Holland.

Hjeds, H. & Krogsgaard-Larsen, P. (1976) Synthesis of some 4-aminoalkyl-5-methyl-3-isoxazolols structurally related to muscimol and γ-aminobutyric acid (GABA). *Acta Chem. Scand.* B30, 567–573.

Hornykiewicz, O., Lloyd, K. G. & Davidson, L. (1976) The GABA system, function of the basal ganglia, Parkinson's disease. In: *GABA in Nervous System Function*, eds. Roberts, E., Chase, T. N. & Tower, D. B., pp. 479–485, Raven Press, New York.

Johnston, G. A. R. (1971) Muscimol and the uptake of γ-aminobutyric acid by rat brain slices. *Psychopharmacologia* 22, 230–233.

Johnston, G. A. R., Curtis, D. R., Beart, P. M., Game, C. J. A., McCulloch, R. M. & Twitchin, B. (1975a) *cis*- and *trans*-4-Aminocrotonic acid as GABA analogues of restricted conformation. *J. Neurochem.* 24, 157–160.

Johnston, G. A. R., Curtis, D. R., DeGroat, W. C. & Duggan, A. W. (1968) Central actions of ibotenic acid and muscimol. *Biochem. Pharmac.* 17, 2488–2489.

Johnston, G. A. R., Krogsgaard-Larsen, P. & Stephanson, A. (1975b) Betel nut constituents as inhibitors of γ-aminobutyric acid uptake. *Nature* 258, 627–628.

Johnston, G. A. R., Krogsgaard-Larsen, P., Stephanson, A. L. & Twitchin, B. (1976a) Inhibition of the uptake of GABA and related amino acids in rat brain slices by the optical isomers of nipecotic acid. *J. Neurochem.* 26, 1029–1032.

Johnston, G. A. R., Stephanson, A. L. & Twitchin, B. (1976b) Uptake and release of nipecotic acid by rat brain slices. *J. Neurochem.* 26, 83–87.

Krogsgaard-Larsen, P. (1977) Muscimol analogues. II. Synthesis of some bicyclic 3-isoxazolol zwitterions. *Acta Chem. Scand.* B31, 584–588.

Krogsgaard-Larsen, P. (1978) GABA agonists and uptake inhibitors of restricted conformations: structure-activity relations. In: *Amino Acids as Neurotransmitters*, ed. Fonnum, F. Plenum Press. In press.

Krogsgaard-Larsen, P. & Christensen, S. B. (1974) Organic hydroxylamine derivatives. XII. Structural analogues of γ-aminobutyric acid (GABA) of the isoxazole enol-betaine type. Synthesis of some 3-hydroxy-5-(1-aminoalkyl)isoxazole zwitterions. *Acta Chem. Scand.* B28, 636–640.

Krogsgaard-Larsen, P. & Hjeds, H. (1974) Organic hydroxylamine derivatives. X. Structural analogues of γ-aminobutyric acid (GABA) of the isoxazole enol-betaine type. Synthesis of 5,6,7,8-tetrahydro-4*H*-isoxazolo[4,5-*d*]azepin-3-ol zwitterion and 4,5,6,7-tetrahydroisoxazolo[4,5-*c*]pyridin-3-ol zwitterion. *Acta Chem. Scand.* B28, 533–538.

Krogsgaard-Larsen, P. & Johnston, G. A. R. (1975) Inhibition of GABA uptake in rat brain slices by nipecotic acid, various isoxazoles and related compounds. *J. Neurochem.* 25, 797–802.

Krogsgaard-Larsen, P. & Johnston, G. A. R. (1978) Structure-activity studies on the inhibition of GABA binding to rat brain membranes by muscimol and related compounds. *J. Neurochem.* 30, 1377–1382.

Krogsgaard-Larsen, P., Johnston, G. A. R., Curtis, D. R., Game, C. J. A. & McCulloch, R. M. (1975) Structure and biological activity of a series of conformationally restricted analogues of GABA. *J. Neurochem.* 25, 803–809.

Krogsgaard-Larsen, P., Johnston, G. A. R., Lodge, D. & Curtis, D. R. (1977a) A new class of GABA agonists. *Nature* 268, 53–55.

Krogsgaard-Larsen, P., Larsen, A. L. N. & Thyssen, K. (1978) GABA receptor agonists. Synthesis of muscimol analogues including (*R*)- and (*S*)-5-(1-aminoethyl)-3-isoxazolol and (*RS*)-5-aminomethyl-2-isoxazolin-3-ol. *Acta Chem. Scand.* In press.

Krogsgaard-Larsen, P., Natova, L. & Christensen, S. B. (1977b) Muscimol analogues. I. Synthesis of 4- and 8-aminocyclohepteno[1,2-*d*]isoxazol-3-ols and 4-(3-aminopropyl)-5-methyl-3-isoxazolol. *Acta Chem. Scand.* B31, 577–583.

Lloyd, K. G., Dreksler, S. & Bird, E. D. (1977a) Alteration in ^{3}H-GABA binding in Huntington's chorea. *Life Sci.* 21, 747–753.

Lloyd, K. G., Möhler, H., Heitz, Ph. & Bartholini, G. (1975) Distribution of choline acetyltransferase and glutamate decarboxylase within the substantia nigra and in other brain regions from control and parkinsonian patients. *J. Neurochem.* 25, 789–795.

Lloyd, K. G., Shemen, L. & Hornykiewicz, O. (1977b) Distribution of high affinity sodium independent ^{3}H-gamma-aminobutyric acid (^{3}H-GABA) binding in the human brain: alterations in Parkinson's disease. *Brain Res.* 127, 269–278.

Martin, D. L. (1976) Carrier-mediated transport and removal of GABA from synaptic regions. In: *GABA in Nervous System Function,* eds. Roberts, E., Chase, T. N. & Tower, D. B., pp. 347–386, Raven Press, New York.

McGeer, P. L. & McGeer, E. G. (1976a) The GABA system and function of the basal ganglia: Huntington's disease. In: *GABA in Nervous System Function,* eds. Roberts, E., Chase, T. N. & Tower, D. B., pp. 487–495, Raven Press, New York.

McGeer, P. L. & McGeer, E. G. (1976b) Enzymes associated with the metabolism of catecholamines, acetylcholine and GABA in human controls and patients with Parkinson's disease and Huntington's chorea. *J. Neurochem.* 26, 65–76.

Naik, S. R., Guidotti, A. & Costa, E. (1976) Central GABA receptor agonists: comparison of muscimol and baclofen. *Neuropharmacology.* 15, 479–484.

Ott, J., Wheaton, P. S. & Chilton, W. S. (1975) Fate of muscimol in the mouse. *Physiol. Chem. Physics.* 7, 381–384.

Pauling, L. (1944) *The Nature of the Chemical Bond,* p. 175. Cornell University Press, New York.

Pullman, B. (1976) Quantum-mechanical studies on the effect of water on the conformation of two biologically important zwitterionic systems: polar head of phospholipids and GABA. In: *Environmental Effects on Molecular Structure and Properties,* ed. Pullman, B., pp. 55–80. D. Reidel Publ. Comp., Dordrecht–Holland.

Pullman, B. & Berthod, H. (1975) Molecular orbital studies on the conformation of GABA (γ-aminobutyric acid). *Theoret. Chim. Acta* (Berl.) 36, 317–328.

Quilico, A. (1962) Isoxazoles and related compounds. In: *The Chemistry of Heterocyclic Compounds,* ed. Weisberger, A., pp. 1–230, John Wiley & Sons, New York.

Roberts, E. (1974) γ-Aminobutyric acid and nervous system function – A perspective. *Biochem. Pharmac.* 23, 2637–2649.

Schousboe, A., Krogsgaard-Larsen, P., Svenneby, G. & Hertz, L. (1978) Inhibition of the high affinity, net uptake of GABA into cultured astrocytes by β-proline, nipecotic acid and other compounds. *Brain Res.* 153, 623–626.

Theobald, W., Büch, O., Kunz, H. A., Krupp, P., Stenger, E. G. & Heimann, H. (1968) Pharmakologische und experimentalpsykologische untersuchungen mit 2 inhaltsstoffen des fliegenpilzes (Amanita muscaria). *Arzneimittelforsch.* 18, 311–315.

Van Kammen, D. P. (1977) γ-Aminobutyric acid (GABA) and the dopamine hypothesis of schizophrenia. *Am. J. Psychiat.* 134, 138–143.

Wong, D. T. & Horng, J. S. (1977) Sodium-independent binding of GABA to the Triton X-100 treated synaptic membranes from cerebellum of rat brain. *Life Sci.* 20, 445–451.

Subcellular Localization of GABA-Receptors; Visualization of Specific Synaptic Components

Helmut Bittiger

The molecular mechanism of neurotransmission is still incompletely understood. In this context the synaptic area is not sufficiently well characterized by specific high resolution histochemistry. Classical centrifugational methods have been fully exploited to subfractionate a number of synaptic elements for their biochemical analysis. Due to principal technical limits of these methods, further subfractionations were not possible, e.g. the separation of presynaptic from postsynaptic membranes, which is of utmost importance for the localization of binding sites in the newly developed radio-receptor assays.

In the present paper the problems are approached by a combination of three different methods: 1. The subcellular distribution of particulate anionic sites and of covalently bound carbohydrates was studied in the electron microscope at a resolution of about 100 Å by using derivatives of the marker ferritin, a ferroprotein containing several thousand iron atoms (Crichton 1973). 2. The specific distributions of these synaptic anionic sites and carbohydrates were exploited to separate synaptic elements by using suitable affinity gels. Fractions enriched in postsynaptic elements were obtained. 3. An ^{3}H-muscimol assay was developed for the study of GABA-receptors; the binding sites were localized on the different subcellular fractions.

Ad 1. The distribution of membrane and particle bound anionic sites in the synaptic area was of interest, as electrical properties of synaptic structures may play a role in neurotransmission. According to histochemical studies, carbohydrates seem to be enriched in the synaptic cleft, at the axon hillock and at the

Research Department, Pharmaceuticals Division, CIBA-GEIGY Ltd. Basle, Switzerland.

"GABA-NEUROTRANSMITTERS", Alfred Benzon Symposium 12, Munksgaard 1978

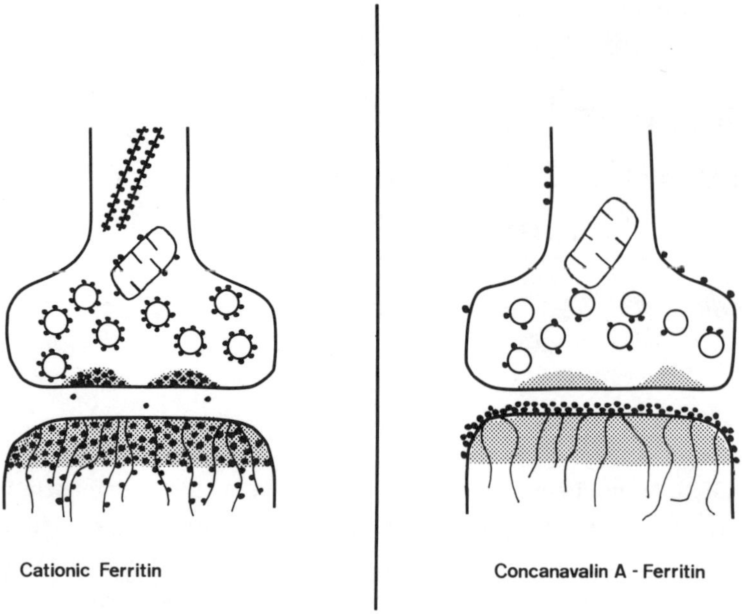

Fig. 1. Schemes of the staining patterns of cationic ferritin and concanavalin A-ferritin at synapses. Cationic ferritin binds also within the synaptic cleft to structures which can be removed by 1 M Nacl (not demonstrated).

Node of Ranvier, places where membrane potentials are generated (Pfenninger 1973). The electron microscopic studies have already been published (Bittiger & Schnebli 1974, Bittiger & Heid 1977). In short, ferritin derivatized with a high number of quaternary ammonium groups – and thus representing a highly cationized probe for the detection of anionic sites – was used to study the distribution of clusters of negative charges on neuronal membranes and other particulate components of the brain (see Scheme in Fig. 1). Such clusters could *not* be detected on the inner or outer surfaces of synaptic membranes; large concentrations were observed on synaptic vesicles, within pre- and postsynaptic densities, on microtubules, microfilaments and other cytoplasmic components and also on the surface and within the lamellae of myelin. Mitochondria were not heavily stained. Cationic ferritin was also bound within the synaptic cleft. The density, however, varied from synapse to synapse. The binding was drastically reduced when the membrane fractions were exposed to 1 M NaCl before incubation with cationic ferritin (under isotonic conditions). Therefore these anionic sites appear to be weakly bound within the cleft.

Lectins which specifically bind to carbohydrates were covalently linked to ferritin and used to study the distribution of mannosides or glucosides (concanavalin A) and galactosides (ricin) on neuronal elements (Bittiger & Schnebli, 1974, 1976) (Scheme in Fig. 1). A low density, well - dispersed distribution of lectin-ferritin was observed on most subcellular structures except mitochondria, which were devoid of any stain; a very high density of label, however, was accumulated on the postsynaptic membranes just along the postsynaptic density of any type of synapse. These findings were also reported by Cotman & Taylor (1974) and Matus & Walters (1976); the latter observed also binding of concanavalin A at the cytoplasmic site of Gray type II postsynaptic membranes.

Ad. 2 The specific distributions of anionic sites and carbohydrates were exploited to subfractionate further synaptic elements by affinity gels carrying cationic groups or lectins. Fractions enriched in postsynaptic structures were obtained by affinity binding on Concanavalin A-Sepharose (Bittiger 1976a,b). The method has been meanwhile improved by inclusion of an ionic exchange step and other modifications and will be described in detail in this paper.

EXPERIMENTAL

^{3}H-Muscimol radioreceptor-assay

Preparation of cerebellar membranes. Rat brain cerebella were homogenized in 6 volumes of 0.32 M sucrose in a glass-Teflon homogenizer. The suspension was sedimented at 1000 x g for 10 min and the resulting supernatant at 8000 x g for 15 min at 4°C. The pellets were resuspended in 1 mM Tris-HCl pH 7, containing 2 mM EDTA and left for 40 min at 4°C. The material was centrifuged twice at 30.000 x g for 20 min; the pellets were suspended in 50 mM Tris-citrate buffer pH 7.1, at 20°C. This was the standard preparation.

Radio-receptor assay. A centrifugational assay was used. Membranes (about 300–500 μg) were incubated in 1 ml 50 mM Tris-citrate buffer pH 7.1, containing ^{3}H-Muscimol (12 Ci/mmol, New England Nuclear) and unlabeled compounds for 7 min at room temperature and then centrifugated for 8 min at 12,000 x g. The supernatants were aspirated and the tips of the tubes containing the pellets were cut off and transferred into counting vials containing 1 ml Soluene (Packard). After dissolution of the pellets, 10 ml of Instagel was added and the

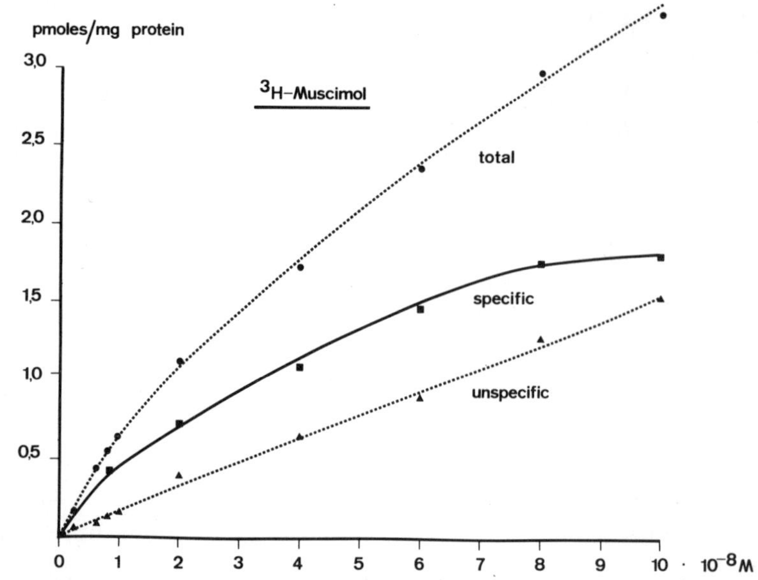

Fig. 2. Binding of ^{3}H-muscimol to cerebellar membranes.

probes were counted at an efficiency of 39% in an Intertechnique liquid scintillation counter.

Preparation of postsynaptic fractions

In the following a standard procedure is described.

Crude mitochondrial fractions. Twenty rat cortices (about 20 g) were homogenized in a glass-Teflon homogenizer in 6 volumes 1 mM phosphate buffer pH 7 containing 0.32 M sucrose and 1 mM $MgCl_2$. The suspension was centrifugated at 1000 x g for 15 min and the procedure was repeated with the resuspended pellet. The pooled supernatants were sedimented at 30,000 x g for 20 min (about 150 mg protein).

Ion exchange step. The pellets were homogenized in 50 ml 10 mM Tris-HCl pH 6.5, containing 0.15 M NaCl, and mixed with 50 ml QAE Sephadex (Pharmacia) equilibrated in the same buffer and shaken for 5 min. The whole suspension was filtered on nylon gauze (30 μ mesh) and washed with 20–30 ml buffer. The filtrate was sedimented at 30,000 x g for 20 min (about 70 mg protein). All these procedures were performed at 4°C.

Affinity-binding. This pellet was resuspended in 50 ml 100 mM acetate buffer pH 6.5 containing 0.3 M NaCl, 1 mM each $MnCl_2$, $MgCl_2$ and $CaCl_2$, mixed with 50 ml Concanavalin A-Sepharose (Pharmacia) in the same buffer at 20°C. The suspension was shaken for 15 min, filtered on nylon gauze and washed with 1–2 l buffer. The Concanavalin A-Sepharose gel trapped on the gauze was suspended in acetate buffer containing 0.2 M of the competitive inhibitor α-methyl mannoside (total volume 100 ml) and kept for at least 3 h at 4°C. The suspension was filtered and washed on nylon gauze. The filtrate was sedimented at 50,000 x g for 20 min. This material is considered as the fraction enriched in postsynaptic particles (about 2 mg protein). Standard procedures were used in electron microscopy. Protein was determined according to Lowry.

RESULTS

^{3}H-Muscimol radio-receptor assay

In Fig. 2 the binding characteristic of ^{3}H-Muscimol to cerebellar membranes is presented. Values are the means of two typical experiments performed in

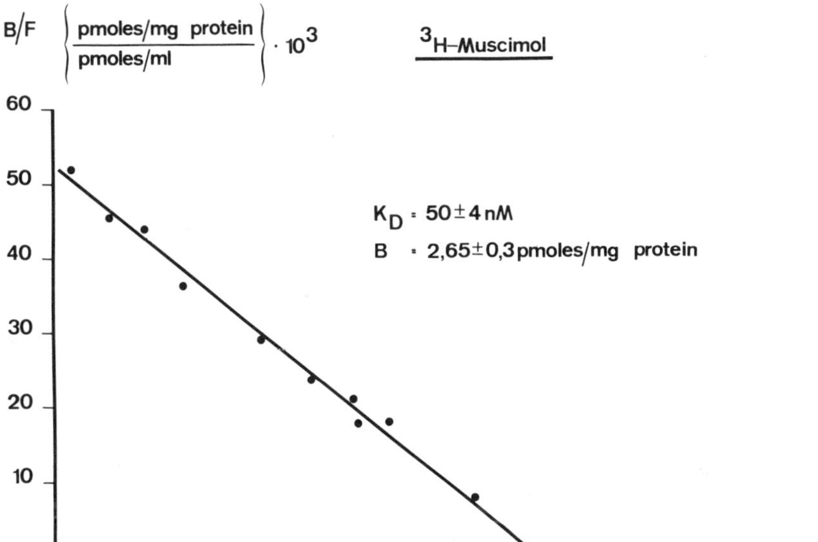

Fig. 3. Scatchard plot of the binding of ^{3}H-Muscimol to cerebellar membranes (K_D=dissociation constant, B=^{3}H-muscimol specifically bound to cerebellar membranes).

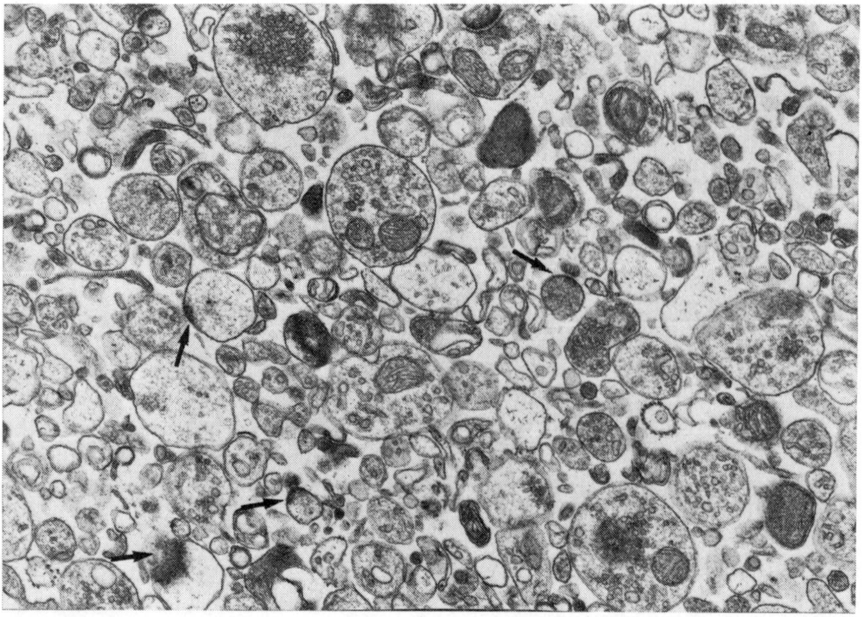

Fig. 4. Electron micrograph of a crude mitochondrial fraction of cerebral cortex; Magnification 21500 x. Postsynaptic particles marked by arrows.

triplicates, which varied less than 10%. Unspecific binding was determined in the presence of 10^{-4}M muscimol. Specific binding ranged from 80% to 50% of total binding. The association time at 20°C is estimated to be less than 3 min, as the binding was already saturated after this time.

From the corresponding Scatchard plot (between 1×10^{-10}M and 3×10^{-7}M) in Fig. 3 a K_D of : 50±4 nM and a density of receptor sites of 2.65±0.3 pmoles/mg protein were calculated. Binding experiments with frozen membranes (−18°C for at least 12 h) or in the presence of 100 mM Na^+ showed only minor differences when compared to those with fresh membranes. Pretreatment of membranes with 0.2% Triton, however, increased the specific binding in the range of 1–10 nM ^{3}H-muscimol by a factor of 2–3, indicative of new binding sites. A careful analysis has not yet been performed.

Inhibition of binding of 5 nM ^{3}H-muscimol by different compounds was also studied. The corresponding K_i values were calculated from the IC_{50} values according to the equation $K_i = IC_{50}/(1 + C/K_D)$ where C is the doncentration of the radioactive ligand and K_D is the dissociation constant.

The values found were: Muscimol 35 nM, GABA 110 nM, Bicuculline 5000 nM and bicuculline methiodide 40,000 nM. Concanavalin A at 10^{-5}M did not interfere with the binding.

Postsynaptic fractions

Electron microscopy. In Fig. 4 an electron micrograph of the crude mitochondrial fraction and in Fig. 5 one of the postsynaptic fractions are presented. Both micrographs are at the same magnification. Fig. 4 shows typical large synaptosomes in high number, but also some isolated postsynaptic particles (arrows). Synaptosomes are the predominant structures in these fractions. A different composition is seen in Fig. 5. Vesicle-containing structures are rare and of small size (arrows). However, a high number of postsynaptic particles is recognized by their postsynaptic web and the absence of vesicles (stars). There are difficulties in identifying postsynaptic structures detached from their presynaptic counterparts. This holds especially for particles originating from Gray type II synapses (Gray 1959) which show barely any postsynaptic differentiation. The membrane structures in the postsynaptic fractions appear to be fully preserved.

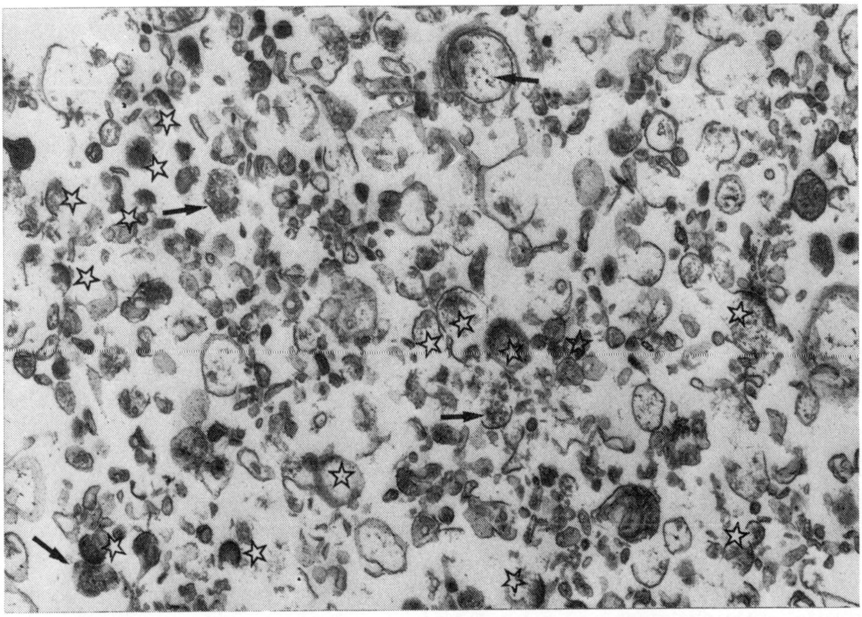

Fig. 5. Electron micrograph of a postsynaptic fraction from cerebral cortex; Magnification 21500 x. Presynaptic particles marked by arrows, postsynaptic particles by stars.

Direct biochemical methods are not available for a straightforward identification of postsynaptic material.

Radio-receptor assay. Specific binding in the fractions was usually compared at a concentration of 5 nM ^{3}H-muscimol. The assay was performed in the same way as with cerebellar membranes. Possible release of endogenous GABA from the different fractions was tested and apparently did not occur. At 5 nM ^{3}H-muscimol about 2000 cpm/mg protein were bound in the crude mitochondrial fraction, about 6000 cpm/mg in the supernatant of the ionic exchange step and 30,000–40,000 cpm in the postsynaptic fraction. The figures were comparable for cerebral cortex and cerebellum, but somewhat higher in the latter. According to these data the enrichment of GABA-receptors from the crude mitochondrial fraction to the postsynaptic fraction would be about 15.

DISCUSSION

A specific staining pattern of cationic ferritin was observed in the environment of the synaptic cleft. Vesicular membranes have completely different electric properties from synaptosomal membranes. A mere fusion of vesicular with synaptosomal membranes during transmitter release without any change in membrane composition is hard to imagine. The highly anionic properties of both vesicles and presynaptic densities would suggest a mutual repulsion of these subcellular entities, which is obviously in contrast to morphological findings. However, it is conceivable, that these negatively charged units are cross-linked by cationic species, e.g. Ca^{2+}. Binding sites for cationic ferritin seem to be relatively loosely fixed within the synaptic cleft, as they can mostly be removed in 1 M NaCl. One may speculate about a possible modulatory role of these sites in neurotransmission.

Carbohydrates – in contrast to anionic sites – seem to be very strongly bound within the synaptic cleft, most probably they are anchored within the postsynaptic density, as the binding of lectin-ferritin is fully preserved after destruction of the postsynaptic membranes by the detergent Triton X-100 (Bittiger & Schnebli 1974). The function of these covalently bound carbohydrates in neurotransmission is still unknown.

Nevertheless the specific accumulation of these compounds allowed to enrich postsynaptic structures by affinity techniques, which is at present the only method to obtain such fractions in a nondestructive way. Purification of intact postsynaptic densities cannot be achieved by conventional centrifugation methods, since there are no exploitable differences in densities between these postsynaptic and other components of crude mitochondrial or synaptosomal fractions. Only by solubilizing synaptosomal membranes with detergents and subsequently separating the postsynaptic densities – which are more resistant to that treatment – by density-gradient centrifugation, can postsynaptic material be isolated (Cotman & Taylor 1974). Exposure to detergents solubilizes more than 50% of the membrane-bound proteins (Cotman *et al.* 1971). Therefore the structural and functional integrity of the postsynaptic membrane by detergent procedures is likely to be severely impaired.

The ^{3}H-muscimol assay for GABA-receptors can be performed at 20°C with fresh untreated membranes. When using ^{3}H-GABA as a ligand, membranes have to be frozen or treated with Triton X-100 and the assay is usually performed at 4°C. The dissociation constant for the binding of ^{3}H-muscimol to fresh cerebellar membranes is very similar to the inhibitory constants of muscimol found in the ^{3}H-GABA radio-receptor assays with frozen membranes, i.e. 50 nM (Enna & Snyder 1977) and 40 nM (Olsen *et al.* 1978) or 58 nM in the ^{3}H-bicuculline methiodide assay (Möhler & Okada 1977). Bicuculline inhibits the ^{3}H-muscimol binding in fresh and the ^{3}H-GABA binding in frozen membranes with K_i values of 4–5 μM (Enna & Snyder 1977, Olsen *et al.* 1978). The K_i value of 110 nM for GABA in the ^{3}H-muscimol assay is somewhat lower than corresponding figures in ^{3}H-GABA assays. Thus the described ^{3}H-muscimol binding seems to fulfill the criteria of an GABA-radio-receptor assay. Treatment of membranes with Triton X-100 changed the binding characteristics of ^{3}H-muscimol and ^{3}H-GABA; sites with higher affinity to these ligands were induced. These findings suggest a pronounced stability of GABA-receptors as with the detergent concentrations used, already membrane proteins are dissolved and at least part of postsynaptic membranes are damaged according to electron microscopic studies (Cotman & Taylor 1974, Bittiger & Schnebli 1974). Thus, despite the high stability of GABA-receptors, a change in the membrane environment or even a loss of important components such as ionophores may be expected.

In our postsynaptic fractions GABA-receptors appear to be already significantly enriched. A density of 40–60 pmoles/mg protein receptor sites was calculated. Assuming a molecular weight of 50000 dalton for the GABA-receptor, about one out of 500 protein weight units would represent one receptor. The figures in enrichment from the crude mitochondrial fraction to the postsynaptic fraction would suggest a mostly postsynaptic localization of the GABA-receptors.

Postsynaptic fractions can obviously also be used to study the localization of ligands for other types of receptors, e.g. those of biogenic amines or diazepam.

ACKNOWLEDGMENT

The excellent technical assistance of J. Heid and W. Hofacher is gratefully acknowledged.

REFERENCES:

Bittiger, H. & Schnebli, H. P. (1974) Binding of concanavalin A and ricin to synaptic junctions of rat brain. *Nature* 249, 370–371.

Bittiger, H. & Schnebli, H. P. (1976) *Concanavalin A as a Tool*, pp. 95–122, John Wiley & Sons, London, New York.

Bittiger, H. (1976a) Fractionation of rat brain by affinity binding on Concanavalin A-Sepharose: separation of mitochondria and postsynaptic densities. *Exp. Brain Res.* 24, 1–23.

Bittiger, H. (1976b) Separation of subcellular fractions from rat brain. In: *Concanavalin A as a Tool*, ed. Bittiger, H. & Schnebli, H. P., 435–445. John Wiley & Sons, London, New York.

Bittiger, H. & Heid, J. (1977) The subcellular distribution of particle – bound negative charges in rat brain. *J. Neurochem.* 28, 917–922.

Cotman, C. W., Levy, W., Banker, G. & Taylor, D. (1971) An ultrastructural and chemical analysis of the effect of Triton X-100 on synaptic plasma membranes. *Biochim. Biophys. Acta* 249, 406–418.

Cotman, C. W. & Taylor, D. (1974) Localization and characterization of concanavalin A receptors in the synaptic cleft. *J. Cell Biol.* 62, 236–242.

Cotman, C. W., Banker, G., Churchill, L. & Taylor, D. (1974) Isolation of postsynaptic densities from rat brain. *J. Cell Biol.* 63, 441–455.

Crichton, R. R. (1973) Struktur und Funktion von Ferritin. *Angew. Chemie* 85, 53–62.

Enna, S. J. & Snyder, S. H. (1975) Properties of GABA-receptor binding in rat synaptic membrane fractions. *Brain Res.* 100, 81–97.

Enna, S. J. & Snyder, S. H. (1977) Influences of ions, enzymes and detergents on GABA receptor binding in synaptic membranes of rat brain. *Mol. Pharmac.* 13, 277–294.

Gray, E. G. (1959) Axosomatic and axo-dentritic synapses of the cerebral cortex. An electron microscope study. *J. Anat.* 93, 420–433.

Matus, A., de Petris, S. & Raff, M. C. (1973) Mobility of concanavalin A receptors in myelin and in synaptic membranes *Nature* (New Biol.) 244, 278–280.

Matus, A. I. & Walters, B. B. (1976) Type 1 and 2 synaptic junctions: Differences in distribution of concanavalin A binding sites and stability of the junctional adhesion. *Brain Res.* 108, 249–256.

Möhler, H. & Okada, T. (1977) GABA receptor binding with $^{3}H(+)$ bicuculline methiodide in rat CNS. *Nature 267*, 65–67.

Olsen, R. W., Ticku, M. K., Van Ness, P. C. & Greenlee, D. (1978) Effect of drugs on GABA receptors, uptake, release and synthesis *in vitro*. *Brain Res.* 139, 277–294.

Pfenninger, K. H. (1973) Synaptic morphology and cytochemistry. In: *Progress in Histochemistry and Cytochemistry,* vol. 5, pp. 1–86. Gustav Fischer Verlag, Stuttgart, Portland.

Wong, D. T. & Horng, J. S. (1977) Na^+-independent binding of GABA to the Triton X-100 - treated synaptic membranes from cerebellum of rat brain. *Life Sciences* 20, 445–452.

Specific Inhibitors of GABA Metabolism

Robert R. Rando

Highly specific irreversible enzyme inhibitors can be designed by incorporating latent reactive groups into substrates for the target enzyme. The turnover of these molecules generates a reactive intermediate which can directly inactivate the enzyme by reaction with an active-site amino acid, or where relevant, the cofactor (Rando 1974). In this paper inhibitors of this type which inactivate GABA transaminase and glutamate decarboxylase will be discussed.

Gabaculine ((−)-5-amino-1,3-cyclohexadiene carboxylic acid) is a naturally occurring neurotoxin isolated from *Strep toyocaenis* (Mishima *et al.* 1976, Rando & Bangerter 1976). The molecule is a potent irreversible inactivator of

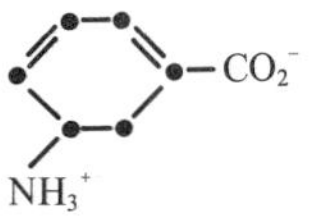

Gabaculine

GABA transaminase (Rando & Bangerter 1976, Rando 1977, Rando & Bangerter 1977a). Pseudo first – order plots for the inactivation of the mouse brain enzyme are shown in Fig. 1. The mode of inactivation is of the "k_{cat}" or suicide type which require catalytic turnover of the drug by the target enzyme prior to inhibition (Rando 1974). The equation appropriate for these inhibitors is shown below. The K_I for the drug binding to the mouse brain enzyme is

$$E + I \underset{K_I}{\rightleftharpoons} E \cdot I \xrightarrow{k_{cat}} E \cdot I' \xrightarrow{k_{cat}} E - I'$$

Department of Pharmacology, Harvard Medical School, Boston, MA 02115 USA

"GABA-NEUROTRANSMITTERS", Alfred Benzon Symposium 12, Munksgaard 1978

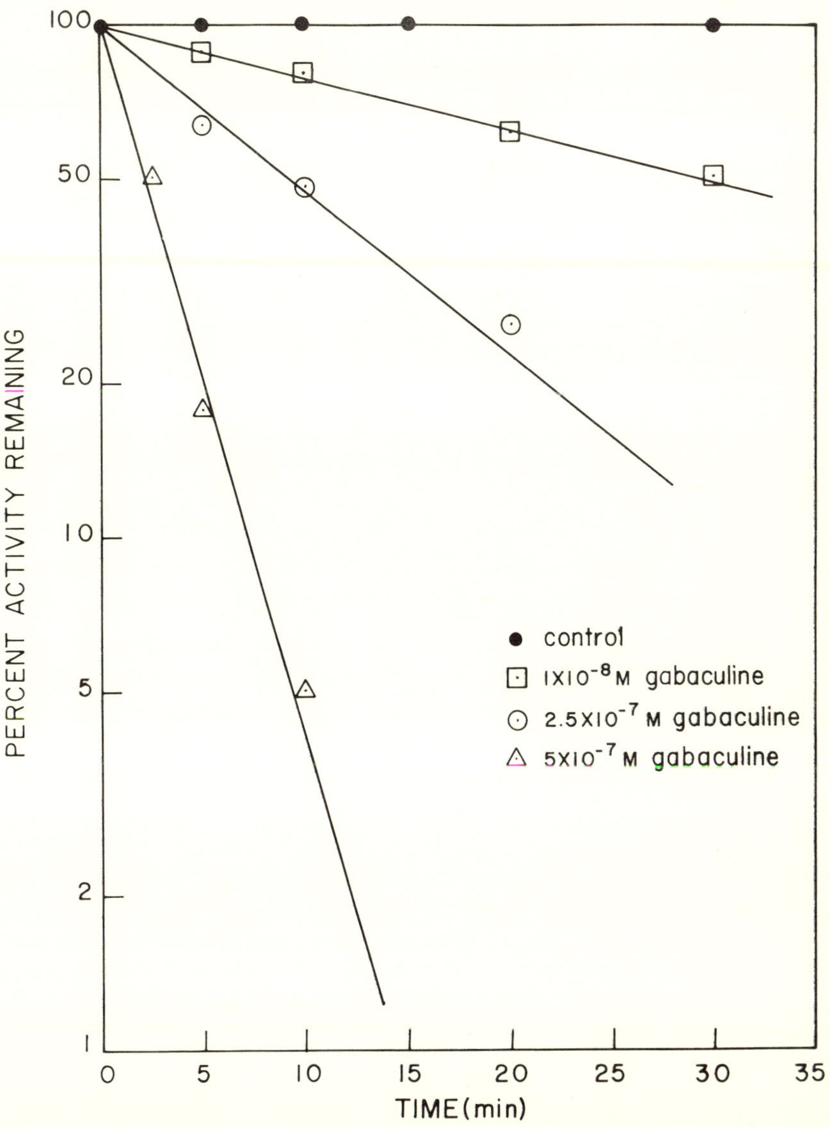

Fig. 1. Irreversible inhibition of GABA-transaminase by gabaculine; 0.05 units of mouse brain enzyme (specific activity=0.03 units/mg) was incubated with gabaculine at the indicated concentrations (based on L-gabaculine) in 0.1 ml of 0.1 M potassium phosphate buffer, pH 8.3 at 37°C. A unit of enzyme is defined as the amount of enzyme required to catalyze the formation of 1 μmol of product per min under standard conditions. At the indicated times aliquots of the enzyme were removed and the remaining activity determined by the standard methods. The activity of the inactive enzyme would not be increased in the slightest by extended dialysis against the phosphate buffer.

5.8×10^{-7}M and the k_{cat} is 1.35×10^{-1}. The half-life of the enzyme at this concentration is 5 min. The K_I for the compound is exceptionally low, being some three orders of magnitude lower than the K_m for GABA. The mechanism of inactivation involves the following sequence of steps.

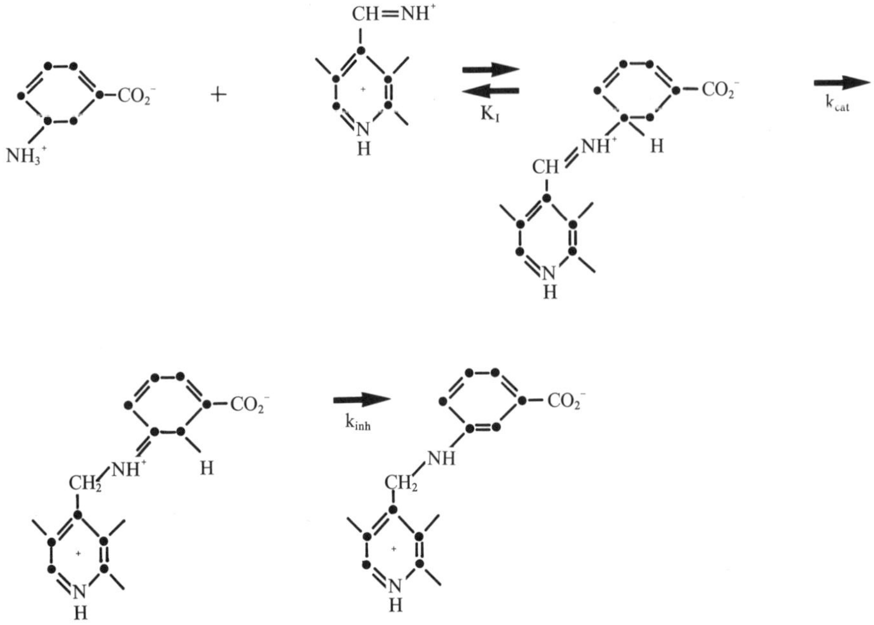

CPP_P

The aromatization mechanism represents a highly novel mode of enzyme inactivation which should be generally applicable to other pyridoxal phosphate – linked enzymes. We demonstrated that this mechanism obtains here by showing that (1) there is a deuterium isotope effect on inhibition with 5-deutero substituted gabaculines, (2) 6-deutero gabaculines show no isotope effect on inhibition even though tracer studies show that the 6-H is lost during inactivation and (3) *meta*-carboxyphenylpyridoxamine phosphate (CPP_P) could be liberated from the enzyme by denaturation after inactivation of the enzyme with ^{3}H-gabaculine (Rando 1977, Rando & Bangerter 1977a). Furthermore, model studies with gabaculine and pyridoxal phosphate and enzymological studies with gabaculine analogs are also wholly consistent with the postulated mechanism (Rando 1977, Rando & Bangerter 1977a).

The enzyme is inactivated because the aromatized cofactor adduct CPP_P binds exceedingly tightly to the active-site of the enzyme and can only be liberated by denaturing conditions. It is noteworthy that only a single turnover of gabaculine by the enzyme is sufficient for inactivation to occur. Since gabaculine requires catalytic turnover by the target enzyme, it is not surprising to find that it is a highly specific inhibitor of GABA transaminase. We have tested gabaculine as a possible inhibitor of a large number of pyridoxal phosphate – linked enzymes including aspartate aminotransferase, alanine aminotransferase, glutamate decarboxylase and ornithine decarboxylase and found it to be inert.

The great specificity of gabaculine can be taken advantage of for *in vivo* studies. When given i.p. to mice, gabaculine inactivates the brain enzyme with a concomitant rise in endogeneous GABA levels (Rando & Bangerter 1977b). At high single doses of gabaculine (100 mg/kg mouse) the brain enzyme is irreversibly inactivated with a $t_{1/2}$ of approximately 1 h. Endogeneous GABA levels rise and after 20 h achieve a level 15–20 times that of the control. Brain aspartate aminotransferase levels are not changed under these conditions. There are several important things to note here. First of all, gabaculine penetrates the blood-brain barrier, albeit not well, whereas GABA does not. This is the reason why relatively high concentrations of the drug must be used *in vivo* to achieve significant inactivation of the brain enzyme. In this context, however, it should be noted that multiple dosing of gabaculine allows the use of much lower concentrations. Secondly, mice treated with gabaculine show behavioral signs quite similar to those reported for the human molecular disease hyper β alanemia (also called hyper-Gabanuria) (Scriver & Perry 1972). The outward signs of this disease are seizures followed by prolonged somnolence. The disease has two names because the GABA transaminase which is lacking or inactive here degrades both GABA and β-alanine. The important point here is that the use of highly specific enzyme inactivators will allow for the creation of models of molecular diseases.

Since GABA transaminase is located in cells other than GABA-ergic neurons in the central nervous system, for example, in the glial cells, the *in vivo* results do not clearly indicate whether inhibition of the neuronal enzyme contributes to the large increase in observed GABA levels. Furthermore, the *in vivo* studies also do not indicate whether the high levels of GABA are functional. That is, can this increased GABA that is formed be released? To answer these and other questions, we have begun a study of the effects of gabaculine on chick embryo spinal cord GABA-ergic neurons in culture. These cultures which lack non-neuronal cells have been developed by Dr. G. D. Fischbach and his associates in the Department of Pharmacology at Harvard Medical School (Fischbach *et al.*, unpublished experiments). We have found that chick spinal cord and brain GABA transaminases are highly sensitive to inactivation by gabaculine. At 9 μM gabaculine the $t_{1/2}$ for the chick embryo enzyme is 5 min in the presence of 6 mM GABA. As expected, when gabaculine is injected into a chick yolk, marked increases in spinal cord and brain GABA are observed (Rando *et al.*, unpublished experiments) (Fig. 2). Treatment of spinal cord cultures containing only neuronal cells leads to a rapid accumulation of GABA. The level of accumulation is dose-dependent, but at 10^{-7}M gabaculine increases of up to 10-fold in neuronal GABA are found after incubating with inhibitor for 0.5 h followed by treatment of the cells with radioactive glutamate for 7 h (Fig. 3). Clearly, gabaculine is exceedingly potent in this system. This increase in GABA

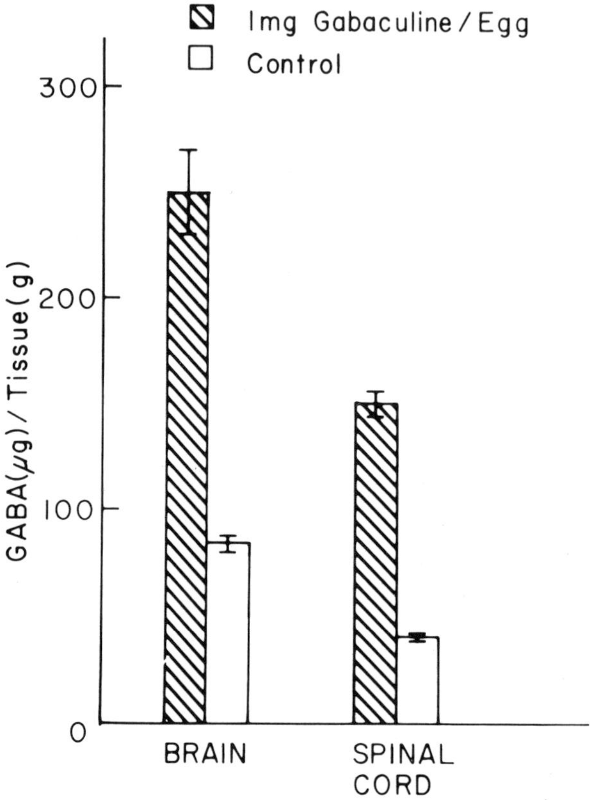

Fig. 2. Increase in chick embryo GABA levels after treatment with gabaculine. 1 mg dl-gabaculine in 0.2 ml saline was injected into 18–day chick embryo yolk sacs. Control animals were injected with 0.2 ml saline. After 24 h the spinal cords and brains were removed and the GABA levels were determined (Rando & Bangerter 1977b).

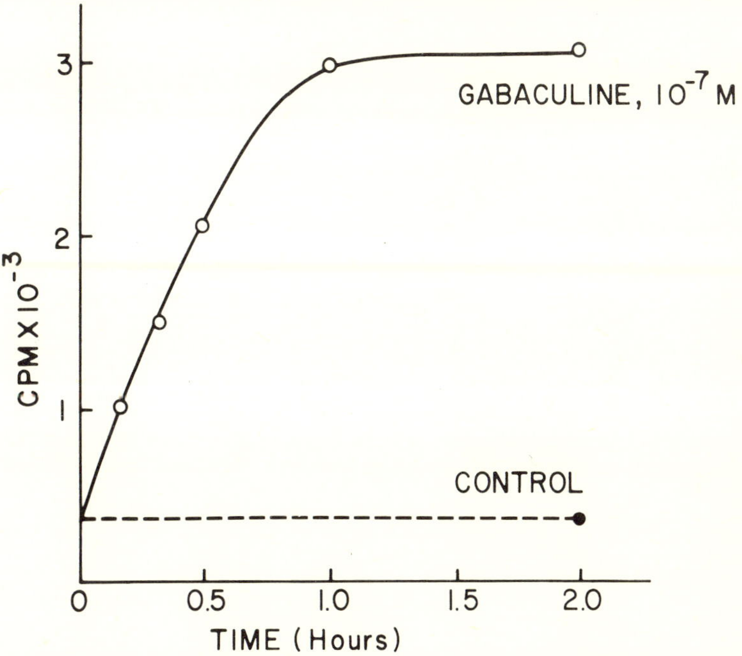

Fig. 3. Time-dependent increase in GABA levels in spinal cord cultures treated with 10^{-7} M gabaculine. 13–day dissociated chick embryo spinal cord cultures (Fischbach *et al.*, unpublished experiments) in minimal essential medium containing 0.25% horse serum (MEM+¼ HS) were incubated with 10^{-7}M dl-gabaculine at 37°C 5% CO_2. At the indicated times the gabaculine was removed by washing with medium twice (2 ml each time). The cultures were then incubated with 8 μl of ^{3}H-glutamate (1 μM SA=50 Ci/mmole) in a total volume of 200 μl for an additional 7 h. The excess glutamate was washed off and the cells were lyophilized. The resulting powder was taken up in 75 μl electrophoresis buffer (25 ml formic acid; 80 ml acetic acid diluted to 1 liter with H_2O) containing 1 mg/ml GABA and 1 mg/ml glutamate. The GABA and glutamate were separated by electrophoresis, eluted from the paper and counted. Each point on the graph represents an average of four experiments.

levels is intracellular because only the cells in this culture were assayed for GABA. It will be of interest to see if these high levels of GABA are releasable. Experiments to decide this point are in progress now.

There are several interesting developmental questions to be answered in this tissue culture system. Long and short-term treatment of these cultures with low levels of gabaculine could have an effect in modulating the levels of GABA-ergic neurons. Short-term electrophysiological experiments can decide whether otherwise silent, non-GABA-ergic cells can be rendered fundamentally GABA-ergic in the presence of gabaculine and in the long-term whether uncomitted cells can be switched to GABA-ergic due to the increased GABA levels. Experiments aimed at deciding these points are currently in progress.

As discussed above, the use of gabaculine allows for the selective increase in GABA levels and in tissue culture. It would, of course, be quite interesting to have a selective irreversible inactivator of pyridoxal phosphate – linked L-glutamate decarboxylase, the enzyme responsible for the biosynthesis of GABA. One such inhibitor is 2-trifluoromethylglutamic acid (Rando *et al.*, unpublished experiments).

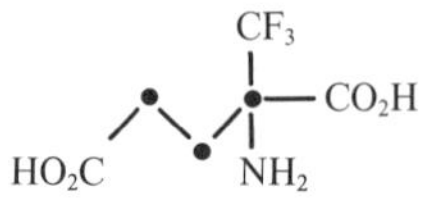

α -trifluoromethyl glutamic acid

This compound inactivates chick embryo brain L-glutamate decarboxylase. The inactivation is first-order in inhibitor. With a $t_{1/2}=3.5$ min at 5×10^{-5} M inhibitor. The molecule seems to be specific in that other pyridoxal linked enzymes such as aspartate aminotransferase, GABA transaminase, alanine aminotransferase and ornithine decarboxylase are not in the least irreversibly inhibited by these molecules in the millimolar ranges. Furthermore, the inhibitor does not inactivate apo-glutamate decarboxylase and the inactivation of the holoenzyme is competitively slowed down by the substrate L-glutamate. A possible mechanism for the inactivation of glutamate decarboxylase by this molecule by analogy with the work of Abeles on the inactivation of various pyridoxal phosphate linked enzymes by trifluoroalanine, is as follows (Silverman & Abeles 1976):

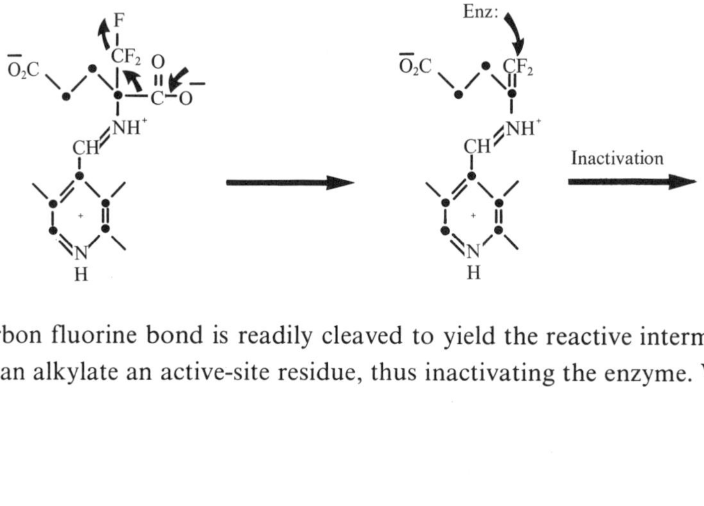

The carbon fluorine bond is readily cleaved to yield the reactive intermediate which can alkylate an active-site residue, thus inactivating the enzyme. We are currently studying the effects of this inhibitor on glutamate decarboxylase in tissue culture. Preliminary experiments suggest a powerful inhibition of the enzyme in these cultures with a concomitant decrease in endogenous GABA levels. It will be of interest to see if the inhibition of glutamate decarboxylase will inhibit GABA-ergic synapse formation in the short- and long-term. Furthermore, since glutamate decarboxylase can be taken as a marker enzyme for GABA-ergic neurons, unlike GABA transaminase, the use of highly radiolabeled α-trifluoromethyl glutamate should enable one to map GABA-ergic connectivity.

REFERENCES

Fischbach, G. D., Farb, D. & Choi, D., unpublished experiments.

Mishima, H., Kurihara, H., Kobayashi, K., Miyazawa, S. & Terahara, A. (1976) Gabaculine: γ-aminobutyrate aminotransferase inhibitor of microbial origin. *Tetrahedron Lett.* 7, 537–539.

Rando, R. R. (1974) The chemistry and enzymology of k_{cat} inhibitors. *Science* 185, 320–324.

Rando, R. R. & Bangerter, F. W. (1976) The irreversible inhibition of mouse brain GABA transaminase by gabaculine. *J. Am. Chem. Soc.* 98, 6762–6764.

Rando, R. R. (1977) The mechanism of the irreversible inhibition of GABA transaminase by the neurotoxin gabaculine. *Biochemistry* 16, 4604–4610.

Rando, R. R. & Bangerter, F. W. (1977a) The reaction of the neurotoxin gabaculine with pyridoxal phosphate. *J. Am. chem. Soc.* 99, 5141–5145.

Rando, R. R. & Bangerter, F. W. (1977b) The *in vivo* inhibition of GABA transaminase by gabaculine. *Biochem. Biophys. Res. commun.* 76, 1276–1281.

Rando, R. R., Bangerter, F. W. & Farb, D., unpublished experiments.

Scriver, C. R. & Perry, T. L. (1972) In: *The Metabolic Basis of inherited Disease*, 3rd ed., ed. Stanbury, J. B., Wyngaarden, D. B. & Fredrickson, D. S. Chapter 25. McGraw – Hill, New York.

Silverman, R. B. & Abeles, R. H. (1976) Inactivation of pyridoxal phosphate-dependent enzymes by mono and polyhaloamines. *Biochemistry* 15, 4718–4723.

γ-Acetylenic GABA and γ-Vinyl GABA – Two Enzyme-Activated Irreversible Inhibitors of GABA Aminotransferase

Brian W. Metcalf, Michel J. Jung, Bruce Lippert, Patrick Casara, Peter Böhlen & Paul J. Schechter

An enzyme inhibitor which requires activation by the target enzyme prior to that enzyme's irreversible inactivation must, by necessity, be extremely specific, because it will inhibit only those enzymes which can accept it as a substrate. Ethanolamine-O-sulfate (EOS), conceived and developed as an irreversible inhibitor of GABA aminotransferase (GABA-T; 4-aminobutyrate: 2-oxoglutarate aminotransferase, E.C.2.6.1.19) is an example of such an inhibitor. EOS is of only limited use, however, since it does not readily penetrate the blood – brain barrier (Fowler & John 1972). We hoped to take advantage of the known mechanisms of action of pyridoxal-phosphate (PyCHO)-dependent enzymes, in order to design potent irreversible inhibitors of GABA-T which would be active when administered peripherally. Inhibition of GABA-T, the enzyme responsible for the catabolism of GABA, has been associated with elevated brain levels of this neurotransmitter (Da Vanzo *et al.* 1964, Kuriyama *et al.* 1966). Furthermore, such an elevation could be expected to have a beneficial effect in several human diseases in which abnormalities in GABA metabolism have been demonstrated or suggested, e.g. Huntington's disease (Bird & Iverson 1974), epilepsy and schizophrenia (Roberts 1974).

Centre de Recherche Merrell International 16, rue d'Ankara, Strasbourg, France.

"GABA-NEUROTRANSMITTERS", Alfred Benzon Symposium 12, Munksgaard 1978

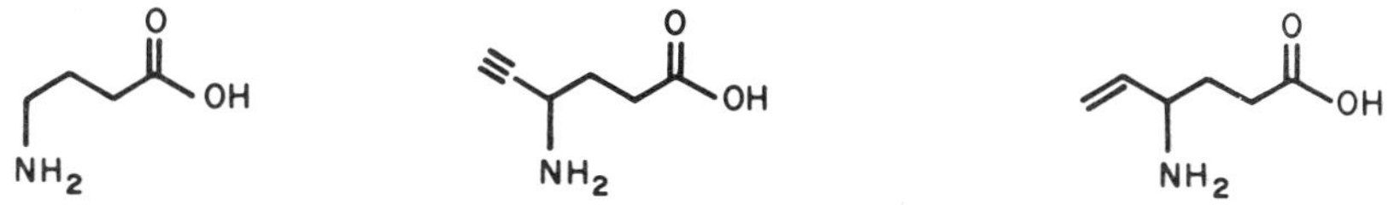

GABA γ-ACETYLENIC GABA γ-VINYL GABA

FIGURE 1

PROPOSED MECHANISMS OF INHIBITION OF GABA-T

γ-Acetylenic GABA (4-aminohex-5-ynoic acid; RMI 71.645) and γ-vinyl GABA (4-aminohex-5-enoic acid; RMI 71.754) are structural analogues of GABA (Fig. 1) in which the flexible GABA structure has been preserved, while the small acetylene or vinyl groups have been added as unreactive appendages to the carbon atom bearing the γ-amino group (Metcalf & Casara 1975, Jung & Metcalf 1975, Lippert *et al.* 1977). By preserving the GABA structure as much as possible, it was hoped that these analogues would be accepted as substrates only by GABA-T.

As shown in Fig. 2, if γ-acetylenic GABA could enter the catalytic cycle in the same manner as GABA itself, then Schiff's base formation with PyCHO could occur. The usual enzymatic proton abstraction of the proton *a* to the pyridoxaldimine function could lead to the tautomeric imine (path a). In this case the acetylene group would enter into conjugation with the newly-generated imine and hence become an alkylating agent. Irreversible inhibition of the enzyme would then result from the covalent linkage of some nucleophilic residue (Nu) in the active site to the transformed inhibitor. Alternatively (path b) the proton abstraction described above could initiate the formation of an allene. Such an allene, being conjugated to the pyridine ring of the coenzyme, would also be an active alkylating agent (Jung & Metcalf 1975). A similar scheme has been proposed to account for the inhibition of plasma amine oxidase by propargylamine (Hevey *et al.* 1973, Rando & Mairena 1974).

Path a suggests that if the acetylene group were to be replaced by a vinyl group, i.e. if γ-vinyl GABA could be accepted as a substrate by GABA-T, then this vinyl group, which was originally an unreactive appendage, would be transformed by the enzyme's own mode of action into an alkylating agent which, once again, could elicit irreversible inhibition (Lippert *et al.* 1977). This process finds analogy in the irreversible inhibition of aspartate aminotransferase by vinyl glycine (Rando 1974), although an alternative mechanism for the action of vinyl glycine has now been found to be operative (Gehring *et al.* 1977).

INHIBITION OF GABA-T *IN VITRO*

When GABA-T, partially purified from pig brain, is incubated for varying time periods with γ-acetylenic GABA, a time-dependent inactivation process is observed which follows pseudo first-order kinetics. Enzymatic half-lives range from 28 min to 9 min with concentrations of inhibitor between 0.029 mM and 0.29 mM. Prolonged dialysis of inhibited preparations against several buffers containing PyCHO (10^{-4}M) do not restore enzyme activity, thus demonstrating the irreversibility of the process (Jung *et al.* 1975).

If GABA is added to the incubation medium, the rate of inactivation induced by γ-acetylenic GABA is dramatically reduced. However, if α-ketoglutarate (α-KG) is also present, this protection against inactivation is lost. Evidently, GABA is able to protect the enzyme against inhibition because the holoenzyme is transformed, in one turnover, to the pyridoxamine form which can no longer bind the inhibitor as Schiff's base formation is no longer possible. In the presence of α-KG, the pyridoxal form is regenerated and inhibition can ensue. Further evidence that the inhibition process requires a catalytically functioning

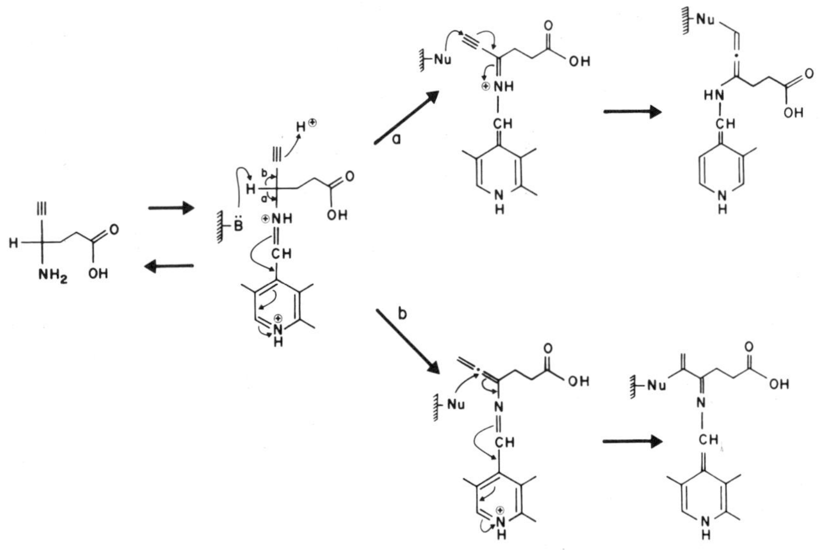

FIGURE 2

enzyme comes from the observation of a primary kinetic isotope effect when the rate of inhibition induced by 4-deuterio-4-aminohex-5-ynoic acid is compared with that induced by the 4-protio compound (Lippert *et al.* 1978). This result confirms that, in analogy to normal transamination with GABA, the enzyme must abstract a proton from carbon 4 of the inhibitor before inhibition can occur.

γ-Vinyl GABA displays a similar activity to that of γ-acetylenic GABA *in vitro* with enzymatic half-lives ranging from 11 min to 1 min with concentrations of inhibitor between 0.05 mM and 1 mM. Appropriate protection experiments using GABA and glutamate as well as the detection of a kinetic isotope effect on the rate of inhibition using 4-deuterio-4-aminohex-5-enoic acid confirm that γ-vinyl GABA is also an active site-directed irreversible inhibitor of GABA-T which requires enzyme activation (Lippert *et al.* 1977).

As far as specificity is concerned, γ-acetylenic GABA also irreversibly inactivates glutamic acid decarboxylase (GAD) *in vitro*, although to a lesser extent than it does GABA-T. γ-Vinyl GABA, however, appears to be a specific inhibitor of GABA-T. No *in vitro* inhibition of GAD or of aspartate aminotransferase has been observed even at 10 mM, although at this concentration there is an inactivation of alanine aminotransferase which is about 1000 times slower than that of GABA-T. γ-Acetylenic GABA, but not γ-vinyl GABA, is also an irreversible inhibitor of bacterial GABA-T (Jung & Metcalf 1975).

In order to probe the mechanism of the unexpected irreversible inhibition of GAD by γ-acetylenic GABA, we have examined the action of this compound on the commercially available bacterial enzyme. A major consideration guiding the choice of the bacterial enzyme rather than the mammalian one for our initial studies was that the stereochemistry of decarboxylation of 2(S)-glutamic acid to GABA has been determined with the bacterial enzyme and found to proceed with retention (Yamada & O'Leary 1978).

Our *in vitro* studies (Jung *et al.* 1978) have shown that γ-acetylenic GABA induces an irreversible time-dependent inactivation of GAD which follows pseudo first-order kinetics. Protection against inactivation is afforded by 2-methylglutamate, and by L-glutamate itself, suggesting that the inhibition process is active site-directed. A kinetic isotope effect of 2.5 at 0.33 mM inhibitor is found using 4-deuterio-4-aminohex-5-ynoic acid, demonstrating that inhibition requires a catalytically functioning enzyme and involves abstraction of the propargylic hydrogen. (±) γ-Acetylenic GABA was resolved and the inhibitory activity found to reside with the (−) isomer. The (−) isomer was assigned the R

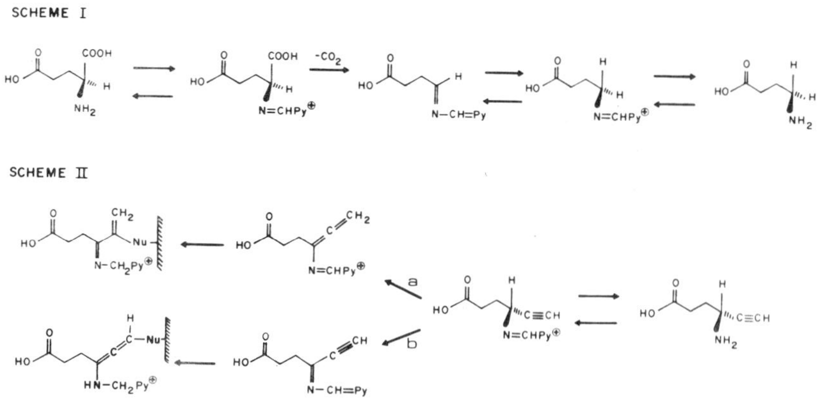

FIGURE 3

absolute configuration as oxidation with RuO_4 yielded R(−)glutamic acid, while the (+) isomer was transformed into S(+)glutamic acid (Jung *et al.* 1978).

As shown in Fig. 3, these results can be rationalized on the basis of the microscopic reversibility principle. Scheme 1 shows the normal enzymatic mechanism for the conversion of 2(S)-glutamic acid to GABA. Bearing in mind that the enzymatic replacement of CO_2 with H occurs with retention of configuration, we suggest that if 4(R)-4-aminohex-5-ynoic acid, which bears a proton stereochemically corresponding to that which replaces CO_2 in 2(S)-glutamic acid, can take the place of GABA in the reverse reaction, then the proton abstraction implicit in the reverse reaction will lead to a propargylic anionic intermediate which would induce irreversible activation of the enzyme by either of paths a or b as shown (Scheme 2).

On the other hand, it is the 4(S)-isomer which irreversibly inhibits mammalian GAD, suggesting that the bacterial and mammalian enzymes function with opposite stereochemical consequences. We believe that the exploition of the microscopic reversibility principle presages a new concept for the irreversible inhibition of amino acid decarboxylases, and have successfully applied this principle to the irreversible inhibition of mammalian ornithine decarboxylase (Metcalf *et al.* 1978).

IN VIVO BIOCHEMISTRY

As shown in Fig. 4, γ-acetylenic GABA (100 mg/kg i.p. in mice) induces an irreversible inhibition of whole brain GABA-T activity which drops to nearly

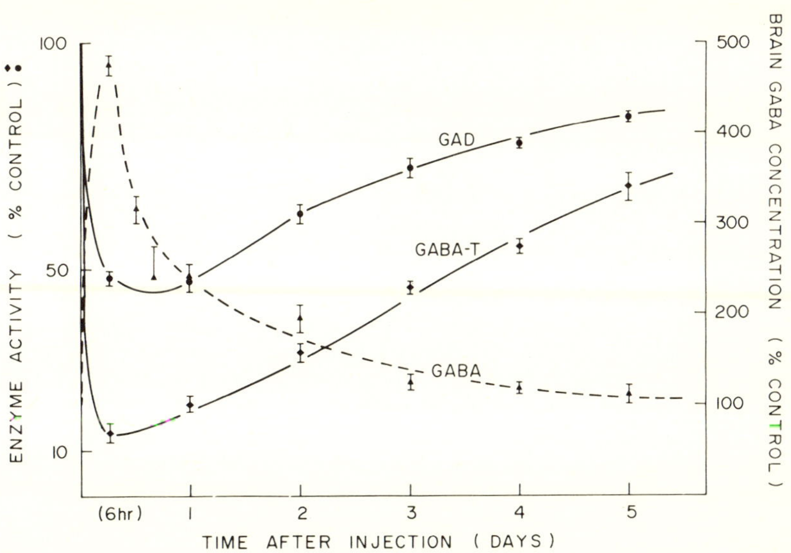

Fig. 4. Effect of a single intraperitoneal dose of γ-acetylenic GABA on mouse brain GABA-T and GAD activities and GABA concentration as a function of time. Mice of the DBA strain were injected intraperitoneally at time zero with 100 mg/kg of γ-acetylenic GABA. At given intervals, the animals were killed and brain GABA levels, GABA-T and GAD activities determined. The enzyme activities are expressed as % of control. Each value is the mean ± S.E.M. of five animals. GABA-T activity ± S.E.M. from pooled control animals is 65.0 μmol/g/h ± 1.5 (n = 34). GAD activity of control animals is 46.5 ± 1.5 μmol/g/h (n = 11). The concentration of GABA in the brain of control animals is 225 ± 6 μ/g, mean ± S.E.M. (n = 24).

zero within 2 h and remains at this level until 8 h. Even at 24 h following injection enzyme activity represents only 15–20% of control. As a result of this blockade of GABA metabolism, and despite the inhibition of GAD, which is at 40% of control activity at 8 h, whole brain concentrations of GABA rapidly increase to about 4 times those of control mice at 8 h. GABA levels then return slowly to those of control values; however, even at 24 h following injection they are still significantly greater than controls (Jung *et al.* 1977a).

Fig. 5 demonstrates the greater specificity and longer duration of action of γ-vinyl GABA compared to γ-acetylenic GABA, although considerably higher doses are required when administered by peripheral routes to achieve a comparable inhibition of GABA-T (Jung *et al.* 1977b). Thus a single dose of 1500 mg/kg i.p. in mice produces a rapid decrease in brain GABA-T activity to approximately 25% of control within 3–4 h after administration, this level of inhibition being maintained for at least 48 h. Brain GABA concentrations increase rapidly to reach a maximum at 3–4 h which represents a five – to sixfold increase over control. This level is maintained for at least 24 h, and even 4 days after injection the brain GABA concentration is still more than twice that of controls. A slow decrease in brain GAD activity is also observed which reaches a minimum of 70% of control 48 h after a single dose of 1500 mg/kg of γ-vinyl GABA. This result was unexpected since γ-vinyl GABA has no inhibitory effect on GAD *in vitro.* The decrease in GAD activity *in vivo* is compatible with a feedback inhibition of new enzyme synthesis. Such a decrease in GAD synthesis induced by accumulation of GABA via GABA-T inhibition has been demonstrated (Sze & Lovell 1970).

ANTISEIZURE ACTIVITY

DBA/2 mice (CNRS, Orleans), genetically susceptible to audiogenically-induced seizures, were chosen as a seizure model, since seizures induced in these animals are quite reproducible (Collins 1972), and changes in seizure susceptibility have been reported with changes in CNS GABA (Simler *et al.* 1973). As shown in Table I, γ-acetylenic GABA protects such mice against seizures

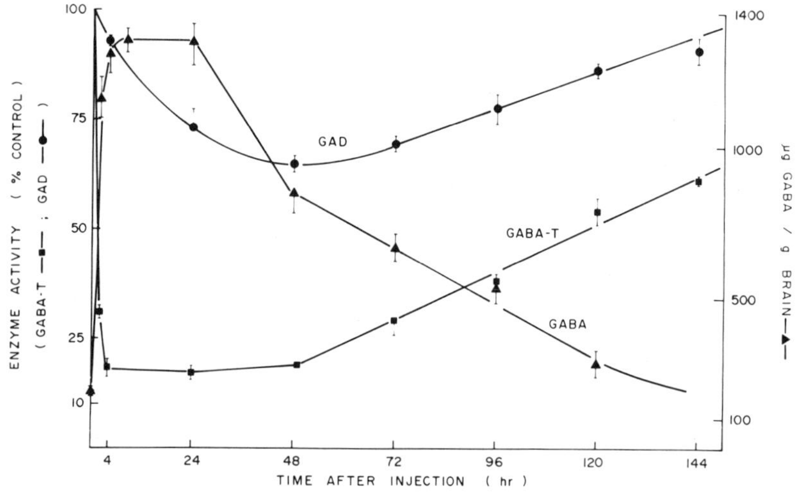

Fig. 5. Effect of a single dose of γ-vinyl GABA on whole brain GABA-T and GAD activities and GABA concentrations. Male mice were injected intraperitoneally with a dose of 1500 mg/kg γ-vinyl GABA. Enzyme activities and GABA concentrations were determined at various time intervals after drug injections. Enzyme activities are expressed as % of control. Each value represents the mean±S.E.M. of five animals. Control levels of enzyme activities are means of pooled controls distributed over the duration of the experiments: GABA-T=77.0 μmol/g/h (mean±S.E.M.; n=20); GAD=45.1±0.6 μmol/g/h (n=20).

Table I

Effect of γ-acetylenic GABA i.p. on audiogenic seizures in susceptible mice (4h post-treatment)

Dose (mg/kg)	No. Tested	% Protected (relative to controls [a])	P^b
12.5	7	2.1	N.S.
25	18	27.8	<0.025
37.5	17	19.0	N.S.
50	8	62.5	<0.05
62.5	6	100	<0.005
75	7	100	<0.005
100	18	94.4	<0.005
125	9	100	<0.005

a Frequency of seizures in controls=97.0±3.0% (mean±S.E.M.; n=36)

b Determined by χ^2 analysis (uncorrected of 2×2 contingency table (Snedecor & Cochran 1967).

induced by a sound stimulus in a dose-dependent manner, the ED50 for protection being 41 mg/kg (Schechter *et al.* 1977a).

γ-Acetylenic GABA also protects mice against the incidence of seizures induced by electroshock as well as seizures induced chemically by thiosemicarbazide, isoniazid and strychnine, but not against those induced by picrotoxin, bicuculline and pentylenetetrazol. The failure of γ-acetylenic GABA to protect against these latter convulsants suggest that its antiseizure properties are not secondary to its sedative effect. The pattern of seizure protection mirrors that of brain GABA elevation. Thus maximum protection occurs by 2 h and seizure inhibition lasts 16 to 24 h after a single dose (Schechter *et al.* 1977a).

γ-Vinyl GABA shows a similar anticonvulsant profile, although, in keeping with its biochemical effects, is less potent, the ED50 being 990 mg/kg. Once again the pattern of seizure protection correlates with that of brain GABA elevation. Hence, complete protection is evident 4 h post-treatment, while at 72 h the level of protection is still 56% relative to control mice (Schechter *et al.* 1977b).

CONCLUSION

We have demonstrated that a consideration of enzyme mechanisms can lead to the conception of new biochemical and pharmacological tools with a relatively specific biological action. Nature, however, is more creative. Recently, Kobayashi *et al.* (1976) isolated gabaculine (5-amino-1,3-cyclohexadienyl carboxylic acid) from a Streptomyces species. This irreversible inhibitor of GABA-T is the most potent reported, and like γ-vinyl GABA, has no *in vitro* effect on GAD (Rando & Bangerter 1976). Professor Rando, in the previous lecture, convincingly demonstrated that the mechanism of this inhibition involves covalent linkage of the transformed inhibitor to the coenzyme, the driving force being aromatization of the cyclohexadiene unit. As other cyclohexadiene derivatives could also be expected to undergo similar enzyme-induced aromatization, we have synthesized 3-amino-1,5-cyclohexadienyl carboxylic acid, an isomer of gabaculine (Metcalf & Jung, unpublished work) which has similar biochemical activity to that reported for gabaculine itself (Rando & Bangerter 1977).

Hence, after a single dose of isogabaculine trifluoroacetate (50 mg/kg, i.p. in mice) there is a progressive decrease of whole brain GABA-T activity to 15–20% of control between 12 and 24 h. On the fifth day post-treatment GABA-T activity is still only 60% of control. GAD activity decreases slowly to a minimum of about 75% of control 24 h after injection. As a consequence of GABA-T inhibition, brain GABA concentrations rise dramatically. Maximal levels occur after 8 h and represent over ninefold control values. After 8 h there is a constant decrease of GABA levels and control values are attained between days 2 and 3 after the single dose administration. Anticonvulsant studies are now in progress.

ACKNOWLEDGMENTS

We thank Benoit Rieger and Yvette Tranier for helpful assistance.

4-Deuterio-4-aminohex-5-ynoic acid and 4-Deuterio-4-aminohex-5-enoic acid were synthesized by Karin Jund.

Fig. 3 is taken from Jung *et al.* (1978), while Fig. 5 is reproduced from Jung *et al.* (1977b).

REFERENCES

Bird, E. D. & Iverson, L. L. (1974) Huntington's Chorea: Post-mortem measurement of glutamic acid decarboxylase, choline acetyltransferase and dopamine in basal ganglia. *Brain* 97, 457–472.

Collins R. L. (1972). In: *Experimental Models of Epilepsy,* ed. Purpura, P., Perry, I. K., Tower, D., Woodbury, D. M. & Walter, R. p. 347. Raven Press, New York.

Da Vanzo, J. P., Matthews, R. J., Young, G. A. & Wingerson, F. (1964) Studies on the mechanism of action of aminooxyacetic acid. *Tox. appl. Pharmac.* 6, 396-401.

Fowler, L. J. & John, R. A. (1972) Active-site-directed irreversible inhibition of rat brain 4-aminobutyrate aminotransferase by ethanolamine O-sulphate *in vitro* and *in vivo. Biochem. J.* 130, 569–573.

Gehring, H., Rando, R. R. & Christen, P. (1977) Active-site labeling of aspartate aminotransferases by the β,γ-unsaturated amino acid vinylglycine. *Biochemistry* 16, 4832–4836.

Hevey, R. C., Babson, J., Maycock, A. L. & Abeles, R. H. (1973) Highly specific enzyme inhibitors. Inhibition of plasma amine oxidase. *J. Am. Chem. Soc.* 95, 6125–6127.

Jung, M. J., Lippert, B., Metcalf, B. W., Schechter, P. J., Böhlen, P. & Sjoerdsma, A. (1977a) The effect of 4-aminohex-5-ynoic acid (γ-acetylenic GABA, γ-ethynyl GABA), a catalytic inhibitor of GABA transaminase, on brain GABA metabolism *in vivo*. *J. Neurochem.* 28, 717–723.

Jung, M. J., Lippert, B., Metcalf, B. W., Böhlen, P. and Schechter, P. J. (1977b) γ-Vinyl GABA (4-aminohex-5-enoic acid), a new selective irreversible inhibitor of GABA-T: Effects on brain GABA metabolism in mice. *J. Neurochem.* 29, 797–802.

Jung, M. J. & Metcalf, B. W. (1975) Catalytic inhibition of γ-aminobutyric acid-α-ketoglutarate transaminase of bacterial origin by 4-aminohex-5-ynoic acid, a substrate analog. *Biochem. Biophys. Res. Commun.* 67, 301–306.

Jung, M. J., Metcalf, B. W., Casara, P., Lippert, B., Schechter, P. J. & Sjoerdsma, A. (1975) Biochemical effects of a unique irreversible inhibitor (RMI 71.645) of γ-aminobutyric acid (GABA) transaminase. The Fifth International Meeting of the ISN, Barcelona, Spain, September 2–6, 1975. Abstracts of Papers.

Jung, M. J., Metcalf, B. W., Lippert, B. & Casara P. (1978) Mechanism of the stereospecific irreversible inhibition of bacterial glutamic acid decarboxylase by (R)-(−)-4-aminohex-5-ynoic acid, an analog of 4-aminobutyric acid. *Biochem.* 17, 2628.

Kobayashi, K., Miyazawa, S., Terahara, A., Mishima, H. & Kurihara, H. (1976) Gabaculine; γ-aminobutyrate amino transferase inhibitor of microbial origin. *Tetrahedron Letts.*, 537–540.

Kuriyama, K., Roberts, E. & Rubinstein, M. K. (1966) Elevation of γ-aminobutyric acid in brain with aminooxyacetic acid and susceptibility to convulsive seizures in mice: A quantitative re-evaluation. *Biochem. Pharmacol.* 15, 221–236.

Lippert, B., Jung, M. J. & Metcalf, B. W. (1978) Unpublished work.

Lippert, B., Metcalf, B. W., Jung, M. J. & Casara, P. (1977) 4-aminohex-5-enoic acid, a selective catalytic inhibitor of 4-aminobutyric acid amino transferase in mammalian brain. *Eur. J. Biochem.* 74, 441–445.

Metcalf, B. W., Bey, P., Danzin, C., Jung, M. J., Casara, P. & Vevert, J. P. (1978) Catalytic irreversible inhibition of mammalian ornithine decarboxylase (E. C. 4.1.1.17) by substrate and product analogues. *J. Am. Chem. Soc.* 100, 2551–2553.

Metcalf, B. W. & Casara, P. (1975) Regiospecific 1,4 addition of a propargylic anion. A general synthon for 2-substituted propargylamines as potential catalytic irreversible enzyme inhibitors. *Tetrahedron Letts.* 3337–3340.

Rando, R. R. (1974) Irreversible inhibition of aspartate aminotransferase by 2-amino 3 butenoic acid. *Biochemistry* 13, 3859–3863.

Rando, R. R. & Bangerter, F. W. (1976) The irreversible inhibition of mouse brain γ-aminobutyric acid (GABA)-α-ketoglutaric acid transaminase by gabaculine. *J. Am. Chem. Soc.* 98, 6762–6764.

Rando, R. R. & Bangerter, F. W. (1977) The *in vivo* inhibition of GABA-transaminase by gabaculine. *Biochem. Biophys. Res. Comm.* 76, 1276–1281.

Rando, R. R. & de Mairena, J. (1974) Propargylamine-induced irreversible inhibiton of nonflavin-linked amine oxidases, *Biochem. Pharmacol.* 23, 463–467.

Roberts, E. (1974) γ-Aminobutyric acid and nervous system function – a perspective. *Biochem. Pharmacol.* 23, 2637–2649.

Schechter, P. J., Tranier, Y., Jung, M. J. & Sjoerdsma, A. (1977a) Antiseizure activity of γ-acetylenic

γ-aminobutyric acid: A catalytic irreversible inhibition of γ-aminobutyric acid transaminase. *J. Pharmacol. Exp. Therap.* 201, 606–612.

Schechter, P. J., Tranier, Y., Jung, M. J. & Böhlen, P. (1977b) Audiogenic seizure protection by elevated brain GABA concentration in mice: Effects of γ-acetylenic GABA and γ-vinyl GABA, two irreversible GABA-T inhibitors. *European J. Pharmacol.* 45, 319–328.

Simler, S., Ciesielski, L., Maitre, M., Randrianarisoa, H. & Mandel, P. (1973) Effect of sodium-n-dipropylacetate on audigenic seizures and brain γ-aminobutyric acid level. *Biochem. Pharmacol.* 22, 1701–1708.

Snedecor, G. W. & Cochran, W. G. (1967). *Statistical Methods,* 6th ed., The Iowa University Press, Ames.

Sze, P. Y. & Lovell, R. A. (1970) Reduction of level of L-glutamic acid decarboxylase by γ-aminobutyric acid in mouse brain. *J. Neurochem.* 17, 1657–1664.

Yamada, H. & O'Leary, M. H. (1978) Stereochemistry of reactions catalyzed by glutamate decarboxylase. *Biochemistry* 17, 669–672.

GABA Uptake Inhibitors and Structurally Related "Pro-Drugs"

L. Brehm, P. Krogsgaard-Larsen & P. Jacobsen

The transport of γ-aminobutyric acid (GABA) across membranes into different nervous tissue elements is of vital importance for the synaptic function of GABA. The tissue localization of these transport systems and the physiological factors which influence this transport have been intensively studied (Martin 1976). However, the knowledge of the physiological role of the transport systems and their mechanism of action at the molecular level is still incomplete. There is evidence to suggest that GABA-mediated synaptic transmission may be terminated by the removal of GABA from the synaptic cleft into the surrounding cells by specific transport systems, and GABA seems to be taken up by neuronal as well as glial elements (Iversen & Kelly 1975).

The GABA transport or uptake systems have been studied with respect to inhibitory effects of various compounds in order to elucidate the structural requirements and substrate specificity of the hypothetic transport carrier(s). The GABA uptake systems may be relevant pharmacological sites of attack in diseases characterized in impaired function of the GABA system, and thus inhibitors of GABA uptake have pharmacological interest.

INHIBITORS OF GABA UPTAKE: DESIGN AND DEVELOPMENT

Simple GABA analogues

A variety of compounds including close structural analogues of GABA have been studied as inhibitors of GABA uptake in rat brain slices, a tissue preparation assumed to represent mainly the neuronal uptake system. The

---

Department of Chemistry BC, Royal Danish School of Pharmacy, 2, Universitetsparken, DK-2100 Copenhagen, Denmark.

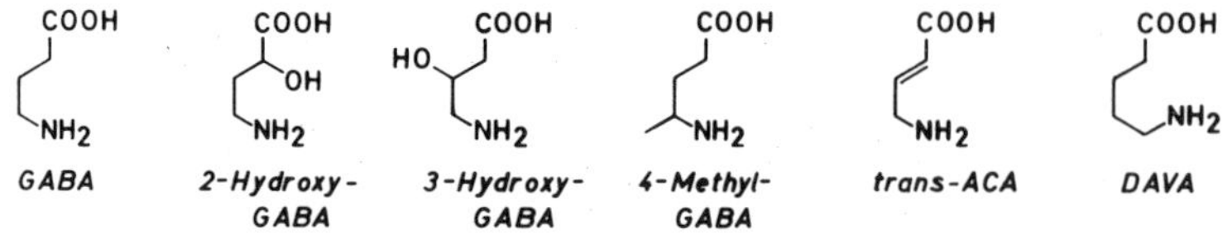

Fig. 1. Schematic diagrams of GABA, *trans*-ACA (*trans*-4-aminocrotonic acid), DAVA (δ-aminovaleric acid), and other GABA analogues.

simple analogues of GABA depicted in Fig. 1 are inhibitors of GABA uptake into rat brain slices (Iversen & Johnston 1971, Beart *et al.* 1972, Beart & Johnston 1973). It has been demonstrated by electrophysiological studies (Curtis & Watkins 1960, Beart & Johnston 1973, Johnston *et al.* 1975a) and receptor affinity binding studies that these compounds also interact with the GABA receptors. This lack of specificity may be a consequence of a certain degree of molecular flexibility of the respective compounds.

The GABA molecule is a very flexible molecule with relatively free rotation around all bonds. The ability to adopt different conformational modes may well be essential to its synaptic activities. Theoretical calculations, spectroscopic studies and crystal structure analyses indicate that GABA can exist in a variety of energetically favorable conformations (Ham 1974, Pullman 1976, Pullman & Berthod 1975, Steward *et al.* 1973a, b, Tomita *et al.* 1973a, Warner *et al.* 1975).

The knowledge of the possible relationship between the conformational mobility of GABA analogues and their affinity for different sites of the GABA synapses is very limited. The availability of substances with different degree of molecular rigidity is of great help in the elucidation of these problems. Pseudorigidity can be conferred on a molecule by, for example steric hindrance and/or the possibility of *intra*molecular hydrogen bonds. In this respect the hydroxylated GABA analogues are of some interest. *Intra*molecular hydrogen bonds may stabilize certain conformations under physiological conditions. The conformation of the 2-hydroxy-GABA cation as determined by X-ray crystallographic methods (Brehm & Krogsgaard-Larsen, unpublished) is illustrated in Fig. 2. It appears that no *intra*molecular hydrogen bond is formed in the crystalline state. The crystal structure is stabilized by *inter*molecular hydrogen bonds, forces which are highly relevant to the interaction of small molecules (substrates) with large biological molecules. The situation in crystals, in solution or under vacuum, may however not reflect "active conformations" of GABA in the biological phase. Nevertheless knowledge of preferred conformations may be a help in the difficult and uncertain game of stereostructure-activity correlations.

A series of compounds, in which the structural characteristics of the GABA analogues depicted in Fig. 1 have been combined, synthesized and tested as inhibitors of binding of ^{3}H-GABA to rat brain membranes (Honoré *et al.* 1978) and as inhibitors of GABA uptake in mouse brain slices (Schousboe *et al.*, unpublished) (Table I). The stereochemical specificities of the GABA receptors and the uptake system appear to be different, and (*R*)- and (*S*)-4-methyl-*trans*-ACA [(*R*)-and (*S*)-4-methyl-*trans*-4-aminocrotonic acid] may prove to be very important tools for studies of the GABA synaptic functions at the molecular level.

Bicyclic muscimol analogues

Using muscimol (5-aminomethyl-3-isoxazolol) as a model compound a number of bicyclic 3-isoxazolol zwitterions have been developed.These compounds have been tested as GABA receptor agonists and as inhibitors of GABA uptake into rat brain slices (Krogsgaard-Larsen *et al.* 1975, 1977, Krogsgaard-Larsen & Johnston 1975, 1978) (Table II). Isoxazole 2 and structurally related cyclic aminocarboxylic acids are potent GABA receptor agonists (see Krogsgaard-Larsen *et al.*, this volume). Isoxazole 3 and 4, on the other hand, are selective but weak inhibitors of GABA uptake in rat brain slices. Considerations of the 3-isoxazolol nucleus as a masked carboxyl group in isoxazole 3 and 4 led to the development of the related amino acids depicted in Fig. 3. Whereas the amino acids containing a 7-membered ring were almost inactive or very weak as inhibitors of GABA uptake, the corresponding amino acids containing 6-membered rings, guvacine (Johnston *et al.* 1975b) and nipecotic acid (Krogs-

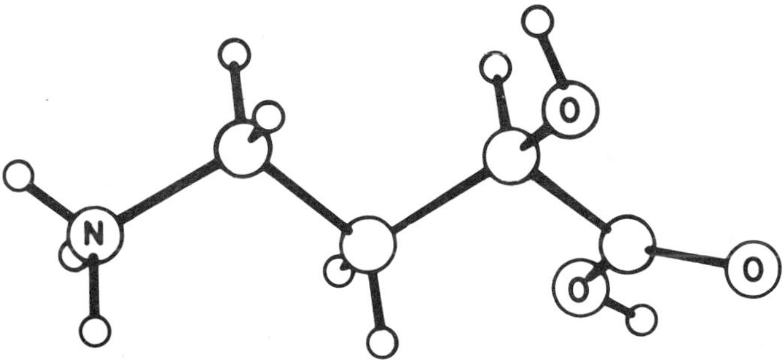

Fig. 2. The molecular structure of the 2-hydroxy-GABA cation as observed in the 2-hydroxy-GABA hydrochloride monohydrate crystals.

Table I

Structurally related GABA analogues as inhibitors of GABA uptake into mouse brain slices and GABA receptor binding *

Compound	Formula	Inhibition of GABA-uptake $IC_{50}(\mu M)$	Inhibition of GABA-binding % at $10^{-4}M$	$IC_{50}(\mu M)$
(S)-4-Methyl GABA	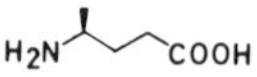	750	91	4.7 ± 0.3
(R)-4-Methyl GABA	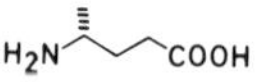	200	91	5.0 ± 0.4
(2RS,4SR)-2-Hydroxy-4-methyl-GABA	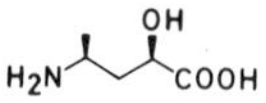	n.t.	11	–
(2RS,4RS)-2-Hydroxy-4-methyl-GABA	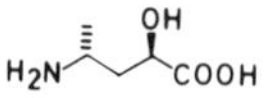	n.t.	6	–
(3RS,4S)-3-Hydroxy-4-methyl-GABA	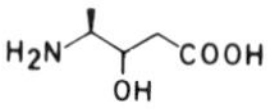	>5000	43	200±15
(3RS,4R)-3-Hydroxy-4-methyl-GABA	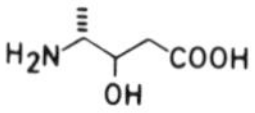	2500	21	–
S-4-Methyl-trans-ACA	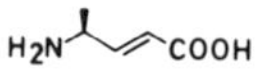	>5000	92	4.1±0.4
R-4-Methyl-trans-ACA	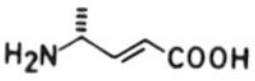	160	48	148±9
trans-5-Amino-2-pentenoic acid	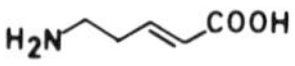	4000	59	48±3
(RS)-3-Hydroxy-DAVA	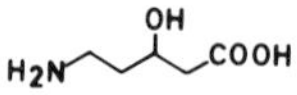	430	73	21±3

* Here and throughout this chapter inhibition of GABA uptake into slices of mouse brain (Schousboe *et al.* 1978) and rat brain (Beart *et al.* 1972), and inhibition of binding of GABA to rat brain membranes (Enna & Snyder 1975) were studied by using published methods.

gaard-Larsen & Johnston 1975, Johnston *et al.* 1976a, b) proved to be very potent inhibitors of GABA uptake into rat brain slices with little or no affinity for the GABA receptor sites (Krogsgaard-Larsen & Johnston 1978).

Nipecotic acid, guvacine, and related compounds

Nipecotic acid (Johnston *et al.* 1976a) and probably also guvacine (Johnston *et al.* 1975b) are substrate-competitive inhibitors of the neuronal uptake of GABA.

Nipecotic acid (Curtis *et al.* 1976) and guvacine (Lodge *et al.* 1977) have been useful means for studying the physiological role of the GABA uptake systems. Microelectrophoretic application of these compounds on single neurones enhance the depressant effect of simultaneously ejected GABA, suggesting that the removal of GABA from the synaptic cleft is retarded by the uptake inhibitors.

A variety of cyclic amino acids related to guvacine and nipecotic acid has been synthesized (Krogsgaard-Larsen *et al.* 1978) and tested as inhibitors of GABA uptake in rat brain slices (Table III) in order to further elucidate the structural specificity of the GABA transport carrier(s). Furthermore these molecular manipulations of guvacine and nipecotic acid have been carried out with the aim of developing inhibitors of GABA uptake, which are not substrates for the transport carrier. Such compounds have interest as tools for physiological and pharmacological studies of the GABA uptake system(s). It is, however, evident from Table III that structural modifications of the compounds concerned result in considerable or almost complete loss of affinity for the uptake system. Studies

Table II

Structurally related muscimol analogues as inhibitors of GABA uptake into rat brain slices and of GABA receptor binding

Isoxazole No.	Formula	Inhibition of GABA-uptake %	Inhibition of GABA-uptake IC_{50} (μM)	Inhibition of GABA-binding % at 10^{-4}M	Inhibition of GABA-binding IC_{50} (μM)
1 (Muscimol)	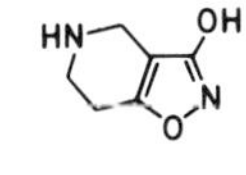	31 (5×10^{-4}M)	–	103	0.024±0.003
2 (THIP)	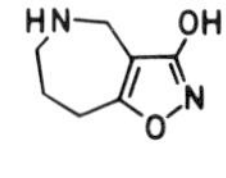	15 (5×10^{-4}M)	–	98	0.130±0.005
3	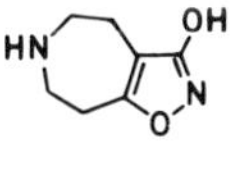	66 (10^{-3}M)	624±55	31	–
4	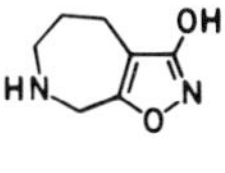	59 (5×10^{-4}M)	402±27	n.s.	
5		17 (10^{-3}M)	–	39	88±22
6		n.s. (5×10^{-4}M)		21	–

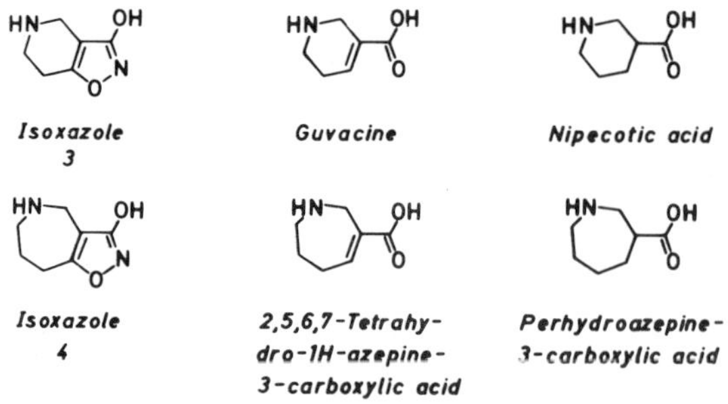

Fig. 3. Schematic diagrams of isoxazole 3 (4,5,6,7-tetrahydroisoxazolo[4,5-*c*]pyridin-3-ol), isoxazole 4 (5,6,7,8-tetrahydro-4*H*-isoxazolo [4,5-*c*]azepin-3-ol), and related cyclic amino acids.

of the optical antipodes of nipecotic acid further indicate stereoselectivity of the GABA uptake system (Tables I and III). Thus, the neuronal GABA uptake system shows a pronounced structural specificity, which leaves the pharmacochemists with a very narrow latitude regarding development of further inhibitors of GABA uptake of pharmacological interest.

cis-4-Hydroxynipecotic acid and related compounds

Ecgonine, the amino acid skeleton of cocaine, is a structural analogue of nipecotic acid with a hydroxy group in the 4-position of the piperidine ring (Table IV). Ecgonine is pharmacologically active after systemic administration to mice (Nieschulz 1971), but the mode of action of this compound is unknown. These findings prompted studies of ecgonine and closely related compounds as inhibitors of GABA uptake in rat brain slices (Johnston *et al.* 1977) and the development of various more simple hydroxylated nipecotic acid analogues. Ecgonine, nor-ecgonine, ψ-ecgonine, and nor-ψ-ecgonine have no affinity for the neuronal GABA uptake system and the GABA receptor sites on rat brain membranes (Table IV). However, *cis*-4-hydroxynipecotic acid is a potent inhibitor of GABA uptake with no affinity for the GABA receptors. From the results listed in Table IV it is evident that even minor structural variations of this amino acid result in compounds which are very weak as inhibitors of GABA uptake. On the other hand the 3-hydroxylated analogue of isonipecotic acid is a selective and relatively potent inhibitor of binding of GABA to its receptor sites (see Krogsgaard-Larsen *et al.*, this volume).

cis-4-Aminonipecotic acid and related compounds

The GABA analogues (*S*)-(+)-2,4-diaminobutyric acid (DABA) (Martin 1976,

Iversen & Kelly 1975) and (±)-*cis*-3-aminocyclohexanecarboxylic acid (*cis*-ACHC) (Beart *et al.* 1972) are inhibitors of the neuronal GABA uptake system and like nipecotic acid, substrate for this GABA transport carrier (Neal &

Table III

Guvacine and nipecotic acid and related compounds as inhibitors of GABA uptake into rat brain slices and GABA receptor binding

Compound	*Formula*	*Inhibition of GABA-uptake*		*Inhibition of GABA-binding*	
		% at 5×10^{-4}M	*IC_{50} (μM)*	*% at 10^{-4}M*	*IC_{50} (μM)*
Guvacine	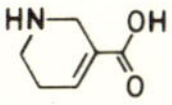	98	8±1	10	
(RS)-5-Methyl guvacine	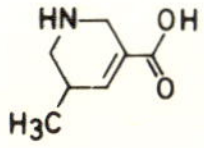	46	547±22	n.s.	
2,5,6,7,-Tetahydro-1H-azepine-3-carboxylic acid	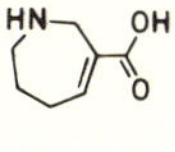	23	–	n.s.	
Isoguvacine	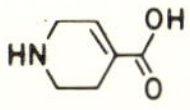	10	–	100	0.015±0.001
Isonipecotic acid	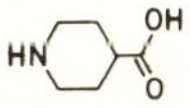	20 †	–	99	0.33±0.02
(R)-Nipecotic acid	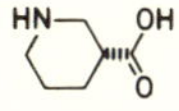	–	5±1	–*	
(S)-Nipecotic acid	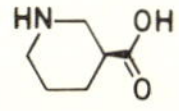	–	30±2	–*	
(RS)-Perhydro-azepine-3-carboxylic acid	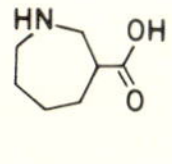	52	502±49	n.s.	
(1R,2R,5R)-Nor-tropane-2-carboxylic acid	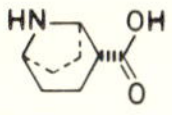	n.s.		n.s.	

† From Beart *et al.* (1972).

* Racemic nipecotic acid was almost inactive as an inhibitor of GABA binding (Krogsgaard-Larsen and Johnston 1978).

Table IV

4-Hydroxynipecotic acid and related compounds as inhibitors of GABA uptake into slices of mouse (*) or rat brains and as inhibitors of GABA receptor binding.

Compound	Formula	Inhibition of GABA-uptake %at 5×10^{-4}M	IC$_{50}$ (µM)	Inhibition of GABA-binding % at 10^{-4}M	IC$_{50}$ (µM)
(3SR,4RS)-4-Hydroxy-nipecotic acid	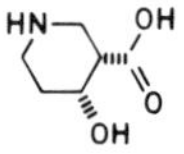	95	12±2	n.s.	
(3SR,4RS,5RS)-4-Hydroxy-5-methyl-nipecotic acid	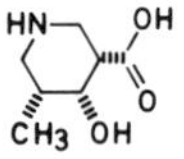	60	260±17	n.s.	
(3SR,4RS,5SR)-4-Hydroxy-5-methyl-nipecotic acid	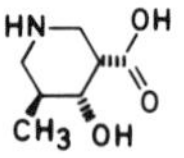	49	349±24	n.s	
4-Hydroxy-isonipecotic acid	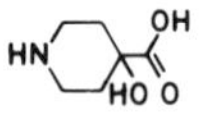		>5000*	45	–
(3RS,4SR)-3-Hydroxy-4-isonipecotic acid	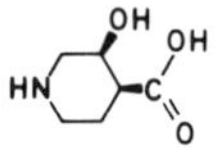		>5000*	85	12±1
Nor-ecgonine	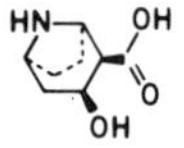	n.s.		n.s.	
Nor-ψ-ecgonine	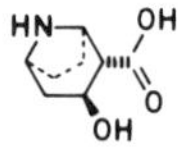	n.s.		n.s.	
Ecgonine	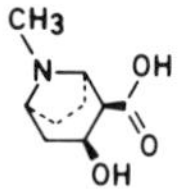	n.s.		n.s.	
ψ-Ecgonine	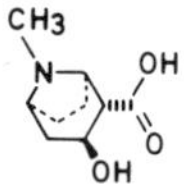	n.s.		n.s.	

Bowery 1977). Furthermore *cis*-ACHC appears to be more selective for neuronal compared to glial uptake of GABA than either DABA or nipecotic acid (Bowery *et al.* 1976).

These selective effects on the neuronal GABA uptake system have made these compounds useful neurochemical tools. Compared with nipecotic acid, DABA and *cis*-ACHC are relatively weak as inhibitors of the neuronal GABA uptake system. As an attemp to develop potent and more specific inhibitors of the neuronal GABA uptake system, a series of compounds which are structural analogues of both DABA and nipecotic acid have been synthesized (Krogsgaard-Larsen & Jacobsen, unpublished). However, these compounds (Fig. 4) are inactive as inhibitors of GABA uptake in mouse brain slices and cultured astrocyte cells (Schousboe *et al.,* unpublished). Furthermore the compounds concerned are weak or inactive as inhibitors of binding of GABA to receptor sites on rat brain membranes.

X-ray and ^{1}H NMR studies on nipecotic acid, cis-4-hydroxynipecotic acid, and nor-ecgonine

It is evident from the above studies that the neuronal GABA transport carrier is characterized in a pronounced substrate specificity. In order to study these aspects in further details, the structures of nipecotic acid, *cis*-4-hydroxynipecotic acid, and nor-ecgonine have been studied in different environments.

The molecular structures as determined by X-ray analyses of (±)-nipecotic acid, (±)-*cis*-4-hydroxynipecotic acid and (−)-nor-ecgonine are shown in Fig. 5. As anticipated from the respective pK_A values, all these compounds crystallize in the zwitterionic forms, and all these crystal structures are stabilized by hydrogen bonds. The piperidine ring of nipecotic acid is in the chair form with the carboxylate group in an equatorial position. The piperidine ring of *cis*-4-hydroxynipecotic acid is also in the chair form, but is slightly more distorted than the piperidine ring of nipecotic acid. The carboxylate group is equatorial and the hydroxy group axial. In each of the compounds the distances from the

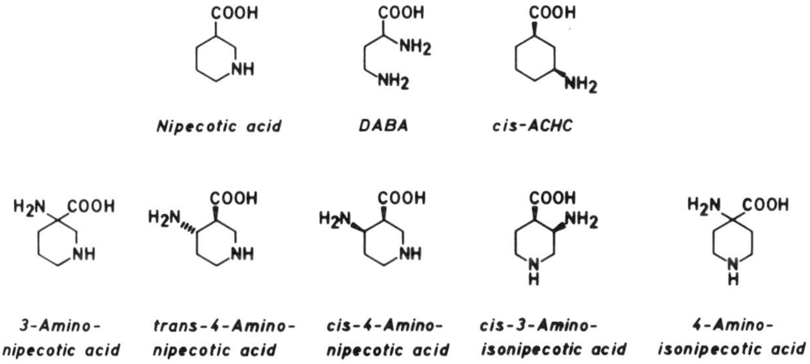

Fig. 4. Schematic diagrams of nipecotic acid, DABA (2,4-diaminobutyric acid), *cis*-ACHC (*cis*-3-aminocyclohexanecarboxylic acid), and related compounds.

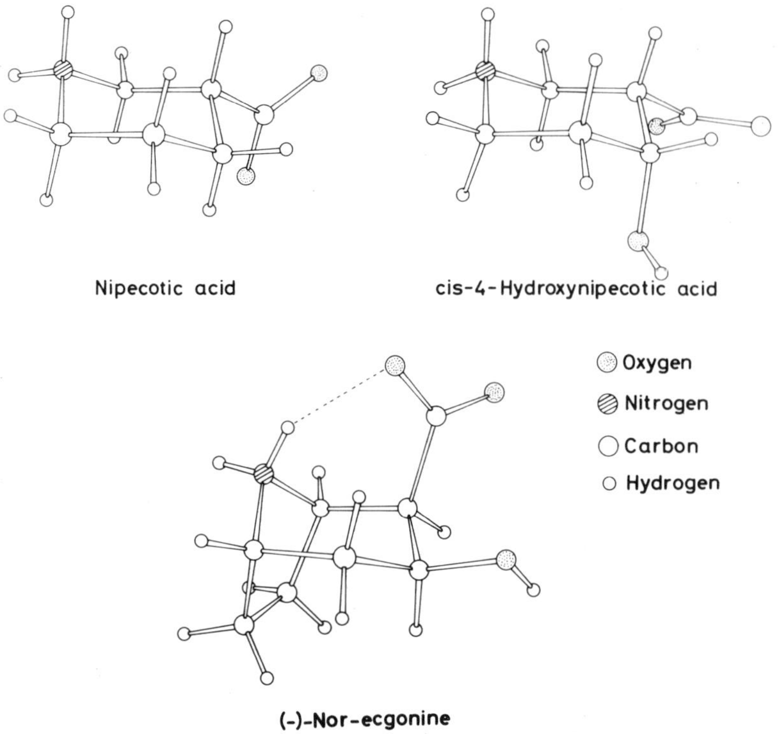

Fig. 5. The molecular structures of nipecotic acid, *cis*-4-hydroxynipecotic acid, and (−)-nor-ecgonine as observed in the respective crystal structures.

nitrogen atom of the aminium group and the oxygen atoms of the carboxylate group are almost the same (4.9 Å and 4.2 Å). Proton magnetic resonance studies indicate that in aqueous solution nipecotic acid exists predominantly in a chair conformation with the carboxylate group equatorial (Brehm *et al.* 1976). *cis*-4-Hydroxynipecotic acid was also shown by ^{1}H NMR spectroscopy to exist in aqueous solution predominantly in a chair conformation with the carboxylate group equatorial and the hydroxy group axial (Brehm *et al.*, unpublished). In agreement with related compounds the X-ray analysis of nor-ecgonine shows that the ethylene bridge deforms the chair type piperidine ring. The carboxylate group is in an axial position and the hydroxy group in an equatorial position, thus these two substituents are *cis* to each other. An *intra*molecular hydrogen bond is formed between the aminium and the carboxylate groups, the distance between the nitrogen and oxygen atoms being 2.7 Å (Brehm *et al.*, unpublished).

It is evident from these studies that specific structural requirements such as essential groups of atoms, stereochemistry, conformation, and charge separa-seem to be factors of importance for inhibitors of and substrates for the neuronal GABA uptake system. The results indicate that GABA is transported in a somewhat folded conformation.

GABA UPTAKE INHIBITORS IN NEUROPHARMACOLOGY

The uptake mechanisms in nerve terminals and glial cells are probably the most important means for terminating the actions of GABA released into the synaptic cleft. Consequently the uptake systems may be relevant pharmacological sites of attack with respect to facilitation of GABA transmission in diseases with impaired function of the GABA system. GABA is directly or indirectly implicated in the pathogenesis of Huntington's chorea (McGeer & McGeer 1976a, b, Enna *et al.* 1977, Lloyd *et al.* 1977a), Parkinson's disease (Hornykiewicz *et al.* 1976, Lloyd *et al.* 1975, Lloyd *et al.* 1977b, McGeer & McGeer 1976b) and possibly of schizophrenia (Roberts 1974, Van kammen 1977) and epilepsy (Meldrum 1975).

The GABA-ergic transmission may be facilitated in a flexible manner by inhibition of GABA uptake (Chase & Walters 1976). A complicating factor in this respect is, however, that the neuronal and glial uptake systems apparently exhibit different structural specificities (Iversen & Kelly 1975, Krogsgaard-Larsen 1978, Schousboe *et al.* 1978). A prerequisite for therapies based on these principles may be the development of compounds capable of blocking both uptake systems. Alternatively a combination of potent inhibitors of both GABA uptake systems might be therapeutically useful.

In this respect nipecotic acid, guvacine, and (±)-*cis*-4-hydroxynipecotic acid are of interest. As previously discussed these compounds are very potent inhibitors of the neuronal GABA uptake mechanisms, which enhance the depressant effect of GABA at the cellular level as established in microelectrophoretic experiments (Krogsgaard-Larsen *et al.* 1975, Curtis *et al.* 1976, Lodge *et al.* 1977). Furthermore these cyclic amino acids have recently proved also to inhibit the uptake of GABA into cultured astrocyte cells (Schousboe *et al.* 1978). (±)-*cis*-4-Hydroxynipecotic acid appears to be equipotent as an inhibitor of both systems with IC_{50} values of about 10 μM, and this compound may be of particular pharmacological interest.

The amino acids concerned apparently do not easily penetrate into the brain after systemic administration. However, derivatives of these compounds, which

Table V

Observed pseudo-first-order rate constants and half-lives for the hydrolysis of some ethyl and methyl esters in 0.1M phosphate buffer solution (pH 7.40, $\mu=0.5$) at 37°C, determined by the hydroxamic acid test (Satterthwait & Jencks 1974).

Compound No	Formula	k_{obs} (h^{-1})	$t_{1/2}$ (h)
7 R-(−)-	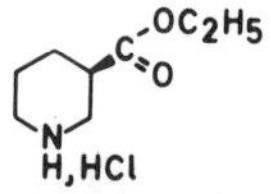	0.37×10^{-2}	187
8 (±)-	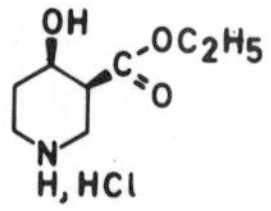	0.39×10^{-2}	178
9	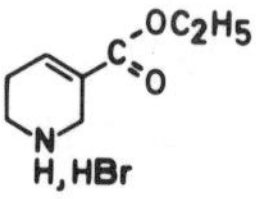	0.12×10^{-2}	578
10 (±)-	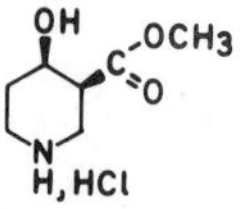	1.44×10^{-2}	48
11 (±)-	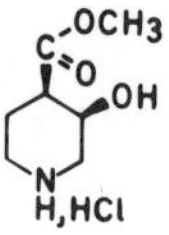	0.75×10^{-2}	92

may be able to penetrate into the brain and subsequently be hydrolyzed to give the parent amino acids may be therapeutically useful "pro-drugs" of nipecotic acid, guvacine, and (±)-*cis*-4-hydroxynipecotic acid. As illustrated in Table V a series of simple esters of the respective amino acids have been synthesized (Krogsgaard-Larsen *et al.*, unpublished), and the time course of their degradation into the parent compounds have been studied *in vitro* under approximate physiologically relevant conditions. The half-lives for hydrolysis of these compounds listed in Table V may be considerably lower *in vivo* due to the presence of esterases in brain tissue.

It has recently been demonstrated that systemic administration of the ethyl esters of (*R*)-(−)- and (*S*)-(+)-nipecotic acids are capable of protecting mice against clonic seizures after pentetrazole treatment (Frey *et al.*, unpublished). The ethyl ester of (*R*)-(−)-nipecotic acid was more powerful as an anticonvulsant than the ester of the corresponding (*S*)-(+)-form. Nipecotic acid could be detected in the brain tissue after this treatment. Since (*R*)-(−)-nipecotic acid is more potent as an inhibitor of neuronal GABA uptake than its optical antipode, these findings together suggest that nipecotic acid generated *in vivo* is responsible for the observed anticonvulsant effects (Frey *et al.*, unpublished). Consequently ethyl nipecotate may be regarded as a "pro-drug" of nipecotic acid.

The ethyl esters of (*R*)-(−)- and (*S*)-(+)-nipecotic acids have weak cholinergic properties (Frey *et al.*, unpublished). These effects combined with the inhibitory effect of especially (*R*)-(−)-nipecotic acid on GABA uptake are of pharmacological interest. In diseases like Huntington's chorea the activities of the acetylcholine (Wastek *et al.* 1976) as well as the GABA transmitter systems are considerable decreased. Thus esters of nipecotic acid, guvacine, or (±)-*cis*-4-hydroxynipecotic acid with proper choice of alkyl groups in the ester functions might be of therapeutical interest for the treatment of Huntington's chorea, based on a certain relationship between cholinergic effect, the rate of hydrolysis of the ester *in vivo,* and the potency of the parent amino acid as an inhibitor of GABA uptake.

ACKNOWLEDGMENTS

This work was supported by grants from The Danish Medical Research Council. We are grateful to Dr. A. Schousboe for his work on GABA uptake into mouse brain slices. Professor D. R. Curtis and Dr. G. A. R. Johnston are gratefully acknowledged for collaboration and helpful discussions. Dr. H. Bundgaard is gratefully acknowledged for experimental work and helpful discussions. We wish to thank our colleagues in the Department of Chemistry BC, Royal Danish School of Pharmacy, for fruitful collaboration.

REFERENCES

Beart, P. M. & Johnston, G. A. R. (1973) GABA uptake in rat brain slices: Inhibition by GABA analogues and by various drugs. *J. Neurochem.* 20, 319–324.

Beart, P. M., Johnston, G. A. R. & Uhr, M. L. (1972) Competitive inhibition of GABA uptake in rat brain slices by some GABA analogues of restricted conformation. *J. Neurochem.* 19, 1855–1861.

Bowery, N. G., Jones, G. P. & Neal, M. J. (1976) Selective inhibition of neuronal GABA uptake by *cis*-1,3-aminocyclohexanecarboxylic acid. *Nature* 264, 281–284.

Brehm, L., Krogsgaard-Larsen, P., Johnston, G. A. R. & Schaumburg, K. (1976) X-ray crystallographic and proton magnetic resonance spectroscopic investigations of nipecotic acid, a potent inhibitor of γ-aminobutyric acid (GABA) uptake. *Acta Chem. Scand.* B30, 542–548.

Chase, T. N. & Walters, J. R. (1976) Pharmacologic approach to the manipulation of GABA mediated synaptic funtion in man. In: *GABA in Nervous System Function*, ed. Roberts, E., Chase, T. N. & Tower, D. B., pp. 497–513, Raven Press, New York.

Curtis, D. R., Game, C. J. A. & Lodge, D. (1976) The *in vivo* inactivation of GABA and other inhibitory amino acids in the cat central nervous system. *Exp. Brain Res.* 25, 413–428.

Curtis, D. R. & Watkins, J. C. (1960) The excitation and depression of spinal neurones by structurally related amino acids. *J. Neurochem.* 6, 117–141.

Enna, S. J. & Snyder, S. H. (1975) Properties of γ-aminobutyric acid (GABA) receptor binding in rat brain synaptic membrane fractions. *Brain Res.* 100, 81–97.

Enna, S. J., Stern, L. Z., Wastek, G. J. & Yamamura, H. I. (1977) Neurobiology and pharmacology of Huntington's desease. *Life Sci.* 20, 205–211.

Ham, N. S. (1974) NMR studies of solution conformations of physiologically active amino acids. In: *Molecular and Quantum Pharmacology,* ed. Bergmann, E. & Pullman, B., pp. 256–263, D. Reidel Publ. Comp., Dordrecht-Holland.

Honoré, T., Hjeds, H., Krogsgaard-Larsen, P. & Christiansen, T. R. (1978) Synthesis and structure-activity studies of analogues of γ-aminobutyric acid (GABA). *Eur. J. Med. Chem.* Submitted.

Hornykiewicz, O., Lloyd, K. G. & Davidson, L. (1976) The GABA system, function of basal ganglia, Parkinson's disease. In: *GABA in Nervous System Function*, ed. Roberts, E., Chase, T. N. & Tower, D. B., pp. 479–485, Raven Press, New York.

Iversen, L. L. & Johnston, G. A. R. (1971) GABA uptake in rat central nervous system: Comparison of uptake in slices and homogenates and the effects of some inhibitors. *J. Neurochem.* 18, 1939–1950.

Iversen, L. L. & Kelly, J. S. (1975) Uptake and metabolism of γ-aminobutyric acid by neurones and glial cells. *Biochem. Pharmacol.* 24, 933–938.

Johnston, G. A. R., Brehm, L. & Krogsgaard-Larsen, P. (1977) Derivatives of nipecotic acid related to cocaine and ecgonine. *Proc. Int. Soc. Neurochem.* 6, 586.

Johnston, G. A. R., Curtis, D. R., Beart, P. M., Game, C. J. A., McCulloch, R. M. & Twitchin, B. (1975a) *cis*- and *trans*-4-Amino-crotonic acid as GABA analogues of restricted conformation. *J. Neurochem.* 24, 157–160.

Johnston, G. A. R., Krogsgaard-Larsen, P. & Stephanson, A. (1975b) Betel nut constituents as inhibitors of γ-aminobutyric acid uptake. *Nature* 258, 627–628.

Johnston, G. A. R., Krogsgaard-Larsen, P., Stephanson, A. L. & Twitchin, B. (1976a) Inhibition of the uptake of GABA and related amino acids in rat brain slices by the optical isomers of nipecotic acid. *J. Neurochem.* 26, 1029–1032.

Johnston, G. A. R., Stephanson, A. L. & Twitchin, B. (1976b) Uptake and release of nipecotic acid by rat brain slices. *J. Neurochem.* 26, 83–87.

Krogsgaard-Larsen, P. (1978) GABA agonists and uptake inhibitors of restricted conformations: Structure-activity relations. In: *Amino Acids as Neurotransmitters*, ed. Fonnum, F. Plenum Press. In press.

Krogsgaard-Larsen, P. & Johnston, G. A. R. (1975) Inhibition of GABA uptake in rat brain slices by nipecotic acid, various isoxazoles and related compounds. *J. Neurochem.* 25, 797–802.

Krogsgaard-Larsen, P. & Johnston, G. A. R. (1978) Structure-activity studies on the inhibition of GABA binding to rat brain membranes by muscimol and related compounds. *J. Neurochem.* 30, 1377–1382.

Krogsgaard-Larsen, P., Johnston, G. A. R., Curtis, D. R., Game, C. J. A. & McCulloch, R. M. (1975) Structure and biological activity of a series of conformationally restricted analogues of GABA. *J. Neurochem.* 25, 803–809.

Krogsgaard-Larsen, P., Johnston, G. A. R., Lodge, D. & Curtis, D. R. (1977) A new class of GABA agonists. *Nature* 268, 53–55.

Krogsgaard-Larsen, P., Thyssen, K. & Schaumburg, K. (1978) Inhibitors of GABA uptake. Syntheses of guvacine, (3*RS*,4SR)-4-hydroxypiperidine-3-carboxylic acid, and related compounds. *Acta Chem. Scand.* B32. In press.

Lloyd, K. G., Dreksler, S. & Bird, E. D. (1977a) Alteration in ^{3}H-GABA binding in Huntington's chorea. *Life Sci.* 21, 747–753.

Lloyd, K. G., Möhler, H., Heitz, Ph. & Bartholini, G. (1975) Distribution of choline acetyltransferase and glutamate decarboxylase within the substantia nigra and in other brain regions from control and parkinsonian patients. *J. Neurochem.* 25, 789–795.

Lloyd, K. G., Shemen, L. & Hornykiewicz, O. (1977b) Distribution of high affinity sodium independent ^{3}H-gamma-aminobutyric acid (^{3}H-GABA) binding in the human brain: Alterations in Parkinson's disease. *Brain Res.* 127, 269–278.

Lodge, D., Johnston, G. A. R., Curtis, D. R. & Brand, J. (1977) Effects of The *Areca* nut constituents arecaidine and guvacine on the action of GABA with cat central nervous system. *Brain Res.* 136, 513–522.

Martin, D. L. (1976) Carrier-mediated transport and removal of GABA from synaptic regions. In: *GABA in Nervous System Function*, ed. Roberts, E., Chase, T. N. & Tower, D. B., pp. 347–386, Raven Press, New York.

McGeer, P. L. & McGeer, E. G. (1976a) The GABA system and function of the basal ganglia: Huntington's disease. In: *GABA in Nervous System Function*, ed. Roberts, E., Chase, T. N. & Tower, D. B., pp. 487–495, Raven Press, New York.

McGeer, P. L. & McGeer, E. G. (1976b) Enzymes associated with the metabolism of catecholamines, acetylcholine and GABA in human controls and patients with Parkinson's disease and Huntington's chorea. *J. Neurochem.* 26, 65–76.

Meldrum, B. S. (1975) Epilepsy and γ-aminobutyric acid-mediated inhibition. In: *Int. Rev. of Neurobiology*, ed. Pfeiffer, C. C. & Smythies, J. R. 17, 1–36, Academic Press, New York.

Neal, M. J. & Bowery, N. G. (1977) *cis*-3-Aminocyclohexanecarboxylic acid: a substrate for the neuronal GABA transport system. *Brain res.* 138, 169–174.

Nieschultz, O. (1971) Psychopharmakologische untersuchungen über cocain und ecgonin. *Arzneim Forsch.* 2, 275–284.

Pullman, B. (1976) Quantum-mechanical studies on the effect of water on the conformation of two biologically important zwitterionic systems: Polar head of phospholipids and GABA. In: *Environmental Effects on Molecular Structure and Properties*, ed. Pullman, B. pp. 55–80. D. Reidel Publ. Comp., Dordrecht-Holland.

Pullman, B. & Berthod, H. (1975) Molecular orbital studies on the conformation of GABA (γ-aminobutyric acid). *Theoret. Chim. Acta* (Berl.) 36, 317–328.

Roberts, E. (1974) γ-Aminobutyric acid and nervous system function – A perspective. *Biochem. Pharmac.* 23, 2637–2649.

Satterthwait, A. C. & Jencks, W. P. (1974) The mechanism of the aminolysis of acetate esters. *J. Am. Chem. Soc.* 96, 7019–7031.

Schousboe, A., Krogsgaard-Larsen, P., Svenneby, G. & Hertz, L. (1978) Inhibition of the high affinity, net uptake of GABA into cultured astrocytes by β-proline, nipecotic acid and other compounds. *Brain Res.* In press.

Steward, E. G., Player, R. B. & Warner, D. (1973a) The crystal and molecular structure of γ-aminobutyric acid determined at low temperature. *Acta Cryst.* B29, 2038–2040.

Steward, E. G., Player, R. B. & Warner, D. (1973b) The crystal structure of γ-aminobutyric acid hydrochloride: a refinement. *Acta Cryst.* B29, 2825–2826.

Tomita, K., Higashi, H. & Fujiwara, T. (1973) Crystal and molecular structure of ω-amino acids, ω-amino sulfonic acids and their derivatives. IV. The crystal and molecular structure of γ-aminobutyric acid (GABA), a nervous inhibitory transmitter. *Bull. Chem. Soc. Japan* 46, 2199–2204.

Van Kammen, D. P. (1977) γ-Aminobutyric acid (GABA) and the dopamine hypothesis of schizophrenia. *Am. J. Psychiat.* 134, 138–143.

Warner, D. & Steward, E. G. (1975) CNDO/2 molecular orbital calculations on the conformational modes of γ-aminobutyric acid. *J. Molecular Structure* 25, 403–411.

Wastek, G. J., Stern, L. Z., Johnson, P. C. & Yamamura, H. I. (1976) Huntington's disease: Regional alteration in muscarinic cholinergic receptor binding in human brain. *Life Sci.* 19, 1033–1039.

Significance of the Glial Transport System for the Inactivation of GABA and Effect of Structural Analogues on the Uptake

Arne Schousboe

GABA which was discovered by Roberts & Frankel (1950) and Awapara *et al.* (1950) in brain extracts is one of the most abundant amino acids in this tissue occurring in concentrations from 1 to 10 mM with great topographical variations (see e.g. Roberts 1962, Baxter 1970). Moreover, this amino acid is unique to the central nervous system being present in only trace amounts in other tissues (Haber *et al.* 1970). There is, however, a recent report (Okada *et al.* 1976) that the GABA content in the islets of Langerhanns in pancreas is comparable to the GABA content in brain.

There is overwhelming experimental evidence that GABA, in addition to being an important constituent of brain metabolism (cf. van den Berg *et al.* 1975), plays a role as a major inhibitory transmitter in the mammalian brain (see e.g. Curtis & Johnston 1970, 1974, Krnjević 1974). Accordingly, there must be an inactivation mechanism and it is generally accepted that this is brought about by transport processes (Curtis & Johnston 1974) which may occur either in neurons or glial cells (Iversen & Kelly 1975, Schousboe *et al.* 1977a, Schousboe 1978a, b). The relative significance of these uptake systems will be discussed below.

In recent years a variety of GABA analogues of restricted conformation has been developed (Krogsgaard-Larsen 1978) and the second part of this paper shall deal with the effect of such compounds on primarily the glial transport

Department of Biochemistry A, University of Copenhagen, Panum Institute, Blegdamsvej 3c, DK-2200 Copenhagen N, Denmark.

"GABA-NEUROTRANSMITTERS", Alfred Benzon Symposium 12, Munksgaard 1978

system, but for the sake of comparison, effects on the neuronal transport system have also been investigated (Brehm *et al.*, this volume).

METHODS

Glial cell preparation

Astrocytes were cultured as described by Booher & Sensenbrenner (1972) with the modifications introduced by Schousboe *et al.* (1975, 1976, 1977a, b). Briefly, cerebral hemispheres from newborn mice (NMRI) were passed through a sterile nylon sieve (80 μm pore size) into a modified Eagle's minimum essential medium containing 20% (v/v) foetal calf serum (Eagle 1959, Schousboe *et al.* 1976), inoculated into plastic T-flasks (NUNC A/S, Denmark) and cultured for 2 weeks in this medium. Subsequently, the cultivation was continued for a third week in an analogous serum-free medium to which 0.1 mM dibutyryl-cyclic-AMP was added. Medium was changed 3 times a week over the entire culture period. In this manner well-differentiated astrocytes with a morphology (Schousboe *et al.* 1976, Hertz *et al.* 1978a) resembling that of their *in vivo* counterparts (Wolff 1970) were obtained. In addition to the morphology, the astrocytic character of the cells is indicated by a high content of the glial fibrillary acidic protein (Bock *et al.* 1975, 1977) which is believed to be specific for astrocytes (Eng *et al.* 1971). Moreover, they have high activities of enzymes such as carbonic anhydrase (Sensenbrenner 1977, Kimelberg *et al.* 1978, Hertz & Sapirstein 1978) and glutamine synthetase (Schousboe *et al.* 1977b) which are glial or astrocyte marker enzymes (Schousboe 1979). For further information of the validity of the cultured astrocytes as models for their *in vivo* counterparts, the reader is referred to discussions by Hertz (1977) and Schousboe (1977).

Brain cortex slices

As a model for the neuronal transport system for GABA mini-slices ('prisms') of brain cortex were used. Experiments by Riddall *et al.* (1976) indicate that the neuronal transport system is preserved whereas the glial transport system is progressively destroyed as the dimensions of a brain slice decrease. 'Prisms' were prepared from 0.5-mm mouse cerebral cortex slices obtained from the outer convexity of each hemisphere using a longitudinally vibrating nylon string (Franck *et al.* 1968, Schousboe 1972). Subsequently the slices were chopped into 0.1-mm 'prisms' by two consecutive choppings (angle 60°) on a McIlwain tissue chopper (McIlwain & Rodnight 1962), and the 'prisms' were suspended in phosphate buffered saline containing 6.0 mM glucose (Schousboe *et al.* 1977a).

GABA uptake and effect of analogues

The kinetics of the GABA uptake in cultured astrocytes were studied as detailed by Schousboe *et al.* (1977a). Briefly, small pieces of the cultures (30–50 μg of protein) were incubated for 5 min at 37°C in phosphate buffered saline containing 6.0 mM glucose and ^{3}H-GABA (specific radioactivity 37 Ci/mmol, New England Nuclear, Boston, Mass.) at different concentrations (5–1000 μM). The incubation was terminated by centrifugation (10 sec) and rapid washing of the pellet (10 sec) with non-radioactive medium. Effects of structural GABA analogues on the high affinity GABA uptake in astrocytes as well as 'prisms' were studied at an external GABA concentration of 1 μM and at analogue concentrations of 10, 50, 100, 500, 1,000 and 5,000 μM (Schousboe *et al.* 1978). From the calculated inhibitions, IC_{50} values were obtained as described by Beart *et al.* (1972). The IC_{50} value is defined as that concentration of analogue which inhibits the GABA uptake (1 μM GABA) 50%. The incubation procedure was similar to the one described for the kinetic studies.

NEURONAL VERSUS GLIAL GABA UPTAKE

Judged from electron microscopic studies (Bloom & Iversen 1971, Iversen & Bloom 1972, Schon & Iversen 1972) of radioautographs of brain sections incubated with ^{3}H-GABA or uptake experiments performed after specific lesions of GABA-ergic pathways (Storm-Mathisen 1975) there is little doubt that GABA is taken up into presynaptic terminals. It is, however, a question as to what extent this uptake may be responsible for the inactivation of GABA, since it has been clearly demonstrated that the major part of the high affinity GABA uptake into synaptosomes is due to a 1:1 homoexchange process (Levi & Raiteri 1974, Raiteri *et al.* 1975) which can be of no physiological importance for removal of GABA from synaptic clefts. Under *in vivo* conditions there may, however, be a concentrative net uptake since the membrane potential is preserved (Sellström *et al.* 1976).

Using bulk-prepared glial cells, Henn & Hamberger (1971) were the first to demonstrate that also this cell type had a high affinity uptake system for GABA. Such a glial transport system has since been demonstrated in peripheral ganglia (Bowery & Brown 1972, Young *et al.* 1973, Schon & Kelly 1974a, b, Roberts

Table I

Kinetic constants for high affinity uptake of GABA into brain slices, synaptosomes and different neuronal and glial preparations

Tissue preparation	K_m (μM)	V_{max} (nmol×min^{-1}×mg^{-1} protein)	Reference
Adult brain slices	11–31	0.36–1.76*	Martin (1976)
Neonatal brain slices	5–43	0.05*	Martin (1976)
Synaptosomes	13	2.2	Levi & Raiteri (1973)
Synaptosomes	4	1.1*	Martin (1976)
Synaptosomes	0.42	–	Henn & Hamberger (1971)
Cerebellar glomeruli	9.6	1.6	Wilkin *et al.* (1974)
Cerebellar glomeruli	10	1.5	Wilson *et al.* (1976)
Cerebellar glomeruli	15	–	Hamberger *et al.* (1976)
Bulk-prepared neurons	0.72	–	Henn & Hamberger (1971)
Cultured cerebellar neurons	0.33	0.21–0.84	Lasher (1975)
Bulk-prepared glial cells	0.27	–	Henn & Hamberger (1971)
Bulk-prepared glial cells	0.6	–	Henn (1976)
Sup. cerv. ganglia	7	0.002*	Bowery & Brown (1972)
Sensory ganglia	10	0.02*	Schon & Kelly (1974b)
Sensory ganglia	9.7	0.03	Roberts (1976b)
Cultured cerebellar glial cells	0.29	0.0005–0.002	Lasher (1975)
C-6 glioma cells	32	0.023	Schrier & Thompson (1974)
C-6 glioma cells	0.22	0.0014	Hutchison *et al.* (1974)
C-6 glioma cells	50	–	Henn (1976)
Cultured astrocytes mouse brain	40	0.35	Schousboe *et al.* (1977a)
Cultured astrocytes mouse brain	45	0.40	Hertz *et al.* (1978b).

Most of the values are quoted verbatim from the literature. The V_{max} for synaptosomes (Levi & Raiteri 1973) is calculated from Fig. 4 in that paper. V_{max} values for brain slices have been recalculated from nmol×min^{-1}×g^{-1} wet wt. on the basis of a protein content of brain cortex slices of 95 mg/g wet wt. (Schousboe 1972). V_{max} values from Lasher (1975) have been converted from nmol/mg DNA on the basis of the DNA content in rat brain reported by Zamenhof *et al.* (1972). In most cases the temperature was 37°. Asterisks indicate that the temperature was 25–27°. The results obtained on superior cervical ganglia and sensory ganglia represents peripheral glial cells since all GABA in the ganglia is located in glial cells (Roberts 1976b).

1976a, b) rat retina (Neal & Iversen 1972, Marshall & Voaden 1974), glioma cell lines (Hutchison *et al.* 1974, Schrier & Thompson 1974, Schubert 1975), spinal cord explant cultures (Hösli *et al.* 1972) and primary cultures of glial cells from cerebellum (Lasher 1975, Burry & Lasher 1975, Hösli & Hösli 1976) and cerebrum (Schousboe *et al.* 1977a, Hertz *et al.* 1978b) but only the latter preparation exhibited a transport with a V_{max} comparable to those previously reported for GABA uptake into brain slices (Table I). From the latter studies of

GABA uptake into cultured astrocytes it could accordingly be concluded that such cells may be involved in the inactivation of GABA. A crucial point in such a conclusion is the existence of a net inward transport and it was demonstrated by Hertz *et al.* (1978b) that the GABA uptake into astrocytes indeed represents a net uptake (Fig. 1) in contrast to what has been found for peripheral ganglia glial cells (Roberts 1976a) and bulk-prepared glial cells (Sellström & Hamberger 1976). In this context it should be mentioned that also GABA uptake into C-6 astrocytoma cells (Schrier & Thompson 1974, Schrier 1977) and rat retina glial cells (Lake & Voaden 1976) seems to represent a net uptake rather than a homoexchange process.

Another difference between the synaptosomal and glial uptake systems for GABA seems to be the sodium dependence. Although both systems are dependent upon sodium, the synaptosomal high affinity transport for GABA requires 2–3 sodium ions per GABA molecule (Martin & Smith 1972, Martin 1973, Sellström *et al.* 1976, Blaustein & King 1976) whereas the corresponding uptake into cultured astrocytes as shown in Fig. 2 requires only one sodium ion per GABA (Hertz *et al.* 1978b). In addition to this it was shown by Hertz *et al.* (1978b) that the GABA uptake into astrocytes did not depend upon external potassium, although this ion inhibits the uptake at concentrations above 10 mM (Schousboe *et al.* 1977a, Schousboe 1978a). On the basis of these findings the maximum tissue/medium ratio that such a transport mechanism can generate may be calculated from the following equation (Martin 1976):

$$\mathrm{GABA_i/GABA_0} = \frac{[\mathrm{N1_0^+}]}{[\mathrm{Na_i^+}]} \times \exp\left(-\mathrm{F} \times \Delta\mathrm{E}/\mathrm{R} \times \mathrm{T}\right)$$

in which F, R and T have their usual meanings. If it is assumed that $[Na_i^+]$ is close to an estimated value for brain slices reported by Schousboe & Hertz (1971) of 50 μmol/g and if a membrane potential (ΔE) of −80 mV (Moonen & Nelson, personal communication) for the cultured astrocytes is used for the calculation, a value of 60 for the equilibrium tissue/medium GABA ratio is obtained. This is close to the actual measured value reported by Hertz *et al.* (1978b), again indicating that GABA is transported in the astrocytes with the mechanism described above. That differences exist between the two transport systems also in terms of structural requirements for the transported molecule (GABA) will be shown in the following.

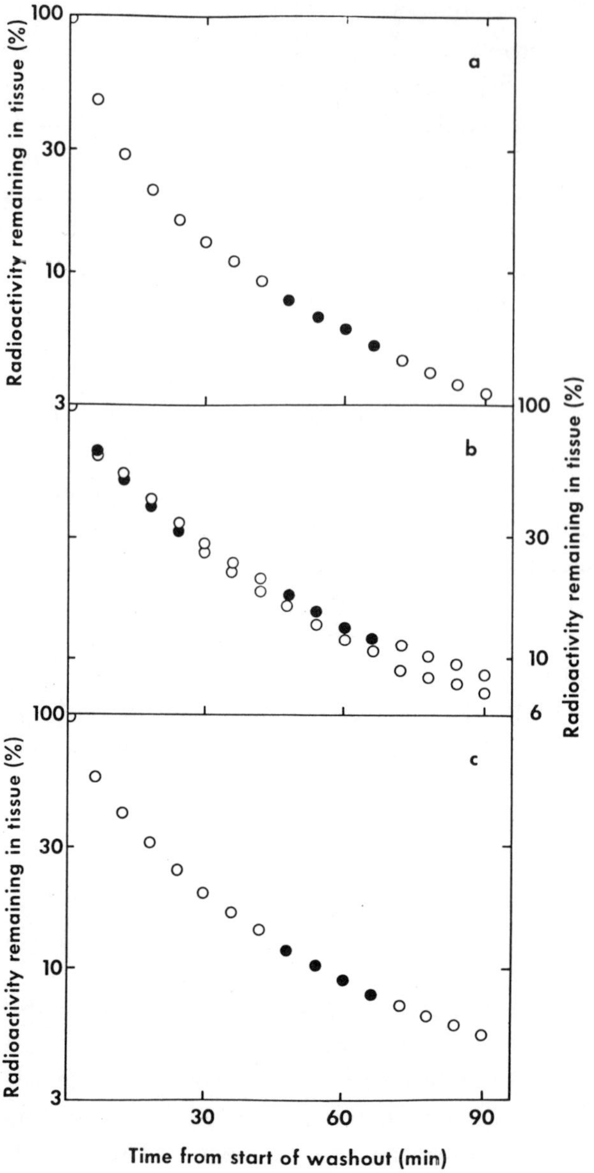

Fig. 1. Washout curves showing, as a function of time, release of radioactivity from astrocyte cultures loaded with ^{14}C-labelled GABA for 30 min. a) The washout medium contained 25 μM (○) GABA except during the period 42–66 min (●) when the GABA concentration was increased to 200 μM. b) The washout medium contained 25 μM (○) GABA except during the period 0–24 or 42–66 min (●) when the GABA concentration was increased to 2,000 μM. c) The washout medium contained 2.5 μM (○) GABA except during the period 42–66 min (●) when the GABA concentration

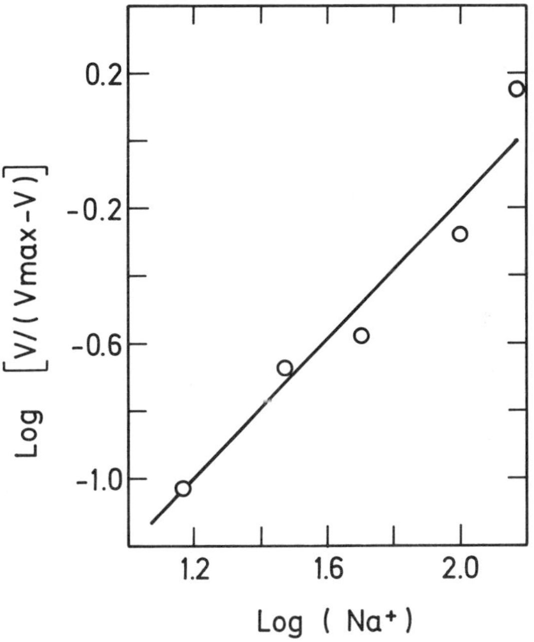

Fig. 2. Hill plot (Hill 1913, Atkinson 1966) showing log $[v/(V_{max}-v)]$ as a function of the logarithm of the sodium concentration; v indicates initial uptake rates at the different sodium concentrations, V_{max} the initial uptake rate at infinitely high sodium concentration and the GABA concentration of 50 μM used in the experiments. From Hertz *et al.* (1978b).

EFFECT OF ANALOGUES ON THE GLIAL TRANSPORT SYSTEM

Aliphatic compounds

The effect of 4-methylated GABA and trans-4-amino-crotonic acid on the high affinity uptake of GABA into cultured astrocytes is shown in Table II. It can be seen that the compounds are much more potent inhibitors in the *R*-configuration than in the *S*-configuration. It is furthermore seen that the difference between the potencies of the *R* and *S* forms is more pronounced in case of the amino-crotonic acid derivatives which represent GABA in its extended conformation than in case of the substituted GABA. For the sake of comparison the inhibitory effect on the GABA uptake in mini-slices ('prisms') is also shown

---

was increased to 200 μM. The lack of effect of nonradioactive GABA under any of these conditions on the efflux of radioactive GABA strongly indicates that the GABA transport is not due to homoexchange. From Hertz *et al.* (1978b).

and it is seen that the same pattern is exhibited in this case (For discussion of the effect on the neuronal transport system, see Brehm *et al.*, this volume). It should, however, be noted that *R*-trans-4-methyl-4-amino-crotonic acid seems to be a more potent inhibitor of the neuronal GABA transport system than of the glial system, although the difference is less pronounced than in case of β-proline which has the opposite preference (cf. below). A more detailed study of the kinetics may show whether this amino-crotonic acid derivative may be useful as a blocker of neuronal GABA transport. This would represent an analogy to 3-aminocyclohexanecarboxylic acid which has been shown to interfere specifically with the neuronal GABA transport (Bowery *et al.* 1976, Neal & Bowery 1977) and which has a structure resembling that of trans-4-methyl-4-amino-crotonic acid. The observed IC_{50} value for *R*-4-methyl-GABA is higher than that previously reported for GABA uptake in mini-slices of rat brain (Beart & Johnston 1973) but these authors used a much lower GABA concentration. Since the inhibition is of the competitive type (Beart & Johnston 1973), such a difference is to be expected and the K_i value reported by Beart & Johnston (1973) is accordingly closer than their IC_{50} to the IC_{50} value obtained in the present study.

It should be pointed out that the stereo selectivity exhibited by the difference in inhibitory potency of the uptake systems between the *R* and *S* forms of the trans-4-methyl-4-amino-crotonic acid is exactly opposite to the selectivity reported for the GABA receptor (Krogsgaard-Larsen *et al.,* this volume).

In addition to these methylated analogues, aminooxyacetic acid, which is an extremely powerful inhibitor of the GABA-transaminase (Schousboe *et al.* 1974) and which has previously been shown to be a relatively weak inhibitor of high affinity transport of GABA in brain cortex slices (Snodgrass & Iversen 1973, Johnston & Balcar 1974), was tested. As shown in Table II it was found to have no effect on the GABA uptake in astrocytes. Also diaminobutyric acid which has previously been classified as a specific inhibitor of the neuronal GABA carrier (Sutton & Simmonds 1974, Schon & Kelly 1974b, Iversen & Kelly 1975, Leach *et al.* 1976) was found to have no effect on the GABA uptake in astrocytes (Schousboe *et al.* 1978). The observed IC_{50} for β-alanine which is believed to be more inhibitory for glial GABA transport than for neuronal GABA transport (Schon & Kelly 1975, Iversen & Kelly 1975, Bowery *et al.* 1976) was higher than the corresponding value reported for GABA uptake into sympathetic ganglia glial cells but relatively close to the value reported for rat retina glial cells (Bowery *et al.* 1976).

Table II

Effect of aliphatic compounds on GABA uptake in astrocytes and cortical mini-slices

Compound		IC_{50} (μM)	
Name	Formula	Astrocytes	Mini-slices
R-4-Methyl-GABA	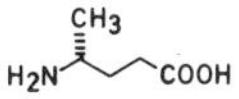	120	200
S-4-Methyl-GABA	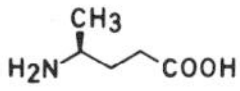	1,000	750
R-Trans-4-methyl-4-amino-crotonic acid	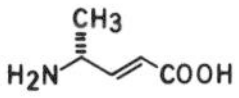	500	160
S-Trans-4-methyl-4-amino-crotonic acid	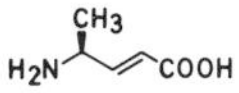	>5,000	>5,000
β-Alaninc	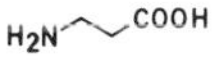	1,000	21,000
S-Diaminobutyric acid	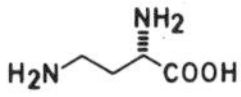	>5,000	50
Aminooxyacetic acid	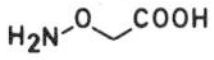	>5,000	-

Values are from unpublished results of Schousboe & Krogsgaard-Larsen and from Iversen & Johnston (1971), Schon & Kelly (1974b) and Schousboe *et al.* (1978).

Table III

Effect of different heterocyclic compounds (five-membered rings) on GABA uptake in astrocytes and cortical mini-slices

Compound		IC_{50} (μM)	
Name	Formula	Astrocytes	Mini-slices
(±) *β*-Proline	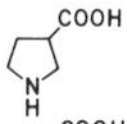	320	>1,000
S-(+) *β*-Proline	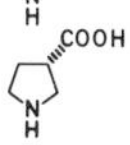	1,900	1,700
3,4-Dehydro-*β*-proline	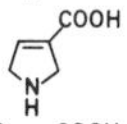	1,200	1,800
(±) Cis-4-OH-*β*-proline	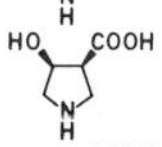	1,800	2,500
(±)-Isoxazolidine-5-carboxylic acid	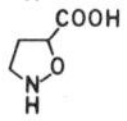	>5,000	1,000
Imidazoleacetic acid	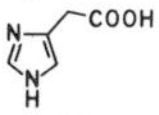	>5,000	-
Muscimol	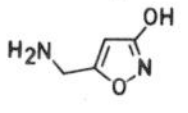	2,000	>1,000
(±) 4,5-Dihydromuscimol	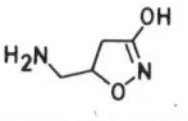	4,000	1,500

Values are from unpublished results of Schousboe & Krogsgaard-Larsen and from Krogsgaard-Larsen & Johnston (1975), Krogsgaard-Larsen (1978) and Schousboe *et al.* (1978).

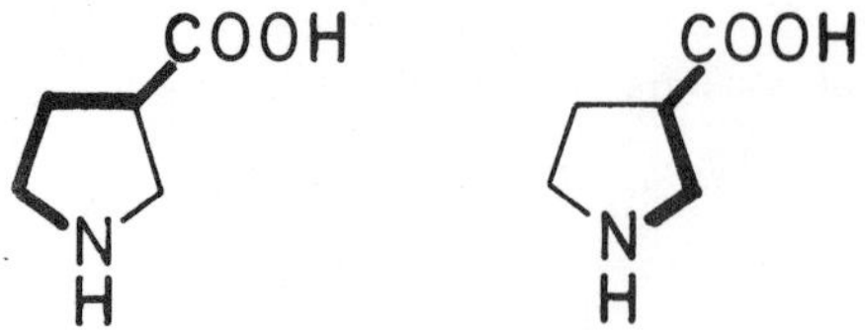

A B

β-Proline

Fig. 3. Formulas of β-proline illustrating its structural relation to GABA (A) and β-alanine (B).

Five membered rings

The effect of different heterocyclic compounds with five membered rings on the high affinity GABA transport is shown in Table III. Of the different derivatives of β-proline the parent compound itself is by far the most potent inhibitor. The loss of effect by the introduction of a double bond (3,4-dehydro-β-proline) may reflect the finding that the amino-crotonic acid derivatives were less potent inhibitors than the corresponding GABA derivatives (cf. Table II). The most interesting finding is that β-proline seems to be specific for the glial transport (Schousboe *et al.* 1978). From the IC_{50} values obtained for (±)β-proline and *S*-(+)β-proline a theoretical IC_{50} value of 100–150 μM for *R*-(−)β-proline may be obtained. This means that the active optical isomer of β-proline is 10 times as potent as β-alanine in the inhibition of GABA uptake into glial cells of central origin. This is interesting since the structure of β-proline combines the structures of GABA and β-alanine (Fig. 3). In this context it should be mentioned that preliminary experiments (Fig. 4) indicate that the inhibition of β-proline is of the competitive type. Further studies will show whether β-alanine interacts with the GABA-carrier in the same manner. In agreement with the finding that aminooxyacetic acid has no effect on GABA uptake, isoxazolidine-5-carboxylic acid which represents the former compound in an extended conformation has no effect on the uptake.

Table III also shows that imidazoleacetic acid and muscimol which are GABA agonists interacting with the bicuculline sensitive postsynaptic receptor or the crustacean slowly adapting stretch receptor (Curtis *et al.* 1971, Enna & Snyder 1975, Enna *et al.* 1977, Krogsgaard-Larsen 1978, Hori *et al.* 1978) and which have the same behavioral effect as GABA when injected into the substantia nigra of rats (Scheel-Krüger *et al.* 1977) have no effect on the glial uptake system. This is also the case for dihydromuscimol which has been found to be a more powerful GABA agonist than muscimol itself (Krogsgaard-Larsen *et al.*, this volume). It is furthermore seen that these compounds have only a slight effect on the GABA uptake into mini-slices ('prisms') which primarily represents neuronal uptake (Schousboe *et al.* 1978).

Six membered rings

The inhibition of the high affinity GABA uptake into astrocytes by nipecotic acid and its derivatives is shown in Table IV. It is seen that (−)nipecotic acid is much more potent than the (+)isomer and that the IC_{50} value corresponds reasonably well with that previously reported for brain slices (Krogsgaard-Larsen & Johnston 1975, Johnston *et al.* 1976). The IC_{50} for (+)nipecotic acid is, however, much higher for the glial transport than for the neuronal transport (Johnston *et al.* 1976). This could mean that the former system is more stereo selective than the latter and further kinetic studies of the mode of action of the

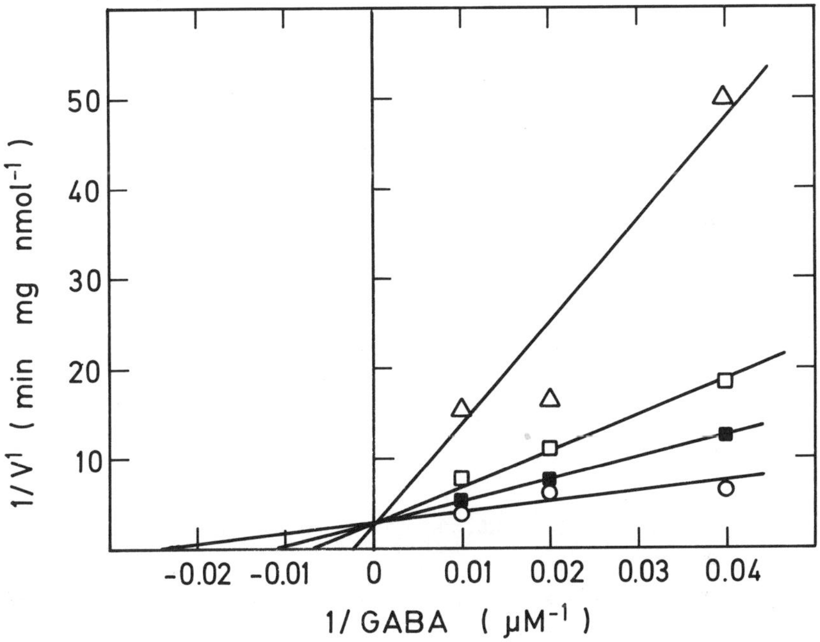

Fig. 4. Double reciprocal plot of the velocity (v′) of the high affinity GABA uptake in astrocytes *versus* the GABA concentration at different concentrations of (±)β-proline. (○) represents the control and (■), (□) and (△) the presence of 0.5 mM, 2.0 mM and 5.0 mM β-proline, respectively. Unpublished experiments of Schousboe & Krogsgaard-Larsen.

Table IV

Effect of different heterocyclic compounds (six-membered rings) on GABA uptake in astrocytes and cortical mini-slices

Compound		IC_{50} (μM)	
Name	Formula	Astrocytes	Mini-slices
S-(+) Nipecotic acid	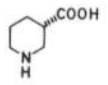	1,000	30
R-(−) Nipecotic acid	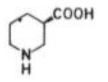	30	5
(±) Cis-4-OH-nipecotic acid	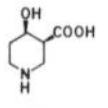	10	12
(±) Cis-2-OH-isonipecotic acid	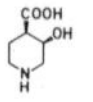	>5,000	>5,000
(±) N-Methyl-nipecotic acid	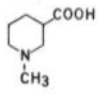	70	46
Guvacine	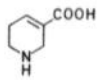	25	8
Isoguvacine	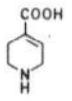	>5,000	>1,000

Values are from unpublished results of Schousboe, Krogsgaard-Larsen & Johnston and from Johnston *et al.* (1975, 1976), Krogsgaard-Larsen *et al.* (1977), Krogsgaard-Larsen (1978) and Schousboe *et al.* (1978).

two stereo isomers of nipecotic acid may well show that the (+)isomer can be used as a specific blocker of neuronal GABA transport. Also the N-methylated derivative of nipecotic acid was a relatively strong inhibitor of GABA uptake both into astrocytes and into neurons. It is interesting to note that whereas 4-OH-nipecotic acid is a very potent inhibitor of GABA uptake both in astrocytes (Schousboe *et al.* 1978) and brain slices (Krogsgaard-Larsen 1978) 3-OH-isonipecotic acid, in which the positions of the carboxylic acid and hydroxy groups have been switched, has no effect on any of the two transport systems.

Table IV also shows the effect of the betel nut *(Areca catechu)* constituent, guvacine, on the uptake systems. It has been shown to be a powerful inhibitor of both the glial (Schousboe *et al.* 1978) and the neuronal transport (Johnston *et al.* 1975). In contrast, isoguvacine which is a strong GABA agonist on the postsynaptic receptor (Krogsgaard-Larsen *et al.* 1977) has no effect on GABA uptake into astrocytes in agreement with what was reported for the neuronal uptake system (Krogsgaard-Larsen *et al.* 1977).

In addition to these compounds a series of amino derivatives of 3- and 4-carboxylic acid piperidine (Fig. 5) were tested as inhibitors of the GABA uptake into astrocytes. As expected from the lack of effect by diaminobutyric acid

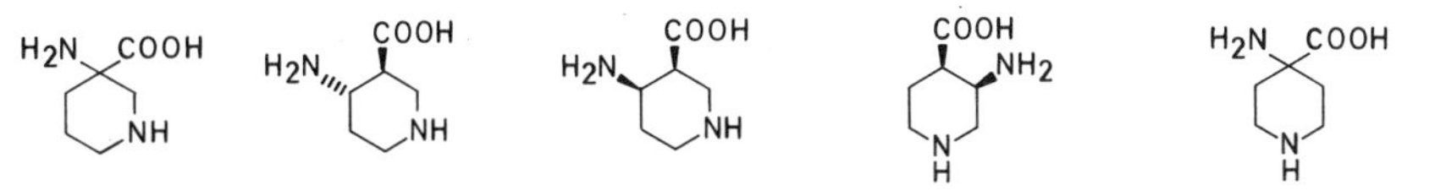

3-Amino-nipecotic acid — *trans-4-Amino-nipecotic acid* — *cis-4-Amino-nipecotic acid* — *cis-3-Amino-isonipecotic acid* — *4-Amino-isonipecotic acid*

Fig. 5. Structural formulas of different amino-derivatives of nipecotic and isonipecotic acid.

(Schousboe *et al.* 1978), none of these compounds had any effect ($IC_{50} > 5{,}000$ μM) on the GABA transport. They were, however, also shown to have no effect on the GABA transport in mini-slices (Brehm *et al.*, this volume).

CONCLUDING REMARKS

It has been shown that astrocytes cultured from mammalian brain hemispheres have a high affinity transport system for GABA which is capable of performing net uptake of GABA at a V_{max} which is comparable with corresponding values reported for brain slices. It may accordingly be concluded that glial cells may well be involved in the inactivation and subsequent metabolism of GABA. The latter conclusion is supported by the relatively high activity of the GABA-transaminase in these cells (Schousboe *et al.* 1977a, Schousboe 1978b).

From a study of a variety of GABA analogues of restricted conformation it can be deduced that derivatives of five membered heterocyclic rings are likely to be specific inhibitors of the glial GABA transport system. Of the compounds tested β-proline was found to be the most potent inhibitor and this analogue may be useful as a specific blocker of the glial transport system. Among the six-membered heterocyclic compounds tested none showed any specificity for the glial transport system. (+)Nipecotic acid may, however, be a specific blocker of neuronal GABA transport. Those compounds which have previously been shown to interact specifically with the bicuculline-sensitive postsynaptic receptor also proved to be without effect when tested on the GABA uptake into astrocytes.

ACKNOWLEDGEMENTS

The expert technical assistance by Miss Hanne Fosmark and Mrs. Inge Damgaard is gratefully acknowledged. Mrs. Grete Rossing is thanked for careful typing of the manuscript.

REFERENCES

Atkinson, D.E. (1966) Regulation of enzyme activity. *Ann. Rev. Biochem.* 35, 85–124.

Awapara, J., Landau, A. J., Fuerst, R. & Seale, B. (1950) Free γ-aminobutyric acid in brain. *J. Biol. Chem.* 187, 35–39.

Baxter, C. F. (1970) The nature of γ-aminobutyric acid. In: *Handbook of Neurochemistry* vol. 3, ed. Lajtha, A., pp. 289–353. Plenum Press, New York.

Beart, P. M., Johnston, G. A. R. & Uhr, M. L. (1972) Competitive inhibition of GABA uptake in rat brain slices by some GABA analogues of restricted conformation. *J. Neurochem.* 19, 1855–1861.

Beart, P. M. & Johnston, G. A. R. (1973) GABA uptake in rat brain slices: Inhibition by GABA analogues and by various drugs. *J. Neurochem.* 20, 319–324.

Blaustein, M. P. & King, C. (1976) Influence of membrane potential on the sodium-dependent uptake of gamma-aminobutyric acid by presynaptic nerve terminals: Experimental observations and theoretical considerations. *J. Membrane Biol.* 30, 153–173.

Bloom, F. E. & Iversen, L. L. (1971) Localizing ^{3}H-GABA in nerve terminals of rat cerebral cortex by electron microscopic autoradiography. *Nature* (Lond.) 229, 628–630.

Bock, E., Jørgensen, O.S., Dittmann, L. & Eng, L. F. (1975) Determination of brain-specific antigens in short term cultivated rat astroglial cells and in rat synaptosomes. *J. Neurochem.* 25, 867–870.

Bock, E., Møller, M., Nissen, C. & Sensenbrenner, M. (1977) Glial fibrillary acidic protein in primary astroglial cell cultures derived from newborn rat brain. *FEBS Lett.* 83, 207–211.

Booher, J. & Sensenbrenner, M. (1972) Growth and cultivation of dissociated neurons and glial cells from embryonic chick, rat and human brain in flask cultures. *Neurobiology* 2, 97–105.

Bowery, N. G. & Brown, D. A. (1972) γ-Aminobutyric acid uptake by sympathetic ganglia. *Nature New Biol.* 238, 89–91.

Bowery, N. G., Jones, G. P. & Neal, M. J. (1976) Selective inhibition of neuronal GABA uptake by cis-1,3-aminocyclohexane carboxylic acid. *Nature* (Lond.) 264, 281–284.

Burry, R. W. & Lasher, R. S. (1975) Uptake of GABA in dispersed cell cultures of postnatal rat cerebellum: an electron microscope autoradiographic study. *Brain Res.* 88, 502–507.

Curtis, D. R. & Johnston, G. A. R. (1970) Amino acid transmitters. In: *Handbook of Neurochemistry,* vol. 4, ed. Lajtha, A., pp. 115–134. Plenum Press, New York.

Curtis, D. R. & Johnston, G. A. R. (1974) Amino acid transmitters in the mammalian central nervous system. *Ergb. Physiol.* 69, 97–188.

Curtis, D. R., Duggan, A. W., Felix, D. & Johnston, G. A. R. (1971) Bicuculline, an antagonist of GABA and synaptic inhibition in the spinal cord of the cat. *Brain Res.* 32, 69–96.

Eagle, H. (1959) Amino acid metabolism in mammalian cell cultures. *Science* 130, 432–437.

Eng, L. F., Van der Haeghen, J. J., Bignami, A. & Gerstl, B. (1971) An acidic protein isolated from fibrous astrocytes. *Brain Res.* 28, 351–354.

Enna, S. J. & Snyder, S. H. (1975) Properties of γ-aminobutyric acid (GABA) receptor binding in rat brain synaptic membrane fractions. *Brain Res,* 100, 81–97.

Enna, S. J., Collins, J. F. & Snyder, H. (1977) Stereospecificity and structure-activity requirements of GABA receptor binding in rat brain. *Brain Res.* 124, 185–190.

Franck, G., Cornette, M. & Schoffeniels, E. (1968) The cationic composition of incubated cerebral cortex slices. *J. Neurochem.* 15, 843–857.

Haber, B., Kuriyama, K. & Roberts, E. (1970) An anion stimulated L-glutamic acid decarboxylase in non-neural tissues. Occurrence and subcellular localization in mouse kidney and developing chick embryo brain. *Biochem. Pharmacol.* 19, 1119–1136.

Hamberger, A., Hansson, H.-A., Lazarewicz, J. W., Lundh, T. & Sellström, Å. (1976) The cerebellar glomerulus: Isolation and metabolic properties of a purified fraction. *J. Neurochem.* 27, 267–272.

Henn, F. A. (1976) Neurotransmission and glial cells: A functional relationship? *J. Neurosci. Res.* 2, 271–282.

Henn, F. A. & Hamberger, A. (1971) Glial cell funtion: Uptake of transmitter substances. *Proc. Natl. Acad. Sci. USA* 68, 2686–2690.

Hertz, L. (1977) Biochemistry of glial cells. In: *Cell Tissue and Organ Cultures in Neurobiology*, ed. Fedoroff, S. & Hertz, L., pp. 39–71, Academic Press, New York.

Hertz, L. & Sapirstein, V. (1978) Carbonic anhydrase activity in astrocytes in primary cultures grown in the presence or abscence of dibutyryl cyclic AMP. *In Vitro*. In press.

Hertz, L., Wu, P. H. & Schousboe, A. (1978b) Evidence for net uptake of GABA into mouse astrocytes in primary cultures. – Its sodium dependence and potassium independence. *Neurochem. Res.* 3, 313–323.

Hertz, L., Schousboe, A., Boechler, N., Mukerji. S. & Fedoroff, S. (1978a) Kinetic characteristics of the glutamate uptake into normal astrocytes in cultures. *Neurochem. Res.* 3, 1–14.

Hill, A. V. (1913) The combinations of haemoglobin with oxygen and with carbon monoxide. *Biochem. J.* 7, 471–480.

Hori, N., Ikeda, K. & Roberts, E. (1978) Muscimol, GABA and picrotoxin: effects on membrane conductance of a crustacean neuron. *Brain Res.* 141, 364–370.

Hutchison, H. T., Werrbach, K., Vance, C. & Haber, B. (1974) Uptake of neurotransmitters by clonal lines of astrocytoma and neuroblastoma in culture. I. Transport of γ-aminobutyric acid. *Brain Res.* 66, 265–274.

Hösli, E. & Hösli, L. (1976) Autoradiographic studies on the uptake of ^{3}H-noradrenaline and ^{3}H-GABA in cultured rat cerebellum. *Exp. Brain Res.* 26, 319–324.

Hösli, E., Ljungdahl, Å., Hökfelt, T. & Hösli, L. (1972) Spinal cord tissue cultures – A model for autoradiographic studies on uptake of putative neurotransmitters such as glycine and GABA. *Experientia* 28, 1342–1344.

Iversen, L. L. & Bloom, F. E. (1972) Studies on the uptake of ^{3}H-GABA and ^{3}H-glycine in slices and homogenates of rat brain and spinal cord by electron microscopic autoradiography. *Brain Res.* 41, 131–143.

Iversen, L. L. & Johnston, G. A. R. (1971) GABA uptake in rat central nervous system: Comparison of uptake in slices and homogenates and the effects of some inhibitors. *J. Neurochem.* 18, 1939–1950.

Iversen, L. L. & Kelly, J. S. (1975) Uptake and metabolism of γ-aminobutyric acid by neurones and glial cells. *Biochem. Pharmacol.* 24, 933–938.

Johnston, G. A. R. & Balcar, V. J. (1974) Amino-oxyacetic acid: a relatively non-specific inhibitor of uptake of amino acids and amines by brain and spinal cord. *J. Neurochem.* 22, 609–610.

Johnston, G. A. R., Krogsgaard-Larsen, P. & Stephanson, A. (1975) Betel nut constituents as inhibitors of γ-aminobutyric acid uptake. *Nature* (Lond.) 258, 627–628.

Johnston, G. A. R., Krogsgaard-Larsen, P., Stephanson, A. L. & Twitchin, B. (1976) Inhibition of the uptake of GABA and related amino acids in rat brain slices by the optical isomers of nipecotic acid. *J. Neurochem.* 26, 1029–1032.

Kimelberg, H. K., Narumi, S., Biddlecome, S. & Bourke, R. S. (1978) Effects of DBcAMP and neurotransmitters on primary rat brain astrocyte cultures. *Trans. Am. Soc. Neurochem.* 9, 63.

Krogsgaard-Larsen, P. (1978) GABA agonists and uptake inhibitors of restricted conformations: Structure-activity relations. In: *Amino Acids as Neurotransmitters*, ed. Fonnum, F. Plenum Press, New York. In press.

Krogsgaard-Larsen, P. & Johnston, G. A. R. (1975) Inhibition of GABA uptake in rat brain slices by nipecotic acid, various isoxazoles and related compounds. *J. Neurochem.* 25, 797–802.

Krogsgaard-Larsen, P., Johnston, G. A. R., Lodge, D. & Curtis, D. R. (1977) A new class of GABA agonist. *Nature* (Lond.) 268, 53–55.

Krnjević, K. (1974) Chemical nature of synaptic transmission in vertebrates. *Physiol. Rev.* 54, 418–540.

Lake, N. & Voaden, M. J. (1976) Exchange versus net uptake of exogenously-applied γ-aminobutyric acid in retina. J. Neurochem. 27, 1571–1573.

Lasher, R. S. (1975) Uptake of GABA by neuronal and nonneuronal cells in dispersed cell cultures of postnatal rat cerebellum. *J. Neurobiol.* 6, 597–608.

Leach, M. J., Riddall, D. R. & Winkley, C. M. (1976) Uptake of L-2,4-diamino [4-^{3}H]butyric acid into slices of rat cerebral cortex. *J. Neurochem.* 27, 1281–1282.

Levi, G. & Raiteri, M. (1973) Detectability of high and low affinity uptake systems for GABA and glutamate in rat brain slices and synaptosomes. *Life Sci.* 12, 81–88.

Levi, G. & Raiteri, M. (1974) Exchange of neurotransmitter and amino acid at nerve endings can simulate high affinity uptake. *Nature* (Lond.) 250, 735–737.

Marshall, J. & Voaden, M. (1974) An investigation of the cells incorporating [^{3}H]GABA and [^{3}H]glycine in the isolated retina of the rat. *Exp. Eye Res.* 18, 367–370.

Martin, D. L. (1973) Kinetics of the sodium-dependent transport of gamma-aminobutyric acid by synaptosomes. *J. Neurochem.* 21, 345–356.

Martin, D. L. (1976) Carrier-mediated transport and removal of GABA from synaptic regions. In: *GABA in Nervous System Function*, ed. Roberts, E., Chase, T. N. and Tower, D. B., pp. 347–386. Raven Press, New York.

Martin, D. L. & Smith III, A. A. (1972) Ions and the transport of gamma-aminobutyric acid by synaptosomes. *J. Neurochem.* 19, 841–855.

McIlwain, H. & Rodnight, R. (1962) *Practical Neurochemistry*, pp. 109–133. Churchill, London.

Neal, M. J. & Bowery, N. G. (1977) Cis-3-aminocyclohexanecarboxylic acid: a substrate for the neuronal GABA transport system. *Brain Res.* 138, 169–174.

Neal, M. J. & Iversen, L. L. (1972) Autoradiographic localization of ^{3}H-GABA in rat retina. *Nature New Biol.* 235, 217–218.

Okada, Y., Taniguchi, H. & Shimada, C. (1976) High concentration of GABA and high glutamate decarboxylase activity in rat pancreatic islets and human insulinoma. *Science* 194, 620–622.

Raiteri, M., Federico, R., Coletti, A. & Levi, G. (1975) Release and exchange studies relating to the synaptosomal uptake of GABA. *J. Neurochem.* 24, 1243–1250.

Riddall, D. R., Leach, M. J. & Davison, A. N. (1976) Neurotransmitter uptake into slices of rat cerebral cortex *in vitro:* Effect of slice size. *J. Neurochem.* 27, 835–839.

Roberts, E. (1962) γ-Aminobutyric acid. In: *Neurochemistry – The Chemistry of Brain and Nerve*, 2nd ed., ed. Elliott, K. A. C., Page, I. H. & Quastel, J. H., pp. 636–656. Charles C. Thomas, Springfield, U.S.A.

Roberts, E. & Frankel, S. (1950) γ-Aminobutyric acid in brain: Its formation from glutamic acid. *J. Biol. Chem.* 187, 55–63.

Roberts, P. J. (1976a) Gamma-aminobutyric acid homoexchange in sensory ganglia. *Brain Res.* 113, 206–209.

Roberts, P. J. (1976b) Amino acid transport in spinal and sympathetic ganglia. In: *Transport*

Phenomena in the Nervous System, ed. Levi, G., Battistin, L. & Lajtha, A. pp. 165–178. Plenum Press, New York.

Scheel-Krüger, J., Arnt, J. & Magelund, G. (1977) Behavioral stimulation induced by muscimol and other GABA agonists injected into the substantia nigra. *Neurosci. Lett.* 4, 351–356.

Schon, F. & Iversen, L. L. (1972) Selective accumulation of [^{3}H]GABA by stellate cells in rat cerebellar cortex *in vivo. Brain Res.* 42, 503–507.

Schon, F. & Kelly, J. S. (1974a) Autoradiographic localisation of [^{3}H]GABA and [^{3}H]glutamate over satellite glial cells. *Brain Res.* 66, 275–288.

Schon, F. & Kelly, J. S. (1974b) The characterisation of [^{3}H]GABA uptake into the satellite glial cells of rat sensory ganglia. *Brain Res.* 66, 289–300.

Schon, F. & Kelly, J. S. (1975) Selective uptake of [^{3}H]β-alanine by glia: Association with the glial uptake system for GABA. *Brain Res.* 86, 243–257.

Schousboe, A. (1972) Development of potassium effects on ion concentrations and indicator spaces in rat brain cortex slices during postnatal ontogenesis. *Exp. Brain Res.* 15, 521–531.

Schousboe, A. (1977) Differences between astrocytes in primary cultures and glial cell lines in uptake and metabolism of putative amino acid transmitters. In: *Cell, Tissue and Organ Cultures in Neurobiology,* ed. Fedoroff, S. & Hertz, L., pp. 441–446. Academic Press, New York.

Schousboe, A. (1978a) Glutamate, GABA and taurine in cultured, normal glia cells. In: *Dynamic Properties of Glia Cells,* ed. Schoffeniels, E., Franck, G., Hertz, L. & Tower, D. B., pp. 173–182. Pergamon Press, Oxford.

Schousboe, A. (1978b) Metabolism and function of GABA in the mammalian brain. Possible role of glia cells. Thesis. University of Copenhagen. pp. 1–83.

Schousboe, A. (1979) Glial marker enzymes. In: *Nervous System Specific Proteins,* ed. Bock, E. *Scand. J. Immunol. Suppl.* In press.

Schousboe, A. & Hertz, L. (1971) Effects of potassium on concentrations of ions and proteins and on pH in brain-cortex slices from new-born and adult rats. *Intern. J. Neuroscience* 1, 235–242.

Schousboe, A., Fosmark, H. & Hertz, L. (1975) High content of glutamate and of ATP in astrocytes cultured from rat brain hemispheres: Effect of serum withdrawal and of cyclic AMP. *J. Neurochem.* 25, 909–911.

Schousboe, A., Fosmark, H. & Svenneby, G. (1976) Taurine uptake in astrocytes cultured from dissociated mouse brain hemispheres. *Brain Res.* 116, 158–164.

Schousboe, A., Hertz, L. & Svenneby, G. (1977a) Uptake and metabolism of GABA in astrocytes cultured from dissociated mouse brain hemispheres. *Neurochem. Res.* 2, 217–229.

Schousboe, A., Svenneby, G. & Hertz, L. (1977b) Uptake and metabolism of glutamate in astrocytes cultured from dissociated mouse brain hemispheres. *J. Neurochem.* 29, 999–1005.

Schousboe, A., Wu, J.-Y. & Roberts, E. (1974) Subunit structure and kinetic properties af 4-amino-butyrate-2-ketoglutarate transaminase purified from mouse brain. *J. Neurochem.* 23, 1189–1195.

Schousboe, A., Krogsgaard-Larsen, P., Svenneby, G. & Hertz, L. (1978) Inhibition of the high affinity, net uptake of GABA into cultured astrocytes by β-proline, nipecotic acid and other compounds. *Brain Res.* 153, 623–626.

Schrier, B. K. (1977) Transmitters, putative transmitters and transmitter-related enzymes studied in cultured cell systems. In: *Cell, Tissue and Organ Cultures in Neurobiology*, ed. Fedoroff, S. & Hertz, L., pp. 423–439. Academic Press, New York.

Schrier, B. K. & Thompson, E. J. (1974) On the role of glial cells in the mammalian nervous system. Uptake, excretion, and metabolism of putative neurotransmitters by cultured glial tumor cells. *J. Biol. Chem.* 249, 1769–1780.

Schubert, D. (1975) The uptake of GABA by clonal nerve and glia. *Brain Res.* 84, 87–98.

Sellström, Å. & Hamberger, A. (1976) γ-Aminobutyric acid release from neurons and glia. *Acta physiol. scand.* 98, 94–102.

Sellström, Å., Venema, R. & Henn, F. (1976) Functional assessment of GABA uptake or exchange by synaptosomal fractions. *Nature* (Lond.) 264, 652–653.

Sensenbrenner, M. (1977) Dissociated brain cells in primary cultures. In: *Cell, Tissue and Organ Cultures in Neurobiology*, ed. Fedoroff, S. & Hertz, L., pp. 191–213. Academic Press, New York.

Snodgrass, S. R. & Iversen, L. L. (1973) Effects of amino-oxyacetic acid on [^{3}H]GABA uptake by rat brain slices. *J. Neurochem.* 20, 431–439.

Storm-Mathisen, J. (1975) High affinity uptake of GABA in presumed GABA-ergic nerve endings in rat brain. *Brain Res.* 84, 409–427.

Sutton, I. & Simmonds, M. A. (1974) The selective blockade by diaminobutyric acid of neuronal uptake of [^{3}H]GABA in rat brain *in vivo. J. Neurochem.* 23, 273–274.

Van den Berg, C. J., Matheson, D. F., Ronda, G., Reijnierse, G. L. A., Blokhuis, G. G. D., Kroon, M. C., Clarke, D. D. & Garfinkel, D. (1975) A model for glutamate metabolism in brain: A biochemical analysis of a heterogeneous structure. In: *Metabolic Compartmentation and Neurotransmission. Relation to Brain Structure and Function*, ed. Berl, S., Clarke, D. D. & Schneider, D., pp. 515–543. Plenum Press, New York.

Wilkin, G., Wilson, J. E., Balázs, R., Schon, F. & Kelly, J. S. (1974) How selective is high affinity uptake of GABA into inhibitory nerve terminals? *Nature* (Lond.), 252, 397–399.

Wilson, J. E., Wilkin, G. P. & Balázs, R. (1976) Metabolic properties of a purified preparation of large fragments of the cerebellar glomeruli: glucose metabolism and amino acid uptake. *J. Neurochem.* 26, 957–965.

Wolff, J. R. (1970) The astrocyte as link between capillary and nerve cell. *Triangle* 9, 153–164.

Young, J. A. C., Brown, D. A., Kelly, J. S. & Schon, F. (1973) Autoradiographic localization of sites of [^{3}H]γ-aminobutyric acid accumulation in peripheral autonomic ganglia. *Brain Res.* 63, 479–486.

Zamenhof, S., Grauel, L., van Marthens, E. & Stillinger, R. A. (1972) Quantitative determination of DNA in preserved brains and brain sections. *J. Neurochem.* 19, 61–68.

Chapter III
Clinical Conditions Relevant for a Therapy with GABA-ergic Drugs and Mode of Action of Anticonvulsive Drugs

GABA System Participation in Human Motor, Cognitive, and Endocrine Function

Thomas N. Chase & Carol A. Tamminga

GABA-containing neurons are widely distributed throughout the mammalian central nervous system (CNS), comprising numerous local neural networks as well as various inter-regional pathways. Attempts to associate GABA system activity with any discrete set of normal behaviors or disease symptoms may thus seem simplistic. Considerable preclinical evidence does, however, suggest that GABA neurons contribute to the regulation of certain motor, cognitive, and endocrine functions. Available biochemical and pharmacologic techniques now permit a preliminary evaluation of such purported GABA mediated functions in man.

A potentially useful biochemical approach to the clinical study of GABA system function is the measurement of GABA levels in cerebrospinal fluid (CSF). Since the limited sensitivity of the ninhydrin procedure hindered GABA detection by conventional amino acid analysis (Perry & Hansen 1976), considerable controversy attended initial attempts to measure GABA in CSF. Recently, however, amino acid analysis using fluorometric detection (Glaeser & Hare 1975), radio receptor assay (Wood *et al.* 1978), or gas chromatographic-mass spectrometric procedures (Huizinga *et al.* 1977, Enna *et al.* 1977) has yielded reasonably consistent and essentially comparable results. Although the possibility that steady state GABA concentrations in lumbar CSF may actually reflect the activity of central GABA systems has yet to be verified, this concept is

---

Intramural Research Program, National Institute of Neurological and Communicative Disorders and Stroke, Bethesda, Maryland, and Department of Psychiatry, University of Chicago, Chicago, Illinois, USA.

"GABA-NEUROTRANSMITTERS", Alfred Benzon Symposium 12, Munksgaard 1978

consistent with the finding of diminished CSF GABA levels in patients with Huntington's disease (Glaeser *et al.* 1975, Enna *et al.* 1977), in whom direct biochemical assay of postmortem tissues has revealed characteristic reductions in brain GABA levels and in glutamic acid decarboxylase (GAD) activity (Perry *et al.* 1973, Bird *et al.* 1973, McGeer *et al.* 1973, Urquhart *et al.* 1975).

The pharmacologic evaluation of GABA system participation in human brain function involves clinical observations during the administration of drugs which selectively influence GABA-mediated synaptic transmission. Although there are a variety of potential sites at which drugs may affect GABA function (Chase & Walters 1976), relatively few agents with the requisite selectivity, potency, and safety are yet available for human use. The present studies are based upon clinical trials with sodium valproate (dipropylacetic acid), a relatively weak GABA transaminase inhibitor (Harvey *et al.* 1975, Anlezark *et al.* 1976), and two putative GABA agonists, imidazole acetic acid (Van Balgooy *et al.* 1972) and muscimol (Curtis *et al.* 1971, Brehm *et al.* 1972, Krogsgaard-Larsen *et al.* 1975, Johnston 1976, Wheal & Kerkut 1976, Naik *et al.* 1976, Beaumont *et al.* 1978, Enna *et al.* This symposium.

MOTOR FUNCTION

A role for GABA neurons in the regulation of certain motor functions in the experimental animal is suggested by anatomic, pharmacologic, and behavioral observations. GABA-containing cells serve as interneurons within the corpus striatum and nucleus accumbens, comprise fibers in a striatonigral tract, and contribute to efferents from the pallidum and accumbens (Walters & Chase 1977, Curtis, this symposium, Fonnum & Walaas, this symposium). Naturally occurring or drug-induced alterations in GABA neuron activity at any of these sites might be expected to influence extrapyramidal motor function. In rodents, unilateral GABA elevations in the zona reticulata of substantia nigra produce ipsilateral rotation in amphetamine-pretreated animals (Dray & Straughan 1976) and contralateral turning in the absence of dopamine agonist pretreatment (Koob *et al.* 1976). Contralateral turning following the unilateral injection of GABA or muscimol into the zona reticulata can be inhibited by the GABA blocking agent, picrotoxin (Oberlander *et al.* 1977, Olpe *et al.* 1977, Scheel-Krüger *et al.* 1977a, Waddington 1977). Systemically administered GABA transaminase inhibitors (Cott & Engel 1977) or muscimol applied to the nucleus accumbens of rats inhibit dopamine agonist-induced hyperactivity, but poten-

Table I
GABA levels in human lumbar CSF

	Number of Patients	p moles/ml
Control subjects	21	544±63
Huntington's disease	17	255±42*
Parkinson's disease	12	191±34*
Tardive dyskinesia	4	139±70**
Adult onset dystonia	7	221±59**

All study subjects were untreated at time of CSF sampling except for three parkinsonian patients who continued to receive L-dopa (Neophytides *et al.* 1978a). GABA assays utilized the high pressure liquid chromatography technique of Meek (1976) as modified by Waniewski & Suria (1977).
* $P<.005$.
** $P<.025$.

tiate dopamine agonist-induced stereotypy (Scheel-Krüger *et al.* 1977b). The various effects of GABA-active drugs on rodent motor behavior appear at least partially independent of the functional state of the dopamine system (Scheel-Krüger *et al.* 1977a, Cott & Engel 1977, Olpe *et al.* 1977, Scheel-Krüger *et al.* 1978).

Biochemical evidence of GABA system dysfunction in human extrapyramidal disease arises from measurements of CNS tissues obtained at autopsy as well as from studies of CSF obtained from the living patient. At present, Huntington's disease is the most thoroughly documented disorder associated with GABA system alteration. As already noted, GABA concentrations and GAD activity in the basal ganglia of Huntingtonian patients are substantially reduced (Perry *et al.* 1973, Urquhart *et al.* 1975, Bird *et al.* 1973, McGeer *et al.* 1973, McGeer & McGeer 1976) and CSF GABA levels are significantly diminished (Table I). Although it is generally assumed that these biochemical changes are a consequence of GABA neuron degeneration, there is no apparent correlation between the duration or severity of Huntington's chorea and the degree of CSF GABA reduction (Neophytides *et al.* 1978a). The finding of lowered GABA values (Table I) in the CSF of parkinsonian patients (Lakke & Teelken 1976) also corresponds with reports of diminished GAD activity in the basal ganglia of individuals dying with this disorder (Lloyd *et al.* 1973, Rinne *et al.* 1974, McGeer & McGeer 1976). The observed reductions in CSF GABA concentrations in patients with tardive dyskinesia or adult onset dystonia (Table I) have as yet no verification in direct biochemical measurements, but are not unexpected in view of observations in the experimental animal. Clearly, biochemical evidence of altered GABA system function does not now appear to be unique to any particular extrapyramidal motor disorder.

If a diminution in GABA system function contributes to the symptoms of any of the aforementioned disorders, then pharmacologic stimulation of GABA-mediated synaptic activity might be expected to ameliorate motor disability. Earlier drug trials in patients with Huntington's chorea involving dipropylacetate (Shoulson *et al.* 1976) or imidazole acetic acid (Shoulson *et al.* 1975) failed to provide symptomatic relief. More recently, muscimol (Table II) has also been found ineffective in the treatment of Huntington's disease (Shoulson *et al.* 1978). Aside from the pharmacodynamic and pharmacologic uncertainties associated with these drugs, although no satisfactory explanation can be offered for these negative results, a disease-associated reduction in the density of postsynaptic GABA receptors could be responsible (Enna *et al.* 1976, Lloyd *et al.* 1977).

A therapeutic trial of muscimol in six schizophrenic patients with tardive dyskinesia has, however, produced more favorable results (Tamminga *et al.* 1978a). In each of these patients, studied under double-blind, placebo controlled conditions, some diminution in involuntary movements was observed at maximum tolerated doses (Table II). Peak clinical effects occurred approximately 2 h after muscimol administration and diminished slowly over the ensuing hours. Although muscimol tended to sedate some patients, reductions in involuntary movements occurred either before or in the absence of this effect. In both Huntington's chorea and tardive dyskinesia patients, diffuse myoclonic twitching commonly supervened as the dose-limiting side effect. Clearly, muscimol's prominent toxicity precludes general clinical usefulness. On the other hand, available results, including those arising from the treatment of tardive dyskinesia with valproate (Linnoila *et al.* 1976), suggest that other GABA agonists might be usefully explored in patients with extrapyramidal motor disorders.

COGNITIVE FUNCTION

Possible GABA system involvement in cognitive function is also suggested by observations in the experimental animal. The mammalian cerebral cortex, including limbic areas, is rich in GABA neurons which appear to exert a predominantly inhibitory influence (Huot *et al.* 1977, Fonum & Walaas, this

Table II
Effect of muscimol on motor function in patients with Huntington's disease (HD) or tardive dyskinesia (TD)

	Number of patients	Rating Score: Placebo	Treatment	Difference	*P*
HD	4	14±1.9	22±5.2	7.7±4.5	$P > .05$
TD	6	6.8±1.6	3.5±.84	−3.3±1.2	$P < .05$

In HD patients, 26 aspects of motor function were rated on a scale of 0 (absent or normal) to 4 (very severe or abnormal) 2 h after a single oral dose of 8–14 mg muscimol (Neophytides *et al.* 1978b). In TD patients, motor function was rated on the same scale following 7–9 mg of muscimol (Tamminga *et al.* 1978a). The study was double-blind, placebo controlled and all subjects were otherwise untreated, except for one TD patient who continued to receive phenytoin.

symposium). GABA system participation in higher integrative cortical function is perhaps suggested by pharmacologic observations such as the ability of muscimol to modify conditioned responses in rats to various stimuli (Theobold *et al.* 1968, Scotti de Carolis *et al.* 1969). In cats, the direct installation of bicuculline into the nucleus accumbens produces behavioral alterations including hypervigilance, automatisms, approach anxiety, waxy flexibility, and motor stereotypies (Stevens *et al.* 1974); these responses are reminiscent of certain behaviors which accompany psychosis in man. Moreover, pharmacologic evidence indicates that stimulation of the GABA system inhibits certain dopaminergic pathways (Hattori *et al.* 1973, Lathi & Losey 1974, Cattabini *et al.*, this symposium, Walters *et al.*, this symposium, Palfreyman *et al.*, this symposium), a pharmacologic attribute shared by all clinically effective antipsychotic drugs.

The hypothesis that GABA system dysfunction attends schizophrenic illness has gained some support from studies of CNS tissues obtained at autopsy. A reduction in GAD activity has been reported in the nucleus accumbens and other brain regions of schizophrenic patients (Bird *et al.* 1977). More recently, however, serious doubt has been cast on the validity of these initial findings (McGeer & McGeer, this symposium, Iverson *et al.*, this symposium). Difficulties in distinguishing disease from premortem drug or postmortem handling effects continue to complicate the interpretation of results from human studies of this type.

In an attempt to evaluate the role of GABA system hypofunction in psychotic illness, six otherwise untreated patients with chronic schizophrenia received muscimol in a double-blind, placebo controlled study (Tamminga *et al.* 1978b). At maximum tolerated dose levels, ranging from 7 to 10 mg, changes in mental status as well as in neurologic function were observed in all patients (Table III). Scores of none of the nine psychotic symptoms rated improved with muscimol. In fact, there was a significant worsening in overall psychosis ratings, with scores for confusion, affect, and thought disorder showing the most consistent deterioration. The behavioral effects of muscimol peaked about 2 h after drug ingestion, and had largely disappeared within 5 h. At dose levels below 5 mg, some patients reported a tranquilizing effect; these individuals described feeling more relaxed, less anxious, and claimed a positive drug experience, despite their lack of relief from psychotic thinking. As found in patients with other disease states, muscimol treatment was associated with a relatively steep dose-effect curve, and adverse effects included transitory myoclonic twitching and somnolence.

Assuming that muscimol acts predominantly as a GABA agonist, it appears that pharmacologic stimulation of the GABA system does not improve psychotic symptoms in patients with chronic schizophrenia. The possibility that the exacerbation of psychosis observed in our patients points to a specific linkage between GABA system hyperfunction and schizophrenic illness would also seem unlikely, since it is known that muscimol can induce complex psychotomimetic effects in normal individuals (Waser 1967, Theobold *et al.* 1968).

ENDOCRINE FUNCTION

Recent preclinical observations indicate that GABA systems may be involved in the neural regulation of certain anterior pituitary hormones. GAD-positive nerve terminals have been found in most hypothalamic nuclei as well as in the median eminence (Hökfelt *et al.* 1978). Biochemical evidence suggests that GABA-containing fibers in the median eminence originate within the hypothalamus, while some GABA terminals in other hypothalamic nuclei arise from cell bodies outside the hypothalamus (Brownstein *et al.* 1976). The intracerebral administration of GABA reportedly elevates serum prolactin and growth hormone levels in rats (Mioduszewski *et al.* 1976, Pass & Ondo 1977, Abe *et al.* 1977). We have observed a biphasic effect of systemically administered muscimol on rat prolactin release (Tamminga & Frohman, 1978); others have noted a prolonged suppression of prolactin secretion following muscimol

Table III
Effect of muscimol on psychotic behavior in schizophrenic patients

	Baseline	2 h	Difference
Placebo	2.5±.2	2.6±.3	0.04±0.1
Drug	2.2±.2	3.0±.2	0.78±0.2*

Scores (mean±SEM) reflect an assessment of nine psychiatric symptoms evaluated on a scale of 0 (normal) to 4 (very abnormal) by a blind observer in a semi-structured interview conducted 2 h after the oral administration of muscimol (7–10 mg) to six otherwise untreated patients (Tamminga *et al.* 1978b).
* $P<.025$.

(Mueller *et al.*, this symposium). Moreover, an increase in circulating prolactin levels has been reported to follow the intravenous injection of bicuculline (Rivier & Vale 1977), while other studies have led to the suggestion that prolactin inhibitory factor (PIF) may be GABA itself (Schally *et al.* 1977). The reasons for these complex and seemingly conflicting results are not yet apparent.

To investigate the possible role of GABA mechanisms in the control of prolactin and growth hormone release in man, serial blood samples were obtained from patients with Huntington's disease and chronic schizophrenia during therapeutic trials of muscimol. All subjects were drug free for at least 1 week prior to study; each was tested on at least three occasions receiving 5 and 9 mg of drug and matching placebo in a double-blind design. All studies began at 9:00 a.m. and were performed on resting patients in a minimal stress environment. Prolactin and growth hormone were measured by a modification of the double antibody radioimmunoassay technique (Sinha *et al.* 1973).

A substantial dose-dependent rise in circulating prolactin values (Table IV) began within 60 min after muscimol administration and persisted for up to 4 h. A comparison of the effects of muscimol in patients with Huntington's disease or schizophrenia revealed no significant differences. In all patients, there was a small, but statistically significant, rise in growth hormone levels following muscimol administration (Table IV); no attendant changes in circulating cortisol or thyroid stimulating hormone (TSH) levels occurred (Tamminga *et al.* 1978c). It is unlikely that these endocrinological effects were stress induced, since no clinical manifestations of stress occurred until high doses of muscimol were administered; in fact, many patients reported tranquilization at the lower dose levels used.

The present results support the view that GABA-containing neurons in man influence the release of prolactin and growth hormone, but are not involved in

Table IV
Effect of muscimol on serum prolactin and growth hormone

	Baseline	60–80 min
Prolactin:		
Placebo	9.2±1.2	6.6 ±0.9
Drug	8.9±1.1	19 ±4.1*
Growth Hormone:		
Placebo	1.2±0.4	0.68±0.8
Drug	0.95±0.3	4.7 ±1.1**

Results are the means±SEM expressed in ng/ml for four choreatic subjects just before and 60 min (growth hormone) or 80 min (prolactin) after oral administration of 9 mg muscimol (Tamminga *et al.* 1978c).
* $P<.025$.
** $P<.01$.

the continuous control of cortisol or TSH. It would appear that the GABA system may affect prolactin secretion by acting within the hypothalamus, since neither GABA (Rivier & Vale 1977) nor muscimol (Szabo & Tamminga, unpublished observations) appear to substantially alter hormone secretion in isolated pituitary cell cultures.

CONCLUDING REMARKS

Available data, although based on indirect biochemical and pharmacologic techniques, support the view that GABA-containing neural systems participate in the regulation of some motor, cognitive, and endocrinologic functions in man. Regarding motor control, stimulation of GABA mediated synaptic function may apparently benefit symptoms in certain hyperkinetic extrapyramidal movement disorders, such as tardive dyskinesia, but not others, such as Huntington's disease. With respect to higher cortical functions, although it appears that the GABA system may be involved in cognitive processes, any link with the pathogenesis of schizophrenia now seems relatively unlikely. Finally, present results suggest that GABA mechanisms, possibly acting within the hypothalamus, facilitate the release of human prolactin and growth hormone. The substantiation and therapeutic exploitation of these tentative views await the development of improved biochemical techniques as well as the discovery of other potent and specific GABA active drugs.

REFERENCES

Abe, H., Kato, Y., Chihara, K., Ohgo, S. & Iwasaki, Y. (1977) Growth hormone release by gamma-amino-butyric(GABA) and gamma-amino-beta-hydroxy-butyric acid (GABOB) in the rat. *Endocrinol. Jpn.* 24, 229–232.

Anlezark, G., Horton, R. W., Meldrum, B. S. & Sawaya, C. B. (1976) Anticonvulsant action of ethanolamine-O-sulphate and di-N-propylacetate and the metabolism of γ-aminobutyric acid (GABA) in mice with audiogenic seizures. *Biochem. Pharmacol.* 25, 413–417.

Beaumont, K., Chilton, W. S., Yamamura, H. I. & Enna, S. J. (1978) Muscimol binding in rat brain: association with synaptic GABA receptors. *Brain Res.* 148, 153–162.

Bird, E. D., MacKay, A. V. P., Rayner, C. N. & Iversen, L. L. (1973) Reduced glutamic-acid decarboxylase activity of postmortem brain in Huntington's chorea. *Lancet* i, 1090–1092.

Bird, E. D., Barnes, J., Iversen, L. L., Spokes, E. G., MacKay, A. V. & Shepherd, M. (1977) Increased brain dopamine and reduced glutamic acid decarboxylase and choline acetyltransferase activity in schizophrenia and related psychoses. *Lancet* ii, 1157–1159.

Brehm, L., Hjeds, H. & Krogsgaard-Larsen, P. (1972) The structure of muscimol, a GABA analogue of restricted conformation. *Acta Chem. Scand.* 26, 1298–1299.

Brownstein, M., Palkovits, M., Tappaz, M. Saavedra, J. & Kizer, J. S. (1976) Effect of surgical isolation of the hypothalamus on its neurotransmitter content. *Brain Res.* 117, 287–295.

Chase, T. N. & Walters, J. R. (1976) Pharmacologic approaches to the manipulation of GABA-mediated synaptic function in man. In: *GABA in Nervous System Function,* ed. Roberts, E., Chase, T. N. & Tower, D. B., pp. 497–513. Raven Press, New York.

Cott, J. & Engel, J. (1977) Suppression by GABA-ergic drugs of the locomotor stimulation induced by morphine, amphetamine, and apomorphine: evidence for both pre- and post-synaptic inhibition of catecholamine systems. *J. Neurol. Trans.* 40, 253–268.

Curtis, D. R., Duggan, A. W., Felix, D. & Johnston, G. A. R. (1971) Bicuculline, an antagonist of GABA and synaptic inhibition in the spinal cord of the cat. *Brain Res.* 32, 69–96.

Dray, A. & Straughan, D. W. (1976) Synaptic mechanisms in the substantia nigra. *J. Pharm. Pharmacol.* 28, 400–405.

Enna, S. J., Bird, E. D., Bennett, J. P., Bylund, D. B., Yamamura, H. I., Iversen, L. L. & Snyder, S. H. (1976) Huntington's Chorea: Changes in neurotransmitter receptors in the brain. *N. Engl. J. Med.* 294, 1305–1309.

Enna, S. J., Stern, L. Z., Wastek, G. J. & Yamamura, H. I. (1977) Cerebrospinal fluid γ-aminobutyric acid variations in neurological disorders. *Arch. Neurol.* 34, 683–685.

Glaeser, B. S. & Hare, T. A. (1975) Measurement of GABA in human cerebrospinal fluid. *Biochem. Med.* 12, 274–282.

Glaeser, B. S., Vogel, W. H., Oleweiler, D. B. & Hare, T. A. (1975) GABA levels in cerebrospinal fluid of patients with Huntington's chorea: a preliminary report. *Biochem. Med.* 12, 380–385.

Harvey, P. K., Bradford, H. F. & Davison, A. N. (1975) The inhibitory effect of sodium n-dipropyl acetate on the degradative enzymes of the GABA shunt. *FEBS Letters* 52, 251–254.

Hattori, T., McGeer, P. L., Fibiger, H. C. & McGeer, E. G. (1973) On the source of GABA-containing terminals in the substantia nigra. Electron microscopic autoradiographic and biochemical studies. *Brain Res.* 54, 103–114.

Hökfelt, T., Edle, R., Fuxe, K., Johansson, O., Ljungdahl, A., Goldstein, M., Luft, R., Efendic, S., Nilsson, G., Terenius, L., Ganten, D., Jeffcoate, S. L., Rehfeld, J., Said, S., Perez de la Mora, M., Possani, L., Tapia, R., Teran, L. & Palacios, R. (1978) Aminergic and peptidergic pathways in the nervous system with special reference to the hypothalamus. In: *The Hypothalamus,* vol. 56, ed. Reichlin, S., Baldessarini, R. J. & Martin, J. B., pp. 69–135. Raven Press, New York.

Huizinga, J. D., Teelken, A. W., Muskiet, F. A. J., v.d. Meulen, J. & Walthers, B. G. (1977) Identification of GABA in human CSF by gas liquid chromatography and mass spectrometry. *N. Engl. J. Med.* 296, 692.

Huot, S., Lippert, B., Palfreyman, M. G. & Schechter, P. J. (1977) Inhibition of dopaminergic activity in the extrapyramidal and limbic systems by γ-acetylenic GABA. *Br. J. Pharmacol.* 60, 264P–265P.

Johnston, G. A. R. (1976) Physiologic pharmacology of GABA and its antagonists in the vertebrate nervous system. In: *GABA in Nervous System Function,* ed. Roberts, E., Chase, T. N. & Tower, D. B., pp. 395–411. Raven Press, New York.

Koob, G., Del Fiacco, M. & Iversen, S. D. (1976) The behavioural effects of EOS induced changes in substantia nigra GABA levels. *Br. J. Pharmacol.* 58, 454P.

Krogsgaard-Larsen, P., Johnston, G. A. R., Curtis, D. R., Game, C. J. A. & McCulloch, R. M. (1975) Structure and biological activity of a series of conformationally restricted analogues of GABA. *J. Neurochem.* 25, 803–809.

Lathi, R. A. & Losey, E. G. (1974) Antagonism of the effects of chlorpromazine and morphine on dopamine metabolism by GABA. *Res. Comm. Chem. Path. Pharmacol.* 7, 31–40.

Lakke, J. P. W. F. & Teelken, A. W. (1976) Amino acid abnormalities in cerebrospinal fluid of patients with parkinsonism and extrapyramidal disorders. *Neurology* 26, 489–493.

Linnoila, M., Viukari, M. & Hietala, O. (1976) Effect of sodium valproate on tardive dyskinesia. *Br. J. Psychiatr.* 129, 114–119.

Lloyd, K. G., Davidson, L. & Hornykiewicz, O. (1973) Metabolism of levodopa in the human brain. *Adv. Neurol.* 3, 173–188.

Lloyd, K. G., Dreksler, S. & Bird, E. D. (1977) Alterations in 3H-GABA binding in Huntington's chorea. *Life Sci.* 21, 747–754.

Meek, J. L. (1976) Application of inexpensive equipment for high pressure liquid chromatography to assays for taurine, γ-aminobutyric acid and 5-hydroxytryptophan. *Anal. Chem.* 48, 375–379.

McGeer, P. L., McGeer, E. G. & Fibiger, H. C. (1973) Choline acetylase and glutamic acid decarboxylase in Huntington's chorea. *Neurology* 23, 912–917.

McGeer, P. L. & McGeer, E. G. (1976) Enzymes associated with the metabolism of catecholamines, acetylcholine and GABA in human controls and patients with Parkinson's disease and Huntington's chorea. *J. Neurochem.* 26, 65–76.

Mioduszewski, R., Grandison, L. & Meites, J. (1976) Stimulation of prolactin release in rats by GABA. *Proc. Soc. Exp. Biol. Med.* 151, 44–46.

Naik, S. R., Guidotti, A. & Costa, E. (1976) Central GABA receptor agonists: Comparison of muscimol and baclofen. *Neuropharmacology* 15, 479–484.

Neophytides, A. N., Suria, A., Waniewski, R. A. & Chase, T. N. (1978a) Cerebrospinal fluid GABA in neurologic disease. In preparation.

Neophytides, A. N., Rosen, L. & Chase, T. N. (1978b) Muscimol treatment of Huntington's disease. In preparation.

Oberlander, C., Dumont, C. & Boissier, J. R. (1977) Rotational behavior after unilateral intranigral injection of muscimol in rats. *European J. Pharmacol.* 43, 389–390.

Olpe, H. R., Schellenberg, H. & Koella, W. P. (1977) Rotational behavior induced in rats by intranigral application of GABA-related drugs and GABA antagonists. *European J. Pharmacol.* 45, 291–294.

Pass, K. A. & Ondo, J. G. (1977) The effects of γ-aminobutyric acid on prolactin and gonadotropin secretion in the unanesthetized rat. *Endocrinology* 100, 1437–1442.

Perry, T. L., Hansen, S. & Kloster, M. (1973) Huntington's chorea: Deficiency of γ-aminobutyric acid in brain. *N. Engl. J. Med.* 288, 337–342.

Perry, T. L. & Hansen, S. (1976) Is GABA detectable in human CSF? *J. Neurochem.* 27, 1537–1538.

Rinne, U. K., Laaksonen, H., Riekkinen, P. & Sonninen, V. (1974) Brain glutamic acid decarboxylase activity in Parkinson's disease. *European Neurol.* 12, 13–19.

Rivier, C. & Vale, W. (1977) Effects of gamma-aminobutyric acid and histamine on prolactin secretion in the rat. *Endocrinology*101, 506–511.

Schally, A. V., Redding, T. W., Arimura, A., Dupont, A. & Linthicum, G. L. (1977) Isolation of gamma-aminobutyric acid from pig hypothalami and a demonstration of its prolactin release inhibiting (PIF) activity *in vivo* and *in vitro. Endocrinology* 100, 681–691.

Scheel-Krüger, J., Arnt, J. & Magelund, G. (1977a) Behavioral stimulation induced by muscimol and other GABA agonists injected into the substantia nigra. *Neuroscience Letters* 4, 351–356.

Scheel-Krüger, J., Christensen, A. V. & Arnt, J. (1978) Muscimol diffentially facilitates stereotypy but antagonizes motility induced by dopaminergic drugs: a complex GABA-dopamine interaction. *Life Sci.* 22, 75–84.

Scheel-Krüger, J., Cools, A. R. & van Wel, P. M. (1977b) Muscimol a GABA agonist injected into the nucleus accumbens increases apomorphine stereotypy and decreases the motility. *Life Sci.* 21, 1697–1702.

Scotti de Carolis, A., Lipparini, F. & Longo, V. G. (1969) Neuropharmacological investigations on muscimol, a psychotrophic drug extracted from *Amanita muscaria. Psychopharmacologica (Berlin)* 15, 186–195.

Shoulson, I., Chase, T. N., Roberts, E. & Van Balgooy, J. N. A. (1975) Huntington's Disease: treatment with imidazole-4-acetic acid. *New Engl. J. Med.* 293, 504–505.

Shoulson, I., Goldblatt, D., Charlton, M. & Joynt, R. J. (1978) Huntington's disease: treatment with muscimol, a GABA-mimetic drug. *Ann. Neurology.* In press.

Shoulson, I., Kartzinel, R. & Chase, T. N. (1976) Huntington's disease: treatment with dipropylacetic acid and gamma-aminobutyric acid. *Neurology* 26, 61–63.

Sinha, Y. N., Selby, F. W., Lewis, V. J. & Vanderlaan, W. P. (1973) A homologous radioimmunoassay for human prolactin. *J. Clin. Endocrinol. Metab.* 36, 509–519.

Stevens, J., Wilson, K. & Foote, W. (1974) GABA blockade, dopamine and schizophrenia: experimental studies in the cat. *Psychopharmacologia* 39, 105–119.

Tamminga, C. A., Chase, T. N. & Crayton, J. W. (1978a) Suppression of involuntary movements in tardive dyskinesia by muscimol, a GABA agonist. *Arch. Gen. Psychiat.* In press.

Tamminga, C. A., Crayton, J. W. & Chase, T. N. (1978b) Muscimol: GABA agonist therapy in schizophrenia. *Am. J. Psychiatry* 135, 746–747.

Tamminga, C. A., Neophytides, A. N., Chase, T. N. & Frohman, L. A. (1978c) Stimulation of prolactin and growth hormone secretion by muscimol, a gamma-aminobutyric acid agonist. *J. Clin. Endocrinol. Metab.* In press.

Tamminga, C. A. & Frohman, L. A. (1978) Muscimol stimulation of rat prolactin and TSH. In preparation.

Theobald, V.W., Büch, O., Kunz, H. A., Krupp, P., Stenger, E. G. & Heimann, H. (1968) Pharmacological and experimental psychologic studies on 2 components of the toadstool (Amanita Muscaria). *Arzneim. Forsch.* 18, 311–315.

Urquhart, N., Perry, T. L., Hansen, S. & Kennedy, J. (1975) GABA content and glutamic acid decarboxylase activity in brain of Huntington's chorea patients and control subjects. *J. Neurochem.* 24, 1071–1075.

Van Balgooy, J. N., Marshall, F. D. & Roberts, E. (1972) Metabolism of intracerebrally administered histadine, histamine and imidazoleacetic acid in mice and frogs. *J. Neurochem.* 19, 2341–2353.

Waddington, J. L. (1977) GABA-like properties of flurazepam and baclofen suggested by rotational behavior following unilateral intranigral injection: a comparison with the GABA agonist muscimol. *Brit. J. Pharmacol.* 60, 263P–264P.

Walters, J. R. & Chase, T. N. (1977) GABA systems and extrapyramidal function. In: Neurotransmitter Function: Basic and Clinical Aspects, ed. Fields, W. S., pp. 193–211. Stratton Intercontinental Medical Book Corporation, New York.

Waniewski, R. A. & Suria, A. (1977) Alterations in γ-aminobutyric acid content in the rat superior cervical ganglion and pineal gland. *Life Sci.* 21, 1129–1141.

Waser, P. G. (1967) The pharmacology of *Amanita Muscaris.* In: *Ethnopharmacologic Search for Psychoactive Drugs.* ed. Efron, D. H., Holmstedt, B. & Kline, N. S., pp. 419–439. U.S. Public Health Service publication.

Wheal, H. V. & Kerkut, G. A. (1976) The action of muscimol on the inhibitory postsynaptic membrane of the crustacean neuromuscular junction. *Brain Res.* 109, 179–183.

Wood, J. H., Glaeser, B. S., Enna, S. J. & Hare, T. A. (1978) Verification and quantification of GABA in human cerebrospinal fluid. *J. Neurochem.* 30, 291–293.

GABA in Relation to Extrapyramidal Diseases, with Particular Relevance to Animal Models

C. D. Marsden

EXTRAPYRAMIDAL DISEASES

First came Parkinson's disease, but there are many other illnesses affecting the extrapyramidal motor system in search of a cause, a cure, or a treatment. Broadly speaking, neurologists distinguish two categories of extrapyramidal disease:

1) *Akinetic-rigid syndromes,* characterized by slowness and poverty of movement with stiff rigid muscles, typified by Parkinson's disease.
2) *Hyperkinetic syndromes,* characterized by abnormal involuntary movements (dyskinesias) such as those of chorea as in Huntington's disease, or those of torsion dystonia as in dystonia musculorum deformans and its variants.

In both the akinetic-rigid syndromes and in those diseases characterized by dyskinesias, the pathology, where known, lies in the basal ganglia. The changes in the brain in idiopathic Parkinson's disease are those of death of the substantia nigra, but a similar akinetic-rigid syndrome can be produced by massive bilateral destruction of the striatum or globus pallidus.

Dyskinesias, on the other hand, are usually associated with *partial* bilateral cell loss and fiber damage in basal ganglia structures. Thus, in Huntington's disease, the characteristic pathological change held to be responsible for the chorea is loss of small interneurons in striatum. However, as the illness

---

University Department of Neurology, Institute of Psychiatry, De Crespigny Park, Denmark Hill, London SE5 8AF, England

"GABA-NEUROTRANSMITTERS", Alfred Benzon Symposium 12, Munksgaard 1978

progresses and more and more striatal cells are lost, the chorea is often replaced by an akinetic-rigid syndrome.

THE 'SIMPLE' PHARMACOLOGY OF EXTRAPYRAMIDAL DISEASE

In the first half of the 1970s, extrapyramidal disease was interpreted in terms of altered dopamine function. Parkinson's disease was due to dopamine deficiency secondary to nigral cell loss, to be relieved by substitution therapy with levodopa. Dyskinesias were provoked in patients with Parkinson's disease by levodopa overdosage (and more recently by directly acting dopamine agonists), and thus were due to dopamine overactivity, to be relieved by neuroleptic drugs which blocked dopamine receptors (see Marsden 1975 for review).

This simple pharmacological model still holds true: dopamine depletion does cause an akinetic-rigid syndrome, dopamine excess does cause dyskinesias. But, as the years have gone by and more information has been gathered, problems over such a simple interpretation have arisen, a few of which may be summarized:

1) Levodopa substitution therapy does not always restore function in Parkinson's disease, nor do its benefits last in many patients (see Marsden & Parkes 1976).
2) Some patients with akinetic-rigid syndromes other than Parkinson's disease have no dopamine deficiency, and do not respond to levodopa therapy (e.g. Wilson's disease, olivopontocerebellar degeneration, etc.).
3) Dopamine excess is not found in many conditions characterized by dyskinesias; for example, in Huntington's chorea where, if anything, striatal dopamine levels are reduced (Bernheimer *et al.* 1973, Bird & Iversen 1974).
4) Dopamine antagonists often have not proved successful in abolishing chorea, and have little useful effect on torsion dystonia (Marsden, personal observations).

These and other observations prompt enquiry into neurotransmitter events occurring subsequent to dopamine action in the basal ganglia. What neurotransmitter systems in the striatum do the nigrostriatal dopaminergic pathways impinge upon? How is the activity of striatal neurons transmitted from striatum to other basal ganglia areas to influence motor mechanisms? Can manipulation of the neurotransmitters involved in these other pathways influence basal ganglia function? If so, will they be useful in extrapyramidal diseases?

WHY GABA IN EXTRAPYRAMIDAL DISEASES?

GABA pathways exist in basal ganglia

The presence of high concentrations of GABA, and its synthesizing enzyme, glutamic acid decarboxylase, in certain basal ganglia structures, especially the globus pallidus and the substantia nigra, in a variety of species is well known (see Fahn 1976). Similarly, there is high affinity sodium - independent binding of GABA to presumed GABA receptors in high concentration in striatum, globus pallidus, and substantia nigra (Enna *et al.* 1975).

In the study of Enna *et al.* (1975) GABA uptake and glutamic acid decarboxylase activity were highly enriched in globus pallidus and substantia nigra, suggesting the presence of GABA terminals in these sites, where GABA receptor concentrations were also high. Indeed, previous studies had established the existence of powerful pallido- and strio-nigral GABA pathways (McGeer *et al.* 1974 Kataoka *et al.* 1974, Fonnum *et al.* 1974) synapsing particularly with nigral dendrites in zona reticulata (Ribak *et al.* 1976). As yet, there is no similar convincing evidence for a GABA striopallidal pathway although physiological studies suggest this as a possibility (Obata & Yoshida 1973) and the biochemical evidence described above may indicate the presence of GABA terminals in globus pallidus. Recent histochemical evidence suggests the presence of a leu-enkephalin striopallidal pathway (Cuello & Paxinos 1978). Finally, there is good evidence, based on ablation studies of afferent inputs into striatum, to suggest that the majority of GABA in that site is contained in intrinsic interneurons (McGeer & McGeer 1975), probably synapsing on corticostriatal and nigro-striatal terminals (Campochiaro *et al.* 1977).

Ascending dopamine pathways innervate not only the striatum, but also mesolimbic areas, such as nucleus accumbens. The latter is, in fact, part of the basal ganglia and is included in the head of the caudate nucleus in man, so may well be involved in extrapyramidal disease. GABA neurones also are present in nucleus accumbens, mainly as intrinsic interneurones, but perhaps, also in a GABA pathway between nucleus accumbens and globus pallidus (see Fonnum & Walaas, this volume).

In summary, GABA pathways throughout the basal ganglia appear likely to have impact on function of the striatum, nucleus accumbens and substantia nigra – areas intimately concerned with dopamine action. Evidence is now available to indicate that dopaminergic activity in nigrostriatal pathways is controlled by GABA, both by the descending GABA pallidonigral and strionigral pathways described above (Okada 1976, Racagni *et al.* 1977, Cattabeni *et al.* this volume, Andén, this volume) and by local control of dopamine release from nerve terminals by intrinsic striatal interneurones (Stoof & Mulder 1977). (Although mesolimbic areas contain a dense GABA innervation, present evidence suggests that there is no accumbens-tegmental GABA pathway controlling the mesolimbic dopamine system (Fonnum & Walaas, this volume)). By these means the functional consequences of dopamine deficiency or dopamine excess may be provoked or modified by GABA action on dopaminergic pathways within the basal ganglia.

In reverse, dopaminergic activity modifies GABA action in both striatal and mesolimbic areas (Perez de la Mora & Fuxe 1977,Fuxe *et al*, this volume, but see Costa *et al.* this volume). Consequently, the expression of dopaminergic deficiency or excess may depend upon subsequent GABA-mediated effects.

For both reasons it is clear that GABA may be involved in, or may modify, extrapyramidal diseases.

Abnormalities of GABA have been found in the brain at postmortem examination in extrapyramidal diseases

Almost all biochemical observations on postmortem brain tissue have been made in patients with Parkinson's disease and Huntington's chorea. Most investigations have concentrated on the enzyme responsible for GABA synthesis, namely, L-glutamic acid decarboxylase (GAD) which resides in GABA neurones and terminals, and more recently, on high-affinity sodium-independent (^{3}H) GABA binding, believed to represent binding to postsynaptic neuronal GABA receptors (Table 1) (see also McGeer & McGeer, this volume).

In Parkinson's disease, GAD is reduced to some 20–50% of normal in striatum, globus pallidus and substantia nigra, while (^{3}H) GABA binding is normal in striatum and globus pallidus, and decreased in nigra. Lloyd & Hornykiewicz (1973) demonstrated that the reduced GAD content in all structures returned to normal after prolonged L-DOPA therapy. These data justify two conclusions, 1) Loss of (^{3}H) GABA binding sites in nigra reflects loss of the nigral dopamine neurones on which they lie, and 2) the reduction in striatal, pallidal and nigral GAD reflects a reversible functional reduction in GABA activity, not loss of GABA cells.

Table I
Abnormalities in GAD and [^3H] GABA Binding

	Parkinson's Disease	Huntington's Disease
STRIATUM (CAUDATE/PUTAMEN)		
GAD	↓1,3,4,5	↓2,5,6
[^{3}H GABA]	N 7	N 6
PALLIDUM		
GAD	↓1,3,4,5,	↓2,5,6,
[^{3}H GABA]	? N 7	N 6
S. NIGRA		
GAD	↓1,3,4,5,	↓2,5,6
[^{3}HGABA]	↓7	↑6

After 1) Lloyd & Hornykiewicz 1973, 2) Bird & Iversen 1974, 3) Rinne *et al.* 1974, 4) Lloyd *et al.* 1975, 5) McGeer & McGeer 1976, 6) Enna *et al.* 1976, 7) LLoyd *et al.* 1977.

In Huntington's chorea, GAD is reduced to some 20–40% of normal in striatum (including accumbens), pallidum and nigra, while (^{3}H) GABA binding is normal in striatum and pallidum and increased in nigra. These data reflect widespread loss of GABA-containing striatal and pallidal neurones, including those of the strio- and pallido-nigral pathways, and preservation of the nigral dopaminergic neurons, whose GABA receptors increase due to denervation.

There have been no comparable large-scale investigations of postmortem material in other extrapyramidal diseases.

INITIAL ATTEMPTS TO MANIPULATE GABA ACTION IN BASAL GANGLIA DISEASE

These have been uniformly unsuccessful, probably not because the concepts are wrong, but because the tools available have been inadequate.

GABA itself has been administered to patients with Parkinson's disease (Barbeau 1973) and Huntington's disease (Barbeau 1973, Fisher *et al.* 1974) with no consistent effects. Drugs with possible GABA-mimetic properties also have been tried. Baclofen had no useful effect in either Parkinson's disease (Barbeau 1973) or Huntington's disease (Barbeau 1973, Andén *et al.* 1973, Paulson 1976), and imidazole-4-acetic acid was of no value in the latter illness (Shoulson *et al.* 1975). Nor has sodium valproate (sodium-n-dipropylacetate) been of value in either Parkinson's disease (Price, *et al.*, unpublished observations), or Huntington's disease (Lenman *et al.* 1976, Shoulson *et al.* 1976, Pearce *et al.* 1976), even when combined with GABA (Shoulson *et al.* 1976).

None of these drugs has had useful effects in either disease, but there are reasons for doubting whether any of them achieve their postulated GABA actions in the brain in the doses used in man.

THEORETICAL CONSIDERATIONS

The necessity for drugs with selective GABA action

Of course, no one neurotransmitter is involved with the various extrapyramidal diseases. A change in function of one will produce secondary changes in others, and the pathological alterations that occur in the various diseases under consideration tend to involve more than one cell type. However, for present purposes, discussion will focus on GABA.

GABA is present throughout the brain, so that drugs affecting GABA action are likely to have widespread effects. Obviously, for diseases such as those affecting the basal ganglia regions, one would hope for agents that might selectively act on GABA synapses in appropriate restricted areas, thereby preventing the unwanted effects of disturbing GABA action elsewhere. A single example emphasises the point. There are reasons to believe that a selective reduction in GABA action in globus pallidus might benefit patients with Parkinson's disease (see below). However, drugs reducing GABA action throughout the brain are likely to provoke epileptic fits in doses that affect pallidal GABA activity (see Meldrum, this volume).

A possible mechanism that might overcome the problem, even with nonselective drugs, is the presence of supersensitivity of GABA receptors provoked by the pathology of the disease. This would focus the effect of low doses of GABA activity drugs onto the appropriate target site. However, in general, the need for site-selective GABA agonists and antagonists is obvious (see Enna *et al.*, this volume), and the necessity for them to enter the brain needs no emphasis.

Parkinson's disease

The practical problem in Parkinson's disease is loss of responsiveness to dopamine agonists during long-term therapy. Among many possible reasons for this is loss of postsynaptic dopamine receptor sites in the striatum. Function might be restored in such patients if the synaptic activity of those cells on which dopamine acts could be enhanced appropriately, or if their action at subsequent synapses could be altered to overcome the effects of dopamine deficiency. GABA action in both striatum and globus pallidus might be involved, but that in substantia nigra is unlikely to be of influence in a disease in which the nigral cells themselves are lost.

Of particular interest is the akinetic-rigid syndrome in rodents provoked by enhanced GABA action in pallidum (see below). This mimics the effects of dopamine depletion in rodents, either by disruption of dopamine stores, or by blockade of dopamine receptors. All produce an animal which is immobile, flexed and rigid, resembling in these respects the human with Parkinson's disease.

The conclusion is that a drug that selectively *inhibits GABA synthesis or postsynaptic action in globus pallidus* may be of benefit in Parkinson's disease.

In contrast, the evidence for a dopaminergic-GABA interaction within the striatum suggests that dopamine receptor striatal activation increases striatal GABA turnover (Perez de la Mora & Fuxe 1977, Costa *et al.*, this volume). On these grounds a drug which *selectively activates GABA action in striatum* might replace dopamine deficiency in Parkinson's disease.

Finally, in view of the apparently inhibitory effect of GABA on nigral dopaminergic neurons, an agent which *selectively inhibits GABA action in nigra* might drive the remaining nigral neurons to produce as much dopamine as possible (although present evidence suggests that this is already the case (Bernheimer *et al.* 1973, Hornykiewicz *et al.* 1976)).

It is certain that present knowledge is incomplete, but even based on that currently available, it is obvious that drugs acting widely on GABA mechanisms given to patients with Parkinson's disease may produce an adverse action at one site and a beneficial effect at another, quite apart from the unwanted effects they may produce from actions elsewhere than in the basal ganglia.

Huntington's disease

In the case of Huntington's disease, the theoretical aim of manipulating GABA in different sites in the basal ganglia would seem to be the same, namely to increase GABA action in striatum, substantia nigra, and globus pallidus.

The loss of GABA neurons in caudate and putamen, which is characteristic of the basal ganglia chemical pathology of Huntington's disease, might be overcome by a directly-acting GABA agonist specific to the site, particularly as GABA receptor binding is unchanged in this area (Enna *et al.* 1976, but see Iversen *et al.*, this volume).

Similarly, a directly acting GABA agonist operating in substantia nigra would decrease nigrostriatal dopaminergic activity with benefit to the chorea that appears to be due to dopaminergic overactivity.

Finally, GABA stimulation in globus pallidus theoretically should provoke a decrease in dyskinetic phenomena in that it produces an akinetic-rigid syndrome.

In conclusion, *a directly acting GABA agonist affecting striatum, nigra and globus pallidus* should provide the ideal therapy for the chorea of Huntington's disease.

Other extrapyramidal diseases

Since so little is known about the chemical pathology of other basal ganglia diseases, such as torsion dystonia and its variants, or drug-induced tardive dyskinesias, that it is fruitless to speculate on the possible roles of GABA in these conditions. Further biochemical information on human postmortem brain material is required urgently.

ANIMAL MODELS OF SELECTIVE GABA ACTION AT DIFFERENT SITES IN THE BASAL GANGLIA

All these data point to the need to develop GABA – acting drugs with *site-selective* action. Such drugs should enter the brain freely, but should act preferentially at specified target sites. To this end, we began some years ago a series of studies designed to develop animal models of GABA action in different regions of the basal ganglia of rodents.

Striatum

Blockade of GABA action in one caudate nucleus of the rat provokes a reproducible myoclonus of the contralateral limbs and trunk (Tarsy *et al.* 1978). We have concluded that this behavioral effect is due to focal inhibition of GABA receptor sites in the caudate, for it is produced by focal injection of picrotoxin, bicuculline, and DL-allylglycine into one striatum, and once established, it is abolished by intrastriatal injection of GABA. Recently, intrastriatal injection of 2-keto-4-pentenoic acid, a main metabolite of allylglycine, has been found to provoke similar myoclonus (Horton *et al.* 1978).

The contralateral myoclonus produced by intrastriatal picrotoxin depends on the presence of a concurrent cortical scar, and is associated with spike discharges first in striatum, then in cortex. This suggests that this model is one of Epilepsia partialis continua, not chorea. It is not substantially influenced by drugs manipulating cerebral dopamine, noradrenaline, serotonin or acetylcholine mechanisms.

Nucleus accumbens

Direct bilateral injection of dopamine into nucleus accumbens in the rat provokes a prolonged locomotor hyperactivity. This response can be prevented by increasing GABA concentrations in this area of the basal ganglia using the GABA transaminase inhibitor ethanolamine-O-sulphate (Pycock & Horton 1976a). Simultaneously, the locomotor hyperactivity provoked by systemic amphetamine is suppressed, but not spontaneous activity and exploration, nor apomorphine-induced stereotypy. Similar results have been obtained using γ-acetylenic GABA, another GABA transaminase inhibitor (Palfryman *et al.*, this volume). Ethanolamine-O-sulphate diffuses widely after intracerebral injection, causing GABA elevations in distant structures, but the effects of γ-acetylenic GABA may be more restricted.

Muscimol, the GABA agonist, also has been found to prevent hyperactivity produced by bilateral injection of ergometrine into nucleus accumbens (Scheel-Krüger *et al. 1977, Scheel-Krüger et al.*, this volume). Muscimol in higher doses injected bilaterally into nucleus accumbens of naive rats causes reduced locomotion, as did GABA and baclofen (see also Andén, this volume).

Globus pallidus

We have found that a bilateral increase of GABA concentration in the region of the globus pallidus of rats by direct injection of ethanolamine-O-sulphate causes a profound reduction in locomotor activity amounting to complete akinesia, accompanied by a flexed posture and rigidity (Pycock *et al.* 1976). Amphetamine-induced hyperactivity is abolished during this phase, but this profound akinesia can be reversed partially by intrapallidal injection of picrotoxin or DL-allylglycine. There is a striking resemblance of such akinetic-rigid animals to reserpine-treated rats or animals with bilateral destruction of the globus pallidus, which is a major source of out put from the strio-pallidal complex.

Substantia nigra

Our early studies suggested that blockade of GABA action in substantia nigra by unilateral focal injection of picrotoxin in the rat could provoke contraversive circling (Tarsy *et al.* 1975). Such injections were confirmed histologically to have been placed in zona compacta, and the effect was abolished by prior destruction of nigral dopamine pathways with 6-hydroxydopamine. We concluded that this was evidence consistent with GABA-mediated inhibition of nigral dopaminergic neurons, as had been suggested by other data.

Subsequently, the picture has become somewhat confused, for other workers have described both ipsiversive and contraversive circling after unilateral blockade of GABA action in substantia nigra, or unilateral increase in GABA at that site (Dray *et al.* 1975, Waddington 1977, Oberlander *et al.* 1977, Olpe *et al.* 1977). However, such discrepancies have been clarified by Scheel-Krüger *et al.* (1977) who established that unilateral stimulation of GABA action (with muscimol or GABA) in the zona reticulata of the substantia nigra provokes contraversive turning, while antagonists, such as picrotoxin or bicuculline, cause ipsiversive circling, and in confirmation of Tarsy *et al.* (1975), picrotoxin injected more rostally into zona compacta provokes contraversive circling. Concurrently, we had undertaken similar experiments with similar results, but can add that injection of muscimol into zona compacta provokes ipsiversive circling (Reavill *et al.*, unpublished observations).

Thus the effects of GABA on nigral activity depend on its site of action. Unilateral injection of GABA agonists inhibit nigral cells in zona compacta to cause ipsiversive circling and we have found this to be antagonized by haloperidol or by destruction of the dopaminergic pathways with 6-hydroxydopamine. Accordingly, it seems that there exists a GABA input inhibiting dopaminergic nigral cells in zona compacta. (^{3}H) leucine studies suggest that this arises from the globus pallidus (Hattori *et al.* 1975).

In contrast, the contraversive circling provoked by unilateral muscimol injections into zona reticulata are insensitive to haloperidol (Reavill *et al.* unpublished observations), or to pretreatment with reserpine and α-methylparatyrosine (Scheel-Krüger *et al.* 1977). The latter workers also found that the stereotyped behavior provoked by bilateral injection of muscimol into zona reticulata was not prevented by reserpine and α-methylparatyrosine, nor by haloperidol or perphenazine. The conclusion is that there exists a second GABA pathway synapsing with dendrites of nondopaminergic nigral neurons in zona reticulata, perhaps arising from the caudate and putamen (Hattori *et al.* 1975). This nondopaminergic nigral pathway might project to midbrain tectum or thalamus. Our present data suggest the latter (see also Scheel-Krüger *et al.* this volume, Di Chiara & Gessa, this volume).

CONCLUSIONS

While there is no doubting the important role of a variety of GABA pathways in basal ganglia function, tools for manipulating specific GABA systems are not yet available for clinical use in extrapyramidal diseases. The various rodent models described of GABA action in different regions of the basal ganglia may provide means of screening compounds for such site-selective action. The information they provide, in conjunction with regional biochemical studies, may allow the development of rational drug therapy aimed at correcting specific GABA abnormalities in diseases of the basal ganglia.

REFERENCES

Andén, N-E. (1978) Functional and chemical effects of GABA and GABA-like drugs in the central nervous system. this volume.

Andén, N-E., Dalén, P. & Johansson, B. (1973) Baclofen and lithium in Huntington's chorea. *Lancet* ii, 93.

Barbeau, A. (1973) GABA and Huntington's chorea. *Lancet* ii, 1499–1500.

Bernheimer, H., Birkmayer, W., Hornykiewicz, O., Jellinger, K. and Seitelberger, F. (1973) Brain dopamine and the syndromes of Parkinson and Huntington: clinical, morphological and neurochemical correlations. *J. Neurol. Sci.* 20, 415–455.

Bird, E. D. & Iversen, L. L. (1974) Huntington's chorea: postmortem measurement of glutamic acid decarboxylase, choline acetyltransferase and dopamine in basal ganglia. *Brain* 97, 457–472.

Campochiaro, P., Schwarcz, R. & Coyle, J. T. (1977) GABA receptor binding in rat striatum: localization and effects of denervation. *Brain Res.* 136, 501–511.

Cattabeni, F., Bugatti, A., Groppetti, A., Maggi, A., Parenti, M. & Racagni, G. (1978) GABA and dopamine (DA): their mutual regulation in the nigro-striatal system. This volume.

Costa, E., Cheny, D. L., Moroni, F. & Peralta, E. (1978) Turnover rate of GABA (TR_{GABA}) in brain nucleus of rats: pharmacological implications. This volume.

Cuello, A. C. & Paxinos, G. (1978) Evidence for a long leu-enkephalin striopallidal pathway in rat brain. *Nature* 271, 178–180.

Di Chiara, G. & Gessa, G. L. (1978) GABA-ergic pathways mediating striatal dopaminergic output. This volume.

Enna, S. J., Kuhar, J. & Snyder, S. H. (1975) Regional distribution of postsynaptic receptor binding for gamma-aminobutyric acid (GABA) in monkey brain. *Brain Res.* 93, 168–174.

Enna, S. J., Bennett, J. P., Bylund, D. B., Snyder, S. H., Bird, E. D. & Iversen, L. L. (1976) Alterations of brain neurotransmitter receptor binding in Huntington's chorea. *Brain Res.* 116, 531–537.

Enna, S. J., Ferkany, J. & Krogsgaard-Larsen, P. (1978) Pharmacological characteristics of GABA receptors in human brain. This volume.

Fahn, S. (1976) Regional distribution studies of GABA and other putative neurotransmitters and their enzymes. In: *GABA in nervous system function,* ed. Rooberts, E., Chase, T. N. & Tower, D. B. pp. 169–186. Raven Press, New York.

Fonnum, F. & Walaas, I. (1978) Neurotransmitters in the mesolimbic system. This volume.

Fonnum, F., Grofová, I., Rinvik, E., Storm-Mathisen, J. & Walberg, F. (1974) Origin and distribution of glutamate decarboxylase in substantia nigra of the cat. *Brain res.* 71, 77–92.

Fuxe, K., Perez de la Mora, M., Schwarcz, R., Andersson, K., Hökfelt, T., Ljungdahl, Å., Agnati, L. F., Possani, L., Tapia, R., Teran, L. & Palacios, R. (1978) GABA neurons and their interaction with monoamine neurons. An anatomical, pharmacological and functional analysis. This volume.

Hattori, T., Fibiger, H. C. & McGeer, P. L. (1975) Demonstration of a pallido-nigral pathway innervating dopaminergic neurons. *J. Comp. Neurol.* 162, 487–504.

Hornykiewicz, O., Lloyd, K. & Davidson, L. (1976) The GABA system and function of the basal ganglia and Parkinson's disease. In: *GABA in nervous system function.* ed. Roberts, E., Chase, T. N. & Tower, D. B. pp. 479–486. Raven Press, New York.

Horton, R. W., Jenner, P., Marsden, C. D., Meldrum, B. S. & Reavill, C. (1978) Behavioural effects of allylglycine (2-amino-4-pentenoic acid) and 2-keto-4-pentenoic acid following focal injection into the rat cerebellum and caudate nucleus. *Brit. J. Pharmacol.,* 63, 381 P.

Iversen, L. L., Spokes, E. & Bird. E. (1978) Agonist specificity of GABA binding sites in human brain and GABA in Huntington's disease of schizophrenia. This volume.

Kataoka, K., Bak, I. J., Hassler, R., Kim, J. S. & Wagner, A. (1974) L-glutamate decarboxylase activity in the substantia nigra and striatum after surgical interruption of the strio-nigral fibers of the baboon. *Exp. Brain. Res.* 19, 217–227.

Lenman, J. A. R., Ferguson, I. T., Fleming, A. M., Herzberg, Robb, J. E. & Turnbull, M. J. (1976) Sodium valproate in chorea. *Brit. Med. J.* ii, 1107–1108.

Lloyd, K. & Hornykiewicz, O. (1973) L-glutamic acid decarboxylase in Parkinson's disease: Effect of L-dopa therapy. *Nature* 243, 521–523.

Lloyd, K. G., Shemen, L. & Hornykiewicz, O. (1977) Distribution of high affinity sodium-independent [^{3}H] gamma-aminobutyric acid ([^{3}H]) GABA) binding in the human brain: alterations in Parkinson's disease. *Brain Res.* 127, 269–278.

Lloyd, K. G., Mohler, H., Heitz, Ph. & Bartholini, G. (1975) Distribution of choline acetyltransferase and glutamate decarboxylase within the substantia nigra and other brain regions from control and Parkinsonian patients. *J. Neurochem.* 25, 789–795.

Marsden, C. D. (1975) The neuropharmacology of abnormal involuntary movement disorders (the dyskinesias). In: *Modern Trends in Neurology,* ed. Williams, D., vol. 6, pp. 141–166. Butterworths, London.

Marsden, C. D. & Parkes, J. D. (1977) Success and problems of long-term levodopa therapy in Parkinson's disease. *Lancet* i, 345–349.

McGeer, P. L. & McGeer, E. G. (1975) Evidence for glutamic acid decarboxylasecontaining interneurones in the neostriatum. *Brain Res.* 91, 331–335.

McGeer, P. L. & McGeer, E. G. (1976) Enzymes associated with the metabolism of catecholamines, acetylcholine and GABA in human controls and patients with Parkinson's disease and Huntington's chorea. *J. Neurochem.* 26, 65–76.

McGeer, E. G. & McGeer, P. L. (1978) GABA-containing neurons in schizophrenia, Huntington's chorea and normal aging. This volume.

Meldrum, B. S. (1978) Convulsants, anticonvulsants and GABA. This volume.

Obata, K. & Yoshida, M. (1973) Caudate-evoked inhibition and actions of GABA and other substances on cat pallidal neurons. *Brain Res.* 64, 455–459.

Oberlander, C., Dumont, C. & Boissier, J. R. (1977) rotational behaviour after unilateral intranigral injection of muscimol in rats. *Europ. J. Pharmac.* 43, 389–390.

Okada, Y. (1976) Role of GABA in the substantia nigra. In: *GABA in nervous system function.* ed. Roberts, E., Chase, T. N. & Tower, D. B. pp. 169–186. Raven Press, New York.

Olpe, H. R., Schellenberg, H. & Koella, W. P. (1977) Rotational behaviour induced in rats by intranigral application of GABA-related drugs and GABA antagonists. *Europ. J. Pharmac.* 45, 291–294.

Palfreyman, M. G., Huot, S., Lippert, B. & Schechter, P. J. (1978) GABA-dopamine interactions: studies using a new irreversible catalytic inhibitor of GABA-transaminase, γ-acetylenic GABA. This volume.

Paulson, S. W. (1976) Lioresal in Huntington's disease. *Dis. Nerv. Syst.* 37, 465–467.

Pearce, I., Heathfield, K. W. G. & Pearce, J. M. S. (1977) Valproate sodium in Huntington's chorea. *Arch. Neurol.* 34, 308–309.

Pérez de la Mora, M. & Fuxe, K. (1977) Brain GABA, dopamine and acetylcholine interactions. 1. Studies with oxotremorine. *Brain Res.* 135, 107–122.

Pycock, C. J. & Horton, R. W. (1976) Possible GABA-mediated control of dopamine-dependent behavioural effects from nucleus accumbens of the rat. *Psychopharmacol.* 49, 173–178.

Pycock, C. & Horton, R. (1976) Evidence for an accumbens-pallidal pathway in rat and its possible GABA-minergic control. *Brain Res.* 110, 629–634.

Pycock, C., Horton, R. W. & Marsden, C. D. (1976) The behavioural effects of manipulating GABA function in the globus pallidus. *Brain Res.* 116, 353–359.

Ribak, C. E., Vaughn, J. E., Saito, K. Barber, R. & Roberts, E. (1976) Immunocytochemical localization of glutamate decarboxylase in rat substantia nigra. *Brain res.* 116, 287–298.

Rinne, U. K., Sonninen, V., Riekkinen, L. & Laaksonen, H. (1974) Dopaminergic nervous transmission in Parkinson's disease. *Med. Biol.* 52, 208–217.

Scheel-Krüger, J., Arnt, J. & Magelund, G. (1977) Behavioural stimulation induced by muscimol and other GABA agonists injected into the substantia nigra. *Neuroscience Letters* 4, 351–356.

Scheel-Krüger, J., Cools, A. R. & Honig, W. (1977) Muscimol antagonists the ergometrine-induced locomotor activity in nucleus accumbens: evidence for a GABA-dopaminergic interaction. *Europ. J. Pharmac.* 42, 311–313.

Scheel-Krüger, J., Arnt, J., Braestrup, C., Christensen, V. & Magelund, G. (1978) Development of new animal models for GABA-ergic actions using muscimol as control. This volume.

Shoulson, I., Chase, T. N. & Roberts, E. (1975) Treatment with imidazole-4 acetic acid. *New Eng. J. Med.* 293, 504–505.

Shoulson, I., Kartzinel, R. & Chase, T. N. (1976) Huntington's disease: treatment with dipropylacetic acid and gamma-aminobutyric acid. *Neurol.* (Minneap.) 26, 61–63.

Stoof, J. C. & Mulder, A. H. (1977) Increased dopamine release from rat striatal slices by inhibitors of GABA-adminotransferase. *Europ. J. Pharmac.* 46, 177–180.

Tarsy, D., Pycock, C., Meldrum, B. & Marsden, C. D. (1975) Rotational behaviour induced in rats by intranigral picrotoxin. *Brain Res.* 89, 160–165.

Tarsy, D., Pycock, C. J., Meldrum, B. S. & Marsden, C. D. (1978) Focal contralateral myoclonus produced by inhibition of GABA action in the caudate nucleus of rats. *Brain* 101, 143–162.

Waddington, J. L. (1977) Induction of rotational behaviour by intranigral baclofen suggests possible GABA agonist activity. *Experientia* 33, 1345–1346.

Pharmacological Profile of SL 76002, a New GABA-Mimetic Drug

K. G. Lloyd, P. Worms, H. Depoortere & G. Bartholini

GABA-ergic neurons have been implicated in the pathophysiology of various neuropsychiatric disorders including Huntington's chorea (Enna *et al.* 1977, Lloyd *et al.* 1977a), Parkinson's disease (Lloyd *et al.* 1976, 1977b), epilepsy (Meldrum 1975) and schizophrenia (Bird *et al.* 1977, Roberts 1976). Thus it is evident that pharmacological agents which alter the activity of GABA neurons or which have an affinity for GABA receptors are interesting not only in elucidating the function of these neurons, but may also be useful at a clinical level. To date, only a very limited number of substances are available which exhibit specificity for GABA-ergic synapses. Many of these compounds which exhibit activity upon microiontophoresis or *in vitro* studies of GABA receptors do not cross the blood-brain barrier (Johnston 1976, Krogsgaard-Larsen 1978). Of the putative agonists available to date (which enter the brain) muscimol appears to have the greatest affinity for the GABA receptor. Other GABA agonists appear to be indirect, acting via diverse mechanisms such as inhibition of GABA metabolism (e.g. aminooxyacetic acid, dipropylacetate, gamma-acetylenic GABA, gamma-vinylGABA, etc.), inhibition of GABA uptake (e.g. diaminobutyric acid, nipecotic acid, beta-alanine) or by as yet unspecified mechanisms (benzodiazepines, pyrrolidinone, baclofen) (Bloom 1977, Iversen 1978, Schechter *et al.* 1977, Pinder *et al.* 1977, Johnston 1976, Perez de la Mora & Tapia 1973, Krjnevic 1977). Bicuculline is the only GABA antagonist readily available which appears to act directly at the postsynaptic GABA receptor site (Johnston 1976); however bicuculline also inhibits acetylcholinesterase, although at concentrations higher than that needed for blockade of GABA receptors (Breuker & Johnston 1975). Other GABA antagonists appear to act via

Synthélabo-L.E.R.S., Research Department, 58, Rue de la Glacière, 75013 Paris, France.

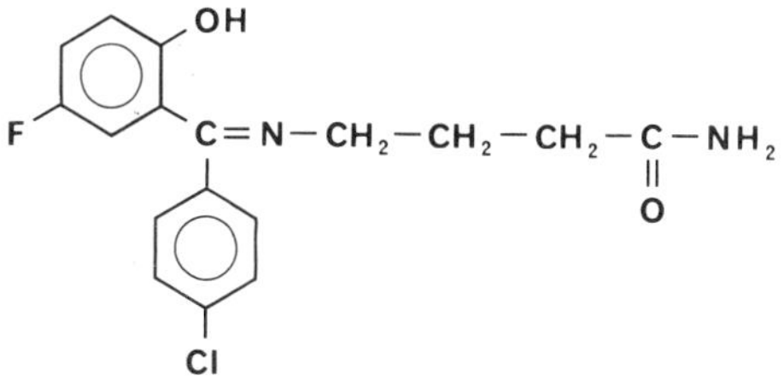

SL 76002

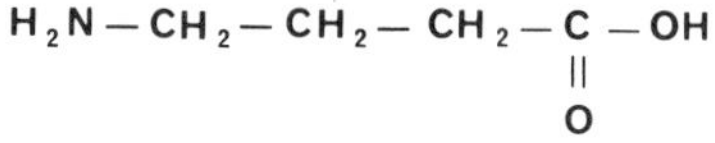

GABA

Fig. 1. Structural formula of SL 76002, {alpha-(chloro-4′-phenyl)fluoro-5-hydroxy-2-benzylidene-amino}-4-butyramide.

blockade of sites distal to the GABA receptor (e.g. picrotoxin, Takeuchi & Takeuchi 1969), or by the inhibition of GABA synthesis (higher doses of aminooxyacetic acid, thiosemicarbazide, glutamyl hydrazide) (Tapia 1974). Most of these compounds cannot be used in man because of convulsant effects (antagonists) or other toxic properties (e.g. hallucinations induced by muscimol) (Chase & Walters 1976).

It is apparent that the availability of a non-toxic agent with specific effects on GABA synapses would be of interest to both clinical and basic research disciplines. SL 76002, {alpha-(chloro-4′phenyl)fluoro-5-hydroxy-2-benzylidene-amino}-4-butyramide (Fig. 1) appears to fulfill these criteria. The present report provides a profile of the pharmacological activity of SL 76002 indicating that this drug is a GABA-mimetic with therapeutic potential as a broad-spectrum anti-convulsant in epilepsy and useful also in neuropsychiatric disorders such as Huntington's chorea and possibly schizophrenia.

METHODS AND MATERIALS

SL 76002 and dipropylacetate were synthesized by Dr J. Kaplan and muscimol was synthesized by Dr N. Tien-Duc of the Chemistry Department, Synthélabo-L.E.R.S. All other products were obtained from normal commercial sources. Mice utilized were CD-1 strain from Charles River (France) weighing 18–22 g.

Male albino rats (CD-COBS, Charles River, France) weighed 150–200 g. All experiments were performed in temperature controlled (20±1°C) sound-attenuated laboratories with constant lighting.

The following methods were used for biological testing:

Acute Toxicity, Anticonvulsant Activity, Locomotor Activity, Barbital Potentiation, Myorelaxant Effect and Interaction with Neuroleptics

See Table I for details.

Table I

Pharmacological methods utilized in determining the profile of SL 76002

Test (reference)	Response measured M=Mice R=Rats	Expression of results
Acute toxicity	Mortality (M)	LD50
Anti-bicuculline (0.45 mg/kg, i.v.) (Perez de la Mora & Tapia 1973)	Convulsions (M)	ED50
Anti-bicuculline (0.9 mg/kg, i.v.) (Perez de la Mora & Tapia 1973)	Mortality (M)	ED50
Anti-metrazole (130 mg/kg, s.c.) (Everett & Richards 1944)	Mortality (M)	ED50
Anti-strychnine (0.5 mg/kg, i.v.)	Mortality (M)	ED50
Anti-picrotoxinin (2.0 mg/kg, i.v.)	Convulsions (M)	ED50
Anti-electroshock (Cornea; 10 mA; 0.5 sec; 50 Hz) (Swinyard *et al.* 1952)	Convulsions (M)	ED50
Actimetry (Apelab Photocell Actimeter) (Boissier & Simon 1965)	Locomotion (M)	ED50
Barbital (140 mg/kg, i.p.) potentiation (Boissier 1959)	Righting Reflex (M)	ED50
Myorelaxant (loaded grid) (Fleury 1957)	Weight Supported (M)	ED50
Neuroleptic potentiation (4 cork test) (Worms & Lloyd 1978)	Catalepsy (R)	% Cataleptic
Neuroleptic potentiation (anti-apomorphine) (Worms & Lloyd 1978)	Stereotypies (R)	ED50

1. LD50s and ED50s (percent of control animals exhibiting syndrome) were determined on log-probit paper (Miller & Tainter 1944).

Multi-Unit Activity in Dorsal Deiters' Nucleus

Cats of either sex (2.0–3.0 kg) were initially anesthetized with diethylether and then intubated and cannulated in the femoral vein. Local anesthetic (Xylocaine,

2%) was infiltrated at all surgical and pressure points. Gallamine was injected and the cat maintained on artificial ventilation at a constant body temperature (37°) and pCO_2 (3–4% in expired air). The multi-unit activity of the neurons in the dorsal Deiters' nucleus (stereotaxic coordinates: posterior 8.8, lateral 4.2, depth 4.2, with aid of the atlas of Berman 1968) was recorded (Depoortere *et al.*, in preparation) by means of a bipolar coaxial electrode (David Kopf, 250 μ diameter). The point of entry anterior to lambda and the electrode inclination of 38° allowed the cerebellum and the descending cerebellar tracts to remain intact. The position of the electrodes was verified histologically. The multi-unit activity was amplified with a Grass Model 79D polygraph and analyzed with an automated spike counter (L.E.R.S.) and the activity recorded every minute. The frequencies analyzed were 0.1–10 kHz. The activity was averaged over periods of 30 min and expressed as a percentage of the first 30-min period.

Statistical Analysis

For the studies on the anticonvulsant and cataleptic properties of the compounds utilized, a nonparametric analysis of variance was utilized (Kruskall-Wallis test, Sokal & Rohlf 1969). For the multi-unit activity in the dorsal Deiters' nucleus, the two-tailed student's t-test was used.

RESULTS

Anticonvulsant Effects of SL 76002 and Reference Compounds (Table II)

SL 76002 was found to be an effective anticonvulsant agent in all of the test systems utilized. Thus, this compound reversed the convulsions and/or the mortality induced by bicuculline, metrazole, strychnine, picrotoxinin or electroshock treatment. In contrast, muscimol protected the animals only against the convulsions elicited by bicuculline or picrotoxinin and prevented the strychnine-induced lethality. Muscimol, even at high doses, did not protect the animals against bicuculline- or metrazole- induced mortality nor did it prevent the electroshock-induced convulsions. Chlordiazepoxide was active against all of the convulsive agents tested. Diphenylhydantoin prevented the convulsions and/or mortality due to bicuculline, electroshock or strychnine treatment, whereas dipropylacetate exhibited a protective effect against bicuculline and strychnine, but not metrazole.

Table II

Anticonvulsant profile of SL 76002 and various reference compounds

	ED50 (mg/kg, i.p.)					
	Anti-bicuculline		Anti-electroshock	Anti-metrazole	Anti-strychnine	Anti-picrotoxinin
Drug	Convulsions	Lethality	Convulsions	Lethality	Lethality	Convulsions
SL 76002	20±3 (3)	65±8 (6)	75±8 (3)	160±23 (3)	75±19 (3)	105±12 (2)
Muscimol	0.25±0.11 (3)	>2 (2)	>2 (2)	>2 (2)	0.90±0.14 (3)	1.1±0.2 (2)
Chlordiazepoxide	0.75±0.17 (3)	2.0±0.3 (3)	6.5±0.9 (2)	2.1±0.3 (5)	3.8±0.4 (4)	—
Dipropylacetate	—	130±22 (3)	—	>200 (2)	160±18 (3)	—
Diphenylhydantoin	12.5±3.9 (3)	50±13 (5)	14±2 (4)	>200 (3)	16±5 (3)	—

1. All data expressed as mean±S.E.M. Number of experimental groups (10 animals per dose per group, three to five doses per dose-response-curve) in parentheses.

Table III

Hypomotility and myorelaxation induced by SL 76002 and other anticonvulsant agents[1]

Drug	Hypomotility (ED50, mg/kg, i.p.)	Myorelaxation (ED50, mg/kg, i.p.)	Ratio $\frac{ED_{50}\text{ Myorelaxation}}{ED_{50}\text{Hypomotility}}$
SL 76002	120±25(3)	200±75(3)	1.67
Muscimol	0.65±0.07(3)	0.45±0.03(3)	0.69
Chlordiazepoxide	26±3(5)	4.5±0.5(5)	0.21
Diphenylhydantoin	25±10(3)	55±21(2)	2.20

1. All data expressed as mean±S.E.M. Number of experimental groups (10–15 animals per group; three to four doses per dose-response curve) in parentheses.

Hypomotility and Myorelaxant Effects (Table III)

All of the agents tested induced myorelaxation and hypomotility, although the relative doses at which these effects appeared varied greatly between the compounds. SL 76002 induced hypomotility at doses which tended to be lower than those for the myorelaxant effect. Muscimol and chlordiazepoxide induced myorelaxation at doses lower ($P<0.05$) than those which produced hypomotility.

These compounds also potentiated barbital-induced sleep. For SL 76002 this effect was seen at doses ($ED_{50}=100$ mg/kg, i.p.) significantly greater than that for antibicuculline lethality (Table II); in contrast the barbital potentiation by chlordiazepoxide ($ED_{50}=3$ mg/kg, i.p.) occurred at doses which were not significantly different than those for the antibicuculline effect (Table II).

Acute Toxicity and Therapeutic Ratios (Table IV)

SL 76002 is a compound with very low toxicity which results in very favorable therapeutic ratios. The therapeutic ratio with respect to the anticonvulsant (bicuculline) effect is superior to that of muscimol, dipropylacetate or diphenylhydantion. The therapeutic ratio for SL 76002 with respect to the myorelaxant effect is superior to any of the other drugs tested; with respect to sedation (hypomotility) SL 76002 is superior to muscimol or diphenylhydantoin.

Effect on Multi-Unit Activity in the Dorsal Deiters' Nucleus

The activity of SL 76002 on the firing rate of neurons in the dorsal Deiters' nucleus was examined and compared with the effect of several reference

Table IV

Acute toxicity and therapeutic ratios for SL 76002 and other anticonvulsant drugs

Treatment	Acute toxicity LD50 mg/kg, i.p.	LD50 / ED50 anti-bicuculline Lethality	Myorelaxant ED50 / ED50 anti-bicuculline Convulsions	Hypoactivity ED50 / ED50 anti-bicuculline Convulsions
SL 76002	900	14	10	6
Muscimol	2.5	<1.3	1.8	2.6
Chlordiazepoxide	270	135	6	35
Dipropylacetate	383[1]	6	—	—
Diphenylhydantoin	200	4	4.4	2

1. From Pinder *et al.* (1977).

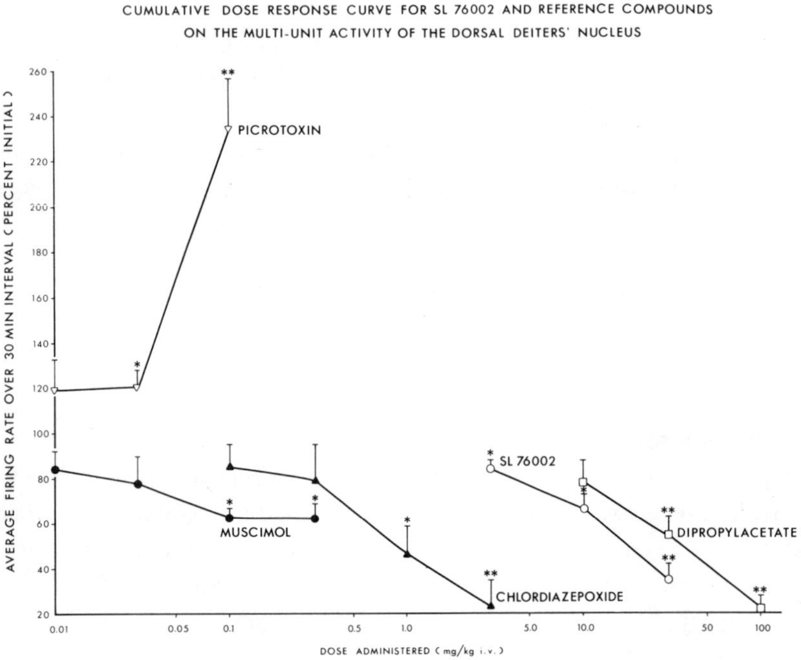

Fig. 2. Cumulative dose response curves for SL 76002 and reference compounds on the multi-unit activity of the dorsal Deiters' nucleus.

Results are expressed as mean with S.E.M., three to five cats per experiment $*P<0.05$ vs control (saline injection); $**P<0.01$ vs control.

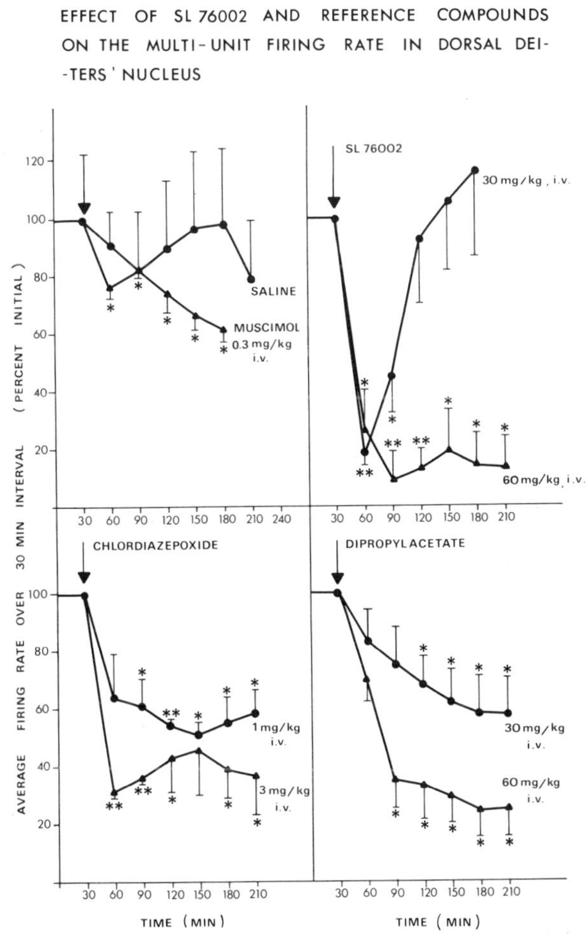

Fig. 3. Effect of SL 76002 and reference compounds on the multi-unit firing rate in dorsal Deiters' nucleus.

Results are expressed as mean with S.E.M. for three to five cats per dose. *$P<0.05$ vs saline injection; **$P<0.01$ vs saline injection.

compounds (Fig. 2). SL 76002 decreased the multi-unit activity measured in this nucleus in a dose-dependent manner with an ED_{50} of 17 mg/kg, i.v. Dipropylacetate (ED_{50}=35 mg/kg, i.v.) and chlordiazepoxide (ED_{50}= 0.8 mg/kg, i.v.) also exhibited a similar dose-dependent effect. Muscimol even at relatively high doses (0.3 mg/kg, i.v.) did not induce a 50% reduction of activity (maximum inhibition occurring at 0.1 mg/kg, i.v.). At subconvulsant doses, picrotoxin markedly enhanced the multi-unit activity of the dorsal Deiters' neurons.

The decrease in activity of the dorsal Deiters' neurons induced by 60 mg/kg of SL 76002 lasted for at least 3 h postinjection (Fig. 3), whereas 90 min after 30 mg/kg of SL 76002 the activity had returned to within the control range. The effect of muscimol (0.3 mg/kg, i.v.) lasted for at least 2.5 h whereas that for chlordiazepoxide (3 mg/kg) or dipropylacetate (30 or 60 mg/kg, i.v.) continued undiminished for at least 3 h postadministration.

The enhanced multi-unit activity induced by picrotoxin (0.1 mg/kg, i.v.) lasted for at least 1.5 h postinjection (Fig. 4). This effect was immediately reversed by either SL 76002 (30 mg/kg) or chlordiazepoxide (3 mg/kg) (Fig. 4). Upon a second injection of SL 76002, the multi-unit activity was reduced to considerably below that of the control (pre-picrotoxin) period. This level was similar to that seen after SL 76002 alone (Fig. 3). Chlordiazepoxide returned the multi-unit activity to that of the control level, but did not further decrease it, even upon a second injection (Fig. 4).

Interaction of SL 76002 with Neuroleptics

SL 76002 significantly enhanced the catalepsy induced by haloperidol, chlorpromazine or thioridazine (Table V). Alone, SL 76002 (or muscimol, chlor-

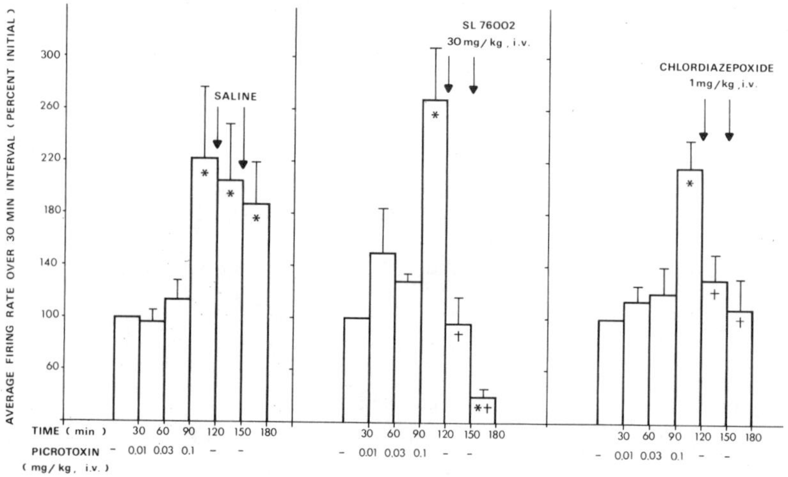

Fig. 4. Reversal of picrotoxin-induced increase in multi-unit activity of dorsal Deiters' nucleus by SL 76002 and chlordiazepoxide.

Data expressed as mean with S.E.M. for five cats per group. *$P<0.01$ versus pre-picrotoxin activity; †$P<0.01$ vs picrotoxin-injected animals.

Table V

Effect of SL 76002, muscimol, chlordiazepoxide and aminooxyacetic acid on the catalepsy induced by various neuroleptic drugs[1]

Neuroleptic	SL 76002		Muscimol		Aminooxyacetic Acid		Chlordiazepoxide	
	Drug Dose (mg/kg, i.p.)							
(mg/kg, i.p.)	0	100	0	1.0	0	2×12.5	0	15
Saline	0	0	0	0	0	0	0	0
Haloperidol								
0.3	14±2	43± 3**	16= 2	37±3*	32±3	62±11*	26±2	22±6
0.6	35±3	66±12*	30=10	57±9*	48±5	82± 6**	38±6	56±6*
Chlorpromazine								
6.0	14±3	31± 6*	10= 3	26±4*	20±7	46± 9*	—	—
9.0	46±6	68± 4**	28= 6	50±4	34±6	62± 3**	—	—
Thioridazine								
10	8±4	12± 4	4= 2	20±6	4±2	25± 7**	—	—
30	32±4	58± 6**	16= 2	48±8**	43±9	64± 9*	—	—
Sulpiride								
30	0	0	0	0	0	0	—	—
100	0	0	0	0	0	0	—	—

1. Data expressed as mean±S.E.M. of the percent of animals which became cataleptic; three to five experiments (6 animals per experiment).

* $P<0.05$ versus neuroleptic alone;

** $P<0.01$ vs neuroleptic alone.

diazepoxide or aminooxyacetic acid) did not induce catalepsy. In addition to SL 76002, neuroleptic-induced catalepsy was potentiated by muscimol, chlordiazepoxide and aminooxyacetic acid. In contrast, after sulpiride- a noncataleptogenic neuroleptic (Table V), neither SL 76002, muscimol nor aminooxyacetic acid induced any degree of catalepsy.

At subconvulsant doses bicuculline exhibited a biphasic effect on haloperidol-induced catalepsy (Fig. 5), at the lower dose potentiating, and at the higher dose

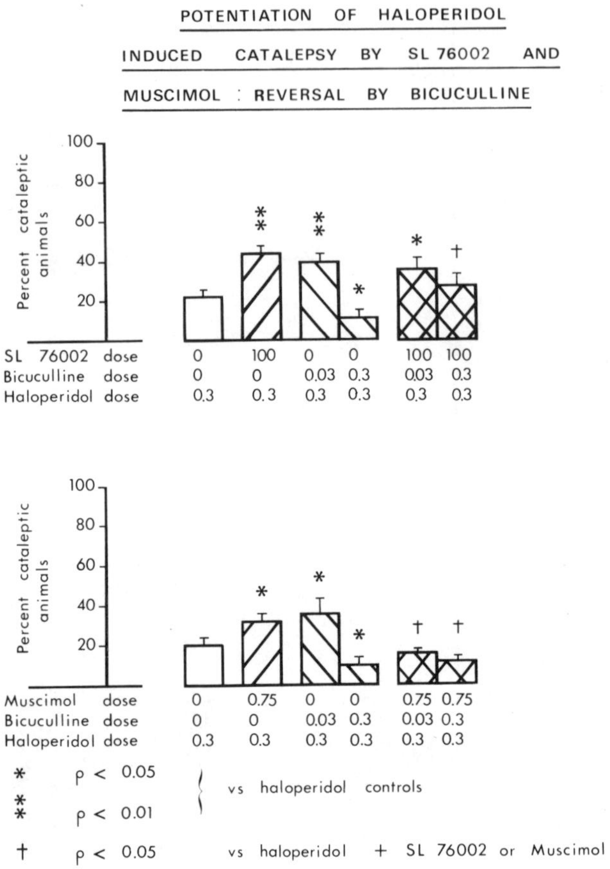

Fig. 5. Potention of haloperidol-induced catalepsy by SL 76002 and muscimol: reversal by bicuculline.

All doses are expressed as mg/kg, i. p. Results are expressed as means with S.E.M. for three to five experiments (6 rats per dose per drug per experiment). *$P<0.05$ vs haloperidol alone; **$P<0.01$ vs haloperidol alone; †$P<0.05$ vs combination of haloperidol plus SL 76002 or muscimol.

reversing the haloperidol catalepsy. Bicuculline blocked the potentiating effect of SL 76002 or muscimol on the haloperidol-induced catalepsy (Fig. 5).

In addition to its cataleptic action, haloperidol also blocks the stereotypies induced by apomorphine (0.5 mg/kg, s.c.) in rats, with an ID_{50} of 0.1 mg/kg, i.p. In addition to their effect on haloperidol-induced catalepsy, both SL 76002 and muscimol potentiated the haloperidol antagonism of apomorphine stereotypies.

DISCUSSION

From its pharmacological profile, SL 76002 appears to be a broad spectrum anticonvulsant agent with an action against bicuculline, picrotoxinin, metrazole, strychnine and electroshock at doses very much below those at which toxic effects are noted. Moreover, at anticonvulsant (e.g. antibicuculline) doses this compound does not produce signs of sedation or myorelaxation. In this light SL 76002 has a therapeutic ratio (LD_{50}:ED_{50} for bicuculline) considerably superior to that of diphenylhydantoin, or dipropylacetate, two other anticonvulsant agents (Pinder *et al.* 1977, Woodbury & Fingl 1975). SL 76002 was also relatively less myorelaxant (ED_{50} myorelaxation:ED_{50} bicuculline) than either diphenylhydantoin or chlordiazepoxide. In addition to being less toxic than diphenylhydantoin, SL 76002 exhibited antimetrazole and antipicrotoxinin actions, whereas diphenylhydantoin is devoid of these activities (Table II, Woodbury & Fingl 1975).

It is very likely that the anticonvulsant action of SL 76002 is mediated via a GABA-mimetic effect. Thus the compound is structurally closely related to GABA (Fig. 1) and the amide only needs to be hydrolyzed and the Schiff base link broken in order to form GABA. Both of these reactions occur *in vivo* (Bartholini *et al.*, this symposium). In addition, the compound itself and also the acid derivative (SL 75102) are likely direct-acting GABA mimetics as both displace ^{3}H-GABA binding *in vitro* (Bartholini *et al.*, this symposium). This explains the immediate onset of the anticonvulsant action of the compound (unpublished data). However, the anticonvulsant profile of SL 76002 is unlike that of muscimol (the latter does not exhibit anti-electroshock or antimetrazole activity, see below). The difference in anticonvulsant profiles between SL 76002 and muscimol may be related to the observation that the latter is metabolized very rapidly after administration (Enna *et al.*, this symposium) and the nature of the metabolites is unknown. It is very likely that these metabolites are pharmacologically active, as the effect of muscimol is longlasting (e.g. Fig. 3).

The anticonvulsant properties of the other compounds studied are generally well known (Pinder *et al.* 1977, Woodbury & Fingl 1975), except for those of muscimol. Thus it is interesting that this compound blocked bicuculline-induced convulsions (but not lethality), strychnine lethality and picrotoxinin-induced convulsions, but was inactive versus electroshock or metrazole. The anti-strychnine effect of muscimol has also been observed by Naik *et al.* (1976).

These results correlate with the observation that muscimol has a high affinity but relatively low intrinsic activity for the GABA receptor, as indicated by the decrease in Deiters' activity by low doses of muscimol, but with a weak maximum effect. The high affinity of muscimol is confirmed by its extremely low K_i in displacing ^{3}H-GABA binding (10nM, Lloyd & Dreksler 1978). Thus, it may be postulated that compounds with low intrinsic activity but high affinity (e.g. muscimol) will preferentially reverse GABA receptor blockers (e.g. bicuculline or picrotoxinin) whereas drugs with a high intrinsic activity (such as SL 76002) will also block seizure states of diverse origins (e.g. electroshock or metrazole).

This proposed GABA-mimetic effect of SL 76002 is consistent with its decrease in the basal level of, and reversal of, the picrotoxin-induced increase in the multi-unit activity of the dorsal Deiters' nucleus. As this activity is to a large part controlled by a GABA-mediated input from the cerebellar Purkinje cells (Ito 1976, Obata 1976), this system seems to be both sensitive and convenient for testing putative GABA agonists or antagonists. Indeed, also muscimol, dipropylacetate, chlordiazepoxide and diazepam (Depoortere *et al.* 1978), in addition to SL 76002, reduced Deiters' activity which is consistent with the hypothesis that these compounds all increase the activation of a GABA receptor (by either direct or indirect means; Bloom 1977, Johnston 1976, Schechter *et al.* 1977). The GABA-mimetic effect of SL 76002 is also confirmed by the potentiation of the neuroleptic-induced catalepsy, an action which is also seen with muscimol, chlordiazepoxide (Table V), aminooxyacetic acid (Table V and Kääriäinen 1976), diaminobutyric acid (Worms *et al.* 1978) and pyrrolidinone (Worms & Lloyd, unpublished). This potentiation is blocked by bicuculline (Fig. 5) which, similarly to metrazole, picrotoxinin or allylglycine (Worms *et al.* 1978) also reverses the haloperidol catalepsy. The common link for all of these compounds is their interference with GABA-mediated receptor events (Iversen 1978, Johnston 1976, Orlowski *et al.* 1977).

From this it appears that the activation of DA neurons by neuroleptics involves the reduction in activity of a GABA-mediated synapse, as previously proposed (Lloyd 1977). Reinstatement or augmentation of this GABA function (e.g. by direct-acting GABA-mimetics such as SL 76002 and muscimol or by inhibiting GABA metabolism) would reduce or block the activation of the nigral DA neuron therefore preventing the compensatory increase of DA synthesis and release. As a consequence, a greater degree of catalepsy is produced. Supporting this hypothesis are the observations that: (1) SL 76002 decreases the release of dopamine into the push-pull perfusate of the cat caudate nucleus (Bartholini *et al.,* this symposium); (2) SL 76002 blocks the activation of striatal tyrosine hydroxylase induced by neuroleptics (Bartholini *et al.,* this symposium); and (3) that ^{3}H-GABA binding sites occur on the nigral DA cell bodies (Lloyd *et al.* 1977b). The observation that in the inverse manner the catalepsy induced by haloperidol is reduced following the administration of drugs which decrease GABA neuron function (for instance bicuculline, vide supra) may indicate that this reduction increases the activation of the nigro-striatal DA neuron.

Bicuculline however shows a biphasic effect on haloperidol catalepsy (Fig. 5); this is also observed with picrotoxinin (Worms *et al.* 1978) suggesting that both the potentiation (at very low doses) and the reversal of catalepsy at moderate (subconvulsive) doses of these compounds are GABA-mediated events. The biphasic effect may be explained by several mechanisms: (a) the compounds exert a partial agonist effect; (b) more than one GABA receptor is involved, the effects of which are opposite in sign, with different sensitivities for activation; and (c) there is a presynaptic GABA receptor (autoreceptor) which is preferentially blocked at low doses of these compounds resulting in an enhanced release of GABA (Johnston & Mitchell 1971).

The potentiation of haloperidol catalepsy by SL 76002 and other GABA-mimetics probably involves a striatal mechanism. Thus, there is some evidence that the cataleptic action of neuroleptics is located in the striatum and the stereotypic action in the limbic system. In fact, SL 76002 (or muscimol) potentiates the cataleptic actions of the "classical" neuroleptics (e.g. haloperidol, chlorpromazine) which preferentially enhance DA turnover in the striatum (Scatton *et al.* 1977). In contrast SL 76002 does not induce catalepsy in the presence of non-cataleptogenic antipsychotic agents (sulpiride, Table V or clozapine, data not shown) which are less effective in the striatum than in the limbic system (Bartholini 1976, Scatton *et al.* 1977). Furthermore, SL 76002 alone or in combination with neuroleptics alters striatal more markedly than limbic DA turnover (Bartholini *et al.,* this symposium).

The observation that neither SL 76002, muscimol, nor any of the other

GABA-mimetic compounds induced catalepsy *per se* yet potentiated neuroleptic induced catalepsy may indicate that increased GABA synaptic activity is insufficient to functionally impair motor activity; a concomitant inhibitory mechanism (e.g. blockade of DA receptors) is necessary in order to provoke extrapyramidal dysfunction. Finally, the influence of GABA on DA function is probably not only limited to the regulation of the activity of DA neurons. Indeed both SL 76002 and muscimol enhanced the haloperidol-induced blockade of apomorphine stereotypies (in preparation), suggesting that neurons postsynaptic to the DA receptors are affected by GABA-ergic synapses.

SUMMARY AND CONCLUSIONS

1. SL 76002 is a novel GABA-mimetic drug with a broad spectrum of anticonvulsant activity, inhibiting seizures and/or lethality induced by bicuculline, strychnine, picrotoxinin, metrazole or supramaximal electroshock.

2. SL 76002 has a low degree of toxicity and a low incidence of sedation or myorelaxation. The therapeutic ratio ($LD_{50}:ED_{50}$) is considerably greater than that for diphenylhydantoin or dipropylacetate.

3. SL 76002, and also several reference compounds, decrease both the resting multi-unit activity of dorsal Deiters' neurons and reverse the increased activity due to picrotoxin.

4. SL 76002, muscimol and aminooxyacetic acid enhance the catalepsy due to "classical" neuroleptics, an affect which is reversed by subconvulsant doses of bicuculline. In combination with sulpiride or clozapine, neither SL 76002 nor muscimol induce catalepsy.

5. SL 76002 and muscimol enhance the effects of haloperidol with regard to the reversal of apomorphine-induced stereotypies.

6. From its range of activities the use of SL 76002 seems to be indicated in several clinical conditions. The most evident of these is epilepsy for which there is good evidence for GABA involvement (Meldrum 1975) and for which an indirect GABA-mimetic (sodium dipropylacetate) has shown therapeutic success (Jeavons 1977, Pinder 1977). There are preliminary clinical indications that SL 76002 will indeed be useful in cases of epilepsy refractory to medication (Bartholini *et al.*, this symposium). Another clinical condition responsive to SL 76002 may be Huntington's chorea (Bartholini *et al.*, this symposium), in which striatal GABA neuron function is greatly decreased (Enna *et al.* 1977, Lloyd *et al.* 1977a) and DA neuron activity relatively increased (Bernheimer *et al.* 1973).

To date, the limited range of GABA agonists tried in this disease have been without therapeutic success (Enna *et al.* 1977).

REFERENCES

Bartholini, G. (1976) Differential effect of neuroleptic drugs on dopamine turnover in the extrapyramidal and limbic system. *J. Pharm. Pharmac.* 28, 429–443.

Berman, A. L. (1968) *The Brainstem of the Cat. A Cytoarchitectonic Atlas with Stereotaxic Coordinates.* The University of Wisconsin Press, Madison.

Bernheimer, H., Birkmayer, W., Hornykiewiz, O., Jellinger, K. & Seitelberger, F. (1973) Brain dopamine and the syndroms of Parkinson and Huntington. *J. Neurol. Sci.* 20, 415–435.

Bird, E. D., Barnes, J. A., Iversen, L. L., Spokes, E. G., Mackay, A. V. P. & Shephard, M. (1977) Increased brain dopamine and reduced glutamic acid decarboxylase and choline acetyl transferase activity in schizophrenia and related psychoses. *Lancet* ii, 1157–1159.

Bloom, F. E. (1977) Neural mechanisms of benzodiazepine actions. *Am. J. Psychiat.* 134, 669–672.

Boissier, J. R. (1959) Experimental pharmacology of neuroleptics and tranquilizers. *Actual. Pharmacol.* 12, 1–69.

Boissier, J. R. & Simon, P. (1965) Action de la caféine sur la motilité spontanée de la souris. *Arch. Int. Pharmacodyn.* 158, 212–221.

Breuker, E., Johnston, G. A. R. (1975) Inhibition of acetylcholinesterase by bicuculline and related alkaloids. *J. Neurochem.* 25, 903–904.

Chase, T. N. & Walters, J. R. (1976) Pharmacologic approaches to the manipulation of GABA-mediated synaptic function in man. In: *GABA in Nervous System Function* ed. Roberts, E., Chase, T. N. & Tower, D. B., pp. 497–513, Raven Press, New York.

Cools, A. R. (1977) Two functionally and pharmacology distinct dopamine receptors in the rat brain. In: *Advances in Biochemical Psychopharmacology.* vol. 16, ed. Costa, E. & Gessa, G. L., pp. 215–225, Raven Press, New York.

Depoortere, H., Lloyd, K. G. & Bartholini, G. (1978) Neuropharmacology of neurons in Deiters' nucleus in the cat. *Abstracts, 11th C.I.N.P. Congress,* p. 375,Vienna.

Enna, S. J., Stern, L. Z., Wastek, G. J. & Yamamura, H. I. (1977) Neurobiology and pharmacology of Huntington's disease. *Life Sci.* 20, 205–212.

Everett, G. M. & Richards, R. K. (1944) Anticonvulsive action of 3, 5, 5,trimethyloxazolidine (tridione), dilantin and phenobarbital. *J. Pharmac. Exp. Therap.* 81, 402–407.

Fleury, C. (1957) Nouvelle technique pour mesure l'effort musculaire de la souris, dite test de l'agrippement. *Arch. Sci.* (Genèva) 10, 107–113.

Ito, M. (1976) Roles of GABA neurons in integrated function of the vertebrate CNS. In: *GABA in Nervous System Function,* ed. Roberts, E., Chase, T. N. & Tower D. B., pp. 427–448. Raven Press, New York.

Iversen, L. L. (1978) Biochemical psychopharmacology of GABA. In: *Psychopharmacology: A Generation of Progress,* ed. Lipton, M. A., DiMascio, A. & Killam, K. F., pp. 25–38, Raven Press, New York.

Jeavons, P. M. (1977) Choice of drug therapy in epilepsy. *Practitioner* 219, 542–556.

Johnston, G. A. R. (1976) Physiologic pharmacology of GABA and its antagonists in the vertebrate nervous system. In: *GABA in Nervous System Function,* ed. Roberts, E., Chase, T. N. & Tower, D. B., pp. 395–411, Raven Press, New York.

Johnston, G. A. R. & Mitchell, J. F. (1971) The effect of bicuculline, metrazol, picrotoxin and strychnine on the release of {^{3}H} GABA from rat brain slices. *J. Neurochem.* 18, 2441–2446.

Kääriäinen, I. (1976) Effects of aminooxyacetic acid and baclofen on the catalepsy and on the increase of mesolimbic and striatal dopamine turnover induced by haloperidol in rats. *Acta Pharmac. Toxicol.* 39, 393–400.

Krnjevic, K. (1977) Effects of substance P on central neurons in cats. In: *Substance P, Nobel Symposium,* Vol. 37, pp. 217-230, ed. Von Euler, U. S., Pernow, B., Raven Press, New York.

Krogsgaard-Larsen, P. (1978) GABA agonists and uptake inhibitors of restricted conformation: structure-activity relationships. In: *Amino Acids as Chemical Transmitters,* ed. Fonnum, F. In Press. Pergamon Press, New York.

Lloyd, K. G. (1977) Neurochemical compensation in Parkinson's disease. In: *Parkinson's Disease: Concepts and Prospects,* ed. Lakke, J. P. W. F., Korf, J. & Wesseling, H., pp. 61–72. Excerpta Medica International Congress Series No 429, Amsterdam.

Lloyd, K. G. & Dreksler, S. (1978) ^{3}H-GABA binding to membranes prepared from post-mortem human brain: pharmacological and pathological investigations. In: *Amino Acids as Chemical Transmitters,* ed. Fonnum, F. In Press. Pergamon Press, New York.

Lloyd, K. G., Dreksler, S. & Bird, E. D. (1977a) Alterations in ^{3}H-GABA binding in Huntington's chorea. *Life Sci.* 21, 747–754.

Lloyd, K. G., Möhler, H., Bartholini, G. & Hornykiewicz, O. (1976) Pathological alterations in glutamic acid decarboxylase activity in Parkinson's disease. In: *Advances in Parkinsonism,* ed. Birkmayer, W. & Hornykiewicz, O., pp. 186–192. Editions Roche, Basle.

Lloyd, K. G., Shemen, L. & Hornykiewicz, O. (1977b) Distribution of high affinity sodium-independent {^{3}H} gamma-aminobutyric acid ({^{3}H}-GABA) binding in the human brain: alterations in Parkinson's disease. *Brain Res.* 127, 269–278.

Lloyd, K. G., Shibuya, M., Davidson, L. & Hornykiewicz, O. (1977c) Chronic neuroleptic therapy: tolerance and GABA systems. In: *Advances in Biochemical Psychopharmacology,* Vol. 16, ed. Costa, E. & Gessa, G. L., pp. 409–415, Raven Press, New York.

Meldrum, B. S. (1975) Epilepsy and γ-aminobutyric acid mediated inhibition. *Int. Rev. Neurobiol.* 17, 1–36.

Miller, L. C. & Tainter, M. L. (1944) Estimation of the ED_{50} and its error by means of logarithmic-probit graph paper. *Proc. Soc. Exp. Biol. Med.* 57, 261–264.

Naik, S. R., Guidotti, A. & Costa, E. (1976) Central GABA receptor agonists: comparison of muscimol and baclofen. *Neuropharmacol.* 15, 479–484.

Obata, K. (1976) Association of GABA with cerebellar purkinje cells: single cell analysis. In: *GABA in Nervous System Function,* ed. Roberts, E., Chase, T. N. & Tower, D. B., pp. 217–222, Raven Press, New York.

Orlowski, M., Reingold, D. F. & Stanley, M. E. (1977) D- and L-stereoisomers of allylglycine: convulsive action and inhibition of brain L-glutamate decarboxylase. *J. Neurochem.* 28, 349–353.

Perez de la Mora, M. & Tapia, R. (1973) Anticonvulsivant action of 5-ethyl, 5-phenyl, 2-pyrrolidinone and its possible relationship to γ-aminobutyric acid-dependent inhibitory mechanisms. *Biochem. Pharmacol.* 22, 2635–2639.

Pinder, R. M., Brogden, R. N., Speight, T. M. & Avery, G. S. (1977) Sodium valproate: a review of its pharmacological properties and therapeutic efficacy in epilepsy. *Drugs* 13, 81–123.

Roberts, E. (1976) Disinhibition as an organizing principle in the nervous system – the role of the GABA system. Application to neurologic and psychiatric disorders. In: *GABA in Nervous System Function,* ed. Roberts, E., Chase, T. N. & Tower, D. B., pp. 515–539. Raven Press, New York.

Scatton, B., Bischoff, S., Dedek, J. & Korf, J. (1977) Regional effects of neuroleptics on dopamine metabolism and dopamine-sensitive adenylate cyclase activity. *Eur. J. Pharmac.* 44, 287–292.

Schechter, P. J., Tranier, Y., Jung, M. J. & Bohlen, P. (1977) Audiogenic seizure protection by elevated brain GABA concentration in mice: effects of γ-acetylenic GABA and γ-vinyl GABA, two irreversible GABA-t inhibitors. *Eur. J. Pharmac.* 45, 319–328.

Sokal, R. R. & Rohlf, F. J. (1969) Biometry. In: *The Principles and Practice of Statistics in Biological Research,* ed. Sokal, R. R. & Rohlf, F. S., pp. 387–395, W. A. Freeman, San Francisco.

Swingard, E. A., Brown, W. C. & Goodman, L. S. (1952) Comparative assays of antiepileptic drugs in mice and rats. *J. Pharmac. Exp. Therap.* 106, 319–330.

Takeuchi, A. & Takeuchi, N. (1969) A study of the action of picrotoxin on the inhibitory neuromuscular junction of the crayfish. *J. Physiol.* (Lond.) 205, 377–391.

Tapia, R. (1974) The role of γ-aminobutyric acid metabolism in the regulation of cerebral excitability. In: *Neurohumeral Coding of Brain Function.* ed. Myers, R. D. & Drucker-Colin, R. R., pp. 3–26. Plenum Publishing Corporation, New York.

Woodbury, D. M. & Fingl, E. (1975) Drugs effective in the therapy of the epilepsies. In: *The Pharmacological Basis of Therapeutics,* ed. Goodman, L. S. & Gilman, A., pp. 201–226. MacMillan, New York.

Worms, P. & Lloyd, K. G. (1978) Predictability and specificity of behavioural screening tests for neuroleptics. In: *Pharmacological Methods in Toxicology,* ed. Zbinden, G. & Gross, F. In Press. Pergamon Press, London.

Worms, P., Willigens, M. T. & Lloyd, K. G. (1978) GABA involvement in neuroleptic-induced catalepsy. *J. Pharm. Pharmac. In Press.*

On the Mode of Action of SL 76 002, a New GABA Receptor Agonist

G. Bartholini, B. Scatton, B. Zivkovic & K. G. Lloyd

According to pharmacological data (Lloyd *et al.*, this symposium), SL 76 002 {α(chloro-4 phenyl)fluoro-5 hydroxy-2 benzilidene-amino}-4-butyramide, Fig. 1) appears to increase GABA-ergic transmission. The action of the compound most likely involves changes in availability of GABA at, and/or direct stimulation of, GABA receptors. The pharmacological results, however, do not provide evidence as to which molecular mechanism accounts for the action of SL 76 002. We have therefore investigated the influence of this compound on cerebral neurotransmitters; in particular, since GABA participates in the regulation of dopamine (DA) neuron activity, we have studied the effect of SL 76 002 on dopaminergic transmission. The present paper discusses neurochemical results together with preliminary kinetic, metabolic and clinical data.

METHODS

Experiments were carried out on male Sprague-Dawley rats (Charles-River, France) weighing 125–150 g and on cats of either sex (3–4 kg). Brain levels of DA, noradrenaline (NA), 5-hydroxytryptamine (5HT) and 5-hydroxyindole-acetic acid were measured fluorimetrically according to Korf *et al.* (1976) and Westerink & Korf (1977). DOPA was measured by the method of Kehr *et al.* (1972) in rats treated with NSD 1015, an inhibitor of L-aromatic aminoacid decarboxylase. Tyrosine hydroxylase activity was assayed by the method of Waymire *et al.* (1971), as modified by Zivkovic *et al.* (1975a). GABA binding was assessed by the method of Enna *et al.* (1975), as modified by Lloyd *et al.*

Research Department, Synthélabo-L.E.R.S., 58 rue de la Glacière, 75013 Paris, France.

"GABA-NEUROTRANSMITTERS", Alfred Benzon Symposium 12, Munksgaard 1978

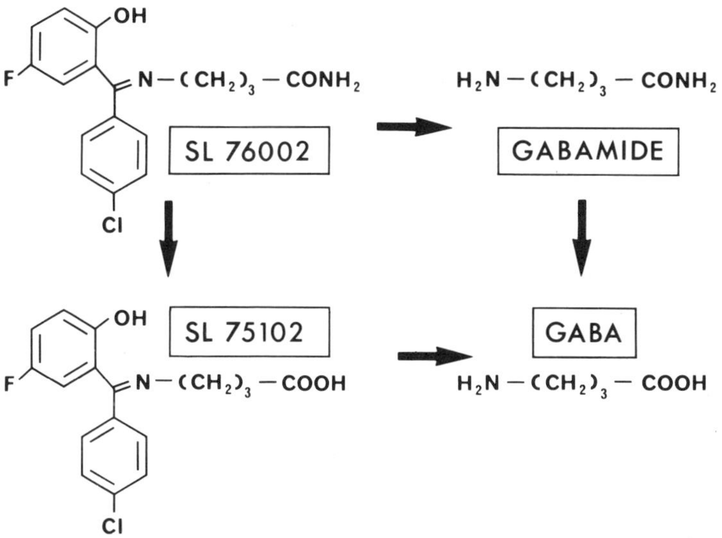

Fig. 1. Possible metabolic routes of SL 76 002.

(1977). The effect of compounds on GABA transaminase activity was estimated on a partially purified enzyme preparation (Wu *et al.* 1973). Endogenous DA released in brain regions of the cat was collected by means of the push-pull cannula and measured radioenzymatically (Bartholini & Stadler 1977). For statistical analysis the two-tailed Student's t-test was used.

METABOLISM AND EFFECT OF SL 76 002 ON GABA FUNCTION

Increase in GABA-ergic activity induced by drugs can occur via direct action on receptors, inhibition of GABA transaminase, blockade of neuronal and/or glial GABA uptake, or stimulation of GABA release.

The chemical structure of SL 76 002 – which contains the GABA moiety – and the nature of the metabolites formed *in vivo*, suggest that stimulation of GABA receptors is the mechanism by which SL 76 002 increases GABA transmission. Chemical structures as well as possible metabolic routes are shown in Fig. 1. Thus, SL 76 002 is a Schiff's base derived from GABAMIDE and an ortho-hydroxybenzophenone; after administration to rats, it is partially transformed into the free GABAMIDE, the acid derivative SL 75 102 and GABA; SL 76 002 and the above-mentioned metabolites appear in the circulation and the brain a few minutes after administration. Since GABA and GABAMIDE virtually do

Table I

Displacement of ^{3}H-GABA from membranes of rat brain and human cerebellum

Compound	IC_{50} (M) Rat	Human
SL 76 002	$3.5 \cdot 10^{-5}$	$3.9 \cdot 10^{-5}$
GABAMIDE	$1.7 \cdot 10^{-5}$	–
SL 75 102	$1.4 \cdot 10^{-6}$	$8.3 \cdot 10^{-7}$
GABA	$5.6 \cdot 10^{-8}$	$2.5 \cdot 10^{-7}$
Muscimol	$9.0 \cdot 10^{-9}$	$1.4 \cdot 10^{-8}$
Bicuculline	$1.0 \cdot 10^{-5}$	$1.8 \cdot 10^{-5}$
Baclofen	$>1.0 \cdot 10^{-3}$	$>1.0 \cdot 10^{-3}$

Rat brain membranes were prepared utilizing 0.05% Triton × 100 which was omitted from the human cerebellar preparation (see Lloyd *et al.* 1977).

not cross the blood-brain barrier, it must be concluded that hydrolysis of SL 76 002 takes place within the central nervous system. In addition, besides its possible cerebral origin, SL 75 102 is formed in extracerebral tissues and penetrates into the brain (Durand & Dring, in preparation).

Interaction with GABA receptors of SL 76 002 and its metabolites is confirmed by their property of displacing ^{3}H-GABA from binding sites of membrane preparations from rat brain and human cerebellum (Table I), the order of potency being GABA>SL 75 102>GABAMIDE≥SL 76 002.

According to these results, SL 76 002 can be considered as both a precursor of GABA receptor agonists and a receptor stimulant itself.

The effect of SL 76 002 on endogenous GABA is not yet clear. SL 76 002 or SL 75 102 does not inhibit *in vitro* GABA transaminase (Table II); however, *in vivo*

Table II

Effect of SL 76 002 and SL 75 102 on GABA-transaminase activity

Concentration of test compounds (M)	nMoles glutamate/90 min/assay SL 76 002	SL 75 102
10^{-4}	107±3	115±3
10^{-5}	119±2	127±3
10^{-6}	117±7	115±1
10^{-7}	123±4	115±3

The activity of GABA transaminase was measured in a partially purified mouse brain enzyme preparation. Each value is the average with S.E.M. of four determinations carried out in two experiments.

Control values: 112±2 nmoles/90 min/assay.

Table III

Effect of SL 76 002 on dopamine and noradrenaline utilization in striatum and limbic areas (nucleus accumbens+olfactory tubercle) of the rat

Treatment (mg/kg ip.)	Dopamine Striatum $\mu g/g$	%	Dopamine Limbic Areas $\mu g/g$	%	Noradrenaline Limbic Areas $\mu g/g$	%
Saline	8.57 ± 0.30	100	4.06 ± 0.21	100	0.73 ± 0.05	100
αMT (250)	2.73 ± 0.16^{a}	32	1.49 ± 0.11^{a}	37	0.45 ± 0.03^{a}	62
αMT (250) +						
SL 76 002 (100)	2.87 ± 0.12	33	1.44 ± 0.06	35	0.38 ± 0.04	52
(200)	3.30 ± 0.19^{a}	39	1.44 ± 0.14	35	0.35 ± 0.03^{c}	48
(600)	3.51 ± 0.19^{b}	41	1.35 ± 0.11	33	0.36 ± 0.02^{c}	50
(1200)	3.50 ± 0.24^{b}	41	1.56 ± 0.09	38	0.33 ± 0.04^{c}	45

α-methyl-p-tyrosine (αMT) and SL 76 002 were injected 4 and 3 h before sacrifice, respectively. The values represent averages with S.E.M. of results obtained in two to four experiments, each of them carried out on six animals per group.

Significance: [a] vs saline $P<0.001$; [b] vs αMT $P<0.01$; [c] vs αMT $P<0.05$

inhibition of the enzyme by other metabolite(s) of SL 76 002 can not be excluded as yet. In addition, SL 76 002 does not seem to block GABA uptake in cortical slices of rat brain (S. Z. Langer, personal communication). Finally, based on preliminary experiments of the *in vivo* perfusion of the cat Deiter's nucleus by means of the push-pull cannula, SL 76 002 does not appear to alter the release of endogenous GABA for at least 1 h.

SL 76 002 AND DA FUNCTION

Ample evidence has been provided that the activity of nigrostriatal and mesolimbic DA neurons is regulated by an inhibitory GABA-ergic influence (Mc Geer *et al.* 1977, Scheel-Krüger 1978). For the nigrostriatal DA neurons, the GABA influence appears to be mediated by a striato-nigral and pallido-nigral GABA-ergic pathway (Mc Geer *et al.* 1977) which likely participates in the feedback regulation originating from striatal postsynaptic DA receptors (Kim *et al.* 1971). Thus, DA neurons provide a convenient and sensitive system to test putative GABA-ergic compounds.

The effect of SL 76 002 on DA neurons has been therefore investigated in extrapyramidal and limbic systems of the rat. SL 76 002 does not modify the levels of DA in either system, for instance, 1 h following 600 mg/kg ip. SL 76 002, the DA concentrations were (μg/g) 8.53$\pm$0.35 in the striatum (controls 7.42$\pm$0.46) and 5.27$\pm$0.26 in nucleus accumbens + olfactory tubercle (controls 5.14$\pm$0.33). Similar negative results were obtained 4 and 6 h after administration of the compound.

In contrast, SL 76 002 reduces the rate of utilization of striatal DA as estimated by measuring the disappearance of the amine induced by α-methyl-p-tyrosine (αMT, Table III) the maximum effect being achieved with 200 mg/kg SL 76 002. Moreover, the effect of SL 76 002 on the liberation of DA is directly demonstrated by results from the *in vivo* perfusion of the cat caudate nucleus by means of the push-pull cannula: intravenous injection of the compound (50 mg/kg) reduces for at least 3 h the liberation of the transmitter (Fig. 2). In addition, SL 76 002 reduces the synthesis of DA in the striatum: thus, the compound, injected to rats, diminishes the *in vivo* DOPA accumulation following NSD 1015 (Table IV) as well as the *in vitro* formation of labelled CO_2 from 1–^{14}C-tyrosine in striatal slices (Scatton, in preparation). In the limbic system (nucleus accumbens + olfactory tubercle) SL 76 002, even in high doses, does not significantly decrease the αMT-induced disappearance of DA (Table

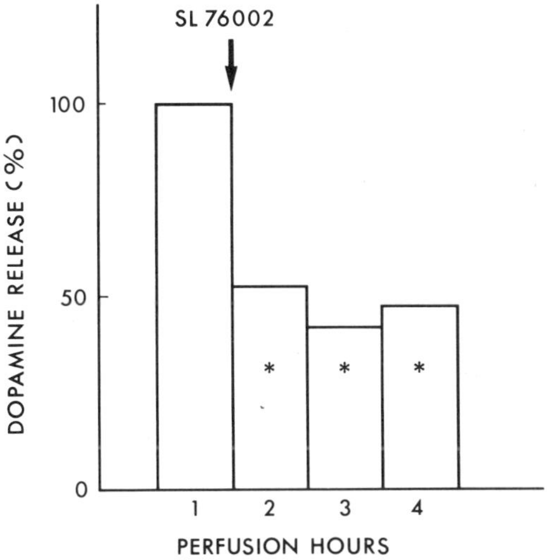

Fig. 2. Effect of SL 76 002 on the release of dopamine in the cat caudate nucleus.

The caudate nucleus of the gallamine-immobilised cat was perfused by means of the push-pull cannula. SL 76 002 (50 mg/kg) was injected iv. 1 h after beginning of the perfusion. The dopamine released per hour is expressed as percentage of control values (preinjection period, 85.5 ± 6.9 pg/hour). Averages of results from three cats.

* $P<0.01$ vs preinjection period.

III), although in histofluorescent studies the compound partially reverses the effect of the synthesis inhibitor (Constantinidis *et al.*, in preparation). This difference may be accounted for by the relative sensitivity of the methods. In addition, SL 76 002 reduces limbic DOPA accumulation (Table IV) and diminishes the spontaneous release of DA in the septal area perfused by means of the push-pull cannula (in preparation). These results indicate that SL 76 002 decreases both release and synthesis and, therefore, the turnover of DA.

Furthermore, the effect of SL 76 002 was investigated under conditions in which the activity of DA neurons was increased by haloperidol. Table V demonstrates that SL 76 002 counteracts in a dose-dependent manner the haloperidol-induced increase in DA utilization in both striatum and limbic areas of the rat. However, as in the absence of haloperidol, the striatum appears to be more sensitive than the limbic regions investigated. Also, the haloperidol-induced increase in tyrosine hydroxylase activity is more sensitive to reversal by different doses of SL 76 002 in the striatum ($ED_{50}=450$ mg/kg) than in the olfactory tubercle ($ED_{50}>1000$ mg/kg) (Fig. 3,A and B). However, when

Table IV

Effect of SL 76 002 on accumulation of DOPA in striatum and limbic areas (nucleus accumbens + olfactory tubercle).

Treatment (mg/kg ip)	DOPA concentration μg/g Striatum	Limbic areas
Saline	1.10±0.06	0.93±0.03
SL 76 002 200	0.84±0.02[a]	0.80±0.05
400	0.78±0.03[a]	0.84±0.04
1000	0.73±0.02[a]	0.75±0.05[b]

Rats received NSD 1015 (100 mg/kg ip.) 30 min after saline or after various doses of SL 76 002 and were sacrificed 30 min thereafter. Each value is the mean with S.E.M. of data from 10 rats (two different experiments).

[a] $P<0.001$; [b] $P<0.01$; as compared to corresponding control (saline).

Table V

Antagonism by SL 76 002 of the haloperidol-induced increase in dopamine utilization in striatum and limbic areas (nucleus accumbens+olfactory tubercle) of the rat.

Treatment	Dose of SL 76 002 (mg/kg ip.)	Dopamine Striatum μg/g	%	Limbic areas μg/g	%
Saline		7.06±0.20	100	4.20±0.19	100
αMT		3.16±0.13[a]	45	1.92±0.10[a]	46
αMT+Haloperidol		2.30±0.08[b]	32	1.45±0.09[b]	35
αMT+Haloperidol+ SL 76 002	100	2.40±0.23	34	1.26±0.06	30
	200	2.57±0.10[c]	36	1.52±0.05	36
	400	2.68±0.10[d]	38	1.48±0.08	35
	800	2.84±0.17[d]	40	1.72±0.13	41
	1000	2.93±0.15[d]	41	1.72±0.15	41
	1200	3.18±0.22[d]	45	1.88±0.04[d]	45

α-Methyl-p-tyrosine (αMT, 250 mg/kg), SL 76 002 and haloperidol (0.5 mg/kg) were injected ip. 2.5, 2 and 1.5 h before sacrifice, respectively.

The values represent averages with S.E.M. of results obtained in two to five experiments, each of them carried out on six animals per group.

Significance: [a] vs saline and [b] vs αMT, $P<0.001$; [c] vs αMT+haloperidol, $P<0.05$; [d] vs αMT+haloperidol, $P<0.01$

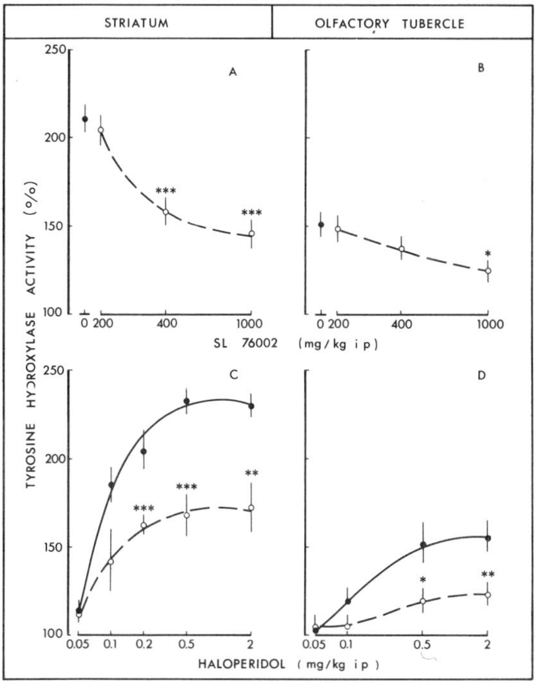

Fig. 3. Antagonism by SL 76 002 of haloperidol-induced activation of tyrosine hydroxylase in striatum and olfactory tubercle of the rat.

A, B: Various doses of SL 76 002 and 0.5 mg/kg haloperidol were injected ip. 60 and 30 min before sacrifice, respectively.

C. D: Various doses of haloperidol and 1000 mg/kg SL 76 002 were injected ip. 30 and 60 min before sacrifice, respectively. ●–● haloperidol; O–O haloperidol+SL 76 002.

The values are expressed in percent of controls (=100) and represent average with S.E.M. of results from two experiments, each of them carried out on five rats per group.

Control values (nmoles $^{14}CO_2$/hour/mg protein): Striatum 3.68±0.11; olfactory tubercle 3.92 ±0.12.

* $P<0.05$; ** $P<0.01$; *** $P<0.001$ as compared to rats treated with haloperidol alone.

varying doses of haloperidol were tested at a constant level of SL 76 002 (1000 mg/kg), the activation of tyrosine hydroxylase was inhibited to a similar extent in both striatum and olfactory tubercle (Fig. 3,C and D). Therefore, SL 76 002 does not change the potency (ED_{50}=0.1 mg/kg) but rather decreases the efficacy of haloperidol, indicating that the interaction of the neuroleptic with DA receptors has not been changed by SL 76 002. Thus, SL 76 002 and haloperidol have different sites of action with respect to the DA neuron activation. Similar results were obtained with other neuroleptic drugs such as butaclamol and sulpiride.

All of these results indicate that SL 76 002 decreases the activity of dopaminergic neurons. This is probably related to an increase in the inhibitory GABA activity involved in the regulation of firing of DA cells. SL 76 002 is more effective when the firing rate of DA neurons is enhanced as, for instance, after neuroleptics. These results correlate with the pharmacological data (Lloyd *et al.*, this symposium), showing that SL 76 002 potentiates the neuroleptic-induced catalepsy: probably, this is due to reduction of DA release and thus the competition of the amine with the neuroleptics for the receptor sites. Finally, a more marked effect of SL 76 002 is observed in the striatum as compared to the limbic system. The reason for this regional difference is not yet known; it may be connected with an uneven distribution of the drug within the brain and/or with a more effective GABA-ergic control of DA neurons in striatum than in limbic system; a difference in affinity of SL 76 002 and/or its metabolites for limbic and striatal receptors can not be excluded.

EFFECT OF SL 76 002 ON THE METABOLISM OF 5-HT AND NA

SL 76 002 (600 mg/kg ip.) does not affect, for at least 4 h, the steady state concentrations of 5-HT in striatum or limbic regions, nor does it change the levels of limbic NA. However, the compound increases striatal 5-hydroxyindoleacetic acid levels (control: 0.37 ± 0.02; SL 76 002, 1 h: 0.51 ± 0.04 μg/g) and accelerates the αMT-induced disappearance of NA in limbic areas (Table III). This indicates that SL 76 002 enhances the turnover of both 5-HT and NA. These results are coherent with previous data (Carlsson *et al.* 1977) showing that injection of GABA enhances the accumulation of 5-hydroxytryptophan in various brain areas and of DOPA in NA-rich regions. Together with the modification of the activity of DA neurons, alteration in 5-HT and NA may be involved in the changes in mood and behavior observed in patients treated with SL 76 002 (see section 7).

COMPARISON OF SL 76 002 WITH OTHER PUTATIVE GABA RECEPTOR AGONISTS

Similarly to SL 76 002, other putative GABA-mimetic compounds, such as muscimol and γ-hydroxybutyrate (γOH, for which however the GABA-ergic action is seriously questioned), produce a decrease in DA utilization. Thus, muscimol (Scatton, in preparation) and γOH (Stock *et al.* 1973) decrease the rate of αMT-induced DA disappearance in striatum and counteract the activation of striatal and limbic tyrosine hydroxylase due to haloperidol (Zivkovic *et al.* 1975b, Zivkovic *et al.*, in preparation). This indicates that the compounds decrease the firing of DA neurons as directly demonstrated for γOH in electrophysiological experiments (Walters *et al.* 1972). Concomitantly with the decrease in the firing rate, a reduction in DA synthesis should be expected. This holds true for SL 76 002 and muscimol (in preparation), which decrease DOPA accumulation after NSD 1015 and do not change the levels of DA. In contrast, γOH enhances both the synthesis and concentration of the amine (Spano *et al.* 1971, Gessa *et al.* 1966). Therefore, one can assume that the decrease in the firing of DA neurons and the increase in the synthesis of the neurotransmitter by γOH are mediated by two different actions of the drug, whereas the effect of SL 76 002 or muscimol on DA synthesis is probably mediated by the decreased firing of DA neurons. However, the possibility can not be excluded that γOH completely blocks, whereas SL 76 002 and muscimol only partially inhibit, the firing of dopaminergic neurons and the release of the amine. This difference may involve changes in the regulation of DA synthesis by autoreceptors. However, this remains a speculation as yet.

PRELIMINARY CLINICAL RESULTS WITH SL 76 002*

The potential alteration of GABA function in neuropsychiatric disorders together with the enhancement of GABA-ergic transmission by SL 76 002 and its virtual lack of toxicity (subchronic trials in two animal species at doses 30–50 times higher than those showing an effect in pharmacological tests), provide a strong rationale for the therapeutic utilization of the compound in various pathological conditions.

Epilepsy

The inhibitory action of GABA on neuronal excitability and the antagonism by SL 76 002 of not only bicuculline – but also metrazole – strychnine – and electroshock-induced seizures (see Lloyd *et al.*, this symposium) predict a broad

---

* L. P. Morselli and E. Zarifian (Clinical Research Dept. Synthélabo-L.E.R.S., Paris), personal communication.

therapeutic action of the compound in epilepsy. So far, SL 76 002, in oral doses of 20–30 mg/kg and in the absence of relevant side effects, has led to a virtual disappearance of seizures in several epileptic patients suffering from complex partial or generalized seizures with 1–4 fits per week and 'resistant' to the commonly used antiepileptic medication; significant clinical amelioration of other subjects, EEG modifications and mood changes (see below) have also been observed.

Huntington's chorea

The reduction in dopaminergic activity by SL 76 002 via a GABA-ergic mechanism (see section 4) – particularly evident in the striatum – suggests the therapeutic use of this compound in patients suffering from Huntington's chorea. In this condition, a relative exaggeration of DA, and a reduction of GABA, function appears to be a pathogenetic factor of the neurological syndrome (Klawans & Weiner 1976). In preliminary clinical trials, SL 76 002 seems to significantly ameliorate patients with Huntington's chorea at an early stage (3–4 years), both at neurological and psychic levels; as it was to be expected, however, the compound is ineffective in advanced cases (over 5 years), most probably due to the progression of the cerebral degenerative alterations, proper to this condition. Obviously, on the basis of the observations to date, it can not be predicted whether or not SL 76 002 will affect the evolution of the disease.

Schizophrenia

Reduction of dopaminergic transmission in the limbic system is thought to be involved in the therapeutic action of neuroleptic drugs (Matthysse 1973). In this light, it might be expected that SL 76 002 improves schizophrenic symptoms since the compound reduces DA function in limbic areas. However, preliminary clinical trials with schizophrenic patients not treated with neuroleptics show no amelioration of the psychotic syndrome by SL 76 002. The possibility exists that SL 76 002 has not caused a sufficient reduction in limbic DA function, since the mesolimbic DA neurons are inhibited to a lower extent than nigrostriatal cells (see section 4). Possibly, the association of SL 76 002 with neuroleptics will lead to a potentiation of the latter and allow a reduction in their posology: indeed, animal experiments (see above) indicate that GABA-mediated inhibition of DA neurons is more effective in blocking activated than normal cells.

SUMMARY AND CONCLUSIONS

According to its pharmacological spectrum, SL 76 002 is a new GABA-mimetic compound (see Lloyd *et al.,* this symposium) which rapidly penetrates into the circulation and the brain after oral administration and is transformed into GABAMIDE, GABA and the acid derivative SL 75 102; these metabolites, together with the parent drug, displace ^{3}H-GABA from binding sites indicating a direct action on GABA receptors. *In vitro,* SL 76 002 and SL 75 102 do not block GABA transaminase nor do they affect GABA uptake; however, it can not be excluded that these effects are caused *in vivo* by other metabolite(s) of SL 76 002.

SL 76 002 inhibits DA activity in the striatum, which correlates with the potentiation of neuroleptic-induced catalepsy (Lloyd *et al.,* this symposium) and represents the rationale for the use of the compound in Huntington's chorea. Also, limbic DA release is reduced by SL 76 002, although less markedly than in the striatum. Since schizophrenia may be ameliorated by reduction of DA transmission, possibly in limbic areas, SL 76 002 might, alone or in association with neuroleptics, improve the psychosis. Finally, the broad anticonvulsant spectrum of SL 76 002 (Lloyd *et al.,* this symposium) suggests a therapeutic activity in epilepsy. Preliminary clinical trials show that SL 76 002 is indeed effective in epilepsy and Huntington's chorea. The results in schizophrenia are not yet conclusive. SL 76 002 might be therapeutically useful in other conditions. For instance, preliminary observations suggest that the compound has a beneficial effect in spasticity of different origins. In addition, a psychic effect of SL 76 002 can be envisaged; in fact, in both Huntington's chorea and epileptic patients, the drug causes mood elevation, sometimes euphoria and increases environmental integration; in two epileptic children, reduction of hyperreactive and aggressive behavior was observed. These changes appeared several days prior to, and therefore were unlikely the consequence of, the amelioration of the neurological syndrome, suggesting that they originate from a primary action of SL 76 002.

ACKNOWLEDGMENTS

The synthesis of SL 76 002 and SL 75 102 was carried out by Dr. J. Kaplan, that of muscimol by Dr. N. Tien-Duc, Chemistry Department, Synthelabo-L.E.R.S., Paris.

REFERENCES

Bartholini, G. & Stadler, H. (1977) Evidence for an intrastriatal GABA-ergic influence on dopamine neurons of the cat. *Neuropharmacology* 16, 343–347.

Carlsson, A., Biswas, B. & Lindqvist, M. (1977) Influence of GABA and GABA-like drugs on monoaminergic mechanisms. In: *Advances in Biochemical Psychopharmacology*, vol. 16, ed. Costa, E. & Gessa, G. L. pp. 471–475. Raven Press, New–York.

Enna, S. J. & Snyder, S. H. (1975) Properties of γ-aminobutyric acid (GABA) receptor binding in rat brain synaptic membrane fractions. *Brain Res.* 100, 81–97.

Gessa, G. L., Vargiu, L., Crabai, F., Boero, C. G., Caboni, R. & Camba, R. (1966). Selective increase of brain dopamine induced by gamma-hydroxybutyrate. *Life Sci.* 5, 1921–1930.

Kehr, W., Carlsson, A. & Lindqvist, M. (1972). A method for the determination of 3,4-dihydroxyphenylalanine (DOPA) in brain. *Naunyn-Schmiedeberg's Arch. Pharmacol.* 274, 273–280.

Kim, J. S., Bak, I. J., Hassler, R. & Okada, Y. (1971) Role of γ-aminobutyric acid (GABA) in the extrapyramidal motor system. 2. Some evidence for the existence of a type of GABA-rich strionigral neurons. *Exptl. Brain Res.* 14, 95–110.

Klawans, H. L. & Weiner, W. J. (1976) The pharmacology of choreatic movement disorders. In: *Progress in Neurobiology*, vol. 6, pp. 49–80, Pergamon Press, Great Britain.

Korf, J., Sebens, J. B., Venema, K. & Van Praag, H. M. (1976) Serum levels of 5-hydroindole derivatives after administration of 5-hydroxytryptophan ethyl ester. *Res. Comm. Chem. Pathol. and Pharmacol.* 15, 171–182.

Lloyd, K. G., Shemen, L. & Hornykiewicz, O. (1977) Distribution of high affinity sodium-independant (^{3}H) gammaaminobutyric acid (^{3}H-GABA) binding in the human brain. Alterations in Parkinson's disease. *Brain Res.* 127, 269–278.

Matthysse, S. (1973) Antipsychotic drug action: A clue to the neuropathology of schizophrenia. *Fed. Proc.* 32, 200–205.

McGeer, P. L., Mc Geer, E. G. & Hattori, T. (1977) Dopamine-acetylcholine – GABA neuronal linkages in the extrapyramidal and limbic systems. In: *Advances in Biochemical Psychopharmacology*, vol. 16, ed. Costa, E. & Gessa, G. L., pp. 397–402. Raven Press, New York.

Scheel-Krüger, J., Christensen, A. V. & Arnt, J. (1978) Muscimol differentially facilitates stereotypy but antagonizes motility induced by dopaminergic drugs: a complex GABA-dopamine interaction. *Life Sci.* 22, 75–84.

Spano, P. F., Tagliamonte, A., Tagliamonte, P. & Gessa, G. L. (1971) Stimulation of brain dopamine synthesis by gammahydroxybutyrate. *J. Neurochem.* 18, 1831–1836.

Stock., G. T., Magnusson, T. & Andén, N.-E. (1973) Increase in brain dopamine after axotomy or treatment with gammahydroxybutyric acid due to elimination of the nerve impulse flow. *Naunyn-Schmiedeberg's Arch. Pharmacol.* 278, 347–361.

Walters, J. R., Aghajanian, G. K. & Roth, R. H. (1972) Dopaminergic neurons: Inhibition of firing by gammahydroxybutyrate. In: *Proc. Fifth Internatl. Cong. Pharmacol.* Abst. 1472, p. 246.

Waymire, J. C., Bjur, R. & Weiner, N. (1971) Assay of tyrosine hydroxylase by coupled decarboxylation of DOPA formed from 1–^{14}C-L-tyrosine. *Analit. Biochem.* 43, 588–600.

Westerink, B. H. C. & Korf, J. (1977) Rapid concurrent automated fluorimetric assay of noradrenaline, dopamine, 3-4-dihydroxyphenylacetic acid, homovanillic acid and 3-methoxytyramine in milligram amounts of nervous tissue after isolation on Sephadex G–10. *J. Neurochem.* 29, 697–706.

Wu, J. Y., Matsuda, T. & Roberts, E. (1973) Purification and characterisation of glutamate decarboxylase from mouse brain. *J. Biol. Chem.* 248, 3029–3034.

Zivkovic B., Guidotti, A., Revuelta, A. & Costa, E. (1975a) Effect of thioridazine, clozapine and other antipsychotics on the kinetic state of tyrosine hydroxylase and on the turnover rate of dopamine in striatum and nucleus accumbens. *J. Pharmacol. Exp. Ther.* 194, 37–46.

Zivkovic, B., Guidotti, A. & Costa, E. (1975b) The regulation of striatal tyrosine hydroxylase: effects of gammahydroxybutyric acid and haloperidol. *Naunyn-Schmiedeberg's Arch. Pharmacol.* 291, 193–200.

GABA-Containing Neurons in Schizophrenia, Huntington's Chorea and Normal Aging

E. G. McGeer & P. L. McGeer

γ-Aminobutyric acid (GABA), as is clear from the existence of this symposium, is now recognized as an important central nervous system neurotransmitter. Indeed, its powerful inhibitory action, its relatively uniform distribution and its presence in a concentration some 200–1000 fold greater than that of transmitters such as dopamine, noradrenaline, acetylcholine or serotonin, suggest that GABA may be the principal inhibitory neurotransmitter in brain. Similar considerations of concentration, widespread distribution and physiological activity suggest that glutamic acid, the immediate precursor of GABA, may have an equally important role in its own right as the common excitatory neurotransmitter of brain.

It is clearly important to establish the roles of GABA in normal brain function and in brain pathology. This paper reviews our findings on glutamic acid decarboxylase (GAD), in some normal and pathological human brains. We chose to study the activity of this key synthetic enzyme rather than the neurotransmitter itself because the activity of the enzyme can be measured reliably on small tissue samples and, in our hands at least, seems somewhat less subject to postmortem changes and pharmacological manipulations than are the levels of the neurotransmitter amino acid.

Some data will also be presented on the possible neuronal localization of glutaminase activity in rat neostriatum since this enzyme is another possible indicator of the integrity of glutamergic or gabergic neurons.

Kinsmen Laboratory of Neurological Research, Department of Psychiatry, University of British Columbia, Vancouver, B.C. V6T 1W5, Canada.

"GABA-NEUROTRANSMITTERS", Alfred Benzon Symposium 12, Munksgaard 1978

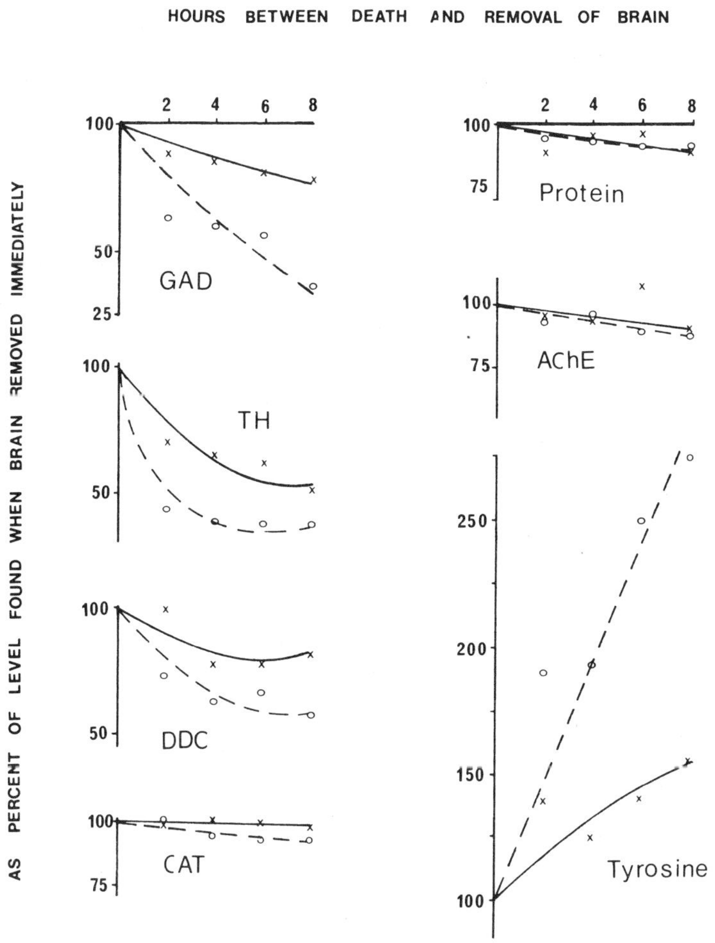

Fig. 1. Postmortem changes in some enzyme activities, protein and tyrosine concentrations in rat brain. Rats were sacrificed and left at either 4°C (x–) or 20°C (o---) for indicated number of hours before removal of the brain.

GAD ACTIVITY IN HUMAN MATERIAL

The Effect of Postmorten Delay

The time from death to autopsy varies considerably in human cases. It is an uncontrollable factor which could conceivably mask any premortem changes associated with age or disease. One approach in judging the importance of postmortem delay has been to carry out studies on rats, waiting for different periods of time between sacrifice and enzyme measurement. Fig. 1 shows decrements in enzyme levels with postmortem delay for gabergic, cholinergic and catecholaminergic neuronal systems. Also shown are decrements in acetylcholinesterase (AChE) and total protein, and the increase in tyrosine. Inspection of the figure shows the anticipated more rapid decline in enzymes when the animals are left at room temperature (dotted lines) as opposed to 4° C (solid lines).

It is evident that there is a fairly severe loss in GAD but the principal decline is during the first 2 h. Such data suggest that postmortem delay can not be ignored in human studies. However, experience in several laboratories has indicated that postmortem delays of 2–48 h have little significant effect upon the results obtained with humans (Bird & Iversen 1974, Grote *et al.* 1974, McGeer & McGeer 1976b). In particular, in the case of GAD, measurement of the activity in human samples obtained by biopsy in both our laboratory (McGeer & McGeer 1976b) and that of Spillane *et al.* (1977) indicates that the values obtained on such biopsy specimens are surprisingly close to what would be anticipated from postmortem studies (Table I).

Premortem condition

Experiments suggest that a much more significant factor contributing to scatter in normal human data is the immediate premortem condition of the patient. Studies performed in our laboratory (McGeer & McGeer 1976b) suggest that a state of coma prior to death, particularly if the patient has been supported by an artificial respirator, can lead to very major declines in many enzyme levels. Two causes of coma were included in the cases in our series: coma due to severe head injury and coma as a terminal state of a lingering nonmetabolic illness. There

Table I.

*Measured activities of GAD in (μmoles/h – 100 mg protein) on biopsy samples removed during operations for epilepsy as compared to autopsy samples corrected for age**

Age	Area	Measured activity	Calculated activity
63	Thalamus	1.6	2.6
37	Cortex	6.6±0.8 (3)	5.4
18	Cortex	8.5±0.6 (3)	6.8
16	Cortex	6.4±1.4 (4)	7.8
16	Caudate	5.5	5.6
13	Cortex	5.1±0.4 (6)	7.2

* Spillane *et al.* (1977) report normal GAD levels in cortical biopsy samples from two cases of presenile dementia.

were no cases of diabetic coma or coma due to kidney or liver failure. GAD (and CAT) seemed to be sharply reduced in cases of coma due to head injury, while TH and AChE were relatively unaffected. Coma from illness, on the other hand, resulted in lesser but significant losses in GAD (and CAT) but sharp losses in TH and DDC. There was little effect on AChE. Not all areas were equally affected and the regional effects of coma obviously need to be considered in future work. The reductions in GAD were on the average to about 31% and 64% of values obtained in noncomatose controls.

Similar deleterious effects of coma are implied in the work by Bowen *et al.* who initially (1974) reported an average reduction of 72–90% in both GAD and dopa decarboxylase activity in seven brain regions from cases of senile dementia (frontal grey matter, medial thalamus, putamen, globus pallidus, caudate nucleus, substantia nigra and temporal lobe). In a later paper (Spillane *et al.* 1977), however, this group pointed out that the changes might well reflect the preterminal state since most of the demented patients died from severe bronchial pneumonia and probably had a defective respiratory reflex with reduced cerebral blood flow. In biopsy samples from dementia cases, the GAD activities were within normal limits.

Normal Distribution of GAD in the Human

GAD is widely and rather evenly distributed in the grey matter of brain with a range of less than 12 fold in the 56 areas analyzed in our series of 28 humans dying without neurological illness (Table II). The relatively even distribution of GAD contrasts with the uneven distribution of enzymes such as choline acetyltransferase and tyrosine hydroxylase. It must be remarked, however, that occasional samples of subcortical white matter we have analyzed have shown very low to negligible GAD activity.

As has been found in a variety of species, the highest concentrations of GAD were in the substantia nigra in the human. In five brains, the zona reticulata was analyzed in comparison with the zona compacta and the latter showed a significantly higher concentration.

In this series, the nucleus accumbens showed an activity equal to that of the substantia nigra as a whole. Other areas which showed relatively high GAD concentrations were the globus pallidus, pre-optic area, the hypothalamus and some regions of the cortex (Table II).

In almost all human brains, a number of caudate and putamen samples, taken at different coronal levels, were analyzed. The data, however, showed no

Table II.
*Relative distribution of GAD in control human brains and apparent effect of age**

	Activity as percent of that in caudate (Mean±S.E.)	Apparent effect of age*		
		Equation(GAD=)	N	r/σ_r
Cortex				
Overall	119±9	4.08±4.87/age	25	4.8
Frontal lobe				
Insula (34)**	125±15			
Motor (4)	136±12			
Premotor	122±22	5.00+69.6/age	8	3.8
Broca's area (44)	158±15			
Frontal pole (11)	165±28			
Straight gyrus	134±28			
Orbital gyrus (13)	107±31			
Parietal lobe				
Somatic sensory (1)	136±10	5.68+37.0/age	18	3.3
Parietal (7)	131±20			
Angular gyrus (39)	102±9			
Temporal lobe				
Acoustic receiving (41)	105±20			
Acoustic assocn. (42)	105±11			
Temporal tip (38)	113±29			
Middle temporal (21)	115±16			
Post inf. temporal (37)	97±10	3.61+59.4/age	9	4.2
Superior temporal	155±21			
Occipital lobe				
Visual assocn. (19)	131±25			
Visual receiv. (197)	125±29			
Calcarine fissure (18)	147±23	4.99+97.6/age	13	3.5
Internal capsule	28±11			
Splenius corpus callosum	33±7			
Genu. corpus callosum	26±12			
Rhinencephalon				
Hippocampus	66±4	1.99+29.1/age	24	4.3
Uncus	129±41			
Amygdala	59±4	1.84+32.3/age	24	6.5
Ant. perf. substance	124±11	4.08+50.0/age	15	4.1
Nucleus accumbens	213±21			
Septal area	116±22			
Posterior cingulate	98±17			

Table II. *(cont.)*

	Activity as percent of that in caudate (Mean±S.E.)	Apparent effect of age*		
		Equation(GAD=)	N	r/σ_r
Olfactory tubercle	135±25			
Fornix	44±15			
Preoptic area	151±25			
Basal ganglia				
Caudate		4.03+25.3/age	22	3.5
Putamen	105±10	3.78+35.6/age	22	4.4
Ant. external G.P.	182±22			
Lat. external G.P.	147±12			
Internal G.P.	168±19			
Overall G.P.	163±11	4.75+57.8/age	21	4.6
Claustrum	56±3			
Diencephalon				
Hypothalamus	141±11	4.65+54.3/age	15	3.0
Mammillary body	67±10	1.68+30.0/age	12	3.9
Subthalamic nuc.	81±7			
Medial geniculate	85±10			
Lateral geniculate	53±8	4.49−0.043 (age)	15	4.2
Pulvinar	60±6	1.83+48.2/age	18	4.6
Ant. thalamus	101±16	6.72−0.066 (age)	18	3.4
V.L. thalamus	74±9	0.03+93.4/age	15	7.5
V.P. thalamus	32±2			
Dorso-med. thalamus	56±12			
C.M. thalamus	69±13	2.67+55.0/age	14	3.4
Dorso-lat. thalamus	76±12			
Post-lat. thalamus	46±13			
Overall thalamus	68±8	1.68+58.4/age	20	6.2
Pons-Midbrain				
Superior colliculus	99±18	1.95+79.4/age	14	8.8
Inferior colliculus	93±10	2.75+63.5/age	12	8.5
S. nigra-overall	214±20	6.83+88.6/age	22	5.3
Zona reticulata	159±32			
Zona compacta	306±44			
Locus coeruleus	97±22	2.55+39.4/age	8	6.6
Red nucleus	59±7	0.86+29.0/age	13	4.7
Raphe area	54±11			
Inferior olive	34±7	68.0/age−0.58	8	4.3

Table II. *(cont.)*

	Activity as percent of that in caudate (Mean±S.E.)	Apparent effect of age*		
		Equation(GAD=)	N	r/σ_r
Cerebellum				
Lat. cortex	99±14	2.90+62.3/age	16	5.9
Vermis	133±22			
Dentate	145±28	4.57+67.2/age	10	4.1

* Absolute mean caudate activities were 4.51±0.53 μmole/h per 100 mg protein for GAD; the corresponding value for rat striatum using the same assay was about 15 μm/h per 100 mg protein. Where no equation for age is given, no significant correlation was found.

significant difference in the concentration of GAD at various levels. Somewhat similar results have been obtained in the rat both by us and by Fonnum *et al.* (1978); the relatively even distribution probably reflects the high concentration of gabergic interneurons.

Various distinct areas of the thalamus were analyzed and the posterior lateral thalamus and the pulvinar seemed to have lower GAD activity than the anterior thalamus. Other nuclei of the thalamus assayed (lateral thalamus, dorso-medial thalamus, centro-medial thalamus and latero-dorsal thalamus) did not differ significantly one from the other.

In the cortex there seems to be considerable variability from region to region and from brain to brain in GAD activity. The only regions, however, which appear to be consistently higher than others were Broca's area (Brodman 44) and the frontal pole (Brodman 11). No significant difference was found between left and right sides in a study of 24 separate areas of cortex from five normal human brains and in 16 areas from five baboons of a species *(Papio papio)* subject to idiopathic epilepsy. In these studies in baboons, as in the few data obtained by us on human biopsy material (Table I), no evidence was found of any abnormality in GAD correlatable with the epileptic phenomenon.

Effect of Aging

Of the 56 areas in our series of humans where five or more samples were available, almost half showed a significant decline of GAD with age (Table II). The best fit for the data was almost always curvilinear, indicating a more severe loss in the younger age groups (Fig. 2). There were equally significant losses with age in other enzymes such as tyrosine hydroxylase and choline acetyltransferase (McGeer & McGeer 1976a). It is interesting, however, that the areas showing the

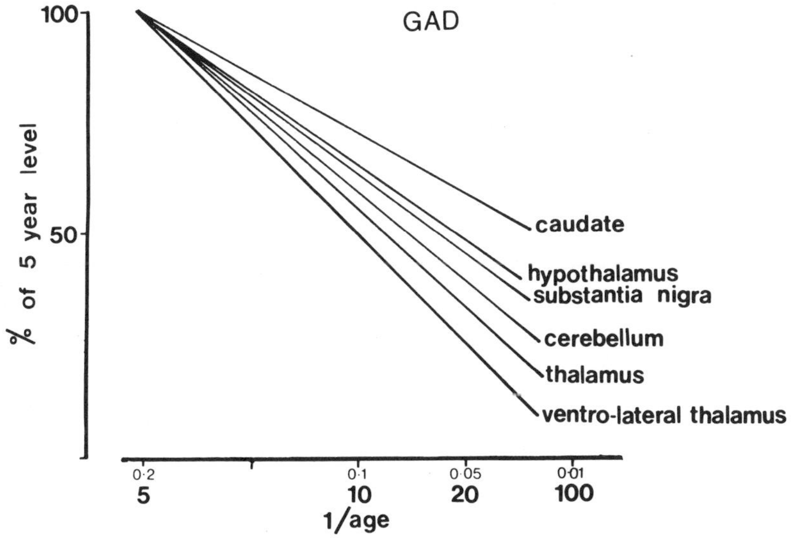

Fig. 2. Representative calculated lines of correlations for GAD activity as a function of age in various brain regions of humans dying without neurological or psychiatric illness.

most significant and greatest loss in GAD were not the same as those showing the greatest losses in TH or CAT. In general, the thalamic areas show the greatest declines in GAD followed by cortical and rhinencephalic areas. The basal ganglia showed relatively less decline of GAD with age. The sharpest drops in CAT, on the other hand, were in cortical areas while those in TH were in the caudate, putamen, and nucleus accumbens.

Perry *et al.* (1977) recently reported data which also indicate loss of GAD with age in many human brain areas. Further studies are needed to confirm and extend these data and there is as yet no indication of what they may mean with relation to brain functioning. It is clear, however, that this is an area of extreme importance, particularly when one considers the ever increasing number of aged individuals in our population.

GAD Activity in Schizophrenic Patients

The activity of GAD, as well as activities of choline acetyltransferase, tyrosine hydroxylase, dopa decarboxylase and acetylcholinesterase, were studied in 50 regions from the brains of 11 chronic schizophrenics for comparison with our control data. The only areas in which there was a significant difference between the average GAD activity in the schizophrenic and control populations were three areas of the cortex (Table III), although a few other areas (Table III) showed a tendency towards lower activity as evidenced by a comparison of the means calculated for the "relative activities" (enzyme activity of a particular region in a given brain expressed as a percentage of that in the caudate of the same brain). There were many areas, including a number of cortical areas, in which the GAD activity in the schizophrenic population appeared to be within normal limits and it was difficult for us to fit the data in Table III into any reasonable hypothesis of the schizophrenic process. We, therefore, have given more emphasis to the increases in choline acetyltransferase we found in the same brains in the nucleus accumbens, caudate and putamen (McGeer& McGeer 1977). These "abnormalities" in choline acetyltransferase have not, however, been confirmed in other studies of schizophrenic versus normal populations (Bird *et al.* 1978, Domino *et al.* 1973). On the other hand, Bird *et al.* have reported variable losses in GAD from the basal ganglia, nucleus accumbens and hippocampal tissue of schizophrenic patients but they have suggested that much of this is due to the premortem condition. Only the reduction in the nucleus accumbens was significant when tissue from control or schizophrenic patients

Table III.
Areas of significant difference between schizophrenic and normal means for glutamic acid decarboxylase activity

Area	Schizophrenic Mean±S.E. (N)	Normal Mean±S.E. (N)	*P* for difference
On both unadjusted and age-adjusted absolute data (unadjusted data in μmoles/hr/100 mg of protein)			
Sensory association [7]†	4.36±0.52 (8)	6.76±0.72 (9)	<0.02
Calcarine fissue [18]	3.97±0.44 (7)	6.99±1.05 (11)	<0.05
Insula [34]	3.66±0.45 (8)	5.99±0.67 (11)	<0.02
On relative activity (enzyme activity in a given brain expressed as a % of that in the caudate of the same brain)			
Anterior perforating substance	78±8%(9)	143±11%(8)	<0.01
Hypothalamus	95±14%(11)	142±11%(12)	<0.02
Substantia nigra	147±18%(11)	219±21%(16)	<0.05
Visual receiving [17]†	89±16%(9)	174±41%(7)	<0.05

† Brodmann numbers given in brackets.

Table IV.
Biochemical changes reported in rats given intrastriatal injections of kainic acid and in Huntington's chorea

<table>
<tr><th>Area and biochemical index</th><th>Striatal kainic acid</th><th>Huntington's chorea</th></tr>
<tr><td>In Neostriatum</td><td></td><td></td></tr>
<tr><td>Gabergic indices*</td><td>– Decreased</td><td>markedly – decreased</td></tr>
<tr><td>Cholinergic indices*</td><td>– Decreased</td><td>markedly – decreased</td></tr>
<tr><td>Dopaminergic indices*</td><td colspan="2">– Normal or elevated –</td></tr>
<tr><td>Serotonergic indices*</td><td colspan="2">Normal</td></tr>
<tr><td>Noradrenergic indices*</td><td colspan="2">Normal</td></tr>
<tr><td>Angiotension converting enzyme</td><td>– Decreased</td><td>markedly – decreased</td></tr>
<tr><td>Receptors* for:</td><td></td><td></td></tr>
<tr><td>AcCh (muscarinic)</td><td>– Decreased</td><td>markedly – decreased</td></tr>
<tr><td>Serotonin</td><td>– Decreased</td><td>markedly – decreased</td></tr>
<tr><td>GABA</td><td>Increased or decreased</td><td>Normal or decreased</td></tr>
<tr><td>In substantia nigra</td><td></td><td></td></tr>
<tr><td>Gabergic indices*</td><td>– Decreased</td><td>markedly – decreased</td></tr>
<tr><td>Substance P levels</td><td>– Decreased</td><td>markedly – decreased</td></tr>
<tr><td>Tyrosine hydroxylase levels</td><td colspan="2">Normal</td></tr>
</table>

* Neuronal indices used include activity of the synthetic enzyme and levels, uptake and release of transmitter. "Receptor" activity refers to sodium-independent binding in synaptic membrane fractions and does not imply pre- or postsynaptic localization or physiological activity.

who suffered sudden death was compared. In our series, the GAD activity in the schizophrenic population in the nucleus accumbens was 6.15 ± 1.24 (11 cases) as compared with 9.26 ± 1.37 for 18 controls. The difference was not statistically significant.

Gabergic Systems in Huntington's Chorea

Perry *et al.* (1973) were the first to report abnormal levels of GABA in Huntington's chorea. In a study of eight cases, compared with a similar number of age-matched controls, they found significant reductions in GABA levels in the caudate, putamen, globus pallidus, substantia nigra and occipital cortex. Homocarnosine, a dipeptide formed from GABA, was also significantly reduced in the extrapyramidal structures. Glycerophosphoethanolamine, on the other hand, was significantly higher. A number of investigators have since studied GAD, as well as other enzyme activities, in the brains of Huntington's chorea patients and have reported highly similar findings (McGeer & McGeer 1976b, Bird 1976, Enna *et al.* 1976, Urquhart *et al.* 1975). By the end of 1975, it was generally accepted that there were severe losses of GABA and GAD in the extrapyramidal nuclei in choreic patients, with no change or elevation in tyrosine hydroxylase activity in these structures; choline acetyltransferase activity was specifically reduced in the caudate with lesser and sometimes insignificant losses in the putamen. The decrements in GAD and CAT activity appeared to be area rather than neuronal specific since the same enzymes showed normal activities in other brain regions studied.

This initial demonstration of a biochemical pathology in Huntington's chorea led to clinical trials of various cholinergic and gabergic agonists. The lack of success in such trials is now understandable in view of the recent reports indicating that the defects in cholinergic and gabergic systems are only two aspects of a complicated biochemical pathology (Table IV) which seems to indicate a generalized loss of neurons with their perikarya in the caudate/putamen and, to a lesser extent, the globus pallidus. A similar morphological and chemical picture can be produced in rats by intrastriatal injections of kainic acid, an analog of glutamate, and this has led to the hypothesis that the destruction of neostriatal neurons in Huntington's chorea may be due to a functional overactivity of the cortico-striatal glutamergic tract (Coyle *et al.* 1978). This possibility has been enhanced by recent evidence that the kainic acid neurotoxicity is dependent upon the integrity of this cortico-striatal tract, the glutamergic nature of which has been indicated by both physiological and biochemical studies (Spencer 1976, Kim *et al.* 1977, McGeer *et al.* 1977, Divac *et al.* 1977).

Intracerebral injections of kainic acid are believed to destroy neurons with their perikarya in the injected area while sparing axons of passage and afferent nerve endings (McGeer *et al.* 1978a). The biochemical changes found in rats after intrastriatal injections of kainic acid, including the severe losses of GAD and other gabergic indices seen in the neostriatum and substantia nigra, are consistent with the hypothesized biochemical anatomy of the extrapyramidal system (Fig. 3).

The existence of a large population of GAD-containing striatal interneurons was indicated by lesion studies showing that severing the known afferents to the neostriatum does not result in significant decreases in neostriatal GAD (McGeer & McGeer 1975, McGeer *et al.* 1971). Evidence supporting gabergic pathways from the globus pallidus and from the caudal portion of the caudate-putamen to the substantia nigra has been derived from lesion studies showing substantial losses in nigral GAD following hemitransections at the level of the anterior

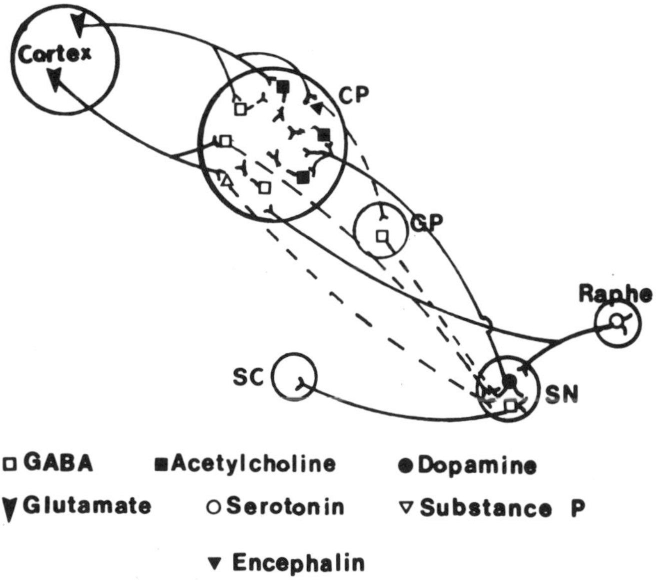

Fig. 3. Hypothesized biochemical neuroanatomy of extrapyramidal system, with dashed lines indicating systems affected by intrastriatal injections of kainic acid. GP=globus pallidus, CP=caudateputamen, SN=substantia nigra, SC=superior colliculus.

hypothalamus (Kataoka *et al.* 1974, Hattori *et al.* 1973, Fonnum *et al.* 1978), lesions of the globus pallidus (McGeer *et al.* 1971) or rostral caudate-putamen (Kim *et al.* 1971, Fonnum *et al.* 1974, 1978). Axonal transport studies indicate that the pallidal-nigral tract provides heavy innervation of dopaminergic nigrostriatal neurons while the striato-nigral tract(s) do not appear to provide a large number of synapses on this dopaminergic system. Early studies of the uptake of ^{3}H-GABA showed that GABA primarily enters nerve endings in the substantia nigra but it is taken up into both cell bodies and nerve endings (Hattori *et al.* 1973) in the caudate-putamen and globus pallidus. Of the three structures, the globus pallidus had the greatest tendency to take GABA into its cell bodies.

The gabergic nature of the nigrotectal projection indicated in this figure is based on biochemical studies indicating a significant fall in GAD activity in the superior colliculus after lesion of the substantia nigra (Table V, Vincent *et al.* 1978). The morphology of nerve endings in the superior colliculus labelled by axoplasmic transport of radioactive protein from the substantia nigra is highly similar to that of gabergic terminals identified in other areas by immunocytochemical and other methods. Preliminary studies on thalamic GAD activity suggest that the nigro-thalamic tract may also use GABA as a neurotransmitter. These data are consistent with the paper by Anderson *et al.* (1977) suggesting that some nigrotectal neurons send collaterals to the ventromedial thalamus and showing that substantia nigral stimulation results in monosynaptic inhibition in the thalamus.

The enkephalin path in Fig. 3 has been suggested recently by Cuello & Paxinos (1978) on the basis of lesion experiments; evidence for the other pathways shown has been reviewed recently (McGeer *et al.* 1978b).

GLUTAMINASE LOCALIZATION IN GABA NEURONS

Much of the glutaminase activity of brain has been reported to be localized in the synaptosomal fraction (Bradford & Ward 1976) and compartmentation studies suggest that some of it must be in gabergic nerve endings where it serves to transform glutamine to glutamate for use as a precursor of GABA. No data appear to exist, however, which indicate whether a significant proportion of the glutaminase activity in brain might be in glutamergic nerve endings where it could serve for the maintenance of the transmitter pool of glutamate. A considerable portion of the gabergic systems of the neostriatum can be selectively destroyed by intrastriatal kainic acid injections which do not affect the integrity of the cortico-striatal glutamergic nerve endings, as indicated by glutamate uptake studies (Fig. 4). Lesions of the corticostriatal tract, on the other hand, can reduce the glutamate uptake in the neostriatum by approximately 40% without any effect upon GAD activity in that region (Fig. 4). These data suggest that this system might be used to explore the relative amount of glutaminase associated with these neuronal types. Glutaminase activity in the neostriatum was therefore measured in rats which had received intrastriatal

Table V.

Biochemical changes in the superior colliculus after lesions of the substantia nigra

	n	Control	Lesion	Per cent of control
Glycine uptake	6	209±27	223±29	107
Aspartate uptake	6	352±40	302±30	86
Choline acetyltransferase	12	18.2±1.3	18.5±1.2	102
Glutamate decarboxylase	8	221±5.7	132±14	60*

Uptake expressed as pmole/mg protein/5 min. Enzyme activity as nmole/mg protein/h.
* $P<0.001$; Student's t-test.

injections of kainic acid or lesions of the cortico-striatal tract at least 10 days before sacrifice.

Fig. 5 illustrates typical results on the animals injected with varying amounts of kainic acid. The decrement in glutaminase correlated significantly with the decrement in GAD and the intercept on the x axis was such as to suggest that some 60% of the glutaminase activity in the neostriatum is located in gabergic structures (or a least some structures destroyed by the kainic acid injection), while 40% is in some unaffected compartment(s). Of the systems so far known to be affected by kainic acid (Table IV), only the gabergic system would appear likely to contain glutaminase. The glutamate uptake in these kainic acid-injected striata was not depressed and indeed, in some, was raised somewhat above the contralateral control striatum. An attempt to take the individual glutamate uptakes into account by calculating for the data a line of correlation of the form: glutaminase activity=a+b (GAD activity)+c (glutamate uptake) was unsuccessful; the coefficient of correlation was much lower than for the line of regression shown in Fig. 5.

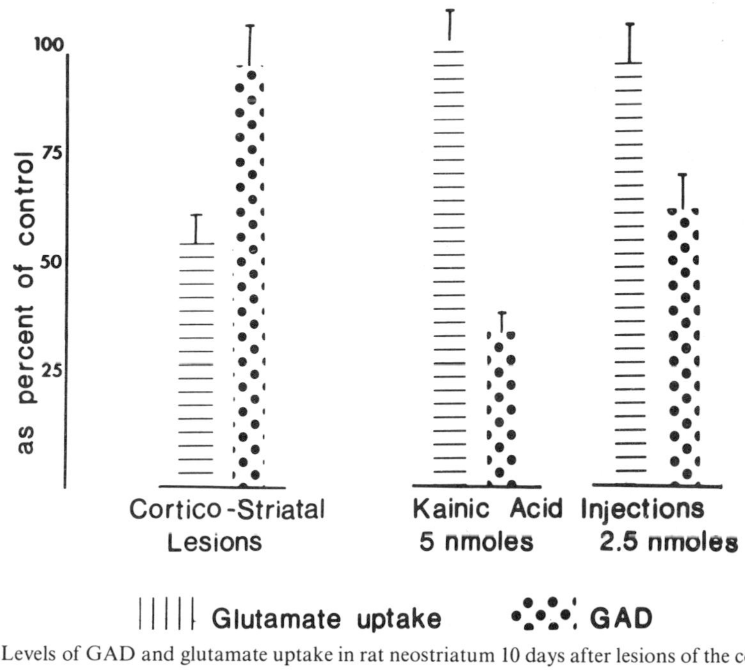

Fig. 4. Levels of GAD and glutamate uptake in rat neostriatum 10 days after lesions of the cortico-striatal tract or injections of kainic acid into the neostriatum.

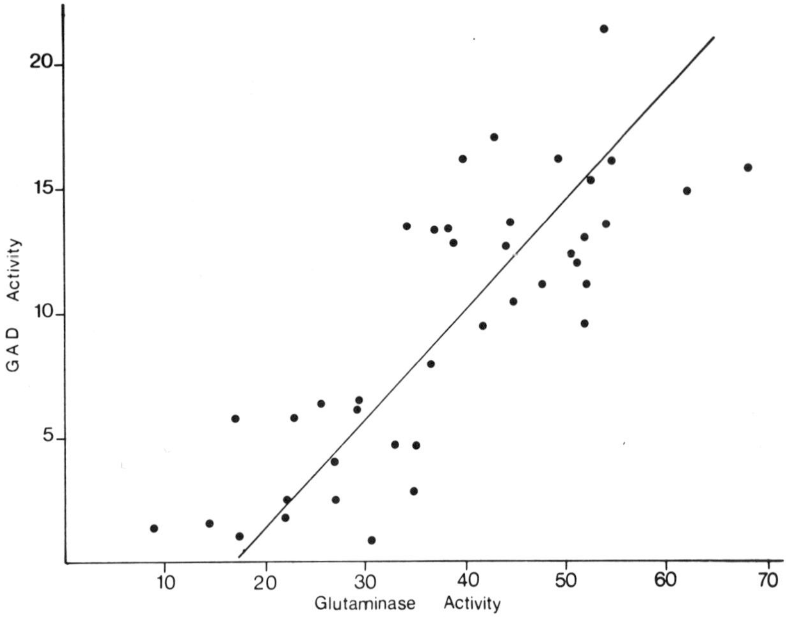

Fig. 5. Glutaminase and GAD activities in rat neostriata following local injection of various amounts of kainic acid.

On the other hand, in animals with lesions of the cortico-striatal tract, we could not demonstrate a significant correlation between glutaminase activity in the neostriatum and glutamate uptake in that structure. In these animals, neither GAD or glutaminase activity was significantly affected by the lesion. These results were disappointing since we had hoped that glutaminase activity might be a convenient index, used alone or together with measurements of GAD, for the integrity of glutamergic systems. These data, however, offer no support for the supposition that the neurotransmitter pool of glutamate may be derived directly from glutamine in the glutamergic nerve endings.

Experiments on the subcellular localization of glutaminase in control rat neostriata indicated that approximately 60% was in the P_2 synaptosomal fraction. This figure is higher than previously reported from other brain areas (Bradford & Ward 1976) but is consistent with the results from kainic acid-injected rats. Taken together, these data suggest that about 40% of the glutaminase in the neostriatum is associated with glia and about 60% with gabergic systems.

CONCLUSION

It is clear that useful measurements can be made on gabergic systems in human autopsy material. Data obtained so far indicate losses in gabergic neuronal activity in normal aging but results in various pathological conditions have either indicated no abnormalities (epilepsy and senile dementia) or losses which are either difficult to relate to present hypotheses of the disease (schizophrenia) or are apparently part of a generalized loss of neurons in the affected brain regions (chorea). Only a few of the many gabergic tracts in brain have been mapped and little is known about their possible role in normal brain functioning. It seems probable that much important information will reward further studies on this neurotransmitter.

REFERENCES

Anderson, M. & Yoshida, M. (1977) Electrophysiological evidence for branching nigral projection to the thalamus and the superior colliculus. *Brain Res.* 137, 361–364.

Bird, E. D. & Iversen, L. L. (1974) Huntington's chorea – Postmortem measurement of glutamic acid decarboxylase, choline acetyltransferase and dopamine in basal ganglia. *Brain* 97, 457–472.

Bird, E. D., Spokes, E. G., Barnes, J., MacKey, A. V. P. & Iversen, L. L. (1978) Glutamic-acid decarboxylase in schizophrenia. *The Lancet* I, 156.

Bowen, D. M., White, P., Flack, R. H. A., Smith, C. B. & Davidsen, A. N. (1974) Brain-decarboxylase activities as indices of pathological change in senile dementia. *Lancet* 1247–1249.

Bradford, H. F. & Ward, H. K. (1976) On glutaminase activity in mammalian synaptosomes. *Brain Res.* 110, 115–125.

Coyle, J. T., McGeer, E. G., McGeer, P. L. & Schwarcz, R. (1978) Neostriatal injections: a model for Huntington's chorea. In: *Kainic Acid,* eds. McGeer, E. G., Olney, J. W. & McGeer, P. L. pp. 139–160. Raven Press, N.Y.

Cuello, A. C. & Paxinos, G. (1978) Evidence for a long Leu-enkephalin striopallidal pathway in rat brain. *Nature* 271, 178–180.

Divac, I., Fonnum, F. & Storm-Mathison, J. (1977) High affinity uptake of glutamate in terminals of corticostriatal axons. *Nature* 266, 377–378.

Domino, E. F., Krause, R. R. & Bowers, J. (1973) Various enzymes involved with putative neurotransmitters. *Arch. Gen. Psychiatry* 29, 195–201.

Enna, S. J., Bennett, J. P., Bylund, D. B., Snyder, S. H., Bird, E. D. & Iversen, L. L. (1976) Alterations of brain neurotransmitter receptor binding in Huntington's chorea. *Brain Res.* 116, 531–537.

Fonnum, F., Gottesfield, Z. & Grofova, I. (1978) Distribution of glutamate decarboxylase, choline acetyltransferase and aromatic amino acid decarboxylase in the basal ganglia of normal and operated rats. Evidence for striatopallidal, striatoentopeduncular and striatonigral gabaergic fibers. *Brain Res.* 143, 125–128.

Fonnum, F., Grofova, I., Rinvik, E., Storm-Mathisen, J. & Waldberg, F. (1974) Origin and distribution of glutamate decarboxylase in substantia nigra of the cat. *Brain Res.* 71, 77–92.

Grote, S. S., Moses, S. G., Robins, E., Hudgens, R. W. & Croninger, A. B. (1974) A study of selected catecholamine metabolizing enzymes: a comparison of depressive suicides and alcoholic suicides with controls. *J. Neurochem.* 23, 791–802.

Hattori, T., McGeer, P. L., Fibiger, H. C. & McGeer, E. G. (1973) On the source of Gaba-containing terminals in the substantia nigra. Electron microscopic autoradiographic and biochemical studies. *Brain Res.* 54, 103–114.

Kataoka, K., Bak, I. J., Hassler, R., Kim, J. S. & Wagner, A. (1974) L-Glutamate decarboxylase and choline acetyltransferase activity in the substantia nigra and the striatum after surgical interruption of the strio-nigral fibers of the baboon. *Exp. Brain Res.* 19, 217–227.

Kim, J. S., Bak, I. J., Hassler, R. & Okada, Y. (1971) Role of γ-aminobutyric acid (GABA) in the extra-pyramidal motor system. *Exp. Brain Res.* 14, 95–104.

Kim, J. S., Hassler, R., Hang, P. & Paik, K. S. (1977) Effect of frontal cortex ablation on striatal glutamic acid level in rat. *Brain Res.* 132, 370–374.

McGeer, E. G. & McGeer, P. L. (1976) Neurotransmitter metabolism in the aging brain. In: *Aging,* vol. 3, eds. Terry, R. D. & Gershon, S. pp. 389–403. Raven Press, N.Y.

McGeer, P. L. & McGeer, E. G. (1975) Evidence for glutamic acid decarboxylase-containing interneurons in the neostriatum. *Brain Res.* 91, 331–335.

McGeer, P. L. & McGeer, E. G. (1976) Enzymes associated with the metabolism of catecholamines, acetylcholine and GABA in human controls and patients with Parkinson's disease and Huntington's chorea. *J. Neurochem.* 26, 65–76.

McGeer, P. L. & McGeer, E. G. Possible changes in striatal and limbic cholinergic systems in schizophrenia. *Arch. Gen. Psychiatry* 34, 1319–1323.

McGeer, P. L., McGeer, E. G. & Hattori, T. (1978a) Kainic acid as a tool in neurobiology. In: *Kainic Acid,* ed. McGeer, E. G., Olney, J. W. & McGeer, P. L. pp. 124–138. Raven Press, N.Y.

McGeer, P. L., McGeer, E. G. & Hattori, T. (1978b) Transmitters in the basal ganglia. In: *Amino Acids as Chemical Transmitters,* ed. Fonnum, F. Raven Press, N.Y. In press.

McGeer, P. L., McGeer, E. G., Scherer, U. & Singh, K. (1977) A glutamatergic cortico-striatal path? *Brain Res.* 128, 369–373.

McGeer, P. L., McGeer, E. G., Wada, J. A. & Jung, E. (1971) Effects of globus pallidus lesions and Parkinson's disease on brain glutamic acid decarboxylase. *Brain Res.* 32, 425–431.

Perry, E. K., Gibson, P. H., Blessed, G., Perry, R. H. & Tomlinson, B. E. (1977) Neurotransmitter enzyme abnormalities in senile dementia – choline acetyltransferase and glutamic acid decarboxylase in necropsy brain tissue. *J. Neuro. Sci.* 34, 247–265.

Perry, T. L., Hansen, S. & Kloster, M. (1973) Huntington's chorea, deficiency of γ-aminobutyric acid in brain. *New Engl. J. Med.* 288, 337–342.

Spencer, H. J. (1976) Antagonism of cortical excitation of striatal neurons by glutamic acid diethyl ester: evidence for glutamic acid as an excitatory transmitter in the rat striatum. *Brain Res.* 102, 91–101.

Spillane, J. A., White, P., Goodhardt, M. J., Flack, R. H. A., Bowen, D. M. & Davidson, A. N. (1977) Selective vulnerability of neurons in organic dementia. *Nature* 266, 558–559.

Urquhart, N., Perry, T. L., Hansen, S. & Kennedy, J. (1975) GABA content and glutamic acid decarboxylase activity in brain of Huntington's chorea patients and control subjects. *J. Neurochem.* 24, 1071–1075.

Vincent, S. R., Hattori, T. & McGeer, E. G. (1978) The nigrotectal projection: a biochemical and ultrastructural characterization. *Brain Res.* In press.

Facilitation of GABA-ergic Transmission by Drugs

W. Haefely, P. Polc, R. Schaffner, H. H. Keller, L. Pieri, H. Möhler

GABA-ergic neurons occupy strategic sites in the CNS. 1) One type of GABA-ergic interneurons mediates presynaptic inhibition (Fig. 1). Incoming impulses in first order neurons (spinal and cranial nerves) are subject to presynaptic modulation by impulses in other afferents or from central structures before being transmitted to second order neurons. 2) Other GABA-ergic interneurons are involved in postsynaptic (collateral and recurrent) inhibition (Fig. 1). GABA-ergic interneurons in these circuits are parts of local feedforward and feedback inhibitory loops on principal neurons (e.g. in cerebral and cerebellar cortex, basal ganglia, hippocampus, hypothalamus, and brainstem). Both mechanisms allow the first excitatory impulses in a train to fully activate a principal neuron, whereas subsequent signals encounter a target cell made less excitable by the preceding volleys. These circuits are inbuilt local devices to prevent excessive excitation of neurons. 3) GABA-ergic projection neurons directly transmit inhibitory influences from one central structure to a distant one (Fig. 1), e.g. the cerebellar Purkinje cells, which carry the total (inhibitory) output from the cerebellar cortex, and the strio-nigral pathway, inhibitory for dopamine cells.

It is a most tempting idea to increase by drugs these physiological inhibitory GABA-ergic mechanisms, although the rather ubiquitous occurrence of GABA-ergic synapses within the CNS might reduce the possibility of selective and useful pharmacological actions. So far, very limited efforts have been made to develop drugs that selectively enhance GABA-ergic transmission. However, agents, already long in use, were shown recently to enhance GABA-ergic transmission. Five classes of such compounds (Fig. 2) will be briefly reviewed.

Pharma Research Department, F. Hoffmann-La Roche & Co. Ltd., Basle, Switzerland.

"GABA-NEUROTRANSMITTERS", Alfred Benzon Symposium 12, Munksgaard 1978

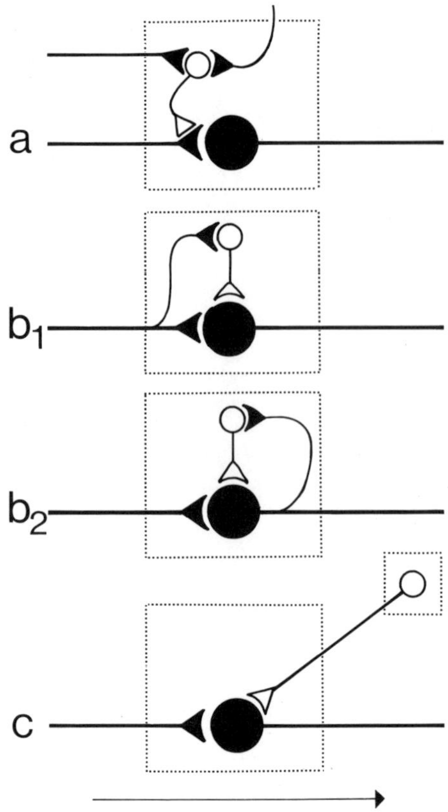

Fig. 1. Schematic diagram of four types of GABA-ergic synapses: presynaptic inhibition (a), collateral inhibition (b_1), recurrent inhibition (b_2), postsynaptic inhibition by projection neurons (c).

BENZODIAZEPINES

The concept proposed a few years ago by ourselves (Polc *et al.* 1974, Haefely *et al.* 1975b, Costa *et al.* 1975) that benzodiazepines facilitate GABA-ergic synaptic transmission seems, by now, solidly supported by ample additional experimental evidence. This facilitatory action is at present known to occur at nine different mammalian GABA-ergic synapses.

GABA-ergic interneurons

The original observation that diazepam enhances *presynaptic inhibition in the spinal cord* (Schmidt *et al.* 1967) has been confirmed and extended (Schlosser 1971, Stratten & Barnes 1971, Chanelet & Lonchampt 1971, Chin *et al.* 1974,

Polc *et al.* 1974, Nicot *et al.* 1976, Polzin & Barnes 1976). Benzodiazepines dose-dependently enhance all signs of presynaptic inhibition (dorsal root potential, DRP; dorsal root reflex, DRR; inhibition of monosynaptic VRRs, increased excitability of primary afferent terminals) with a plateau reached at approximately 10 times the threshold doses (Fig. 3). Benzodiazepines increase mainly the peak of inhibition produced by an activation of a presynaptic inhibitory pathway, but only slightly affect the time constant of presynaptic inhibition. The relative potencies of benzodiazepines in facilitating presynaptic inhibition reflect their potencies as tranquillizers. There is a mutual surmountable antagonism between the facilitatory effect of benzodiazepines and the depressant effect of presumed blockers of GABA receptors or Cl^- channels. The abolition of presynaptic inhibition after inhibitors of GABA synthesis cannot be reversed by benzodiazepines.

Presynaptic inhibition in the cuneate nucleus (Polc & Haefely 1976) is affected by benzodiazepines in essentially the same way as in the spinal cord. After depletion of endogenous GABA (Banna & Jabbur 1971), the drugs are no longer active.

Postsynaptic inhibition in the spinal cord was found to be unaffected by diazepam (Schmidt *et al.* 1967), which is of particular interest, because this inhibition is not mediated by GABA, but probably by glycine. In contrast,

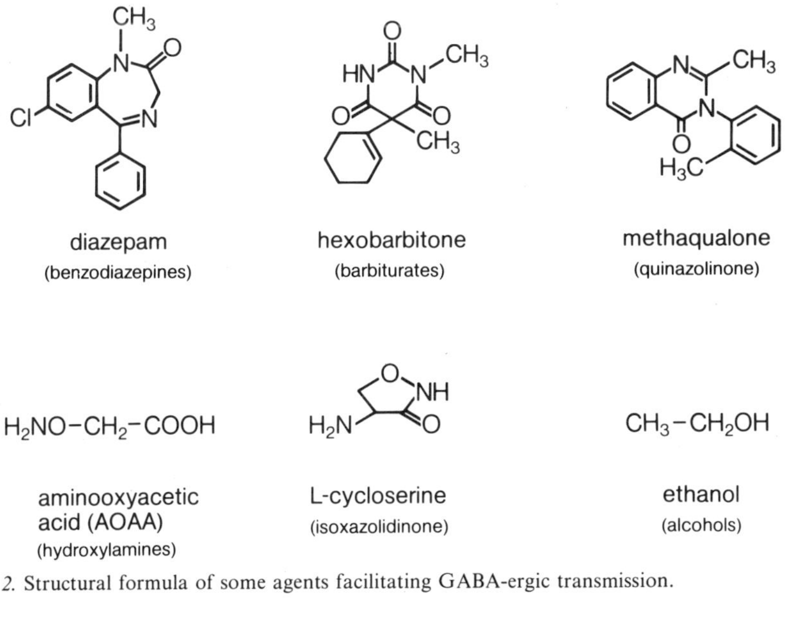

Fig. 2. Structural formula of some agents facilitating GABA-ergic transmission.

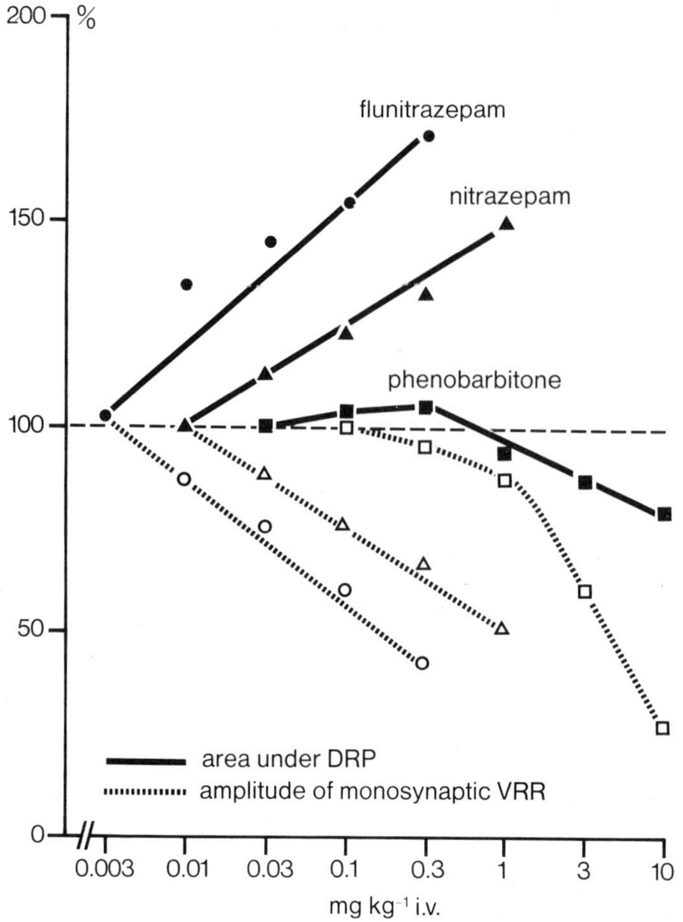

Fig. 3. Effects of two benzodiazepines (flunitrazepam and nitrazepam) and phenobarbitone on presynaptic inhibition (expressed as the area under the dorsal root potential) and the amplitude of the monosynaptic ventral root reflex in spinal cats. The points are the means of at least four cats. (Polc, unpublished results).

postsynaptic inhibition of cuneothalamic relay cells is, at least in part, due to GABA. The finding that benzodiazepines enhance postsynaptic inhibition in the cuneate nucleus (Polc & Haefely 1976) was therefore most relevant for understanding their actions.

The spontaneous firing rate of single *Purkinje cells* is dose-dependently decreased by various benzodiazepines (Pieri & Haefely 1976). This depression affects single spikes and not the complex spikes induced by the climbing fiber input (Mariani & Delhaye-Bouchaud 1978). The assumption that this effect on Purkinje cells is due to enhanced inhibition from stellate and basket cells was shown to be correct by direct studies of the basket cell inhibition (Curtis *et al.* 1976, Geller *et al.* 1978). The electrophysiological findings agree well with neurochemical observations (Costa *et al.* 1975, Guidotti 1978), indicating that the cerebellar content of cGMP reflects activity of Purkinje cells; benzodiazepines decrease the resting level of cerebellar cGMP and counteract its increase by agents which activate these cells. In contrast to the effect of GABA-mimetics, e.g. muscimol, that of benzodiazepines seems to depend entirely on ongoing GABA-ergic activity.

Diazepam enhances *collateral inhibition of cortical pyramidal tract cells* by the GABA-ergic basket cell (Raabe & Gumnit 1977). This effect probably accounts for the enhanced depression of intracortical responses observed after diazepam (Zakusov *et al.* 1975).

Activity of *hippocampal pyramidal cells* is depressed after a preceding orthodromic or antidromic volley; GABA-ergic basket cells which mediate this inhibition are excited by recurrent collaterals of pyramidal cells. Benzodiazepines intensify this recurrent inhibition (Wolf & Haas 1977).

Tuberal hypothalamic cell activity is modulated by recurrent inhibition. Diazepam enhances this evoked inhibition in cultured hypothalamic cells and counteracts the suppressant effect of picrotoxin (Geller *et al.* 1978).

Indirect evidence suggests the existence of a GABA-ergic inhibitory input to *noradrenergic locus coeruleus neurons* in the cat, and the facilitatory action of benzodiazepines on this synapse (Haefely *et al.* 1975a). This action may at least in part underly the prevention of stress-induced activation of central noradrenergic neurons (Corrodi *et al.* 1971).

GABA-ergic projection neurons

The cell bodies of the GABA-ergic *striato-nigral pathway* are distributed diffusely within the caudate-putamen; their axons run through the globus pallidus to impinge on dopamine cells in the substantia nigra (Brownstein *et al.* 1977, Gale *et al.* 1977). Single stimuli in the cat caudate nucleus evoke a simple mass potential in the substantia nigra which is abolished by picrotoxin and bicuculline, but resistant to strychnine. Benzodiazepines have little effect on the amplitude of this evoked potential, however, they very potently antagonize the depressant effect of bicuculline (Haefely *et al.* 1975b, 1978, Schaffner & Haefely 1975). Wolf & Haas (1977) observed a depressant effect of benzodiazepines on

Table I

Facilitation of GABA-ergic transmission by benzodiazepines: possible mechanisms

I POSTSYNAPTIC SITE	
1) *GABA-mimetic action*	
No electrophysiological evidence	Polc *et al.* 1974, Polc & Haefely 1976, 1977, Bowery & Dray 1978
No interaction with GABA and bicuculline binding sites	Möhler & Okada, 1977b, c, Olsen *et al.* 1978
2) *Potentiation of exogenous GABA action*	
Rat hypothalamic tuberal cells in culture	Geller *et al.* 1978
Rat cerebellar Purkinje cells	Geller *et al.* 1978
Cultured mouse spinal cord neurons	Choi *et al.* 1977, MacDonald & Barker 1978
Sensorimotor neurons *in situ*	Kozhechkin & Ostrovskaja 1977
Isolated frog spinal cord	Nistri & Constanti 1978
No potentiation in rat isolated sup. cervical ganglion	Bowery & Dray 1978
No potentiation in lobster muscle	Nistri & Constanti 1978
3) *Postsynaptic reversal of bicuculline antagonism*	
Rat isolated sup. cervical ganglion	Bowery & Dray 1978
Rat medullary neurons *in situ*	Dray & Straughan 1976, Bowery & Dray 1978
4) *Chloride conductance*	
Increase: mammalian skeletal muscle	Vyskočil 1977
No increase: crayfish muscle	Olsen *et al.* 1978
5) *Affinity of GABA to its receptor*	
Increase in fresh brain membranes	Guidotti *et al.* (this symposium)
II PRESYNAPTIC SITE	
1) *GABA uptake*	
No specific effect	Iversen & Johnston 1971, Olsen *et al.* 1978
2) *GABA release*	
By action potentials *in situ*	not investigated
Spontaneous in synaptosomes: increase	Olsen *et al.* 1978
High K^+-induced in synaptosomes: decr.	Olsen *et al.* 1978
Low K^+-induced in synaptosomes: increase	Mitchell & Martin 1978
(Excitation → intracellular Ca^{2+} in muscle)	Moudgil & Pleuvry 1970

the spontaneous firing rate of substantia nigra cells. The conclusion that benzodiazepines enhance GABA-ergic transmission at nigral dopamine neurons is well supported by neurochemical studies. The drugs slightly reduce the turnover of striatal dopamine in normal rats and markedly attenuate its acceleration by neuroleptics (Keller *et al.* 1976). Chéramy *et al.* (1977) observed a mutual antagonism between picrotoxin and diazepam in their effect on the spontaneous release of dopamine within the caudate. Benzodiazepines prevent changes in kinetic properties of striatal tyrosine hydroxylase induced by neuroleptics (Guidotti, personal communication). Functional consequences of increased GABA-ergic inhibition of dopamine neurons are potentiation of neuroleptic-induced catalepsy (Keller *et al.* 1976, Matsui & Deguchi 1977), a rotation after intranigral injection similar to that seen after muscimol and inhibitors of GABA-T (Waddington 1977), and potentiation of the depressant effect of neuroleptics on conditioned avoidance responses (Cumin, unpublished).

GABA-ergic *cerebellar Purkinje cells* project, *inter alia,* to the lateral vestibular nuclei to inhibit Deiter's neurons. Potentials evoked in Deiters' nucleus by single pulses to Purkinje cell axons have a picrotoxin- and bicuculline-sensitive but strychnine-resistant component. Benzodiazepines prevent the depressant effect of GABA antagonists on this component (Haefely *et al.* 1978).

Benzodiazepine receptors

Recent studies show that benzodiazepines bind with high affinity and specificity to proteins in synaptic membranes of the CNS *in vitro* and *in vivo* (Braestrup & Squires 1977, 1978, Braestrup *et al.* 1977, Squires & Braestrup 1977, Möhler & Okada 1977a, b, Speth *et al.* 1978, Chang & Snyder 1978, Bosmann *et al.* 1978, Nielsen *et al.* 1978, Waddington & Owen 1978). These binding sites recognize benzodiazepines according to their tranquillizing potencies but not neurotransmitters or other psychotropic drugs, in particular barbiturates, meprobamate, methaqualone, and phenytoin. These binding sites very likely represent, in part, the pharmacological receptors which benzodiazepines have to trigger, in order to produce their characteristic effects (Haefely 1978b). Distribution of benzodiazepine receptors in the CNS is uneven; whether they are located presynaptically on GABA neurons or postsynaptically on GABA-ceptive neurons is yet unknown. The marked decrease of their number in the striatum along with a fall of GAD activity in brains of Chorea Huntington patients (Okada *et al.* 1978) suggests a presynaptic localization.

Mechanism of facilitation of GABA-ergic transmission

The effects of benzodiazepines on GABA-ergic transmission could be explained equally well by either a post- or presynaptic action. Experimental findings relevant for this question are presented in Table I. Direct activation of GABA receptors by benzodiazepines is excluded by electrophysiological and receptor binding studies. Several authors have observed a potentiation of the effects of exogenous GABA *in vivo* and *in vitro*; in the rat isolated sup. cervical ganglion, however, such an effect is questionable. The positive findings are not conclusive evidence for a postsynaptic site of action of benzodiazepines, unless presynaptic effects can be clearly excluded, e.g. changes in synaptic concentrations of endogeneous GABA or in basal excitatory synaptic activity. Reversal of bicuculline-induced depression of GABA effects, which is less marked than that seen with barbiturates, is very interesting, but difficult to explain, because benzodiazepines do not interfere with the binding of bicuculline (Möhler & Okada 1977c). Increase of the resting Cl^-conduction in skeletal muscle and bicuculline reversal suggest that benzodiazepines somehow modulate the ionic permeability changes induced by GABA. At present, the most spectacular observation is that benzodiazepines enhance the affinity of GABA for its receptor in fresh synaptic membranes; a physiological inhibitor of GABA binding might be involved (Guidotti, this symposium). In spite of suggestive evidence for postsynaptic benzodiazepine actions, a presynaptic site cannot be excluded. Enhancement of the GABA release induced by small increases of extracellular K^+, and increase of twitch responses in skeletal muscle (ascribed to reduced sequestration of intracellular Ca^{2+}) demonstrate the urgent need for a study of benzodiazepines on excitation-secretion coupling in GABA neurones in situ. Reduction of GABA turnover (Haefely *et al.* 1975b, Mao *et al.* 1977, Peričić *et al.* 1977, Bernasconi & Martin 1978) is no compelling evidence against an improved stimulus-induced release of GABA; enhanced efficiency of GABA cell activity should reduce the number of discharges of principal neurons and, thereby, also recurrent activation of GABA interneurons.

Facilitation of GABA-ergic transmission and profile of pharmacological actions of benzodiazepines

Some possible links between increased GABA-ergic transmission and somatic and psychic actions of benzodiazepines were discussed earlier (Haefely 1977, 1978a, b) as well as the reasons why a selective and quantitatively restricted potentiation of GABA-ergic transmission could underly both the many useful therapeutic actions and the exceptionally good tolerance of these drugs.

BARBITURATES

Besides numerous unspecific effects on artificial and biological nonsynaptic membranes (Blaustein 1968, Seeman 1972, Blaustein & Ector 1975, Frazier *et al.* 1975), barbiturates have specific effects on excitatory (Galindo 1969, Barker 1975, Barker & Gainer 1973) and inhibitory (Nicoll 1978a, b) synaptic mechanisms.

In the *spinal cord*, prolongation of DRPs by pentobarbitone was described as early as 1946 (Eccles & Malcolm). This increase of presynaptic inhibition was confirmed for many barbiturates in mammals and in frogs (Eccles *et al.* 1963, Schmidt 1963, Miyahara *et al.* 1966, Abdelmoumene & Besson 1967, Nicoll 1975a). Postsynaptic inhibition in the spinal cord was found unaffected by pentobarbitone (Weakly *et al.* 1968), but prolonged by hexobarbitone (Larson & Major 1970). In contrast to benzodiazepines, barbiturates only slightly increase the amplitude of DRPs at low doses and depress it at higher doses; however, they prolong the duration of the DRPs over the whole dose range (Polc, unpublished). The area under the DRP, as a measure of the total primary afferent depolarization, is increased in low and decreased in higher doses (Fig. 3). In the *cuneate nucleus*, pentobarbitone slightly increases the amplitude and markedly prolongs the surface P-wave and antagonizes the opposite effect of picrotoxin (Banna & Jabbur 1969). Experiments in our laboratories (Polc & Haefely 1976) show that phenobarbitone (3 mg mg^{-1}) enhances both pre- and postsynaptic inhibition in the cat cuneate nucleus. After 30 mg kg^{-1} the enhancement of inhibition is less marked than after 10 mg kg^{-1}; this decline is clearly correlated with depression of excitation. Recurrent inhibition of *hippocampal pyramidal cells* is prolonged after barbiturates (Nicoll *et al.* 1975, Wolf & Haas 1977). Studies of a very particular type of synapse, the dendrodendritic reciprocal synapse between mitral cells and internuncial granule cells in the *rabbit olfactory bulb*, led Nicoll (1972, 1978a) to conclude that the inhibition of mitral cells by GABA-ergic granule cells is enhanced by various barbiturates at doses which do not yet depress the excitation of granule cells by the mitral cells. In the isolated *olfactory cortex* of the guinea pig recurrent inhibition is intensified by pentobarbitone in subanesthetic concentrations (Scholfield 1978, Pickles & Simmonds 1978). Recurrent inhibition of the *thalamo-cortical relay cells* in the VL and VPL nuclei of the thalamus was found markedly enhanced by very small doses of pentobarbitone (Bremer 1970), as was recurrent inhibition of pyramidal tract neurons in the cortex (Veselyune *et al.* 1971). Thiamylal markedly enhances basket cell-mediated inhibition of cerebellar Purkinje cells (Eccles *et al.* 1971). Phenobarbitone affects cerebellar cGMP levels in a similar way as benzodiazepines, although it is considerably less potent (Guidotti 1978). Inhibition of

Table II
Facilitation of GABA-ergic transmission by barbiturates: possible mechanisms

I POSTSYNAPTIC SITE	
GABA-induced conductance increase	
Tissue cultured mouse spinal neurons: enhanced	Ransom & Barker 1976, Barker & MacDonald 1977
Cat dorsal horn interneurons: enhanced depression by bicuculline reversed	Curtis & Lodge 1977
Isolated rat superior cervical ganglion:	
enhanced	Evans 1977
not enhanced	Bowery & Dray 1978
bicuculline-induced depression reversed	Bowery & Dray 1977, 1978
Isolated frog sympathetic ganglion:	
enhanced	Nicoll 1978a, b
Isolated spinal cord (motoneurons):	
enhanced	Nicoll 1975b
Neurons of rat medulla: depression by bicuculline reversed	Bowery & Dray 1977, 1978
GABA-like conductance increase	
Isolated frog spinal cord: depolarization of primary afferents	Nicoll 1975a
Hyperpolarization of motoneurons	Nicoll 1975a
Isolated frog dorsal root ganglion cells: depolarization	Nicoll 1975a
Isolated frog sympathetic ganglion: depolarization	Nicoll 1978c
^{36}Cl-uptake of crayfish muscle: no increase, GABA effect antagonized	Olsen *et al.* 1978
"GABA receptor binding": no effect	Olsen *et al.* 1978 Jessell & Richards 1977
II PRESYNAPTIC SITE	
Quantum content of endplate potentials increased	Proctor & Weakly 1976 Weakly & Proctor 1977
GABA uptake inhibition: very weak	Olsen *et al.* 1978

neurons in the rat substantia nigra, induced by stimulation of the caudate nucleus, was found to be more marked in animals anesthetized with pentobarbitone than with urethane (Dray *et al.* 1976). Depression by bicuculline of strio-nigral evoked inhibitory potentials is prevented by phenobarbitone (Schaffner, unpublished).

In summary, barbiturates enhance both pre- and postsynaptic inhibition at all GABA-ergic synapses of the CNS studied. In contrast to benzodiazepines, they preferentially prolong the duration of individual or mass IPSP's and the duration of evoked primary afferent depolarizations, but affect to a negligible extent peak hyper- or depolarization.

The mechanisms by which barbiturates affect GABA-ergic transmission are not yet clear (Table II). A number of observations favor a postsynaptic site of action: barbiturates increase the effect of exogenous GABA on various neurons and reverse the antagonism by bicuculline. Higher doses produce a GABA-like effect on Cl^- conductance; however, this effect is unlikely due to a stimulation of GABA receptors. The available evidence suggests to us that barbiturates alter the function of chemically-regulated membrane ionophores at synapses more potently than voltage-dependent ion channels; at low concentrations they may facilitate the interaction between GABA receptor and Cl^- channels, at higher concentrations they open these channels and prevent activation of Na^+ channels by excitatory transmitters. In spite of strong evidence for postsynaptic actions of barbiturates, additional presynaptic mechanisms should not be overlooked, e.g. inhibition of GABA uptake and a possible increase of excitation-secretion coupling in GABA-ergic terminals (as found at the cholinergic motor nerve endings).

Barbiturates superficially resemble benzodiazepines in their facilitatory action on GABA-ergic transmission, but their molecular mechanisms of action clearly differ. Whereas the latter produce very few additional effects on neuronal functions in concentrations that maximally facilitate GABA-ergic transmission, barbiturates depress synaptic excitation with increasing concentrations and produce nonspecific stabilizing effects on membranes. GABA-ergic facilitation may explain the similar pharmacological profile of benzodiazepines and of barbiturates at subanesthetic doses (Haefely 1977).

METHAQUALONE

Methaqualone is a widely used hypnotic of the quinazolidinone class which has moderate anticonvulsant properties, blocks polysynaptic reflexes and, in high doses, produces flaccid paralysis (Swift *et al.* 1960, Weaver *et al.* 1963). Intravenous injections induce short lasting surgical anesthesia in man (Saxena *et al.* 1972). Little is known about the synaptic pharmacology of this drug. In own experiments (Polc, unpublished), the compound enhanced DRPs and DRRs in the spinal cat in doses of 1 and 3 mg kg^{-1}. Although resembling benzodiazepines in this respect rather than barbiturates, methaqualone does not interact with the binding of ^3H-diazepam to benzodiazepine receptors (Möhler, unpublished).

The effect on postsynaptic GABA-ergic inhibition remains to be investigated, before a general facilitation of GABA-ergic transmission can be accepted as relevant for the pharmacology of methaqualone.

ETHANOL

Ethanol produces a bewildering number of partly opposite effects on central nervous functions. The physicochemical properties explain its affinity for biological membranes and favor the general view that its cellular effects are highly unspecific. However, as in the case of barbiturates, ethanol has more specific actions than earlier assumed.

Miyahara *et al.* (1966) observed an enhancement by ethanol of presynaptic inhibition in the cat spinal cord, but similar doses were found by Eidelberg & Wooley (1970) to be inactive on primary afferent terminal excitability, DRPs and DRRs. Later studies, however, confirmed the original findings of Miyahara *et al.* (1966). Thus, in the isolated frog spinal cord, ethanol markedly increases DRPs (Davidoff 1973). In the cuneate and gracile nuclei of cats, peak as well as duration of presynaptic inhibition were increased after i.v. injection (Banna 1969) and after superfusion of the dorsal column nuclei (Davidson & Rix 1972). Primary afferent endings of cutaneous afferents in the spinal trigeminal nucleus were depolarized by ethanol in the unconditioned state and, more markedly, during activation of presynaptic inhibitory pathways descending from the cerebral cortex (Sauerland *et al.* 1970). Preliminary results in our laboratories (Polc, unpublished) show an increase of DRPs and DRRs by ethanol (100 mg kg^{-1} i.v.), along with a tonic depolarization of primary afferent endings, as reflected by an increased excitability in the absence of conditioning volleys in the presynaptic inhibitory pathway. All these effects of ethanol are blocked by bicuculline. The effect of ethanol on GABA-ergic postsynaptic inhibition is being investigated at present.

The available evidence indicates that ethanol either directly stimulates GABA receptors, activates Cl^- channels and/or increases the spontaneous and evoked release of GABA. The latter effect is not unlikely in view of a similar action on cholinergic neurons; in fact, ethanol was found to increase the release of acetylcholine from motoneurons both at their terminals in the muscle endplate (Okada 1967) and at their recurrent collaterals to Renshaw cells (Meyer-Lohmann *et al.* 1972). A depression of the spontaneous firing rate of cerebellar Purkinje cells and of Deiters' neurons in the vestibular nuclei (Eidelberg *et al.*

1971) would be in line with a facilitated release of GABA at postsynaptic inhibitory synapses and explain the motor incoordination occurring after ethanol and high doses of benzodiazepines.

INHIBITORS OF GABA-TRANSAMINASE (GABA-T)

The question how inhibition of GABA-T and increase of GABA levels affect the function of GABA-ergic synapses is of uppermost importance for evaluating the potential usefulness of such inhibitors.

In earlier investigations we studied the facilitating effect of aminooxyacetic acid (AOAA) on presynaptic inhibition in the spinal cord (Polc *et al.* 1974), pre- and postsynaptic inhibition in the cuneate nucleus (Polc & Haefely 1976) and dopamine turnover (Keller *et al.* 1976). In spinal cats, a single dose of 10 mg kg^{-1} i.v. more than doubled the GABA level in the spinal cord after 2 h. At this time, mono- and polysynaptic reflexes were unaltered; however, presynaptic inhibition was enhanced and markedly prolonged. In the cuneate nucleus, a dose of 5 mg kg^{-1} of AOAA slightly increased the amplitude of the surface P-wave and of the dorsal column reflex. Postsynaptic inhibition of cuneo-thalamic relay cells was also increased. Neither in the spinal cord nor in the cuneate nucleus did AOAA increase the excitability of primary afferents in the absence of conditioning volleys in the presynaptic inhibitory pathway.

L-cycloserine inhibits very potently GABA-T without substantially affecting GAD (Bonavita *et al.* 1964, Scotto *et al.* 1963, Wood *et al.* 1978). L-cycloserine blocks conditioned avoidance responses in the rat, an effect which is reversed by pyridoxine and antagonized by isoniazid (Bonavita *et al.* 1964). In rabbits and cats, L-cycloserine synchronizes the EEG and depresses the cortical arousal reaction (La Grutta & Monaco 1962). In man, EEG synchronization, sedation, and sleep induction are observed (Monaco & La Grutta 1961). We have confirmed the marked increase of GABA levels occurring after L-cycloserine. In spinal cats, a dose of 10 mg kg^{-1} increased the amplitude of DRPs with little effect on their duration 90 min after administration; this effect of L-cycloserine was blocked by bicuculline. Excitability of primary afferent terminals was not increased in the absence of conditioning volleys. We have not yet studied the effect of L-cycloserine on GABA-ergic inhibition of dopaminergic neurons with electrophysiological methods, however, biochemical experiments (Keller & Da Prada, unpublished) show that the turnover of striatal dopamine is decreased and its neuroleptic-induced increase depressed. So far, the effects of L-cycloserine on GABA-ergic synaptic transmission look very similar to those of benzodiazepines. We conclude that, at the doses used, cycloserine markedly increases the level of GABA; in the absence of GABA neuron activation this increase apparently does not augment the synaptic concentration of the transmitter sufficiently to tonically depolarize primary afferent endings. However, GABA-T inhibitors are able either to increase the amount of GABA released by action potentials or to depress its rapid removal from the synapse.

CONCLUSIONS

Five groups of compounds which facilitate GABA-ergic synaptic transmission are reviewed. The molecular mechanisms of action are incompletely understood and probably differ for the various compounds. Facilitation of GABA-ergic transmission seems to be the only relevant synaptic action of benzodiazepines and perhaps of GABA-T inhibitors, but is only one of several ways by which the other agents affect the function of the CNS.

REFERENCES

Abdelmoumene, M. & Besson, J. M. (1967) Comparaison de l'action des barbituriques et du chloralose sur les potentiels de racine dorsale chez le chat. *J. Physiol* (Paris) 59, 323–324.

Banna, N. R. (1969) Potentiation of cutaneous inhibition by alcohol. *Experientia* 25, 619–620.

Banna, N. R. & Jabbur, S. J. (1969) Pharmacological studies on inhibition in the cuneate nucleus of the cat. *Int. J. Neuropharmacol.* 8, 299–307.

Banna, N. R. & Jabbur, S. J. (1971) The effects of depleting GABA on cuneate presynaptic inhibition. *Brain Res.* 33, 530–532.

Barker, J. L. (1975) Inhibitory and excitatory effects of CNS depressants on invertebrate synapses. *Brain Res.* 93, 77–90.

Barker, J. L. & Gainer, H. (1973) Pentobarbital: selective depression of excitatory postsynaptic potentials. *Sci.* 182, 720–722.

Barker, J. L. & MacDonald, R. L. (1977) Postsynaptic correlates of barbiturate effects observed in tissue-cultured mammalian neurons. Abstr. 7th Annual Meeting Soc. Neuroscience, vol. III, pp. 403.

Bernasconi, R. & Martin, P. (1978) Effects of diazepam and baclofen on the GABA turnover in various mouse brain regions. *Naunyn-Schmiedeberg's Arch. Pharmacol.,* Suppl. 302, R58.

Blaustein, M. P. (1968) Barbiturates block sodium and potassium conductance increases in voltage-clamped lobster axons. *J. Gen. Physiol.* 51, 293–307.

Blaustein, M. P. & Ector, A. C. (1975) Barbiturate inhibition of calcium uptake by depolarized nerve terminals *in vitro. Mol. Pharmacol.* 11, 369–378.

Bonavita, V., Lettieri, M. & Monaco, P. (1964) Behavioral studies on rats injected with L-cycloserine and other compounds. *Psychopharmacol.* 5, 234–238.

Bosman, H. B., Penney, D. P., Case, K. R., Di Stefano, P. & Averill, K. (1978) Diazepam receptor:

specific binding of [^{3}H] diazepam and [^{3}H] flunitrazepam to rat brain subfractions. *FEBS Letters* 87, 199–202.

Bowery, N. G. & Dray, A. (1977) Barbiturate reversal of amino acid antagonism produced by convulsant agents. *Nature* 264, 276–278.

Bowery, N. G. & Dray, A. (1978) Reversal of the action of amino acid antagonists by barbiturates and other hypnotic drugs. *Br. J. Pharmacol.* 63, 197–215.

Braestrup, C. & Squires, R. F. (1977) Brain specific benzodiazepine receptors in rats characterized by high affinity ^{3}H-diazepam binding. *Proc. Nat. Acad. Sci.* 74, 3805–3809.

Braestrup, C. & Squires, R. F. (1978) Pharmacological characterization of benzodiazepine receptors in the brain. *Europ. J. Pharmacol.* 48, 263–270.

Braestrup, C., Albrechtsen, R. & Squires, R. F. (1977) High densities of benzodiazepine receptors in human cortical areas. *Nature* 269, 702–704.

Bremer, F. (1970) Inhibitions intrathalamiques récurrentielles et physiologie du sommeil. *EEG Clin. Neurophysiol.* 28, 1–16.

Brownstein, M. J., Mroz, E. A., Tappaz, M. L. & Leeman, S. E. (1977) On the origin of substance P and glutamic acid decarboxylase (GAD) in the substantia nigra. *Brain Res.* 135, 315–323.

Chanelet, J. & Longchampt, P. (1971) Action du diazépam sur la moelle épinière du chat. *J. Physiol.* (Paris) 63, 185.

Chang, R. S. L. & Snyder, S. H. (1978) Benzodiazepine receptors: labeling in intact animals with [^{3}H] flunitrazepam. *Europ. J. Pharmacol.* 48, 213–218.

Chéramy, A., Nieoullon, A. & Glowinski, J. (1977) Blockade of the picrotoxin-induced in vivo release of dopamine in the cat caudate nucleus by diazepam. *Life Sci.* 20, 811–816.

Chin, J. H., Crankshaw, D. P. & Kendig, J. J. (1974) Changes in the dorsal root potential with diazepam and with the analgesics aspirin, nitrous oxide, morphine and meperidine. *Neuropharmacol.* 13, 305–315.

Choi, D. W., Farb, D. H. & Fischbach, G. D. (1977) Chlordiazepoxide selectively augments GABA action in spinal cord cell cultures. *Nature* 269, 342–344.

Corrodi, H., Fuxe, K., Lidbrink, P. & Olson, L. (1971) Minor tranquillizers, stress and central catecholamine neurons. *Brain Res.* 29, 1–16.

Costa, E., Guidotti, A., Mao, C. C. & Suria, A. (1975) New concepts on the mechanism of action of benzodiazepines. *Life Sci.* 17, 167–186.

Curtis, D. R. & Lodge, D. (1977) Effect of pentobarbitone on the inhibition of spinal interneurons in the cat by glycine and GABA. *J. Physiol.* 272, 48P–49P.

Curtis, D. R., Lodge, D., Johnston, G. A. R. & Brand, S. J. (1976) Central actions of benzodiazepines. *Brain Res.* 118, 344–347.

Davidoff, R. A. (1973) Alcohol and presynaptic inhibition in an isolated spinal cord preparation. *Arch. Neurol.* 28, 60–63.

Davidson, R. & Rix, K. J. B. (1972) A comparison of the effects of systemic infusion and topical application of ethanol solutions in the rat brain. *J. Physiol.* (Lond.) 227, 24P–26P.

Dray, A. & Straughan, D. W. (1976) Benzodiazepines: GABA and glycine receptors on single neurons in the rat medulla. *J. Pharm. Pharmac.* 28, 314–315.

Dray, A., Gonye, T. J. & Dakley, N. R. (1976) Caudate stimulation and substantia nigra activity in the rat. *J. Physiol.* (London) 259, 825–849.

Eccles, J. C. & Malcolm, J. L. (1946) Dorsal root potentials of the spinal cord. *J. Neurophysiol.* 9, 139–160.

Eccles, J. C., Schmidt, R. F. & Willis, W. D. (1963) Pharmacological studies on presynaptic inhibition. *J. Physiol.* (London) 168, 500–530.

Eccles, J. C., Faber, D. S. & Tábořiková, H. (1971) The action of parallel fiber volley on the antidromic invasion of Purkyně cells of cat cerebellum. *Brain Res.* 25, 335–356.

Eidelberg, E. & Wooley, D. F. (1970) Effects of ethyl alcohol upon spinal cord neurons. *Arch. Int. Pharmacodyn. Ther.* 185, 388–396.

Eidelberg, E., Bond, M. L. & Kelter, A. (1971) Effects of alcohol on cerebellar and vestibular neurons. *Arch. Int. Pharmacodyn. Ther.* 192, 213–219.

Evans, R. H. (1977) GABA-potentiating action of pentobarbitone on the isolated superior cervical ganglion of the rat. *J. Physiol.* (London) 272, 49P–50P.

Frazier, D. T., Murayama, K., Abbott, N. J. & Narahashi, T. (1975) Comparison of the action of different barbiturates on squid axon membranes. *Europ. J. Pharmacol.* 32, 102–107.

Gale, K., Hong, J.-S. & Guidotti, A. (1977) Presence of substance P and GABA in separate striatonigral neurons. *Brain Res.* 136, 371–375.

Galindo, A. (1969) Effects of procaine, pentobarbital and halothane on synaptic transmission in the central nervous system. *J. Pharmacol. Exp. Ther.* 169, 185–195.

Geller, H. M., Taylor, D. A. & Hoffer, B. J. (1978) Benzodiazepines and central inhibitory mechanisms. *Naunyn-Schmiedeberg's Arch. Pharmacol.* In press.

Guidotti, A. (1978) Synaptic mechanisms in the action of benzodiazepines. In: *Psychopharmacology: a generation of progress,* eds. Lipton, M. A., Di Mascio, A. & Killam, K. F., pp. 1349–1357. Raven Press, New York.

Haefely, W. E. (1977) Synaptic pharmacology of barbiturates and benzodiazepines. *Agents and Actions* 7, 353–359.

Haefely, W. E. (1978a) Behavioral and neuropharmacological aspects of drugs used in anxiety and related states. In: *Psychopharmacology: a generation of progress,* eds. Lipton, M. A., Di Mascio, A. & Killam, K. F., pp. 1359–1374. Raven Press, New York.

Haefely, W. E. (1978b) Central actions of benzodiazepines: general introduction. *Brit. J. Psychiatry.* In press.

Haefely, W., Jalfre, M. & Ruch-Monachon, M.-A. (1975a) A pathway and neurotransmitters involved in the control of noradrenergic locus coeruleus neurons. In: *Chemical Tools in Catecholamine Research,* eds. Almgren, O., Carlsson, A. & Engel, J., pp. 135–142. North Holland, Amsterdam.

Haefely, W., Kulcsár, A., Möhler, H., Pieri, L., Polc, P. & Schaffner, R. (1975b) Possible involvement of GABA in the central actions of benzodiazepines. In: *Mechanism of Action of Benzodiazepines,* eds. Costa, E. & Greengard, P., pp. 131–151. Raven Press, New York.

Haefely, W., Keller, H. H., Pieri, L., Polc, P., Schaffner, R. & Zihlmann, R. (1978) Interaction of minor tranquillizers with synaptic processes mediated by GABA. In: *Neuro-Psychopharmacology,* eds. Deniker, P., Radouco-Thomas, C., Villeneuve, A., pp. 907–916, Pergamon Press, Oxford.

Jessel, T. M. & Richards, C. D. (1977) Barbiturate potentiation of hippocampal i.p.s.p.s is not mediated by blockade of GABA uptake. *J. Physiol.* (London) 269, 42P–44P.

Iversen, L. L. & Johnston, G. A. R. (1971) GABA uptake in rat central nervous system: comparison of uptake in slices and homogenates and the effects of some inhibitors. *J. Neurochem.* 18, 1939–1950.

Keller, H. H., Schaffner, R. & Haefely, W. (1976) Interaction of benzodiazepines with neuroleptics at central dopamine neurons. *Naunyn-Schmiedeberg's Arch. Pharmacol.* 294, 1–7.

Kozhechkin, S. N. & Ostrovskaya, R. U. (1977) Are benzodiazepines GABA antagonists? *Nature* 269, 72–73.

La Grutta, G. & Monaco, P. (1962) Mécanisme de l'action centrale de la L-cyclosérine. *Arch. Int. Pharmacodyn. Ther.* 135, 187–196.

Larson, M. D. & Major, M. A. (1970) The effect of hexobarbital on the duration of the recurrent IPSP in cat motoneurons. *Brain Res.* 21, 309–311.

Mao, C. C., Marco, E., Revuelta, A., Bertilsson, L. & Costa, E. (1977) The turnover of γ-aminobutyric acid in the nuclei of telecephalon: implications in the pharmacology of antipsychotics and of a minor tranquilizer. *Bio. Psychiatr.* 12, 359–371.

MacDonald, R. & Barker, J. L. (1978) Benzodiazepines specifically modulate GABA-mediated postsynaptic inhibition in cultured mammalian neurones. *Nature* 271, 563–564.

Mariani, J. & Delhaye-Bouchaud, N. (1978) Effect of diazepam on the spontaneous and harmaline-induced electrical activity of Purkinje cells in the cerebellum of the rat and rabbit. *Neuropharmacol.* 17, 45–51.

Matsui, Y. & Deguchi, T. (1977) Cataleptic action of nitrazepam and brain dopamine function in mice. *Neuropharmacol.* 16, 253–258.

Meyer-Lohmann, J., Hellweg, C. & Benecke, R. (1972) The action of ethyl alcohol on the activity of individual Renshaw cells. *Naunyn-Schmiedeberg's Arch. Pharmacol.* 272, 131–142.

Mitchell, P. R. & Martin, I. L. (1978) The effects of benzodiazepines on K^+-stimulated release of GABA. *Neuropharmacol.* 17, 317–320.

Miyahara, J. T., Esplin, D. W. & Zablocka, B. (1966) Differential effects of depressant drugs on presynaptic inhibition. *J. Pharmacol. Exp. Ther.* 154, 118–127.

Möhler, H. & Okada, T. (1977a) Benzodiazepine receptor: demonstration in the central nervous system. *Science* 198, 849–851.

Möhler, H. & Okada, T. (1977b) Properties of ^{3}H-diazepam binding to benzodiazepine receptors in rat cerebral cortex. *Life Sci.* 20, 2101–2110.

Möhler, H. & Okada, T. (1977c) GABA receptor binding with ^{3}H(+) bicuculline-methiodide in rat CNS. *Nature* 267, 65–67.

Monaco, P. & La Grutta, G. (1961) Analyses des actions centrales du L-4-amino-3-isoxazolidone. Modifications électroencéphalographiques chez l'homme. *Arch. Int. Pharmacodyn. Ther.* 131, 32–38.

Moudgil, G. & Pleuvry, B. J. (1970/II) Diazepam and neuromuscular transmission. *Brit. Med. J.* 734–735.

Nicoll, R. A. (1972) The effects of anesthetics on synaptic excitation and inhibition in the olfactory bulb. *J. Physiol.* (London) 223, 803–814.

Nicoll, R. A. (1975a) Presynaptic action of barbiturates in the frog spinal cord. *Proc. Nat. Acad. Sci.* 72, 1460–1463.

Nicoll, R. A. (1975b) Pentobarbital: action on frog motoneurons. *Brain Res.* 96, 119–123.

Nicoll, R. A. (1978a) Selective actions of barbiturates on synaptic transmission. In: *Psychopharmacology: a generation of progress,* eds. Lipton, M. A., Di Mascio, A. & Killam, K. F., pp. 1337–1348. Raven Press, New York.

Nicoll, R. A. (1978b) Modification of excitatory and inhibitory synaptic mechanisms by minor tranquilizers. In: *Neuro-Psychopharmacology,* eds. Deniker, P., Radouco-Thomas, C., Villeneuve,A., pp. 925–932, Pergamon Press, Oxford.

Nicoll, R. A. (1978c) Pentobarbital: differential postsynaptic actions on sympathetic ganglion cells. *Science* 199, 451–452.

Nicoll, R. A., Eccles, J. C., Oshima, T. & Rubia, F. (1975) Prolongation of hippocampal inhibitory postsynaptic potentials by barbiturates. *Nature* 258, 625–627.

Nicot, G., Decaud, J. & Besson, J.-M. (1976) Action du diazépam et clonazépam sur les phénomènes d'inhibition présynaptique au niveau spinal chez le lapin. *J. Pharmacol.* (Paris) 7, 17–26.

Nielsen, M., Braestrup, C. & Squires, R. F. (1978) Evidences for a late evolutionary appearance of brain-specific benzodiazepine receptors: an investigation of 18 vertebrate and five invertebrate species. *Brain Res.* 141, 342–346.

Nistri, A. & Constanti, A. (1978) Effects of flurazepam on amino acid-evoked responses recorded from the lobster muscle and the frog spinal cord. *Neuropharmacol.* 17, 127–135.

Okada, K. (1967) Effects of alcohols and acetone on the neuromuscular junction of the frog. *Jap. J. Physiol.* 17, 245–261.

Okada, T., Spokes, E. G., Bird, E. D. & Möhler, H. (1978) Huntington's chorea: decrease in benzodiazepine receptor binding in putamen and caudate nucleus. In preparation.

Olsen, R. W., Ticku, M. K., Van Ness, P. C. & Greenlee, D. (1978) Effects of drugs on γ-aminobutyric acid receptors, uptake, release and synthesis *in vitro. Brain Res.* 139, 277–294.

Peričić, D., Walters, J. R. & Chase, T. N. (1977) Effect of diazepam and pentobarbital on aminooxyacetic acid-induced accumulation of GABA. *J. Neurochem.* 29, 839–846.

Pickles, H. G. & Simmonds, M. A. (1978) Field potentials, inhibition and the effect of pentobarbitone in the rat olfactory cortex slice. *J. Physiol.* (London) 275, 135–148.

Pieri, L. & Haefely, W. (1976) The effect of diphenylhydantoin, diazepam and clonazepam on the activity of Purkinje cells in the rat cerebellum. *Naunyn-Schmiedeberg's Arch. Pharmacol.* 296, 1–4.

Polc, P. & Haefely, W. (1976) Effects of two benzodiazepines, phenobarbitone, and baclofen on synaptic transmission in the cat cuneate nucleus. *Naunyn-Schmiedeberg's Arch. Pharmacol.* 294, 121–131.

Polc, P. & Haefely, W. (1977) Effects of systemic muscimol and GABA in the spinal cord and superior cervical ganglion of the cat. *Experientia* 33, 809.

Polc, P., Möhler, H. & Haefely, W. (1974) The effect of diazepam on spinal cord activities: possible sites and mechanisms of action. *Naunyn-Schmiedeberg's Arch. Pharmacol.* 284, 319–337.

Polzin, R. & Barnes, C. D. (1976) The effect of diazepam and picrotoxin on brain stem evoked dorsal root potentials. *Neuropharmacol.* 15, 133–137.

Proctor, W. R. & Weakly, J. N. (1976) A comparison of the presynaptic and postsynaptic actions of pentobarbitone and phenobarbitone in the neuromuscular junction of the frog. *J. Physiol.* (London) 258–268.

Raabe, W. & Gumnit, R. J. (1977) Anticonvulsant action of diazepam: increase of cortical postsynaptic inhibition. *Epilepsia* 18, 117–120.

Ransom, B. R. & Barker, J. L. (1976) Pentobarbital selectively enhances GABA-mediated postsynaptic inhibition in tissue cultured mouse spinal neurons. *Brain Res.* 114, 530–535.

Sauerland, E. K., Mizuno, N. & Harper, R. M. (1970) Presynaptic depolarization of trigeminal cutaneous afferent fibers induced by ethanol. *Exp. Neurol.* 27, 476–489.

Saxena, R. C., Bhatnagar, N. S., Misra, S. C. & Bhargava, K. P. (1972) Intravenous methaqualone: a new nonbarbiturate anaesthetic. *Brit. J. Anaesth.* 44, 83–85.

Schaffner, R. & Haefely, W. (1975) The effects of diazepam and bicuculline on the strio-nigral evoked potential. *Experientia* 31, 732.

Schlosser, W. (1971) Action of diazepam on the spinal cord. *Arch. Int. Pharmacodyn.* 194, 93–102.

Schmidt, R. F. (1963) Pharmacological studies on the primary afferent depolarization of the toad spinal cord. *Pflüger's Archiv* 277, 325–346.

Schmidt, R. F., Vogel, M. E. & Zimmermann, M. (1967) Die Wirkung von Diazepam auf die präsynaptische Hemmung und andere Rückenmarkreflexe. *Naunyn-Schmiedeberg's Arch. Pharmak. Exp. Path.* 258, 69–82.

Scholfield, C. N. (1978) A barbiturate induced intensification of the inhibitory potential in slices of guinea pig olfactory cortex. *J. Physiol.* 275, 559–566.

Scotto, P., Monaco, P., Scardi, V. & Bonavita, V. (1963) Neurochemical studies with L-cycloserine, a central depressant agent. *J. Neurochem.* 10, 831–839.

Seeman, P. (1972) The membrane actions of anesthetics and tranquilizers. *Pharmacol. Rev.* 24, 583–655.

Speth, R. C., Wastek, G. J., Johnson, P. C. & Yamamura, H. I. (1978) Benzodiazepine binding in human brain: characterization using [^{3}H] flunitrazepam. *Life Sci.* 22, 859–866.

Squires, R. F. & Braestrup, C. (1977) Benzodiazepine receptors in rat brain. *Nature* 266, 732–734.

Stratten, W. P. & Barnes, C. D. (1971) Diazepam and presynaptic inhibition. *Neuropharmacol.* 10, 685–696.

Swift, J. G., Dickens, E. A. & Becker, B. A. (1960) Anticonvulsant and other pharmacological activities of tuazolone. *Arch. Int. Pharmacodyn. Ther.* 128, 112–125.

Veselyune, M. A., Gutman, A. M. & Lesene, V. A. (1971) Effect of nembutal upon the inhibitory wave of antidromically evoked potential in the motor cortex of the cat. *Farmakol. i toksik.* 34, 520–522.

Vyskočil, F. (1977) Diazepam blockade of repetitive action potentials in skeletal muscle fibres. A model of its membrane action. *Brain Res.* 133, 315–328.

Waddington, J. L. (1977) GABA-like properties of flurazepam and baclofen suggested by rotational behaviour following unilateral intranigral injection: a comparison with the GABA agonist muscimol. *Br. J. Pharmac.* 60, 263P–264P.

Waddington, J. L. & Owen, F. (1978) Stereospecific benzodiazepine receptor binding by the enantiomers of oxazepam sodium hemisuccinate. *Neuropharmacol.* 17, 215–216.

Weakly, J. N. & Proctor, W. R. (1977) Barbiturate-induced changes in transmitter release independent of terminal spike configuration in the frog neuromuscular junction. *Neuropharmacol.* 16, 507–509.

Weakly, J. N., Esplin, D. W. & Zablocka, B. (1968) Criteria for assessing effects of drugs on postsynaptic inhibition. *Arch. Int. Pharmacodyn. Ther.* 171, 385–393.

Weaver, L. C., Jones, W. R. & Kerley, T. L. (1963) Some central nervous system depressant properties of 2-methyl-3-O-tolyl-4 (3h)-quinazolinone (TR-495). *Arch. Int. Pharmacodyn. Ther.* 143, 119–126.

Wolf, P. & Haas, H. L. (1977) Effects of diazepines and barbiturates on hippocampal recurrent inhibition. *Naunyn-Schmiedeberg's Arch. Pharmacol.* 229, 211–218.

Wood, J. D., Peesker, S. J., Gorecki, D. K. J. & Tsui, D. (1978) Effect of L-cycloserine on brain GABA metabolism. *Canad. J. Physiol. Pharmacol.* 56, 62–68.

Zakusov, V. V., Ostrovskaya, R. U., Markovitch, V. V., Molodavkin, G. M. & Bulayev, V. M. (1975) Electrophysiological evidence for an inhibitory action of diazepam upon cat brain cortex. *Arch. Int. Pharmacodyn.* 214, 188–205.

GABA Convulsants and Their Interactions with Central Depressant Agents

A. Dray & N. G. Bowery

Synaptic function in the mammalian central nervous system appears to be particularly susceptible to barbiturates. Thus, for example, barbiturates alter brain neurotransmitter levels (Richter & Crossland 1949, Anderson & Bonnycastle 1960, Corrodi *et al.* 1966), decrease or enhance transmitter release (Mitchell 1963, Phillis & Chong 1965, Phillis 1968, Weakley 1969, Cutler & Dudzinski 1974, Cutler *et al.* 1974), interfere with the removal of transmitter (Cutler *et al.* 1974) and they can depress the sensitivity of postsynaptic cells to excitatory neurotransmitters such as glutamate (Crawford & Curtis 1966, Crawford 1970, Richards & Smaje 1974) or acetylcholine (Bloom *et al.* 1965, Bradley & Dray 1973). It is unclear at present which, if any, of these actions are related to the hypnotic, anesthetic or anticonvulsant properties of barbiturate. However, perhaps the most recent suggestion that their hypnotic action may be related in part to the prolongation of central inhibitory transmission produced by GABA may be of greater significance (Nicoll *et al.* 1975). Such a possibility stems from the observations that barbiturates, pentobarbitone in particular, increased the duration of pre- and postsynaptic inhibition at spinal and supraspinal sites (Eccles *et al.* 1963, Eccles *et al.* 1971, Nicoll *et al.* 1975). These effects might be accounted for by a direct action of barbiturates on GABA receptors (Nicoll 1975a, b) or by an interaction with the ionic conductance mechanism triggered by GABA (Ransom & Barker 1976).

Department of Physiology, Duke University Medical Center, Durham, N.C. 27710 USA, and Department of Pharmacology, St. Thomas' Hospital Medical School, London SE1 7EH England.

"GABA-NEUROTRANSMITTERS", Alfred Benzon Symposium 12, Munksgaard 1978

We have examined this association of barbiturates with GABA receptors both *in vitro* and *in vivo*. During this study we observed and reported (Bowery 1976, Bowery & Dray 1976, 1978) that barbiturates and other hypnotics prevented or reversed the action of GABA antagonists and to a lesser extent the glycine antagonist strychnine. We felt that these findings provided some insight into the interaction of convulsant agents with amino acid receptors and considered that these effects might also be relevant to the therapeutic actions of barbiturates.

METHODS

The method of preparing and recording from the isolated superior cervical ganglion was essentially that previously described (Bowery & Brown 1974). Briefly, superior cervical ganglia were excised from anesthetized rats, desheathed and suspended vertically with a nonpolarizable Ag^+/AgCl electrode in contact with the post ganglionic trunk and another in contact with the ganglion body. The potential difference between these electrodes was monitored continuously while the tissue was superfused with Krebs' solution in which drugs could be mixed.

The *in vivo* experiments were made in rats anesthetized with urethane and prepared for recording from brain stem as previously described (Bradley & Dray 1973). Multibarrelled glass micropipettes were used to record extracellular activity from single neurons in the medulla and to administer substances close to them by electrophoresis.

RESULTS

Superior cervical ganglia

Pentobarbitone (PB) depolarized the isolated ganglion in a dose-dependent manner (threshold 100–300 μM compared with 0.5–1 μM for GABA-induced depolarization in the same preparation). The response to PB was more prolonged than responses to GABA and the duration appeared to increase with the concentration of the barbiturate. The potency of PB (peak depolarization determined at the GABA ED_{50} level) relative to GABA was 0.0047 ± 0.0008. Quinalbarbitone and phenobarbitone also depolarized the ganglion, but whereas quinalbarbitone was as active as PB, phenobarbitone was only 0.025–0.05 as active. Chlordiazepoxide, promethazine and amitriptyline (up to 2 mM) did not produce depolarization.

Superfusion with bicuculline methochloride (BMC) displaced both the GABA and PB log dose response curves to the right, with a greater shift of the GABA curve. At concentrations (4–80 μM) too low to depolarize the ganglion,

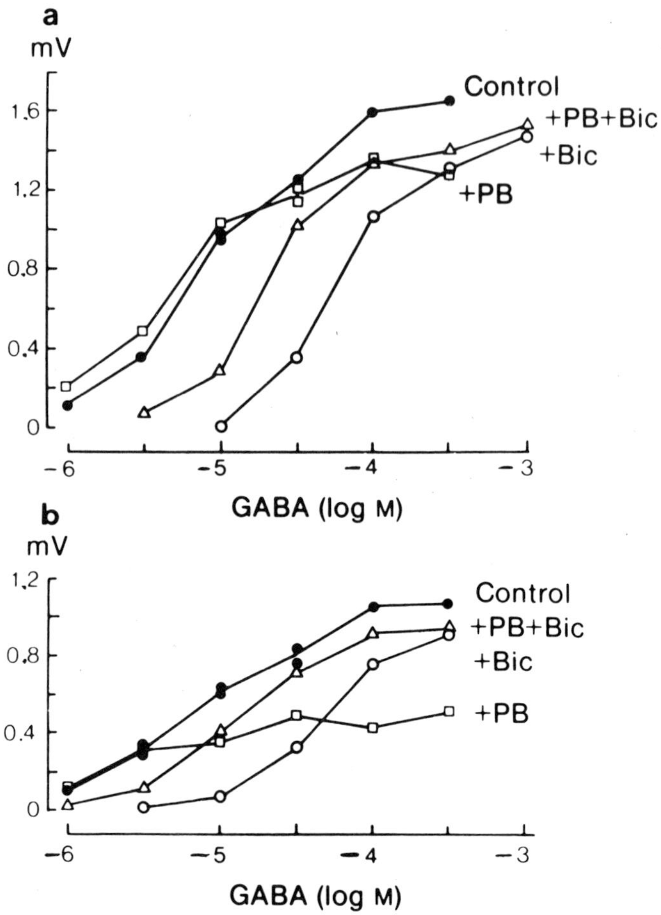

Fig. 1. Effect of pentobarbitone sodium on the dose-response curve to GABA obtained in the presence and absence of bicuculline methochloride. Data obtained from two superior cervical ganglia (a&b). Control (●), plus pentobarbitone (PB 80 μM□), plus bicuculline methochloride (BMC 20 μM○), plus PB (80 μM) and BMC (20 μM) (△). Ordinates: response to GABA (peak depolarization in millivolts). Abscissae: log molar concentration of GABA. Each concentration of GABA was in contact with the tissue for 1 min. 15-min intervals were allowed between doses. After removal of PB (and before the addition of BMC) a recovery curve was obtained in both tissues but these have been omitted as they were superimposed on the control curves. In a) potentiation of the responses of GABA (<30 μM) occurred in the presence of PB whereas in b) no potentiation occurred but there was a marked depression in the responses of GABA at concentrations above 3 μM.

PB generally produced a small potentiation in the response to GABA at doses below the GABA ED_{50} level and either a reduction or no change in the responses to higher GABA concentrations (Fig. 1). The effects of PB were reversed within 30 min of its removal from the superfusate. Subsequent superfusion with BMC (20 μM) in the same preparation displaced the GABA curve as expected but the further addition of PB at this stage now displaced the GABA curve back toward the control. An apparant reversal of the BMC antagonism had occurred. Similarly if superfusion with PB was followed by concomitant superfusion with BMC, then PB reduced or prevented the expected decrease in the response to GABA produced by BMC.

The reversal of BMC antagonism did not appear to result from an increase in the response to GABA in a manner unrelated to the presence of the antagonist. Thus, a) slight PB potentiation occurred only in some experiments while reversal

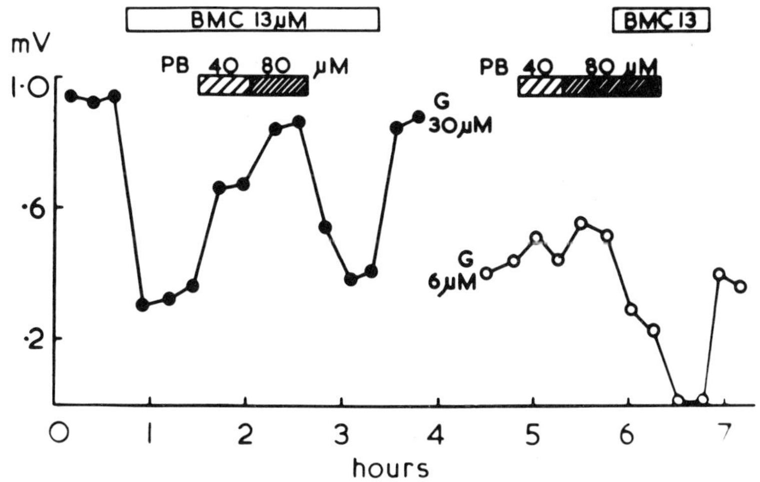

Fig. 2a. Comparison of the effect of pentobarbitone on responses to GABA in the presence and absence of bicuculline methochloride. The solid dots indicate the magnitude of responses of a single superior cervical ganglion to 1-min applications of GABA (30 μM). Bicuculline methochloride (BMC 13 μM) superfused over the tissue during the period indicated by the first open horizontal bar depressed the response to GABA. This depression was overcome by the addition of pentobarbitone (PB 40 & 80 μM) indicated by the hatched bars. After the pentobarbitone and bicuculline methochloride had been removed and the control response to GABA reestablished, the GABA concentration was reduced (to 6 μM) such that the responses (open dots) now matched the previous responses to GABA (30 μM) obtained in the presence of BMC. PB (40 & 80 μM) alone did not potentiate the response to 6 μM GABA, but in the presence of BMC did reduce the expected GABA antagonism which can be seen to occur following the removal of PB. Ordinate: peak depolarization in millivolts. Abscissa: time in hours.

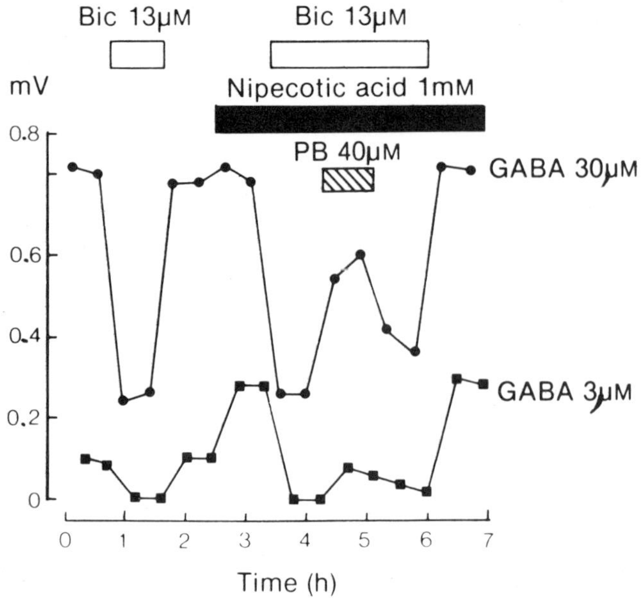

Fig. 2b. The inability of nipecotic acid to prevent or reduce the GABA antagonism produced by bicuculline methochloride. Two concentrations of GABA (3 and 30 μM) were superfused over the ganglia alternately for 1-min periods at 12–15-min intervals. Ordinate: response in millivolts. Abscissa: time in hours. Continuous superfusion with nipecotic acid (1 mM) indicated by the solid horizontal bar, potentiated the responses to 3 μM GABA but had little or no effect on responses to 30 μM GABA (cf. Brown & Galvan 1977). However, the addition of bicuculline methochloride (Bic 13 μM open bars) still antagonized the response to GABA to the same extent as in the absence of nipecotic acid. Pentobarbitone (40 μM hatched bar) decreased the antagonism.

of BMC antagonism occurred in every experiment, b) PB did not enhance responses to GABA which were of equal magnitude to those obtained at higher concentration in the presence of BMC (Fig. 2a), c) nipecotic acid which potentiates the responses to GABA (Brown & Galvan 1977) neither reversed nor prevented the antagonism produced by BMC (Fig. 2b).

Similar interactions could be demonstrated between PB and BMC antagonism of other GABA-mimetics such as muscimol and 3-aminopropanesulphonic acid. Additionally the antagonism of GABA responses by picrotoxin, tetramethylenedisulphotetramine and isopropylbicyclophosphate was also prevented or reversed by PB. As with BMC there was a interdependence between the concentration of the antagonist and that of PB to reverse its effects. Interestingly strychnine also produced a prolonged antagonism of the responses to GABA but this was nonselective as matched responses to carbachol were reduced to the same extent (Bowery & Brown 1974). PB readily reversed the action of strychnine on GABA responses but did not effect, or reduced even further, the responses to carbachol. Moreover, PB did not reverse the antagonism of carbachol by hexamethonium.

Reversal of BMC antagonism was observed with a number of other barbiturates and hypnotics (Fig. 3a). Thiopentone and amylobarbitone were of

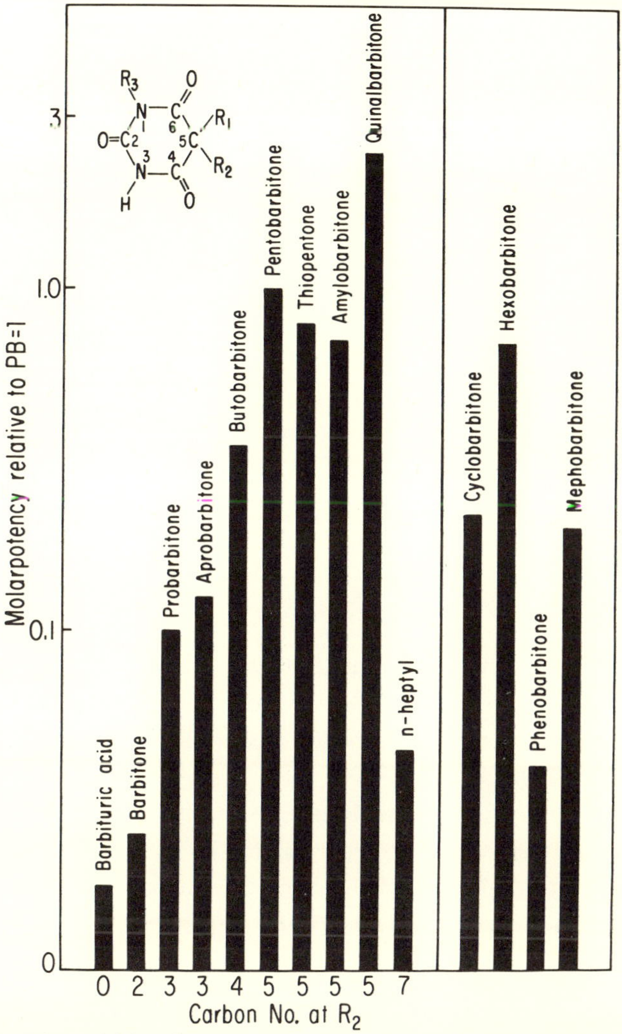

Fig. 3a. Comparative activities of barbiturates in reversing antagonism produced by bicuculline methochloride of responses to GABA in the rat superior cervical ganglion (PB=pentobarbitone).

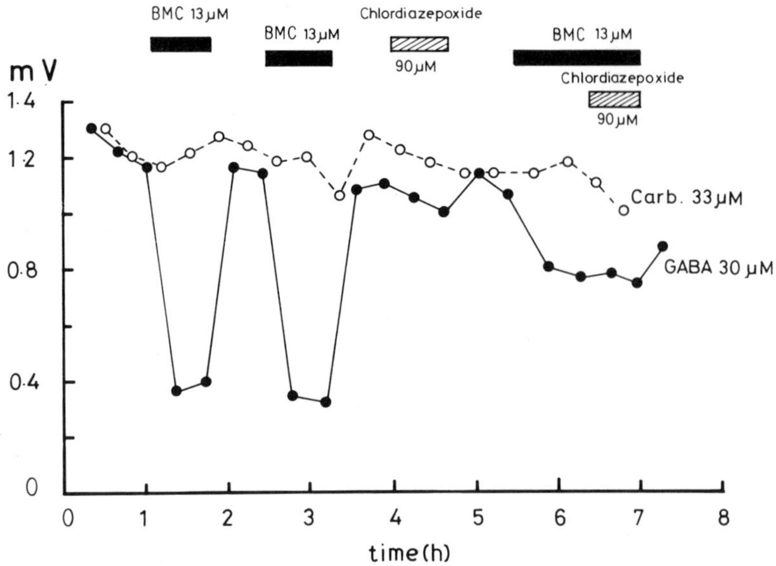

Fig. 3b. Prevention by chlordiazepoxide of the antagonism of responses to GABA produced by bicuculline methochloride (BMC). The solid dots represent the magnitude of depolarizing responses obtained in a single ganglion to GABA (30 μM). The open circles represent responses to carbachol (33 μM). Each agonist was applied alternately at 10-min intervals. During the periods indicated by the horizontal bars BMC 13 μM (solid bars) or chlordiazepoxide 90 μM (hatched bars) were present in the superfusion solution. Chlordiazepoxide produced little or no change in the responses to GABA and carbachol. However even 50 min after removal of the chlordiazepoxide the antagonistic effect of BMC on responses to GABA was markedly reduced. Ordinate: peak depolarization in millivolts. Abscissa: time in hours. Hyoscine (2.6 μM) was present in all superfusion solutions to limit the action of carbachol to nicotinic receptors.

similar activity to PB, whereas quinalbarbitone was 2–3 times more active, but the anticonvulsants phenobarbitone and mephobarbitone were less active. All of the other hypnotics tested were able to reduce BMC-induced antagonism of GABA (Table I). In addition, other classes of drugs showed this property, notably the neuroleptics chlorpromazine and haloperidol, the antihistamine substanced promethazine and mepyramine, and the tricyclic antidepressant amitriptyline. However, the MAO-inhibitor antidepressants tranylcypromine and iproniazid were ineffective as was trifluoperazine. The benzodiazepines were of particular interest since they were active at lower concentrations than any of the barbiturates. However they produced only partial but long lasting reversal of BMC antagonism and this reversal was always less than the maximal effect of PB. In the absence of BMC the benzodiazepines did not affect the

Table I
Reversal of bicuculline methochloride

Effective	Threshold concentration†	Ineffective	Maximum concentration tested
Pentobarbitone	5 μM	Bemegride	645 μM
Chloral hydrate	500 μM	Nikethamide	720 μM
Urethane	1 mM	Leptazol	724 μM
Glutethimide	35 μM	Caffeine	515 μM
Chlordiazepoxide	0.5 μM		
Diazepam	12 μM	Morphine	266 μM
Flurazepam	4 μM		
Clonazepam	0.5 μM	Lignocaine	1 mM
Phenytoin	80 μM	Procaine	10 mM
Chlorpromazine	90 μM	Iproniazid	720 μM
Haloperidol	70 μM	Tranylcypromine	1.5 mM
Promethazine	70 μM	Atropine	273 μM
Mepyramine	100 μM	Hyoscine	260 μM
Amitriptyline	80 μM	Trifluoperazine	208 μM

† The concentration which produced a just-measurable increase in the response to GABA (30 μM) in the presence of bicuculline methochloride (13 μM) in at least three experiments for each substance.

GABA dose-response curve (see also Straughan 1977), but even after prolonged removal from the superfusing fluid they were able to reduce the antagonistic effect of subsequently superfused BMC (Fig. 3b).

Electrophoretic experiments in the rat brain stem

When BMC selectively antagonized the inhibition of spontaneous firing produced by GABA, the occurrent administration of PB from the same micropipette partially (50%) or completely reversed the effects of BMC (Fig. 4a). This reversal occurred in every cell tested, and could be overcome by increasing the expulsion of BMC. For most cells, after reversal of BMC antagonism had been demonstrated, a similar administration of PB in the absence of BMC produced no change in the submaximal response to GABA or glycine (Fig. 4b). However, slight potentiation or reduction of both GABA and glycine responses was observed on a few occasions. Also PB rarely produced any changes in background firing, although expulsion with higher currents (100–150 nA) consistently depressed firing. In some experiments additional reduction of glycine responses was intentionally obtained with BMC: PB always reversed this antagonism sooner than that of GABA.

Strychnine was also tested on neurons where PB had already reversed the effects of BMC. The concurrent administration of PB reversed the selective strychnine antagonism of glycine in one third of the cells tested (Fig. 4a). Moreover, PB also readily reversed any nonselective block of GABA by strychnine (Fig. 4a).

In all cells tested, quinalbarbitone (which was more active than PB *in vitro*) also partially or completely restored GABA responses during the administra-

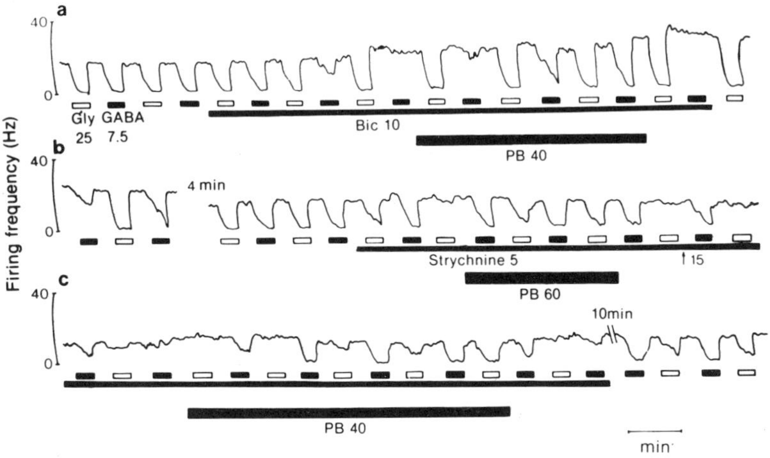

Fig. 4a. The effects of bicuculline and strychnine on responses of GABA and glycine and the interactions of pentobarbitone with these effects. The continuous rate meter records (firing frequency in Hz against time in min) of a spontaneous brain stem neuron showing reproducible depression by glycine and GABA. The top trace shows that the continuous administration of bicuculline methochloride selectively reduced the responses of GABA. The additional continuous administration of pentobarbitone restores the GABA response without producing any significant effect on background firing rate. Shortly after the cessation of pentobarbitone administration the GABA response is again completely blocked by bicuculline. After complete recovery of the responses to GABA a continuous administration of strychnine selectively reduced the glycine response (middle trace). An additional administration of pentobarbitone restores the glycine response which is again blocked after the pentobarbitone current was switched off. Increasing the ejecting current of strychnine to 15 nA produced additional antagonism of the GABA response. A repeated administration of pentobarbitone rapidly restored the GABA response and also that of glycine. Responses to both GABA and glycine were blocked after pentobarbitone was switched off, and recovered some 10 min after the strychnine administration was stopped. In all records the horizontal bars indicate the duration of drug ejection and the ejecting currents are indicated in nA.

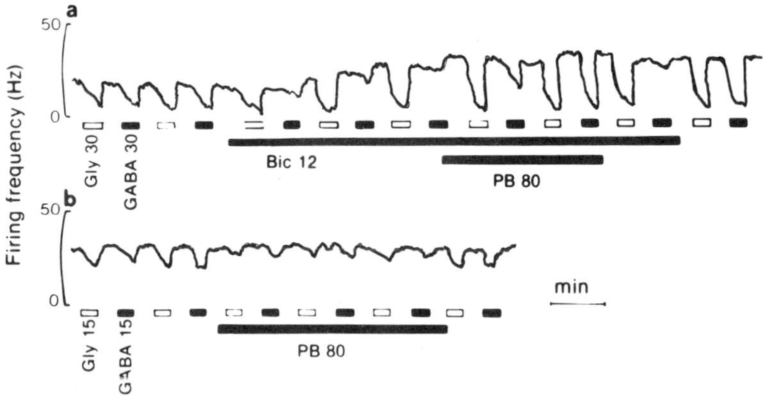

Fig. 4b. The effects of pentobarbitone on GABA and glycine responses in the presence and absence of bicuculline methochloride (Bic). The top trace shows that the selective antagonism of GABA by Bic was reversed by pentobarbitone 80 nA. Following recovery of the responses to GABA after the cessation of Bic ejection the expelling currents for GABA and glycine were reduced from 30 to 15 nA to produce clearly submaximal responses. Pentobarbitone administered with the same current as before but for a longer period had no significant effect on background firing and slightly reduced the effects of GABA and glycine.

tion of BMC. Like PB this barbiturate had no effect on submaximal responses to GABA or glycine in the absence of BMC. On the other hand electrophoretic benzodiazepines were less able to reverse the antagonism of GABA by BMC. Thus chlordiazepoxide restored the effects of GABA in 50% of the cells tested whereas flurazepam produced no significant reversal. Unlike the reversal seen with barbiturates, the effect of chlordiazepoxide was only partial (20–40% reversal).

Further studies with intravenous infusion of barbiturates (0.4–5.5 mg/kg, thiopentone, hexobarbitone and PB) produced short lasting reversal of electrophoretic BMC antagonism of GABA. Also intravenous clonazepam (100–200 μg/kg) produced partial but prolonged reversal of BMC antagonism (Fig. 5).

DISCUSSION

Barbiturates and other central depressants can clearly have a number of actions on postsynaptic membranes (see introduction). The hypnotic and sedative properties have been considered to result in part from an interaction with inhibitory processes mediated by GABA. Our experiments suggest that

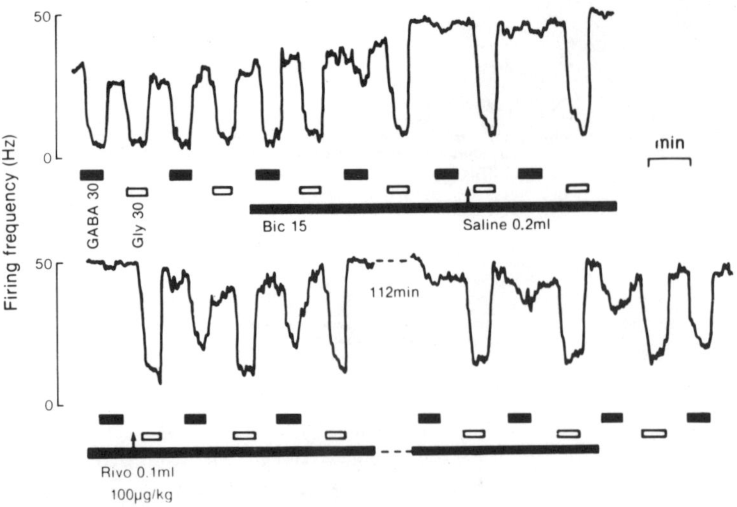

Fig. 5. Effects of intravenous clonazepam (Rivo) on the antagonism of GABA by the continuous electrophoretic administration of bicuculline (Bic). A control injection of saline (0.2 ml) had no effect on the response to GABA. However, the administration of clonazepam (100 μg/kg) partially restored the response to GABA and slightly depressed background firing. A repeat injection of clonazepam at the same dose (not shown) produced no additional improvement of the GABA response. The response to GABA were again blocked by the continued BMC ejection some 112 min after the first injection of clonazepam. The effect of GABA was rapidly restored after the termination of the BMC ejection.

barbiturates interact at postsynaptic sites indirectly associated with inhibitory amino acid receptors. Thus both *in vitro* and *in vivo*, barbiturates reversed the antagonistic effects of BMC and strychnine at concentrations which had no obvious direct effect and at which no significant modification of GABA, glycine or other agonist responses was observed. The reversal of BMC was more easily demonstrable than that of strychnine, especially *in vivo*, possibly because of the difference in the binding affinity of these substances to their site of action (see Zukin *et al.* 1974). Other barbiturates also reversed the action of BMC and there appeared to be a structural requirement for this action (see Fig. 3a and Bowery & Dray 1978). A number of other structurally dissimilar hypnotics/sedatives were also capable of reversing the action of BMC (see Table I) though none appeared to have significant GABA-mimetic actions. In particular the benzodiazepines were effective at lower concentrations than PB but produced only partial, though prolonged reversal of BMC.

It is conceivable that barbiturates and other hypnotics potentiate the action of GABA or possibly increase its receptor affinity (Ransom & Barker 1976, Lodge

& Curtis 1977, Brown & Constanti 1978, Nicoll 1978, MacDonald & Barker 1978) and thereby produce an apparent reversal of its antagonism. However, in our experiments such potentiations were not consistent, whereas reversal of antagonism was. Possibly the concentration range for reversal of an antagonist, potentiation of the agonist or direct effects on neuronal activity may be narrow.

Our observations can be tentatively explained by assuming that amino acids and their antagonists bind to the cell surface at different sites. Thus when an antagonist is present, it prevents access of the amino acid to its receptor, not because of preferential binding but by occluding or distorting it. Barbiturates may have particular affinity for the antagonistic binding site and could therefore displace the antagonist without affecting the receptor. The possibility of differences in agonist and antagonistic sites has been suggested in the case of glycine and strychnine (Young & Snyder 1974). Additionally the binding sites for GABA and ^{3}[H]-α-dihydropicrotoxinin appear to be distinct (Olsen 1978). Furthermore, PB appears not to interfere with ^{3}[H]-GABA binding (Zukin *et al.* 1974, Peck *et al.* 1976, Collins & Cryer 1978) but prevents BMC from displacing GABA (Collins & Cryer 1978) and will displace ^{3}[H]-α-dihydropicrotoxinin from its binding sites (Ticku & Olsen 1978). On the other hand, Möhler & Okada (1977) described specific binding with bicuculline methiodide which was unaffected by PB.

Our results do not necessarily indicate that barbiturates produce their hypnotic effects by interacting with membrane bound-endogenous substanced integrated with amino acid receptor sites but such an interaction appears possible with the benzodiazepines (see Guidotti *et al.*, this symposium). Our observations may however provide an explanation for the efficacy of these drugs in the treatment of acute convulsant poisoning (Esplin & Zablocka-Esplin 1970, Franz 1975). It could also be reasoned that the effects of barbiturates on various conductance mechanisms, e.g. Na^{+}, K^{+}, Ca^{2+} (Blaustein 1968, 1976, Sato *et al.* 1976) and possibly Cl^{-}, does not require a direct interaction with receptors which might operate these ionophores but may be due to effects on closely associated parts of the nerve membrane which are linked to the receptor and/or the ionophore.

ACKNOWLEDGMENT

The authors wish to acknowledge the assistance of Alan Hudson and thank the British Journal of Pharmacology for permission to reproduce some of the figures.

REFERENCES

Anderson, E. G. & Bonnycastle, D. D. (1960) A study of the central depressant action of pentobarbital, phenobarbital, and diethyl ether in relationship to increases in brain 5-hydroxytryptamine. J. Pharmac. exp. Ther. 130, 138–143.

Blaustein, M. P. (1968) Barbiturates block Na^+ and K^+ conductance increases in voltage clamped lobster axons. *J. Gen. Physiol.* 51, 293–307.

Blaustein, M. P. (1976) Barbiturates block calcium uptake by stimulated and potassium-depolarized rat sympathetic ganglia. *J. Pharmac. Exp. Ther.* 196, 80–86.

Bloom, F. A., Costa, E. & Salmoiraghi, G. C. (1965) Anesthesia and the responsiveness of individual neurons of the caudate nucleus of the cat to acetylcholine, norepinephrine and dopamine administered by microelectrophoresis. *J. Pharmac. Exp. Ther.* 150, 244–252.

Bowery, N. G. (1976) Reversal of the action of γ-aminobutyric acid (GABA) antagonists by barbiturates. *Br. J. Pharmac.* 58, 456–457P.

Bowery, N. G. & Brown, D. A. (1974) Depolarizing actions of γ-aminobutyric acid and related compounds on rat superior cervical ganglia *in vitro*. *Br. J. Pharmac.* 50, 205–218.

Bowery, N. G. & Dray, A. (1976) Barbiturate reversal of amino acid antagonism produced by convulsant agents. *Nature* (Lond.) 264, 276–278.

Bowery, N. G. & Dray, A. (1978) Reversal of the action of amino acid antagonists by barbiturates and other hypnotics. *Br. J. Pharmac.* 63, 197–215.

Bradley, P. B. & Dray, A. (1973) Modification of the responses of brain stem neurons to transmitter substances by anaesthetic agents. *Br. J. Pharmac.* 48, 212–224.

Brown, D. A. & Constanti, A. (1978) Interaction of pentobarbitone and γ-aminobutyric acid on mammalian sympathetic ganglion cells. *Br. J. Pharmac.* 63, 217–224.

Brown, D. A. & Galvan, M. (1977) Influence of neuroglial transport on the action of γ-aminobutyric acid on mammalian ganglion cells. *Br. J. Pharmac.* 59, 373–378.

Collins, J. F. & Cryer, G. (1978) A study of the GABA receptor using ^{3}H-bicuculline methobromide. In: *Amino Acids as Chemical Transmitters,* ed. Fonnum, F., Plenum Press. In press.

Corrodi, H., Fuxe, K. & Hokfelt, T. (1966) The effect of barbiturates on the activity of the catecholamine neurones in the rat brain. *J. Pharm. Pharmac.* 18, 556–558.

Crawford, J. M. (1970) Anaesthetic agents and the chemical sensitivity of cortical neurones. *Neuropharmacol.* 9, 31–46.

Crawford, J. M. & Curtis, D. R. (1966) Pharmacological studies on feline Betz cells. *J. Physiol.* (Lond.) 186, 121–138.

Cutler, R. W. P. & Dudzinski, D. S. (1974) Effect of pentobarbital on uptake and release of ^{3}H-GABA and ^{14}C-glutamate on brain slices. *Brain Res.* 67, 546–548.

Cutler, R. W. P., Markowitz, D. & Dudzinski, D. S. (1974) The effect of barbiturates on ^{3}H-GABA transport in rat cerebral cortex slices. *Brain Res.* 81, 189–197.

Eccles, J. C., Faber, D. S. & Taborikova, H. (1971) The action of a parallel fiber volley on the antidromic invasion of Purkyne cells of cat cerebellum. *Brain Res.* 25, 335–356.

Eccles, J. C., Schmidt, R. & Willis, W. D. (1963) Pharmacological studies on presynaptic inhibition. *J. Physiol.* (Lond.) 168, 500–530.

Esplin, D. W. & Zablocka-Esplin, B. (1970) Central nervous system stimulants. In: *The Pharmacological Basis of Therapeutics, 4th ed.* ed. Goodman, L. S. & Gilman, A., London, Macmillan.

Franz, D. N. (1975) Central nervous system stimulants. In: *The Pharmacological Basis of Therapeutics, 5th ed.* ed. Goodman, L. S. & Gilman, A., London, Macmillan.

Lodge, D. & Curtis, D. R. (1977) Pentobarbitone enhancement of the inhibitory action of GABA. *Nature* (Lond.) 270, 543–544.

MacDonalds, R. & Barker, J. L. (1978) Benzodiazepines specifically modulate GABA-mediated postsynaptic inhibition in cultured mammalian neurones. *Nature* 271, 563–564.

Mitchell, J. F. (1963) The spontaneous and evoked release of acetylcholine from the cerebral cortex. *J. Physiol.* (Lond.) 165, 98–116.

Möhler, H. & Okada, T. (1977) GABA receptor binding with ^{3}H(+)bicuculline methiodide in rat CNS. *Nature* (Lond.) 267, 65–67.

Nicoll, R. A. (1975a) Presynaptic action of barbiturates in the frog spinal cord. *Proc. Nat. Acad. Sci.* (USA) 72, 1460–1463.

Nicoll, R. A. (1975b) Pentobarbital: action on frog motoneurons. *Brain Res.* 96, 119–123.

Nicoll, R. A. (1978) Pentobarbital: differential postsynaptic actions on sympathetic ganglion cells. *Science* 199, 451–452.

Nicoll, R. A., Eccles, J. C., Oshima, T. & Rubia, F. (1975) Prolongation of hippocampal inhibitory postsynaptic potentials by barbiturates. *Nature* (Lond.) 258, 625–627.

Olsen, R. W. (1978) Studies on the gamma-aminobutyric acid receptor/ionophore proteins in mammalian brain. In: *Amino Acids as Chemical Transmitters.* ed. Fonnum, F., Plenum Press. In press.

Peck, E. J., Miller, A. L. & Lester, B. R. (1976) Pentobarbital and synaptic high-affinity receptive sites for gamma-aminobutyric acid. *Brain Res. Bull* 1, 595–597.

Phillis, J. W. (1968) Acetylcholine release from the cerebral and cerebellar cortices: its role in cortical arousal. *Brain Res.* 7, 378–389.

Phillis, J. W. & Chong, G. C. (1965) Acetylcholine release from the cerebral and cerebellar cortices: its role in cortical arousal. *Nature* (Lond.) 207, 1253–1255.

Ransom, B. R. & Barker, J. L. (1976) Pentobarbital selectively enhances GABA-mediated post synaptic inhibition in tissue cultured mouse spinal neurones. *Brain Res.* 114, 530–535.

Richards, C. D. & Smaje, J. C. (1974) The actions of halothane and pentobarbitone on the sensitivity of neurones in the guinea pig prepiriform cortex to iontophoretically applied L-glutamate. *J. Physiol.* (Lond.) 239, 103–105P.

Richter, D. & Crossland, J. (1949) Variation in acetylcholine content of the brain with physiological state. *Am. J. Physiol.* 159, 247–255.

Sato, M., Austin, G. M. & Yai, H. (1967) Increase in the permeability of the postsynaptic membrane to potassium produced by "Nembutal". *Nature* (Lond.) 215, 1506–1508.

Straughan, D. W. (1977) Current views on the mechanism of action of benzodiazepines. *Arch de Farmacol. y Toxicol.* 3, 3–22.

Ticku, M. K. & Olsen, R. W. (1978) Barbiturate interaction with picrotoxinin binding sites in rat brain related to GABA receptor-ionophores. *Fed. Proc.* 37, 907.

Weakly, J. N. (1969) Effect of barbiturates on 'quantal' synaptic transmission in spinal motoneurons. *J. Physiol.* 204, 63–77.

Young, A. B. & Snyder, S. H. (1974) Strychnine binding in rat spinal cord membranes associated with the synaptic glycine receptor: cooperativity of glycine interactions. *Molec. Pharmac.* 10, 790–809.

Zukin, S. R., Young, A. B. & Snyder, S. H. (1974) Gamma-aminobutyric acid binding to receptor sites in the rat central nervous system. *Proc. Nat. Acad. Sci.* (USA) 71, 4802–4807.

Convulsant Drugs, Anticonvulsants and GABA-Mediated Neuronal Inhibition

Brian Meldrum

In most areas of neuropharmacology it is not possible to give a systematic account relating the actions of drugs as demonstrated at the molecular and neuronal level to their behavioural effects in the intact animal. However, recent improvements in our understanding of drug actions on GABA-mediated inhibition at the cellular level (as exemplified in this volume) urge us to renew the attempt to relate convulsant and anticonvulsant drug effects to the synaptic pharmacology of GABA (Meldrum 1975). Such an attempt sharpens awareness of defects in our understanding. Whole animal studies can indicate the need for new interpretations of conclusions derived from 'molecular' or single cell studies.

At present the line of argument from 'molecular' mechanisms to whole body effects is much stronger for convulsant than for anticonvulsant drug effects. It seems almost self-evident that disrupting a system responsible for a large part of the inhibitory activity in higher brain areas would facilitate excessively synchronous or sustained neuronal discharges (i.e. epilepsy). However, 'spontaneous' epileptic discharges have multiple causes and it is not obvious what is required to raise the threshold for their initiation, or to prevent their propagation once begun. The exact details of the interconnections and consecutive interactions of neuronal systems will be important. Inhibitory mechanisms will only be effective at preventing excessive synchronicity of neuronal firing if activated at the right time and in the right place.

CONVULSANT DRUGS

Studies at the molecular and cellular level allow us to classify convulsant drugs

Department of Neurology, Institute of Psychiatry, London SE5 8AF, England.

"GABA-NEUROTRANSMITTERS", Alfred Benzon Symposium 12, Munksgaard 1978

acting on GABA-mediated inhibition into three precise and more or less mutually exclusive groups:

1) drugs impairing the synthesis of GABA
2) drugs blocking the synaptic release of GABA
3) drugs impairing the neuronal inhibitory action of GABA.

There are some convulsant drugs that possibly act on GABA-mediated inhibition that we cannot reliably classify in this system. Thus pentylenetetrazol and bemegride, like bicuculline and picrotoxin, reduce primary afferent depolarization (Banna & Hazbun 1969, Hayes *et al.* 1977). This correlates with presynaptic inhibition in the primary afferent pathway, an effect very probably dependent on GABA (Levy 1977). Our lack of precise cellular data relating to pentylenetetrazol may be a consequence of the general rule that lipid soluble compounds that penetrate the blood-brain barrier well (such as bicuculline hydrochloride and pentylenetetrazol), tend to be poor candidates for iontophoretic studies, where water solubility and ionisation are of critical importance.

The following detailed consideration of these three specific mechanisms reveals further uncertainties.

Drugs impairing the synthesis of GABA (Table 1)

Many compounds that inhibit cerebral glutamic acid decarboxylase (GAD. 4.1.1.15) have been described (Wu & Roberts 1974, Taberner *et al.* 1977) but not all of these have been evaluated as convulsants. Among systemic convulsants three types of GAD inhibition have been identified: a) *Substrate competition* – the best studied example of a compound competing with glutamate is 3-mercaptopropionic acid (3MPA). When systemically administered in rodents or baboons, 3MPA produces generalised seizures, beginning after 2–6 min, continuing for 1–20 min, terminating with either death or rapid recovery (Horton & Meldrum 1973). Electrophysiologically the seizures in baboons begin diffusely in the cortex, closely resembling those seen after picrotoxin (Meldrum & Horton 1974). Inhibition of whole brain GAD activity and reduction of the rate of GABA synthesis *in vivo* occurs with a time course that matches the time course of the generalised seizures (Horton & Meldrum 1973, Adcock & Taberner 1978).

b) *Compounds interfering with the synthesis or coenzymic function of pyridoxal phosphate.* This is a large and diverse group (reviewed in more detail in Meldrum

Table I

Convulsant drugs that inhibit glutamic acid decarboxylase

	Enzyme inhibition	Convulsant Dose mmol/kg Rodents	Convulsant Dose mmol/kg Baboons	Seizure latency (min)	Duration of enhanced photosensitivity (h)
3-Mercaptopropionic acid	competitive	1.1	0.3−0.8	2−6	0.1−0.3
4-Deoxypyridoxine		1.2	0.5−0.9	15−45	1−5
Methyl-dithiocarbazinate	pyridoxal	0.1	—	30−45	—
Isoniazid	phosphate	—	0.7−1.9	7−40	0.5−2
Thiosemicarbazide	antagonists	0.3	0.04−0.1	60−240	3−6
Allylglycine	irreversible	1.0	4	60−120	12+
"2-Keto-pent-4-enoic-acid"	(catalytic)	(10–20μg)*	—	30−60	—

* Focal intracerebral injections inducing seizures in mice or rats.

Data from Meldrum *et al.* 1970, Meldrum & Horton 1971, Horton & Meldrum 1973, Meldrum *et al.* 1975, Horton & Meldrum 1977.

1975), including pyridoxine analogues (e.g. 4-deoxypyridoxine), hydrazides and related compounds (e.g. isoniazid, thiosemicarbazide, methyldithiocabazinate and hydrazine), and other carbonyl-trapping reagents, (e.g. aminooxyacetic acid). These compounds variably inhibit other decarboxylases (including L-aromatic amino acid decarboxylase (which as '3,4 dihydroxy-L-phenylalanine carboxy-lyase, DCA, EC.4.1.1.26' participates in the synthesis of dopamine and noradrenaline, and as '5-hydroxy-L-tryptophan carboxy-lyase, E.C.4.1.1.28' participates in the synthesis of serotonin) (Gey & Georgi 1974). Changes in monoaminergic activity can influence seizure thresholds; however, this decarboxylase is not generally the rate limiting step, and a recent study (Sawaya *et al.* 1978) comparing GAD inhibition, DCA inhibition and monoamine and metabolite concentrations after several pyridoxal phosphate antagonists found little evidence for a major role of reduced monoamine synthesis in epileptogenesis. Pyridoxal phosphate antagonists and carbonyl trapping agents can also inhibit GABA transaminase (4-aminobutyrate: 2-oxoglutarate aminotransferase, E.C.2.6.1.19). Generally, GAD is more strongly inhibited, but after amino oxyacetic acid and hydrazine, the effect on GABA-transaminase predominates.

Seizures after pyridoxal phosphate antagonists typically begin after a long latency (45–300 min), often with a focal onset. The seizures are brief and followed by full neurological recovery, but recur at roughly regular intervals over a period that may extend for several hours. In baboons, electroencephalography commonly indicates a focal onset posteriorly in one cerebral hemisphere (Meldrum *et al.* 1970, Meldrum & Horton 1971). This pattern of seizures is strikingly similar to that seen after DL-allylglycine and suggests that the aetiology is similar in both circumstances.

c) *Compounds leading to irreversible inhibition of GAD.* DL-allylglycine (2-amino pent-4-enoic acid) produces irreversible inhibition of cerebral GAD, apparently through one or more metabolites formed *in vivo*, that act as catalytic inhibitors (Horton & Meldrum 1973, Orlowski *et al.* 1977). *In vitro,* both D- and L-allylglycine are only weakly active as GAD inhibitors (Orlowski *et al.* 1977). Preincubation with brain homogenates enhances the inhibition. Incubation of D- or L-allyglycine with D- or L-aminoacid oxidase leads to the formation of an extremely potent compound which appears to be a catalytic inhibitor of GAD (Horton 1978). With each isomer the primary product of the action of aminoacid oxidase is 2-keto pent-4-enoic acid. This compound is unstable. Products formed from it include 2-keto pent-3-enoic acid and 2hydroxy-pent-3-

enoic acid (see Marcotte & Walsh 1978). Our recent studies (Horton *et al.* 1978a, b) provide evidence for regional cerebral differences in the metabolism, and effects, of the isomers of allylglycine. D- and L-allylglycine induce different patterns of seizures in rodents (Orlowski *et al.* 1977, Horton & Meldrum 1977, Horton *et al.* 1978a). L-allylglycine (1.2mmol/kg, i.p.) is followed by forepaw myoclonus, wild running and tonic seizures repeated two to four times before death or recovery; D-allylglycine (3.75 mmol/kg, i.p.) is followed by irregular trunk and limb jerks, sudden jumps and brief seizures with rotation around the longitudinal axis, repeated 50–100 times over 2–4 h before recovery. In baboons L-allylglycine enhances photosensitive epilepsy (100 mg/kg) and induces seizures (150–200 mg/kg) with a pattern closely resembling that seen after pyroxidal phosphate antagonists (Horton & Meldrum 1973, Meldrum *et al.* 1978), i.e. long latency brief recurrent seizures, commonly with a focal cortical onset. D-allylglycine (up to 780 mg/kg) produces vertical nystagmus but no seizures.

The distinctive effects of D-allylglycine are apparently a consequence of the restricted distribution of D-amino oxidase, which in rodents and primates is virtually confined to the cerebellum, brainstem and spinal cord (Goldstein 1966, Neims *et al.* 1966). Thus GABA content falls with a similar time course in most rat brain regions after L-allylglycine, but declines only in the cerebellum and pons-medulla after D-allylglycine (Horton *et al.* 1978a, b).

If seizures following pyridoxal phosphate antagonists and allylglycine are due to impairment in the rate of synthesis of GABA, it is necessary to explain why minimal convulsant doses lead to intermittent seizures with intervening EEG and neurological recovery. Several mechanisms are possible. The pH optimum for GAD is just below 7.0 so that enhanced P_{CO_2} or lactic acid concentration could enhance GAD activity. ATP inhibits GAD and this effect is relieved by inorganic phosphate (Seligman *et al.* 1978) so that the changes in adenine nucleotides occurring during seizures (Chapman *et al.* 1977) might also enhance GABA synthesis. Depolarization by potassium or veratridine leads to an increase in GAD activity in striatal slices (Gold *et al.* 1978). Hypoxia (through a decrease in NAD^+) is known to increase brain GABA content by decreasing the further metabolism of GABA. Direct proof of the mechanism permitting functional recovery, while GAD inhibition persists, is not yet available.

Drugs blocking the release of GABA

Tetanus toxin acts presynaptically to reduce the physiologically-induced release of GABA (Curtis *et al.* 1973, Davies & Tongroach 1977); the release of glycine is similarly blocked (Curtis & De Groat 1968). In generalised seizures induced by tetanus toxin, the relative importance of spinal, midbrain and cortical actions (or the peripheral neuromuscular blockade – Duchen & Tonge 1973) is not known. However, the focal injection of small quantities of tetanus toxin into the ventral hippocampus induces generalized seizures in the rat comparable to those seen after the systemic administration of much larger quantities (Mellanby *et al.* 1977).

Drugs blocking the inhibitory action of GABA

The list of convulsant drugs that can be shown to block the inhibitory actions of GABA has grown steadily since Curtis *et al.* (1970) described the action of bicuculline on spinal seizures. However, the potency of the different antagonists varies markedly according to the test system. Blockade of the inhibition of neuronal firing produced by the iontophoretic application of GABA or by activation of a GABA-ergic pathway is the most appropriate 'physiological' test system. Competition with ^{3}H-GABA or with (^{3}H) α-dihydropicrotoxinin (DHP) for binding sites in brain membrane preparations is the most informative at the 'molecular' level. Blockade of the depolarizing action of GABA on the isolated rat superior cervical ganglion is a very convenient *in vitro* test system. In Table II, results with these test systems are compared with the effects in baboons, of picrotoxin, bicuculline, 4-isopropyl bicyclophosphate (IPBP) and tetramethylenedisulphotetramine (TETS). Picrotoxin IPBP and TETS all compete with DHP for membrane binding sites (Olsen *et al.* 1978). Interference with the inhibitory process at a later stage than GABA recognition seems to correlate with a prolonged enhancement of photosensitive epilepsy by subconvulsant drug doses.

Seizures in baboons after a minimal convulsant dose of TETS sometimes have a diffuse cortical onset and a brief latency (i.e. resembling those after picrotoxin) but a slightly higher dose produces seizures of generalized onset and extremely short latency (i.e. resembling those induced by bicuculline). TETS and picrotoxin also share the capacity to produce a very sustained enhancement of the natural syndrome of photosensitive epilepsy in baboons when given in subconvulsant doses. A cortical site of action would adequately account for the convulsant effects of picrotoxin and TETS, although focal injections of picrotoxin at many levels of the nervous system can induce epileptic discharges or epileptiform motor phenomena (e.g. Tarsy *et al.* 1978).

Table II

Convulsant drugs that are GABA antagonists

	GABA antagonism demonstrated				Convulsions in baboons		Duration of enhanced photosensitivity (h)
	Iontophoretically	On rat sup. cerv. ganglion	By competition for binding sites DHP	GABA	Dose μmol/kg	Latency (min)	
Picrotoxin	++	++	++	0	2.5	2−10	3
Bicuculline	++	++	0	++	0.8	0.1−0.2	—
4-Isopropyl bicyclophosphate	++	++	++	0	0.2	1−2	?
Tetramethylene disulphotetramine	(+?)	++	++	0	0.8	0.1−2	6+

Data from Olsen *et al.* (1978), Bowery *et al.* 1975, 1976, Meldrum & Horton 1974, Meldrum (unpublished).
DHP=α-dihydropicrotoxinin.

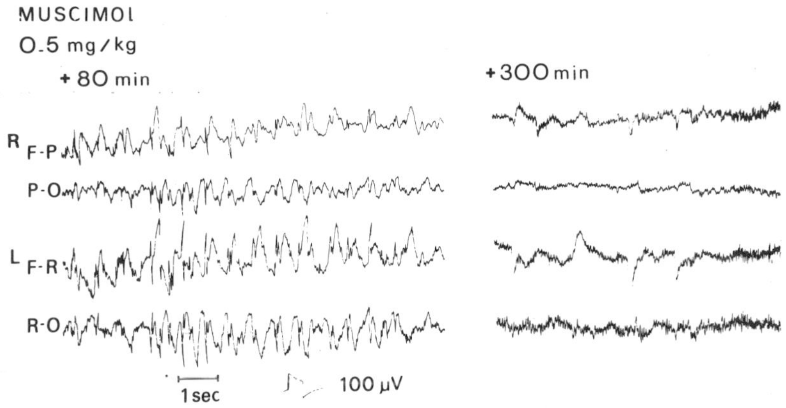

Fig. 1. EEG records from an adult female baboon, *Papio papio* , after the intravenous injection of muscimol, 0.5 mg/kg. Records taken from subcutaneous platinum needle electrodes: R and L, right and left hemispheres, F-P, frontal-parietal, P-O, parietal to occipital. Bilateral spikes and spike and wave disharges (some of which were associated with myoclonic jerks) are seen 80 min after drug injection. After 5 h there is a return to normal EEG appearances (including muscle and eye movement artefacts).

ANTICONVULSANT DRUG ACTION AND GABA

The mechanism of action of anticonvulsant drugs in clinical use in poorly understood. The grounds for believing that benzodiazepines enhance GABA-mediated inhibition have been presented by Haefely (1978) but the mechanism is not yet clear. An interaction with GABA-mediated inhibition has been suggested in the case of di-n-propylacetate, barbiturates and trimethadione (Meldrum 1975) and most recently diphenylhydantoin (Deisz & Lux 1977). Enhancement of presynaptic inhibition in the spinal cord by barbiturates, benzodiazepines and trimethadione has been known for many years (Miyahara *et al.* 1966, Schmidt 1971) but the relationship of this effect to enhancement of GABA-mediated inhibition has become apparent only recently (Levy 1977).

An explanation in molecular and cellular terms of enhancement of GABA-mediated inhibition should, if our current concepts of synaptic function are correct, cover the following three mechanisms:

1) Enhancing the physiological release of GABA
2) a GABA 'agonist' action, which strictly means an action at the GABA receptor site, but may be extended to include an action 'cooperative' with that of GABA, as proposed for benzodiazepines by Haefely (1978)
3) blockade of GABA uptake.

Enhancing the physiological release of GABA

The optimal mechanism would be a drug-induced increase in GAD activity leading to a sustained enhancement of GABA release.

In vitro studies of the stimulated release of labelled GABA have not yet provided a clear conclusion. Diazepam and barbiturates depress the electrically stimulated release from cortical slices (Schacht 1978) and the Ca^{++} stimulated release from synaptosome preparations (Olsen *et al.* 1978). However, the K^+ stimulated release from cortical prisms is facilitated by low concentrations (10^{-6}M) of flurazepam and diazepam (Mitchell & Martin 1978).

Baclofen apparently enhances the stimulated release of GABA from the globus pallidus (Kerwin & Pycock 1978). In cortical slices GABA efflux is unchanged, whereas the release of exicatory amino acids is depressed in the presence of baclofen, 4μM (Potashner 1978).

The possibility that inhibition of GABA-transaminase activity may lead to an increase in the physiological release of GABA is discussed below.

GABA agonists

A true GABA agonist fulfils the following three criteria: (a) it produces a bicuculline-sensitive inhibition of neuronal firing when applied iontophoretically to appropriate neurones in the brain or spinal cord, (b) it competes with ^{3}H-GABA for binding sites in brain membrane preparations, (c) it produces the same neurological or behavioural effects as GABA when injected focally into specific brain regions. The most potent and best authenticated GABA agonist is muscimol. Although some anticonvulsant activity can be demonstrated in a rodent test system (Anlezark *et al.* 1978) studies in progress in photosensitive baboons (Meldrum, Horton & Pedley 1978) show that it is not an effective convulsant drug. Not only does muscimol, 0.5 mg/kg, intravenously, fail to block photically-induced epileptic responses, but it leads to a great enhancement of slow rhythms on the EEG which often take on a paroxysmal appearance, not unlike the discharges associated with 'absence' attacks (Fig. 1). This effect is similar to that of β-(p-chloro)-phenyl-GABA (baclofen) in baboons (Meldrum & Horton 1974). Although neuronal inhibition produced by baclofen could not be blocked by bicuculline (Curtis *et al.* 1974), focally injected baclofen mimics the actions of GABA and muscimol (e.g. Scheel-Krüger *et al.* 1977), so it may be functionally a GABA agonist. A tendency for direct GABA agonists to increase the synchronicity of cortical electrical activity is perhaps not surprising. The simultaneous activation of all GABA receptors may prevent recurrent and other

Table III
Inhibitors of GABA uptake

	Rat brain slices IC_{50} μm	Intracerebroventricular injection blocking audiogenic seizures μ moles	causing convulsions μ moles
(−)-nipecotic acid	5	1.6−3.2	−
S(+)-2,4-diaminobutyric acid	35	0.5−2	0.5−2
cis 1,3-aminocyclohexane carboxylic acid	85	−	3.2
S(−)piperazic acid	21	(4)	−
	Johnston *et al.* 1976, 1977 Lodge *et al.* 1976	Horton *et al.* (unpublished)	

inhibitory pathways functioning normally to terminate excessive discharges.

This problem does not arise with drugs that enhance the action of physiologically released GABA (as proposed for benzodiazepines by Haefely 1978), as the inhibitory action will occur only at the appropriate time and place.

GABA uptake blockade

Inactivation of extracellular GABA is by a high affinity, sodium-dependent uptake system (Iversen & Kelly 1975). Inhibition of this uptake can be produced by a wide range of compounds (see Harris *et al.* 1973, Beart & Johnston 1973, Krogsgaard-Larsen & Johnston 1975) but the specificity of the effect is low (compounds not structurally related to GABA tend to inhibit uptake of many other amino acids and transmitters – GABA analogues tend to interact in other ways with the GABA system). Prolongation of 'physiological' (stimulus-induced) inhibition and of inhibition due to iontophoretically applied GABA has been demonstrated after administration of various inhibitors of GABA uptake (Curtis *et al.* 1976, Lodge *et al.* 1977). Among the most potent and selective compounds, (−)nipecotic acid, (+)−2,4-diaminobutyric acid, arecaidine and guvacine all, when applied iontophoretically, enhance the inhibitory action of β-alanine as well as that of GABA. There is little evidence to indicate a correlation between GABA uptake blockade and anticonvulsant activity of systemically administered drugs, although adequate studies are lacking. We have been studying the effects of the intracerebroventricular administration of drugs known to block high affinity GABA uptake in mice (DBA/2) genetically susceptible to sound-induced seizures (Table III). (−)Nipecotic acid, 3.2 μmoles in 10μl intracerebroventricularly, produced a partial protection against audiogenic seizures, associated with a slight fall in body temperature and some postural changes. Protection was not seen after nipecotic acid, 1.2 mM/kg, intraperitoneally. S(+)−2,4-diaminobutyric acid, 2 μmoles, i.c.v., apparently produced partial protection against audiogenic seizures after 30 min. However, animals at this time showed myoclonic movements of the limbs, which became more severe in the following 30–40 min, progressing to whole body myoclonic jerks and sometimes to tonic seizures. A similar but more sustained epileptic syndrome was seen after i.c.v. injection of putrescine, 2 μmoles, and after *cis* 1,3-aminocyclohexane carboxylic acid, 3,2 μmoles, i.c.v. (S)-piperazic acid, 4 μmoles, produced some slight protection against seizures, associated with ataxia and a reduction in body temperature.

β-alanine (which blocks glial uptake of GABA) caused a significant mortality but no protection against seizures.

The convulsions seen after DABA and ACHC probably result from actions other than inhibition of GABA uptake. DABA, for example, inhibits GABA binding to cortical membranes (Johnston & Twitchin 1977).

Inhibition of the further metabolism of GABA

The relation between inhibition of cerebral GABA-transaminase activity and anticonvulsant drug action has been greatly clarified by the recent introduction of the catalytic inhibitors of GABA transaminase (see Rando 1978 and Metcalf *et al.* 1978). Inhibition of GABA transaminase by amino oxyacetic acid has long been proposed as the mechanism responsible for its anticonvulsant effects (Wallach 1961, Meldrum *et al.* 1970, Meldrum 1975) but it is neither a good experimental tool nor useful therapeutically because of other actions. Inhibition of GABA transaminase by di-n-propylacetate was described by Mandel *et al.* (Simler *et al.* 1973, Godin *et al.* 1969), but the importance of this effect in its anticonvulsant action is not yet established (Anlezark *et al.* 1976, Horton *et al.* 1977).

The studies of gabaculine, γ-acetylenic GABA and γ-vinyl GABA (Table IV) reported here (Rando 1978, Metcalf *et al.* 1978) have extended and confirmed earlier studies with ethanolamine-O-sulphate in rodents (Fowler 1973, Anlezark *et al.* 1976). Inhibition of whole brain or cortical GABA transaminase by more than 50% leads to a marked increase in brain GABA content (up to 10 times control concentration). Seizure thresholds are raised with a similar time course.

Table IV
Drugs inhibiting GABA transaminase

	Rodents anticonvulsant dose (mM/kg)	Baboons anticonvulsant dose (mM/kg)	Latency (min)	Duration (h)
Amino-oxyacetic acid	0.3	0.06−0.17	30−40	6−24
Di-n-propyl acetate	1.2−3.6	0.6 −1.8	5−15	1−3
γ-Acetylenic GABA	0.3	0.8 −1.6	60	24+
γ-Vinyl GABA	7.7	3.5	60	24+
Gabaculine	0.4	—	—	—
	Kuriyama *et al.* 1966, Allen *et al.* 1977, Schechter *et al.* 1977b	Meldrum *et al.* 1970, 1977, Meldrum & Horton 1978		

The anticonvulsant effect of γ-acetylenic GABA and γ-vinyl GABA described in rodents (Schechter *et al.* 1977a, b) has been confirmed in baboons (*Papio papio*) with photosensitive epilepsy (Meldrum & Horton 1978). Complete protection against myoclonic or seizure responses to photic stimulation is seen after γ-acetylenic GABA, 160–200 mg/kg, i.v., or γ-vinyl GABA, 450–950 mg/kg, i.v. The protection is maximal 3–8 h after the injection and continues for 24 h or more. It is not associated with signs of acute neurological toxicity.

The anticonvulsant action of GABA transaminase inhibition needs an explanation in terms of synaptic function. Three possibilities that could be explored in *in vitro* test systems are: a) an increased release of GABA from synaptic terminals, b) a diminished rate of uptake of synaptically released GABA and c) a release of GABA from glial cells, provoked by the increase in extracellular potassium occurring during the initial phase of a seizure discharge.

CONCLUSION: ANTICONVULSANT DRUGS AND GABA

Any GABA analogue or agent acting on GABA receptors or carrier molecules is likely to act on GABA metabolism and GABA-mediated inhibition at more than one point. As scientists we value most highly agents which we think have specific action. We should not forget that the most useful drug in any particular form of epilepsy might be of low specificity, acting partially on any of the following: GABA synthesis and release, GABA receptors and carriers, the further metabolism of GABA, and ionophores or other membrane elements modifying ionic conductance or transport.

ACKNOWLEDGMENTS

It is a pleasure to thank my colleagues, Drs. Anlezark, Chapman, Horton, Pedley and Sawaya for their collaboration, and the following bodies for financial support: The Wellcome Trust, the Medical Research Council, the British Epilepsy Association and the National Fund for Research into Crippling Diseases.

REFERENCES

Adcock, t. & Taberner, P. V. (1978) Measuring changes in cerebral glutamate and GABA metabolism prior to convulsions induced by 3-mercaptoproprionate. *Biochem. Pharmacol.* 27, 246–248.

Allan, R. D., Johnston, G. A. R. & Twitchin, B. (1977) Effects of gabaculine on the uptake, binding and metabolism of GABA. *Neurosci. Letters* 4, 51–54.

Anlezark, G., Collins, J. & Meldrum, B. (1978) GABA agonists and audiogenic seizures. *Neurosci. Letters* 7, 337–340.

Anlezark, G., Horton, R. W., Meldrum, B. S. & Sawaya, M. C. B. (1976) Anticonvulsant action of ethanolamine-O-sulphate and di-n-propylacetate and the metabolism of γ-aminobutyric acid (GABA) in mice with audiogenic seizures. *Biochem. Pharmacol.* 25, 414–417.

Banna, N. R. & Hazbun, J. (1969) Analysis of the convulsant action of pentylenetetrazol. *Experientia* 26, 382–383.

Beart, P. M. & Johnston, G. A. R. (1973) GABA uptake in rat brain slices: inhibition by GABA analogues and by various drugs. *J. Neurochem.* 20, 319–324.

Bowery, N. G., Brown, D. A. & Collins, J. F. (1975) Tetramethylenedisulphotetramine: an inhibitor of γ-aminobutyric acid induced depolarization of the isolated superior cervical ganglion of the rat. *Br. J. Pharmac.* 53, 422–424.

Bowery, N. G., Collins, J. F. & Hill, R. G. (1976) Bicyclic phosphorus esters that are potent convulsants and GABA antagonists. *Nature* 261, 601–603.

Chapman, A. G., Meldrum, B. S. & Siesjö, B. K. (1977) Cerebral metabolic changes during prolonged epileptic seizures in rats. *J. Neurochem.* 28, 1025–1035.

Curtis, D. R., Duggan, A. W., Felix, D. & Johnston, G. A. R. (1970) GABA, bicuculline and central inhibition. *Nature* (Lond.) 226, 1222–1224.

Curtis, D. R., Felix, D., Game, C. J. A. & McCullough, R. M. (1973) Tetanus toxin and the synaptic release of GABA. *Brain Res.* 51, 358–362.

Curtis, D. R., Game, C. J. A., Johnston, G. A. R. & McCulloch, R. M.(1974) Central effects of *β*-(*p*-chlorophenyl)-γ-aminobutyric acid. *Brain Res.* 70, 493–499.

Curtis, D. R., Game, C. J. A. and Lodge, D. (1976) The *in vivo* inactivation of GABA and other inhibitory amino acids in the cat nervous system. *Exp. Brain Res.* 25, 413–428.

Curtis, D. R. & de Groat, W. C. (1968) Tetanus toxin and spinal inhibition. *Brain Res.* 10, 208–212.

Davies, J. & Tongroach, P. (1977) Antagonism of synaptic inhibition in the rat substantia nigra by tetanus toxin. *Br. J. Pharmac.* 59, 589P.

Deisz, R. A. & Lux, H. D. (1977) Diphenylhydantoin prolongs postsynaptic inhibition and iontophoretic GABA action in the crayfish stretch receptor. *Neurosci. Letters* 5, 199–203.

Duchen, L.W. & Tonge, D. A. (1973) The effects of tetanus toxin on neuromuscular transmission and on the morphology of motor endplates in slow and fast skeletal muscle in the mouse. *J. Physiol.* 228, 157–172.

Fowler, L. J. (1973) Analysis of the major amino acids of rat brain after *in vivo* inhibition of GABA transaminase by ethanolamine-O-sulphate. *J. Neurochem.* 21, 437–440.

Gey, K. F. & Georgi, H. (1974) Effect of neurotropic agents on total pyridoxal phosphate and on the activity of the decarboxylase of aromatic amino acids as well as of other pyridoxal phosphate-dependent enzymes in rat brain. *J. Neurochem.* 23, 725–738.

Godin, Y., Heiner, L., Mark, J. & Mandel, P. (1969) Effects of di-n-propylacetate an anticonvulsant compound, on GABA metabolism. *J. Neurochem.* 16, 869–873.

Gold, B. I., Simon, J. R. & Roth, R. H. (1978) Glutamic acid decarboxylase activity in striatal slices: persistent increase following depolarization. *Life Sci.* 22, 187–194.

Goldstein, D. B. (1966) D-aminoacid oxidase in brain: distribution in several species and inhibition by pentobarbitone. *J. Neurochem.* 13, 1011–1016.

Haefely, W. (1978) Facilitation of GABAergic transmission by drugs. In: *GABA-Neurotransmitters,* ed. H. Kofod, P. Krogsgaard-Larsen, J. Scheel-Krüger.

Harris, M., Hopkin, J. M. & Neal, M. J. (1973) Effect of centrally acting drugs on the uptake of γ-aminobutyric acid (GABA) by slices of rat cerebral cortex. *Brit. J. Pharmacol.* 47, 229–239.

Hayes, A. G., Gartside, I. B. & Straughan, D. W. (1977) Effect of four convulsants on the time course of presynaptic inhibition and its relation to seizure activity. *Neuropharmacol.* 16, 725–730.

Horton, R. W. (1978) The role of 2-keto-4-pentenoic acid in seizures induced by allylglycine. *Biochem. Pharmacol.* 27, 1471–1477.

Horton, R. W. & Meldrum, B. S. (1973) Seizures induced by allylglycine, 3-mercaptopropionic acid and 4-deoxypyridoxine in mice and photosensitive baboons, and different modes of inhibition of cerebral glutamic acid decarboxylase. *Brit. J. Pharmac.* 49, 52–63.

Horton, R.W. & Meldrum, B. S. (1977) A comparison of the effects of allylglycine and 2-keto-4-pentenoic acid on cerebral glutamic acid decarboxylase activity and convulsions in mice. *Brit. J. Pharmac.* 61, 477P.

Horton, R.W., Anlezark, G. M., Sawaya, M. C. B. & Meldrum, B. S. (1977) Monoamine and GABA metabolism and the anticonvulsant action of di-n-propylacetate and ethanolamine-O-sulphate. *Europ. J. Pharmacol.* 41, 387–397.

Horton, R.W., Chapman, A. G. & Meldrum, B. S. (1978a) Differential effect of D- and L-allylglycine (2-amino-pent-4-enoic acid) on regional cerebral γ-aminobutyrate concentrations. *Trans. Biochem. Soc.* 6, 115–118.

Horton, R.W., Chapman, A. G. & Meldrum, B. S. (1978b) Regional changes in cerebral GABA concentration and convulsions produced by D- and L-allylglycine. *J. Neurochem.* 30, 1501–1504.

Iversen, L. L. & Kelly, J. S. (1975) Uptake and metabolism of γ-aminobutyric acid by neurones and glial cells. *Biochem. Pharmacol.* 24, 933–938.

Johnston, G. A. R., Krogsgaard-Larsen, P., Stephanson, A. L. & Twitchin, B. (1976) Inhibition of the uptake of GABA and related amino acids in rat brain slices by the optical isomers of nipecotic acid. *J. Neurochem.* 26, 1029–1032.

Johnston, G. A. R., Stephanson, A. L. & Twitchin, B. (1977) Piperazic acid and related compounds as inhibitors of GABA uptake in rat brain slices. *J. Pharm. Pharmac.* 29, 240–241.

Johnston, G. A. R. & Twitchin, B. (1977) Stereospecificity of 2,4-diaminobutyric acid with respect to inhibition of 4-aminobutyric acid uptake and binding. *Brit. J. Pharmacol.* 59, 218–219.

Kerwin, R. & Pycock, C. (1978) Baclofen enhances (^{3}H) GABA release from rat globus pallidus *in vitro. Brit. J. Pharmacol.* 63, 388P.

Krogsgaard-Larsen, P. & Johnston, G. A. R. (1975) Inhibition of GABA uptake in rat brain slices by nipecotic acid, various isoxazoles and related compounds. *J. Neurochem.* 26, 797–802.

Kuriyama, K., Roberts, E. & Rubinstein, M. K. (1966) Elevation of γ-aminobutyric acid in brain with amino-oxyacetic acid and susceptibility to convulsive seizures in mice: a quantitative re-evaluation. *Biochem. Pharmacol.* 15, 221–236.

Levy, R. A. (1977) The role of GABA in primary afferent depolarization. *Progress in Neurobiol.* 9, 211–267.

Lodge, D., Johnston, G. A. R., Curtis, D. R. & Brand, S. J. (1977) Effects of the areca nut constituents arecaidine and guvacine on the action of GABA in the cat central nervous system. *Brain Res.* 136, 513–522.

Lodge, D., Johnston, G. A. R. & Stephenson, A. L. (1976) The uptake of GABA and β-alanine in slices of cat and rat CNS tissue: regional differences in susceptibility to inhibitors. *J. Neurochem.* 27, 1569–1570.

Marcotte, P. & Walsh, C. (1978) The sequence of reactions which follows enzymatic oxidation of propargylglycine and allylglycine. *Biochemistry.* In press.

Meldrum, B. S. (1975) Epilepsy and GABA-mediated inhibition. *Internat. Rev. Neurobiol.* 17, 1–36.

Meldrum, B. S., Anlezark, G. M., Ashton, C. G., Horton, R. W. & Sawaya, M. C. B. (1977) Neurotransmitters and anticonvulsant drug action. In *Post-traumatic epilepsy, pharmacological prophylaxis of epilepsy.* Ed. Majkowski, J., pp. 139–153. Polish Chapter of ILEA, Warsaw.

Meldrum, B. S., Balzano, E., Gadea, M. & Naquet, R. (1970) Photic and drug-induced epilepsy in the baboon (*Papio papio*): the effects of isoniazid, thiosemicarbazide, pyridoxine and amino-oxyacetic acid. *Electroenceph. Clin. Neurophysiol.* 29, 333–347.

Meldrum, B. S. & Horton, R. W. (1971) Convulsive effects of 4-deoxypyridoxine and of bicuculline in photosensitive baboons (*Papio papio*) and in Rhesus monkeys (*Macaca mulatta*). *Brain Res.* 35, 419–436.

Meldrum, B. S. & Horton, R. W. (1974) Neuronal inhibition mediated by GABA, and patterns of convulsions in photosensitive baboons with epilepsy (*Papio papio*). In: *The Natural History and Management of Epilepsy,* ed. Harris, P. & Mawdsley, C., pp. 55–64. Churchill Livingstone, Edinburgh.

Meldrum, B. & Horton, R. (1978) Blockade of epileptic responses in the photosensitive baboon, *Papio papio*, by two irreversible inhibitors of GABA transaminase, γ-acetylenic GABA (4-amino-hex-5-yonic acid) and γ-vinyl GABA (4-amino-hex-5-enoic acid). *Psychopharmacol.* 59.

Meldrum, B. S., Horton, R. W. & Sawaya, M. C. B. (1975) The convulsant action of methyldithiocarbazinate: a comparison with other sulphur containing hydrazides. *J. Neurochem.* 24, 1003–1010.

Meldrum, B. S., Menini, C., Naquet, R., Stutzmann, J. M. & Laurent, H. (1978) Proconvulsant, convulsant and other actions of the D- and L-stereoisomers of allylglycine in the photosensitive baboon, *Papio papio. J. Electroenceph. Clin. Neurophysiol.*

Mellanby, J., George, G., Robinson, A. & Thompson, P. (1977) Epileptiform syndrome in rats produced by injecting tetanus toxin into the hippocampus. *J. Neurol. Neurosurg. Psych.* 40, 404–414.

Metcalf, B. W., Jung, M. J., Lippert, B., Casara, P., Bohlen, P. & Schechter, P. J. (1978) γ-acetylenic GABA and γ-vinyl GABA – two enzyme-activated irreversible inhibitors of GABA aminotransferase. In: *GABA-Neurotransmitters*. Ed. Kofod, H., Krogsgaard-Larsen, P. & Scheel-Krüger, J.

Mitchell, P. R. & Martin, I. L. (1978) The effects of benzodiazepines on K^+ stimulated release of GABA. *Neuropharmacol.* 17, 317–320.

Miyahara, J. T., Esplin, D. W. & Zablocka, B.(1966) Differential effects of depressant drugs on pre-synaptic inhibition. *J. Pharmacol. Exp. Therap.* 154, 119–127.

Neims, A. H., Zieverink, W. D. & Smilack, J. D. (1966) Distribution of D-aminoacid oxidase in bovine and human nervous tissues. *J. Neurochem.* 13, 163–168.

Olsen, R. W., Ticku, M. K., Van Ness, P. C. & Greenlee, D. (1978) Effects of drugs on γ-amino-butyric acid receptors, uptake, release and synthesis *in vitro*. *Brain Res.* 139, 277–294.

Orlowski, M., Reingold, D. F. & Stanley, M. E. (1977) D- andL-stereoisomers of allylglycine: convulsive action and inhibition of brain L-glutamate decarboxylase. *J. Neurochem.* 28, 349–353.

Olsen, R. W., Ticku, M. K., Greenlee, D. & Van Ness, P. (1978) GABA receptor and ionophore binding sites: interaction with various drugs. In: *GABA-Neurotransmitters.*, ed. Kofod, H., Krogsgaard-Larsen, P. & Scheel-Krüger).

Potashner, S. J. (1978) Baclofen: effects on amino acid release. *Can. J. Physiol.* 56, 150–154.

Rando, R. R. (1978) Specific inhibitors of GABA metabolism. In *GABA-Neurotransmitters.* ed. Kofod, H., Krogsgaard-Larsen, P. & Scheel-Krüger, J.

Sawaya, C., Horton, R. & Meldrum, B. (1978) Transmitter synthesis and convulsant drugs: effects of pyridoxal phosphate antagonists and allylglycine. *Biochem. Pharmacol.* 27, 475–481.

Schacht, U. (1978) *In vitro* studies on GABA release. *Brit. J. Clin. Pharmacol.*

Schechter, P. J., Tranier, Y., Jung, M., Sjoerdsma, A. (1977a) Antiseizure activity of γ-acetylenic γ-aminobutyric acid: A catalytic irreversible inhibitor of γ-aminobutyric acid transaminase. *J. Pharmacol. Exp. Therap.* 201, 606–612.

Schechter, P. J., Tranier, Y., Jung, M. J. & Bohlen, P. (1977b) Audiogenic seizure protection by elevated GABA concentration in mice: effects of γ-acetylenic GABA and γ-vinyl GABA, two irreversible GABA-T inhibitors. *Europ. J. Pharmacol.* 45, 319–328

Scheel-Krüger, J., Arnt, J. & Magelund, G. (1977) Behavioural stimulation induced by muscimol and other GABA agonists injected into the substantia nigra. *Neurosci. Letters* 4, 351–356.

Schmidt, R. F. (1971) Presynaptic inhibition in the vertebrate central nervous system. *Ergebn. Physiol. Biol. Chem. Exp. Pharmakol.* 63, 20–101.

Seligman, B., Miller, L. P., Brockman, D. E. & Martin, D. L. (1978) Studies on the regulation of GABA synthesis: the interaction of adenine nucleotides and glutamate with brain glutamate decarboxylase. *J. Neurochem.* 30, 371–376.

Simler, S., Ciesielski, L., Maître, M., Randrianarisoa, H. & Mandel P. (1973) Effect of sodium n-dipropylacetate on audiogenic seizures and brain γ-aminobutyric acid level. *Biochem. Pharmacol.* 22, 1701–1708.

Taberner, P. V., Pearce, M. J. & Watkins, J. C. (1977) The inhibition of mouse brain glutamate decarboxylase by some structural analogues of L-glutamic acid. *Biochem. Pharmacol.* 26, 345–349.

Tarsy, D., Pycock, C. J., Meldrum, B. S. & Marsden, C. D. (1978) Focal contralateral myoclonus produced by inhibition of GABA action in the caudate nucleus of rats. *Brain* 101, 143–162.

Wallach, D. P. (1961) Studies on the GABA pathway. I. The inhibition of γ-aminobutyric acid-α-ketoglutaric acid transaminase. *Biochem. Pharmacol.* 5, 323–331.

Wu, J.-Y. & Roberts, E. (1974) Properties of brain L-glutamate decarboxylase: inhibition studies. *J. Neurochem.* 23, 759–767.

A Molecular Mechanism for the Facilitation of GABA Receptor Function by Benzodiazepines

A. Guidotti, G. Toffano, M. Baraldi, J. P. Schwartz & E. Costa

During the last few years a number of reports from this and other laboratories have suggested that a facilitatory action on the transmitter function of γ-aminobutyric acid (GABA) may be of significance to explain certain therapeutic effects of benzodiazepines (Costa *et al.* 1975, Polc *et al.* 1974, Haefely 1978, Guidotti 1978, Choi *et al.* 1978, McDonald & Barker 1978). Since this facilitation is related to the benzodiazepines potency to bind to their specific brain receptor sites (Squires & Bræstrup 1977, Mohler & Okada 1977), we have decided to search for a unifying mechanism, where a specific diazepam binding site becomes operative in mediating the facilitation of GABA-ergic transmission. This report summarizes the results obtained in support of the view that the specific binding site for benzodiazepines can be associated with the regulation of GABA-ergic transmission. We will show that high affinity binding of benzodiazepines and the regulation of Na^+ independent high affinity binding of GABA depend on the interaction of benzodiazepines with an endogenous membrane constituent which functions as a modulator of high affinity GABA binding.

REGULATION OF Na^+ INDEPENDENT HIGH AFFINITY BINDING OF GABA BY AN ENDOGENOUS PROTEIN

Electrophysiological evidence has shown that specific GABA recognition sites

Laboratory of Preclinical Pharmacology, National Institute of Mental Health, Saint Elizabeths Hospital, Washington, D.C. 20032 USA.

"GABA-NEUROTRANSMITTERS", Alfred Benzon Symposium 12, Munksgaard 1978

Table I.

Kinetic of Na independent ^{3}H-GABA binding to freshly prepared (type A) or frozen+Triton treated (type B) membrane preparations from rat cerebral cortex

	S.B. ^{3}H-GABA kinetic components			
	High affinity		Low affinity	
Crude synaptic membranes	K_{D1}	$Bmax_1$	K_{D2}	$Bmax_2$
Type A	*	*	218	2.4
Type B	20	1.8	111	5.3
Sup. Buff. Type A + Type B	*	*	195	3.9

K_D = Dissociation constant in nM. Bmax = maximal binding sites in pmoles/mg prot. Membranes were prepared according to Enna & Snyder (1977). The S.B. (specifically bound) ^{3}H GABA was measured using 200–250 μg membrane proteins in 1 ml volume with the method described by Enna & Snyder (1977). K_D and Bmax values were determined from Scatchard plot analysis. The kinetic constant were estimated at 0°.

* The high affinity component of ^{3}H-GABA binding became undetectable in the presence of the inhibitor. Supernatant was obtained by centrifuging Type A membrane preparations for 15 min at 30,000 × g.

are located on postsynaptic membranes and their function is associated with a Cl^- ionophore (Roberts 1974). Biochemical experiments have indicated that freshly prepared membranes from rat brain bind ^{3}H-GABA with a Km of about 200 nM (Enna & Snyder 1975). Since this Km value can be lowered by about tenfold by repeated freezing and thawing and Triton X-100 treatment of the membranes (Olsen *et al.* 1977, Enna & Snyder 1977) it was concluded that the function of GABA receptors in postsynaptic membranes is under the control of one or more modulatory factors.

In the organization of the neuronal membranes these modulators may represent an essential structural component in the supramolecular organization of the GABA receptor complex. In order to gain an insight on the presence and nature of the endogenous modulators for GABA receptors our strategy has been that of using measurement of specific ^{3}H-GABA binding to crude synaptic membranes of rat cerebral cortex in a Na^+-free medium.

When ^{3}H-GABA binding was measured in freshly prepared (Type A) or in frozen triton-treated (Type B) repeatedly washed membranes, in agreement with previous reports (Enna & Snyder 1977, Olsen 1978), we noticed a substantial difference in the kinetic characteristics of the binding (Table I). However, when the Type B membranes were reconstituted with the supernatant buffer obtained by centrifuging Type A membranes, the kinetic characteristics of this recombined preparation were similar to that of Type A membranes (Table I). These experiments suggest that an endogenous agent, in the crude synaptic membranes preparation, may modulate the affinity of GABA for its receptor. The next step in our strategy was to define the nature and the subcellular distribution of this modulator, as well as the type of cell it is present in. The modulator is not dialyzable, is thermostable (95°×15 min) and is destroyed by trypsin (4 h at 37°)

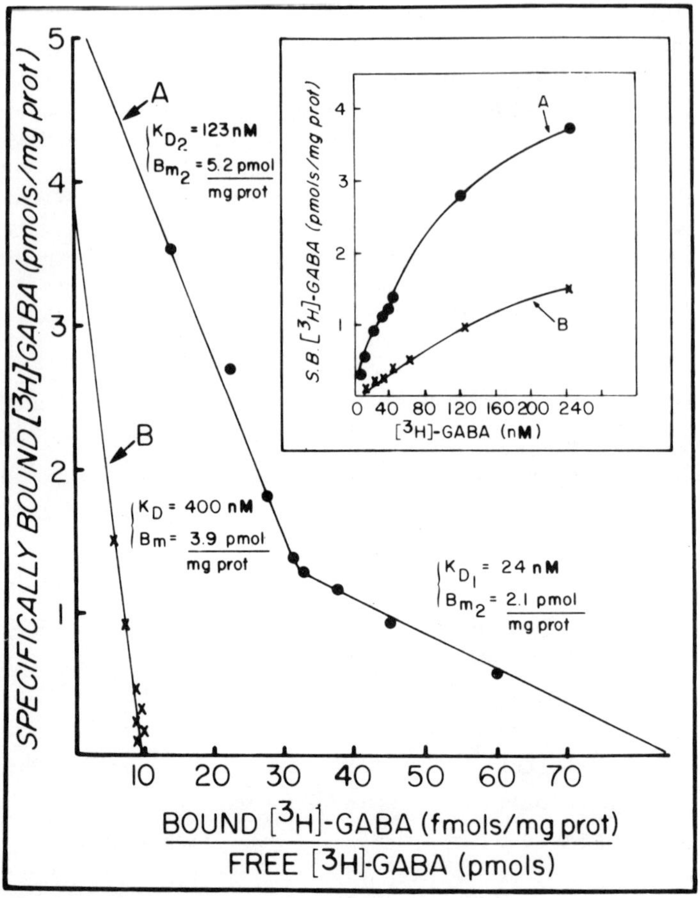

Fig. 1. Effect of purified (500fold) endogenous protein modulator of GABA binding on the Scatchard plot analysis of ^{3}H-GABA binding to type B membranes.

Type B membranes (200 μg prot) were incubated with (curve B) and without (curve A) 15 μg of purified modulator protein. K_D=dissociation constant in nM. B_m,=Total binding sites in pmoles/mg prot. In the insert the values of the specifically bound (S.B.) ^{3}H-GABA are plotted against the concentration of ^{3}H-GABA in the mixture.

Table II.

^{3}H-GABA, ^{3}H-diazepam binding and endogenous protein modulator in crude P_2 membrane fractions from cerebral cortex of rat and from C6 glioma cells

Tissue	Membrane treatment	S.B. ^{3}H-GABA K_D (nM)	S.B. ^{3}H-GABA Bmax (pmoles/mg prot)	S.B. ^{3}H-diazepam K_D (nM)	S.B. ^{3}H-diazepam Bmax (pmoles/mg prot)	Endogenous protein modulator (units/g tissue)
Rat brain cerebral cortex	Fresh	220	1.8	12	0.25	110
	Frozen+ Triton	20	5.3	6.8	0.15	–
C6 glioma cells	Fresh	210	0.45	11	0.35	150
	Frozen+ Triton	26	0.92	–	–	–

Membranes were prepared according to Enna & Snyder (1977) as modified by Toffano *et al.* (1978) The ^{3}H-GABA or ^{3}H-diazepam binding was carried out in Tris-citrate buffer pH 7.1. Endogenous protein modulator was assayed according to Toffano *et al.* (1978). S. B. = Specifically bound ^{3}H-GABA. The glioma cells were grown to confluency in Dulbecco's modified Eagel's medium containing 10% fetal calf serum, as described by Schwartz *et al.*(1977).

(Toffano *et al.* 1978). The modulator was purified by approximately 500fold by a series of procedures including gel filtration and ion exchange column chromatography. The purified modulator has an apparent molecular weight of about 15,000 dalton (Toffano *et al.* 1978). As shown in Fig. 1 the purified modulator added to Type B membranes will decrease the binding of GABA and will mask the presence of an high affinity site for GABA (see Fig. 1). Thus the action of the purified and of the crude modulator are similar (compare Table I and Fig. 1).

An analysis of the data reported in Fig. 1 reveals that the modulator acts noncompetitively to modify the affinity of the receptor for GABA. Among other possibilities we have proposed that this endogenous protein modulator indirectly interacts with some membrane component producing allosteric changes in the conformation of GABA receptors (Toffano *et al.* 1978).

Using ^{3}H-GABA binding to Type B membranes as a simple method to measure the modulator, questions about the distribution, the chemical nature and possible changes in the brain content following drug treatment may be easily explored. However in our opinion, among other problems, one of the points of major interest in interpreting the possible role of this modulator in the GABA receptor function *in vivo* was to know whether the GABA receptor site and the modulator were present in the same membranes. Since our experiments were performed in homogenates of brain, different type of cells could have contributed to the presence of GABA receptors and modulator protein in crude synaptic membranes. We have started, therefore, a search for cell lines which have on their membranes GABA receptors. We have found that the rat C6 glioma cell line possesses a significant amount of specific, saturable and high affinity receptor sites for GABA (Table II).

The sodium independent binding of GABA to these receptors is increased by detergent treatment (Table II). Thus, this cell line contains a receptor for GABA which resembles that measured in homogenates of brain cortex. In addition the supernatant obtained from freshly prepared membranes of C6 glioma cells contains a substantial amount of modulator for GABA receptors (Table II). These experiments indicate that the endogenous modulator protein of the high affinity component of GABA binding is present on the same membranes that contain GABA recognition sites and validate our tenet that this endogenous modulator may represent an important component of the supramolecular structure of GABA receptor complex (GABA receptor site + modulator + ionophore).

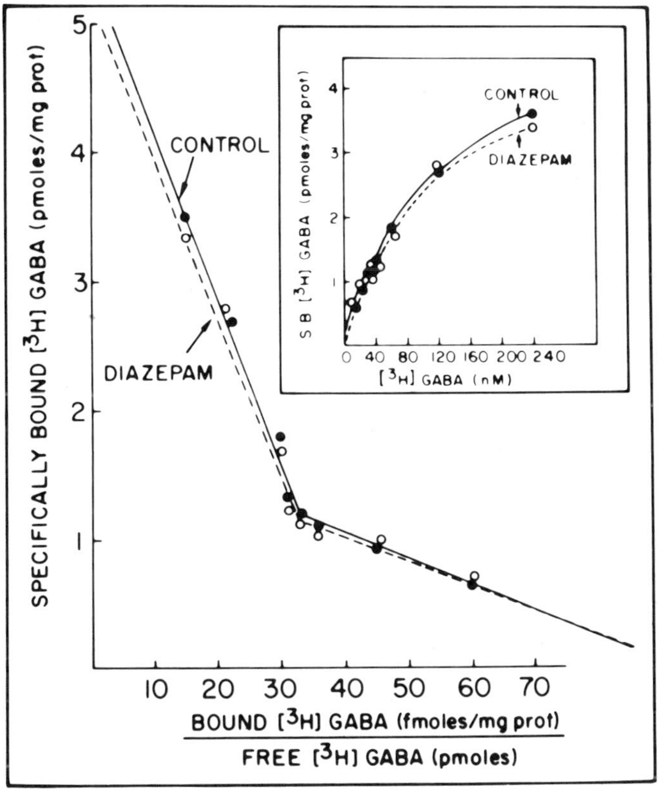

Fig. 2. Scatchard plot analysis for the binding of GABA to type B membranes (200 μg prot) in presence and absence of 5.10^{-7}M diazepam.

In the insert the values of the specifically bound (S.B.) ^{3}H-GABA are plotted against the concentration of ^{3}H-GABA in the mixture.

INTERACTION BETWEEN BENZODIAZEPINES AND ENDOGENOUS MODULATOR OF HIGH AFFINITY Na^+ INDEPENDENT GABA RECEPTORS

In keeping with neuropharmacological and neurophysiological evidence which indicates that benzodiazepines facilitate GABA receptor function by an indirect mechanism (Costa *et al.* 1975, Haefely 1978, Guidotti 1978) and in consideration of recent reports indicating that in various brain areas where benzodiazepine receptors are abundant there is also an abundance of high affinity GABA binding sites (Mohler & Okada 1977), we decided to explore in detail the possible action of benzodiazepines on the function of the GABA receptor complex. We have measured the action of benzodiazepines on ^{3}H-GABA binding in Type A (freshly prepared and rich in modulator) and Type B (frozen+triton treated; repeatedly washed, devoid of modulator) membranes. When benzodiazepines were added to Type B membranes no effect on ^{3}H-GABA binding was observed (Fig. 2). In contrast when Type A membranes were pretreated with benzodiazepines the affinity of the membranes for GABA was increased (Table III). However, addition of diazepam to Type B membranes in the presence of purified modulator prevents the inhibitory action of the modulator on GABA binding by a competitive mechanism (Costa *et al.* 1978, Guidotti *et al.* 1978).

The action of benzodiazepines on Type A membranes is therefore apparently mediated by an interaction between the benzodiazepines and the endogenous protein modulator.

As shown in Table IV the rank-order potency of different benzodiazepines in blocking the inhibition of the endogenous modulator on ^{3}H-GABA binding indicates that the *in vitro* interaction between benzodiazepines and endogenous modulator protein may be relevant to explain the *in vivo* action of benzodiazepines on GABA transmission. This conclusion is upheld by experiments with two benzodiazepine stereoisomers (Table IV).

Of course several questions have to be answered before it can be convincingly proved that benzodiazepines act via their interaction with the endogenous inhibitor. Among other problems it is important to establish whether the

Table III.

Effect of different benzodiazepines on the binding of GABA to freshly prepared crude synaptic membranes from rat cerebral cortex

	Conc (M)	K_{D1} (nM)	K_{D2} (nM)
Control		*	210
Diazepam	5.10^{-9}	*	190
	5.10^{-7}	61	200
	5.10^{-6}	34	321
	5.10^{-5}	26	285
Clonazepam	5.10^{-7}	35	265
Nitrazepam	5.10^{-7}	26	290
Flunitrazepam	5.10^{-7}	31	295
RO-11 3128 (+)	5.10^{-7}	43	315
RO-11 3624 (−)	5.10^{-7}	*	230
Muscimol	4.10^{-8}	*	420

* K_{D1} – undetectable.

Table IV.
Effect of various benzodiazepines on the K_i value for the endogenous protein modulator in comparison with their K_i values for ^{3}H-diazepam displacement

Drug	μg modulator (K_i)	^{3}H-diazepam displacement (K_inM)*
Solvent	1.0	-
RO-5-3027	18.0	1.3
Clonazepam	12.0	1.5
Flunitrazepam	11.0	2.8
RO-11 3128 (+)	3.2	3.6
Diazepam	3.0	6.3
Chlordiazepoxide	2.0	220
Medazepam	1.5	600
RO-5-4864	1.1	<1000
RO-11 3624 (−)	1.2	<1000

The K_i for the inhibitor was measured in presence of 10^{-6}M benzodiazepines. Each benzodiazepine was preincubated with frozen triton-treated membranes × 15 min at 0°.
* The K_i values for ^{3}H benzodiazepine displacement are from Mohler & Okada (1977).

benzodiazepine receptors, GABA receptors and the endogenous protein modulator are located in the same membrane.

This possibility is supported by indirect data such as the finding that freezing, thawing and treatment with Triton X-100 increases the K_D for GABA and the K_D for diazepam binding to brain membranes. Moreover the addition of the endogenous modulator to frozen membranes decreases the K_D for diazepam binding. Recently direct support for the view that the endogenous protein modulator, diazepam and GABA binding site reside in the same membrane came from studies in C6 glioma cells showing that these membranes contain high affinity diazepam binding sites, endogenous modulator and ^{3}H-GABA binding sites (Table II). Moreover when these membranes were frozen, thawed, washed and treated with Triton X-100, the K_D for GABA binding (Table II) was reduced.

CONCLUSION

The evidence presented supports a supramolecular model of the GABA receptor which includes an endogenous modulator that acts as an inhibitor of the high affinity binding sites for GABA. Since the total binding sites increase when the modulator is washed out from the membranes, we suggest that there are two populations of receptors and that the endogenous modulator masks the presence of the high affinity receptors for GABA. This function of the endogenous modulator could extend to other receptor functions in other or in the same cell because we know that a similar if not identical protein is present in many other tissues. We are proposing that diazepam and other benzodiazepines competitively interact with the binding of the endogenous modulator: the rank-order of this competitive interaction compares with that of the anxiolytic activity of these drugs. Since the site for the high affinity binding of diazepam has the same rank-order of the anxiolytic action, it follows that the high affinity binding site of diazepam would be that of the endogenous modulator. Implicit in this proposal is the attempt to explain a specific pharmacological response with an interaction of a drug with a protein, which, as we admit above, regulates GABA receptor function and possibly a number of other functions.

Preliminary work with this protein appears to indicate that it is an inhibitor of protein kinase. Thus, two characteristics should be considered in determining the profile of this modulator protein with regard to its potential as a substrate for drug action. On one hand, the active site for the antienzymatic action and on the other the specific binding to membrane sites. While the specific antienzymatic action would be identical for every endogenous location and function of this modulator protein, its specific binding sites could be "function" specific. We propose that the benzodiazepines would interact with a specific binding site of the endogenous modulator located on the GABA receptor.

As far as we know this is the first time that a specific protein part of a receptor has been isolated, purified and characterized as a site for drug action. The question then arises as to what we have learned as a general concept that we can apply to the mechanism of action of drugs? We have probably learned that the steric configuration which regulates modulator binding to the site of action may be more important for drug modeling than the active site of the molecule. In other words, according to our hypothesis we do not expect that inhibitors of protein kinase modeled after the active site of the endogenous modulators may be pharmacological antagonists of benzodiazepines, because although they may retain the capability of mimicking the endogenous inhibitor their action will not be as specific in competing with benzodiazepines.

The present studies have also opened a new avenue in pharmacology: the study of the antagonists of modulators of receptor function. Perhaps with the evidence presented here, receptor pharmacology has entered a new era.

REFERENCES

Choi, D. W., Ferb, O. H. & Fischbach, G. D. (1977) Chlordiazepoxide selectively augments GABA action in spinal cord cell cultures. *Nature* (London) 269, 342–344.

Costa, E., Guidotti, A., Mao, C. C. & Suria, A. (1975) New concepts on the mechanism of action of benzodiazepines. *Life Sci.* 17, 167–186.

Costa, E., Guidotti, A. & Toffano, G. (1978) Molecular mechanisms mediating the action of diazepam on GABA receptors. *Brit. J. Psychiat.* In press.

Enna, S. J. & Snyder, S. H. (1975) Properties of gamma-aminobutyric acid (GABA) receptor binding in rat brain synaptic membrane fractions. *Brain Res.* 100, 81–97.

Enna, S. J. & Snyder, S. H. (1977) Influence of ions, enzymes and detergents on gamma-aminobutyric acid receptor binding in synaptic membranes of rat brain. *Mol. Pharmacol.* 13, 442–453.

Guidotti, A. (1978) Synaptic mechanisms in the action of benzodiazepines. In: *Psychopharmacology: A generation of Progress,* ed. Lipton, M. A., DiMascio, A. & Killman, K. F. pp. 1349–1357. Raven Press, New York.

Guidotti, A., Toffano, G. & Costa, E. (1978) An endogenous protein inhibits Na^+ independent GABA binding and function as a ligand for benzodiazepine receptors in rat brain. *Nature* (in press).

Haefely, W. E. (1978) Behavioral and neuropharmacology aspects of drugs used in anxiety and related states. In: *Psychopharmacology: A Generation of Progress,* ed. Lipton, M. A., DiMascio, A. & Killman, K. F. pp. 1359–1374. Raven Press, New York.

McDonald, R. & Barker, J. L. (1977) Benzodiazepines specifically modulate GABA mediated postsynaptic inhibition in cultured mammalian. *Nature* 271, 563–564.

Olsen, R. W., Greenlee, D., Van Ness, P. & Ticku, M. K. (1978) Studies on the gamma-aminobutyric acid receptor/ionophore proteins in mammalian brain. In: *Amino Acids As Neurotransmitters,* ed. Fonnum, F., Plenum Press, New York. In press.

Polc, P., Mohler, H. & Haefely, W. E. (1974) The effect of diazepam on spinal cord activities: Possible sites and mechanism of action. *Naunyn-Schmiedeberg's Arch. Pharmacol.* 284, 319–337.

Roberts, E. (1974) Gamma-aminobutyric acid and nervous system function: A prospective. *Biochem. Pharmacol.* 23, 2637–2649.

Schwartz, J. P., Chuang, D. M. & Costa, E. (1977) Increase in nerve growth factor content of C6 glioma cells by the activation of a β-adrenergic receptor. *Brain Res.* 137, 369–375.

Squires, R. F. & Bræstrup, C. (1977) Benzodiazepine receptors in rat brain. *Nature* 266, 732–734.

Toffano, G., Guidotti, A. & Costa, E. (1978) Purification of an endogenous protein inhibitor for the high affinity binding of gamma-aminobutyric acid to synaptic membranes of rat brain. *Proc. Natl. Acad. Sci.* 75, 4024–4028.

Chapter IV
Animal Models for Testing GABA-ergic Drugs

Kainic Acid-Induced Lesion of the Striatum as an Animal Model for Huntington's Disease

Joseph T. Coyle, Kathleen Biziere, Peter Campochiaro, Robert Schwarcz & Robert Zaczek

Huntington's disease (HD) is a neurodegenerative disorder, inherited as an autosomal dominant, that is characterized by psychiatric symptoms, dementia and a movement disorder typically appearing in midlife (Bruyn 1968). The neuropathology of HD is primarily confined to the striatum, which undergoes severe atrophy resulting from degeneration of its intrinsic neurons; but to a lesser and variable extent, neuronal cell loss also occurs in other regions of the brain, in particular the deep layers of the cerebral cortex. With the pioneering studies of Perry *et al.* (1973) who demonstrated a marked reduction in the levels of γ-aminobutyric acid (GABA) in the striata of patients dying with HD, there has been a ferment of interest in identifying the types of neurons affected in this disorder. Studies from several groups have further shown that the striato-nigral GABA-ergic (Bird & Iversen 1974, McGeer & McGeer 1976) as well as substance P pathways degenerate (Kanazawa *et al.* 1977); in addition, striatal cholinergic neurons are affected whereas the nigro-striatal dopaminergic pathway remains relatively intact. Thus, on the basis of these neurochemical results and clinical pharmacologic studies, there is reason to believe that the dyskinesia and possibly the psychiatric symptoms in HD reflect a functional imbalance between the intact dopaminergic projection and the waning population of striatal neurons (Klawans 1970). The loss of striatal GABA-ergic neurons may play a particularly critical role in this equation since they provide

Departments of Pharmacology and Experimental Therapeutics and Psychiatry and the Behavioral Sciences, The Johns Hopkins University School of Medicine, Baltimore, Maryland 21205 USA

"GABA-NEUROTRANSMITTERS", Alfred Benzon Symposium 12, Munksgaard 1978

inhibitory feedback to the substantia nigra (Fonnum *et al.* 1974) as well as have direct influence on the release of dopamine from striatal terminals (Bartholini & Stadler 1977).

Progress in understanding the pathophysiology of HD and in developing more effective drugs to treat the disorder has been severely hampered by the lack of a suitable animal model. Since the symptoms of HD reflect a neuronal imbalance in the striatum, simply ablating the region does not provide an adequate model because this procedure does not create an inter-neuronal imbalance. What is required is a method that selectively kills striatal intrinsic neurons but leaves intact the axons projecting to the region from extra-striatal neuronal perikarya. Although agents such as 6-hydroxydopamine have been synthesized that kill monoaminergic neurons through selective accumulation by their presynaptic transport processes, similar neurotoxins have not been devised for the majority of central neurons including the GABA-ergic neurons. The identification and characterization of a suitable neurotoxin, kainic acid, is the subject of this review.

EXCITOTOXIC AMINO ACIDS

Since the original report of Lucas & Newhouse (1957) two decades ago, considerable evidence has accumulated that excitatory amino acids, of which glutamate is the prototype, can cause neuronal degeneration by excessive activation of receptors localized in the region of the neuronal cell body (Olney *et al.* 1972). The lesions resulting from systemic treatment with monosodium glutamate, however, are restricted to the arcuate nucleus of the hypothalamus and the neural retina and can be produced only during the early postpartum period for rodents (Perez *et al.* 1976). In order to restrict the lesion to the striatum and to avoid the variety of metabolic processes that inactivate free glutamate in the mature brain, our laboratory examined the effects of stereotaxic injection of the conformationally restricted analog of glutamate, kainic acid, into the adult rat striatum. Kainic acid is a heterocyclic compound containing the sequence of glutamate in its structure and is approximately 50-fold more potent than glutamate in depolarizing neurons in the mammalian central nervous system (Biscoe *et al.* 1976). Kainate is not, however, taken up by the glutamate high affinity transport process (Simon *et al.* 1976). Because of the localization of excitatory receptors on the neuronal dendrites and their absence from axons (Curtis *et al.* 1972), we hypothesized that the intrastriatal injection of kainic acid would kill neurons with cell bodies near the infusion site but spare axons from extrastriatal neurons.

NEUROCHEMISTRY OF THE STRIATAL KAINATE LESION

Stereotaxic injection of 10 nmoles of kainic acid diluted in 1 μl of artificial CSF into the rat striatum caused a degeneration of neurons with cell bodies in the region (Coyle & Schwarcz 1976). The presynaptic neurochemical markers for the cholinergic neurons – choline acetyltransferase, endogenous acetylcholine and the synaptosomal high affinity uptake of choline – were reduced by 60–70% at 10 days after injection (Table I). The presynaptic markers for the GABA-ergic

Table I

Neurochemical sequelae of striatal kainate injections in rat

Parameter	Units	Control	Injected	Δ%
		Striatum		
GABA-ergic neurons				
GAD	nmoles/mg/h	12.9±0.9	4.1±0.8	−68
GABA	nmoles/mg	2.2±0.2	0.7±0.1	−67
GABA uptake	pmoles/mg/4 min	16.5±1.3	7.1±1.2	−57
Cholinergic neurons				
CAT	nmoles/mg/h	20±1	6±1	−70
ACh	pmoles/mg	68±4	20±4	−71
Ch uptake	pmoles/mg/4 min	0.12±0.01	0.05±0.01	−60
Dopaminergic neurons				
TH	pmoles/mg/h	232±21	340±25	+47
DA	pmoles/mg	60±4	52±4	−13
DA uptake	pmoles/mg/4 min	2.4±0.3	3.1±0.3	+29
Non-specific				
MAO	pmoles/mg/h	17±2	15±1	−10
COMT	pmoles/mg/h	31±2	42±2	+35
Wet weight	mg	49±2	48±2	−2
Protein	μg/mg/tissue	173±7	165±9	−5
		Substantia nigra		
GABA-ergic neurons				
GAD	nmole/mg/h	35±1	15±1	−57
GABA	nmole/mg	10.5±0.3	4.4±0.4	−58
Dopaminergic				
TH	pmole/mg/h	96±14	88±13	−8

Rats received a unilateral injection of 10 nmoles of kainic acid in the striatum 5–10 days prior to sacrifice for neurochemical assays. The results are expressed as mean±S.E.M. of 6–12 separate preparations assayed in duplicate (from Schwarcz & Coyle 1977a, b).

neurons – glutamate decarboxylase, endogenous GABA and synaptosomal high affinity uptake of GABA – were similarly reduced. In contrast, the presynaptic markers for the dopaminergic terminals innervating the injected striatum – tyrosine hydroxylase, endogenous dopamine and synaptosomal high affinity uptake of dopamine – were not reduced. The neurochemical alterations evolved rapidly with significant reductions in the activities of choline acetyltransferase and glutamate decarboxylase detectable at 6 h postinjection, and maximal deficits achieved by 48 h. Notably, nonspecific enzymatic markers in the region such as monoamine oxidase and catechol–0–methyl transferase were not reduced as a result of the lesion. The neurochemical alterations were not restricted to the striatum, because a selective reduction in the presynaptic markers for the GABA-ergic nerve terminals in the substantia nigra also occurred (Schwarcz & Coyle 1977a); this is consistent with a degeneration of the striato-nigral GABA-ergic pathway.

NEUROPATHOLOGY OF THE STRIATAL KAINATE LESION

The neuropathologic alterations in the striatum were apparent as early as 2 h after injection (Coyle *et al.* 1978). Neuronal perikarya in the injected striatum first exhibited aggregation of cytoplasmic Nissl-substance with edematous changes in the neuropil; this progressed to severe shrinkage and angulation of the perikarya with chromatin clumping and pycnosis of the neuronal nuclei by 24 h after injection. Between 24 and 48 h after injection, the affected neurons underwent autolysis and only occasional clumps of nuclear chromatin remained at this time. Although virtually all striatal neuronal perikarya within a 1.5 mm radius of the injection site degenerated, at the periphery of the lesion the large striatal neurons appeared less vulnerable than the much more numerous small interneurons; this selectivity was especially apparent in the monkey caudate (DeLong & Coyle, in preparation). Between 4 and 14 days after injection, there was a marked proliferation of reactive astrocytes (Figs. 1A and B); electron photomicrographs revealed numerous Gitter-cells ingesting the remnants of the degenerated neurons. The myelinated bundles of internal capsule fibers that project from the cerebral cortex were spared by the neurotoxin; and glyoxylic acid histofluorescence microscopy confirmed the integrity of the nigro-striatal dopaminergic terminals in the lesioned striatum (Fig. 1C). Over several months, a progressive atrophy of the injected striatum took place resulting in hydrocephalus *ex vacuo*; notably, the severe astrocytic reaction also resolved to a considerable degree (Zaczek *et al.* 1978). These neurochemical and neuroanatomic studies provide compelling evidence that the striatal kainate injection causes degeneration of neurons with cell bodies near the infusion site but spared axons of passage or of termination derived from extra-striatal neurons.

BEHAVIORAL EFFECTS OF THE STRIATAL KAINATE LESION

The unilateral striatal kainate injection produced a characteristic behavioral syndrome in the rats (Schwarcz & Coyle 1977a). Upon awakening from anesthesia, the rats commenced spontaneous contraversive turning that lasted up to 24 h after injection. Between 2 and 6 days after injection, the rats were hypoactive and suffered from moderate adipsia and aphagia resulting in a 20% weight loss; this behavior is reminiscent of the ingestive abnormalaties following nigral 6-hydroxydopmine lesions (Ungerstedt 1971). During the subacute period, the rats also exhibited spontaneous ipsiversive rotation; but by 10 days after injection, the feeding abnormalities and the spontaneous motor asymmetry had largely resolved. However, a pharmacologic challenge of the chronically lesioned rats with indirectly or directly acting dopamine agonists precipitated ipsiversive rotation; this result is consistent with the loss of postsynaptic dopamine receptors measured biochemically in the lesioned striatum (Schwarcz *et al.* 1978a). Although lesioned rats do not develop dyskinesia, a monkey that had received multiple kainate lesions of the caudate, putamen and globus pallidus exhibited disturbances of fine motor coordination and repetitive adventitious movements of the contralateral extremities for several days after lesion (DeLong & Coyle, in preparation).

GABA RECEPTORS AND STRIATAL KAINATE LESION

The selective neuronal degeneration produced by striatal kainate lesion offers a method for determining the localization of neurochemical parameters since only neurons with cell bodies near the infusion site are destroyed and axons from extrinsic neurons and glia are spared. Since GABA is thought to exert synaptic influences both at the dendritic level as well as at axonal sites, the effects of striatal kainate lesion on the putative GABA receptor binding site were examined. The striatal kainate lesion caused a rapid increase in GABA receptor binding to 100% above control by 24 h after injection and to 200% above control by 48 h at which level it remained for 10 days after lesion (Campochiaro

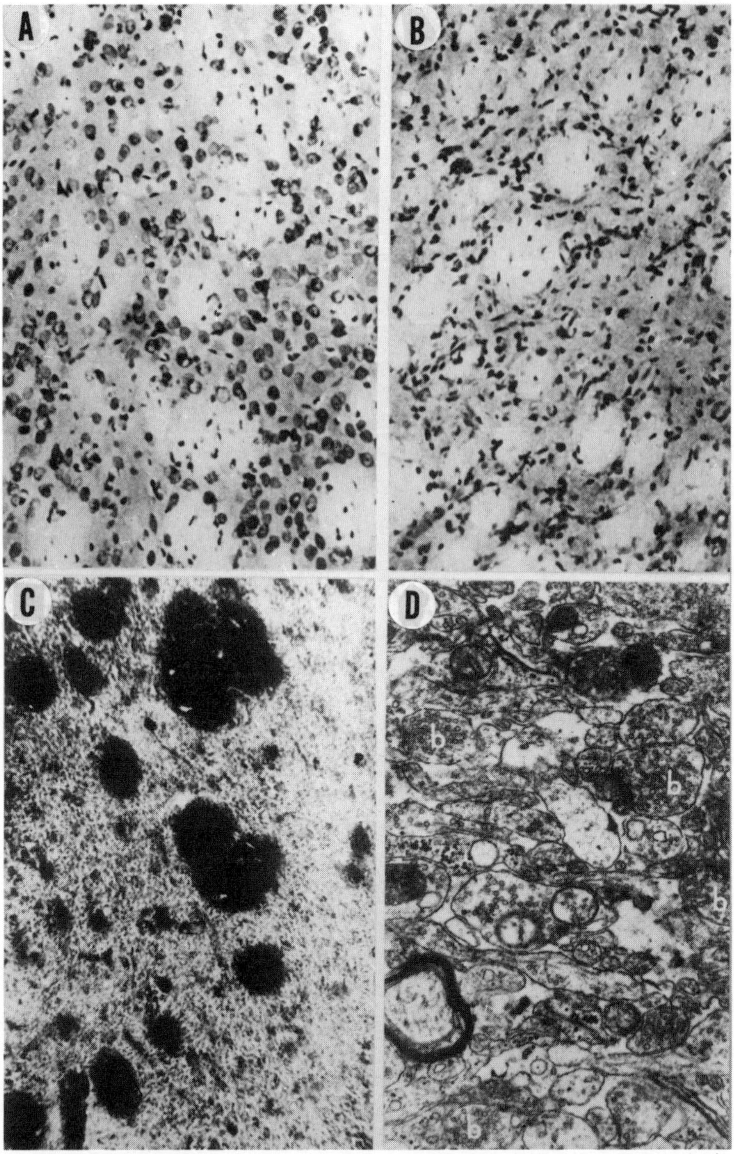

Fig. 1. A. Nissl-stained section of control striatum. Note the intrinsic neuronal perikarya surrounding the bundles of internal capsule fibers.

B. Nissl-stained section through the striatum 10 days after injection of kainic acid. Note the absence of intrinsic neuronal perikarya and the dense gliotic reaction that spares the internal capsule fibers.

C. Glyoxylic acid histofluorescence photomicrograph through the kainate-injected striatum. Note the dense field of catecholamine containing fluorescent fibers pierced by the uninnervated

et al. 1977). The time course of the increase in receptor binding was a mirror image of the reduction in the striatal levels of the presynaptic GABA-ergic markers, glutamate decarboxylase and endogenous GABA. The elevation in receptor binding did not appear to be due to an artifact of differential contamination of the membranes with endogenous GABA since extensive dialysis of the membranes prior to assay did not reverse the effect. Scatchard analysis of GABA binding in normal striatum revealed two components; a high affinity site with a K_D of 7.5 nmolar and B_{max} at 10.6 fmole/mg and a low affinity site with a K_D of 56 nmolar and B_{max} of 41 fmole/mg. In the kainate lesioned striatum, a single receptor site with a K_D of 19 nmolar and a B_{max} of 43 fmole/mg was observed.

Since striatal intrinsic neurons had degenerated following kainate injection, these results suggested that GABA receptor binding may have a presynaptic localization on axons of extrinsic neurons that survive the lesion. In support of this hypothesis, lesioning of the nigral dopaminergic cell bodies with 6-hydroxydopamine, which caused degeneration of the nigro-striatal dopaminergic pathway, significantly reduced GABA receptor binding in control striata by 22% and attenuated the increase in the kainate-lesioned striata by 33%. The conclusion that GABA receptors have an exclusively presynaptic localization in the striatum, however, must be tempered because electronmicroscopic studies have shown prolonged survival of postsynaptic densities adherent to surviving terminal boutons (Coyle *et al.* 1978). The postsynaptic membrane specializations are thought to be the regions enriched with neurotransmitter receptors (Fig. 1D). Furthermore, assay of striata 9 months after kainate lesion, in which these postsynaptic membrane specializations are no longer present revealed a marked 80% reduction in GABA receptor binding (Zaczek *et al.* 1978). Thus, the enhanced receptor binding for GABA appears to be restricted to the subacute period after lesion and dramatizes the complex alterations in neurochemical parameters that occur as the lesion evolves.

HUNTINGTON'S DISEASE AND STRIATAL KAINATE LESION

The numerous similarities between the neurochemical alterations in the rat

---

internal capsule fibers; Nissl-stained adjacent section reveals a complete absence of intrinsic neuronal perikarya.

D. Electronphotomicrograph through the neuropil of the kainate-injected striatum 10 days after kainate injection. Note several terminal boutons (b) that remain associated with degenerated postsynaptic processes. An intact myelinated axon is also visible. (from Coyle *et al.* 1978).

striatal kainate lesion and those occurring in the caudate, putamen and nigra of patients dying with HD have previously been described in detail (Coyle *et al.* 1977). In both conditions, the presynaptic GABA-ergic indices are reduced in the striatum and substantia nigra, and the cholinergic markers are depressed in the striatum whereas dopaminergic presynaptic markers appear relatively intact in both the striatum and substantia nigra. With regard to neurotransmitter receptors, muscarinic cholinergic and serotonin receptor binding are similarly depressed in both conditions (Schwarcz & Coyle 1977b, Schwarcz *et al.* 1977a). GABA receptor binding has been reported as normal or reduced in the striatum in HD and, depending upon the time after lesion, is elevated or reduced in the striatal kainate lesion. In terms of the neuropathology, in both conditions, a loss of neuronal perikarya in the striatum with sparing of the substantia nigra occurs; in the chronic kainate lesion, the striatal atrophy with hydrocephalus *ex vacuo* closely resembles that of HD. A notable difference between the two conditions involves the absence of cortical neuronal degeneration in the striatal kainate lesion. The symptoms of HD usually appear in midlife, rarely in childhood and never in infancy (Bruyn 1968); in this regard, it is noteworthy that striatal vulnerability to kainate is absent in the neonatal rat but develops between the second and third week after birth (Campochiaro & Coyle 1978). The relationship between the behavior in the kainate-lesioned rat and the neurologic and psychiatric symptoms of HD remains problematic because of major differences between rat and man in striatal circuitry and function; however, preliminary studies in the primate show promise of possible parallels.

PHARMACOLOGIC AUGMENTATION OF GABA

An advantage of an animal model for HD is that it offers an opportunity for testing drugs that may be of therapeutic value in HD. Because of the GABA-ergic deficit in the disorder, it seems reasonable that correction of this deficit may reduce the extrapyramidal symptoms. Since GABA is inactivated by deamination by GABA-aminotransferase (GABA-T), drugs that inhibit this enzyme elevate brain GABA levels. Two such drugs, γ-acetylenic GABA (GAG) and sodium valproate (VAL), were examined (Schwarcz *et al.* 1977b). Acute treatment with GAG (100 mg/kg) caused a dramatic increase in the GABA levels in the kainate-lesioned striatum and ipsilateral substantia nigra; this dose, however, was associated with marked sedation (Table II). Chronic administration of low doses of GAG (20 mg/kg) which did not grossly impair animal

Table II

Effects of GABA-T inhibitors on endogenous GABA

Treatment	Striatum	Substantia nigra
	nmoles/mg tissue	
Control	2.68±0.09	10.5±0.3
Ka-lesion	1.35±0.13*	4.4±0.4*
Ka-lesion & acute GAG (100 mg/kg)	4.10±0.25*	15.2±1.2*
Ka-lesion & acute VAL	1.97±0.08*	ND
Ka-lesion & chronic GAG (20 mg/kg)	2.82±0.35	ND

Rats received a unilateral injection of kainic acid (Ka) in the striatum 10 days prior to drug treatment. For acute treatments, the rats received an intraperitoneal injection of γ-acetylenic GABA (GAG), 100 mg/kg, or sodium valproate (VAL), 400 mg/kg, 4 h prior to sacrifice. For chronic treatment, rats received a daily injection of 20 mg/kg of GAG for 1 week. All values are the mean±S.E.M. of at least six animals (from Schwarcz *et al.* 1977a).

* $P<0.001$ vs control

ND=not determined.

behavior, restored striatal GABA levels in the kainate lesion to normal. In contrast, an extremely high dose of the reputed GABA-T inhibitor, sodium valproate (400 mg/kg), caused only a modest 40% increase in GABA levels in the kainate-lesioned striatum. Whereas GAG profoundly inhibited the activity of GABA-T extracted from the striata of treated rats, VAL did not affect the activity of the enzyme. Although it remains to be established whether the increased GABA levels after GAG treatment potentiate GABA-ergic neurotransmission in the surviving GABA-ergic processes, suicide substrates for GABA-T appear promising as new agents potentially effective in the treatment of HD.

MECHANISM OF NEUROTOXICITY OF KAINATE

Because of the number of similarities in the neuropathology and neurochemical alterations in the nigro-striatal circuit in the striatal kainate lesion and in HD, it is tempting to speculate that kainate's neurotoxicity may provide some insight into the primary defect in HD. Accordingly, it is imperative to understand better the mechanism of neurotoxic action of kainic acid. The selection of kainic acid as a potential neurotoxin was posited on the assumption that it was a potent glutamate agonist. A number of recent observations have called this hypothesis into question. Most importantly, we have been unable to demonstrate specific

Table III

Effects of decortication on the neurotoxicity of kainate and glutamate in the striatum

Lesion	Injection	CAT	GAD	TH
		Percent of Control		
None	none	100±2	100±2	100±5
None	Ka	28±5*	27±3*	145±8
Decortication	none	77±5*	103±5	118±8
Decortication	Ka	71±6*	96±5	118±8
Decortication	Glu	95±7	109±10	138±13
Decortication	Ka+Glu	41±5*†	73±7*†	135±10

Rats received a unilateral decortication 7 days prior to the injection of kainate (Ka, 10 nmoles) or glutamate (Glu, 1 μmole) into the striatum on the lesioned side. Three days after injection, the striata were assayed for the activities of choline acetyltransferase (CAT), glutamate decarboxylase (GAD) and tyrosine hydroxylase (TH). Results are presented in terms of percent (±S.E.M.) of unlesioned control and derived from six or more preparations assayed in duplicate (Biziere & Coyle 1978b).

* $P<0.01$ vs nonlesioned, noninjected

† $P<0.01$ vs decorticate, noninjected.

neurotoxicity of glutamate injected into the striatum at doses 500-fold greater than the threshold dose of kainic acid (Schwarcz *et al.* 1978); Nadler *et al.* (1978) have similarly reported that glutamate is virtually devoid of neurotoxic action in the hippocampus. If the potency of kainate simply reflected the restricted conformation of the carboxyl and nitrogen moities of the glutamate sequence, then dihydrokainate, which maintains this conformation, should be neurotoxic. To the contrary, dihydrokainate is inactive at 50 times the threshold dose of kainic acid. *In vitro* studies have revealed that kainic acid differs considerably from glutamate in terms of effects on the uptake of rubidium and water and on the levels of ATP in striatal slices (Biziere & Coyle 1978a). Taken together, these results do not support the original hypothesis that kainate is simply a potent analog of glutamic acid.

Electrophysiologic studies in invertebrates indicate that kainate is a weak neuroexcitant but potentiates the depolarizing action of glutamate by activating a distinctly different set of receptors (Daoud & Usherwood 1975, Walker 1976). In light of the association between glutamatergic innervation and neuronal vulnerability to kainate demonstrated in the cerebellum (Herndon & Coyle 1977), the possibility of an interaction between synaptically released glutamate and injected kainate was examined (Biziere & Coyle 1977b). The glutamatergic cortico-striatal projection was lesioned by removal of the parietal and frontal cortex overlying the striatum (Table III). The lesion was associated with 48% reduction in the synaptosomal uptake of glutamate and 55% reduction in endogenous glutamate in the ipsilateral striatum; in contrast, the presynaptic markers for the GABA-ergic neurons in the striatum were unaffected although choline acetyltransferase activity was slightly but significantly reduced. Prior cortical ablation completely blocked the neurotoxic action of 10 nmoles of kainate injected into the striatum; as is the case in the intact striatum, 1 μmole of glutamate was also devoid of neurotoxicity. However, co-injection of 10 nmole of kainate with 1 μmole of glutamate restored to a considerable degree the neurotoxic action of kainate on the striatal cholinergic and GABA-ergic neurons. These results indicate that kainate's potent neurotoxicity requires the integrity of cortical afferents to the striatum and may involve a cooperative interaction between synaptically released glutamate and the injected kainic acid.

CONCLUSION

These studies demonstrate numerous parallels between the neurochemical and neuropathologic alterations in HD and those occurring after injection of nanomole quantities of kainic acid into rat striatum. This animal model for HD allows for detailed neurochemical and neurophysiologic studies of the sequelae of striatal neuronal degeneration that are not possible in human subjects. With the animal model, drugs can be screened to determine whether they correct the neurotransmitter imbalances thought to be responsible for the symptoms of HD. The numerous similarities between the striatal kainate lesion and HD suggest that a better understanding of the neurotoxic action of kainic acid may shed light on the underlying defect that results in the progressive neuronal degeneration in HD. On a more basic level, the kainic acid lesion technique, although not specific for GABA-ergic neurons, nevertheless does offer a method for pharmacologically lesioning GABA-ergic neuronal perikarya. Studies in the striatum, retina (Schwarcz & Coyle 1977a), and cerebellum (Herndon & Coyle 1977) indicate that GABA-ergic neurons with cell bodies in these regions of the CNS are vulnerable to kainic acid. However, because the mechanism of neurotoxicity of kainic acid remains to be clarified, its application to lesion GABA-ergic neurons in other regions of the brain must be carefully assessed by neurochemical and histological techniques.

ACKNOWLEDGMENT

This research was supported by USPHS Grants MH 26654 and NS 13584 and RSDA K02–MH00125 to JTC and grants from the National Foundation and the McKnight Foundation.

REFERENCES

Bartholini, G. & Stadler, H. (1977) Evidence for an intrastriatal GABA-ergic influence on dopamine neurons of the cat. *Neuropharmacol.* 16, 343–349.

Bird, E. D. & Iversen, L. L. (1974) Huntington's chorea: postmortem measurement of glutamic acid decarboxylase, choline acetyltransferase and dopamine in basal ganglia. *Brain* 97, 457–472.

Biscoe, T. J., Evans, R. H., Headley, P. M., Martin, M. R. & Watkins, J. C. (1976) Structure-activity relations of excitatory amino acids on frog and rat spinal neurons. *Br. J. Pharmacol.* 58, 373–382.

Biziere, K. & Coyle, J. T. (1978a) Effects of kainic acid on ion distribution and ATP levels of striatal slices incubated *in vitro*. *J. Neurochem.* 31, 513–520.

Biziere, K. & Coyle, J. T. (1978b). Influence of cortico-striatal afferents on striatal kainic acid neurotoxicity. *Neurosci. Letts.* 8, 303–310.

Bruyn, G. W. (1968) Huntington's chorea: historical, clinical and laboratory synopsis. *Handbook of Clinical Neurology,* Vol. 6, p. 298. North Holland, Amsterdam.

Campochiaro, P., Schwarcz, R. & Coyle, J. T. (1977) GABA receptor binding in rat striatum: localization and effects of denervation. *Brain Res.* 136, 501–511.

Campochiaro, P. & Coyle, J. T. (1978) Ontogenetic development of kainate neurotoxicity: correlates with glutamatergic innervation. *Proc. Natl. Acad. Sci. USA* 75, 2025–2029.

Coyle, J. T. & Schwarcz, R. (1976) Lesion of striatal neurons with kainic acid provides a model for Huntington's chorea. *Nature* 263, 244–246.

Coyle, J. T., Schwarcz, R., Bennett, J. P. & Campochiaro, P. (1977) Clinical, neuropathologic and pharmacologic aspects of Huntington's disease: correlates with a new animal model. *Prog. Neuro-Psychopharmacol.* 1, 13–30.

Coyle, J. T., Molliver, M. E. & Kuhar, M. J. (1978) *In situ* injection of kainic acid: a new method for selectively lesioning neuronal cell bodies while sparing axons of passage. *J. Comp. Neurol.* 180, 301–324.

Curtis, D. R., Ruggan, A. W., Felix, D., Johnston, G. A. R., Trebecis, A. K. & Watkins, J. C. (1972) Excitation of mammalian neurons by acidic amino acids. *Brain Res.* 41, 283–301.

Daoud, A. & Usherwood, P. N. R. (1975) Action of kainic acid on a glutamatergic synapse. *Comp. Biochem. Physiol.* 52C, 51–53.

Fonnum, F., Grofova, I., Rinvik, E., Storm-Mathesin, J. & Walberg, F. (1974) Origin and distribution of glutamate decarboxylase in substantia nigra of the cat. *Brain Res.* 71, 77–92.

Herndon, R. & Coyle, J. T. (1977) Selective destruction of neurons by a transmitter agonist. *Sci.* 198, 71–72.

Kanazawa, I., Bird, E., O'Connell, R. & Powell, D. (1972) Evidence for a decrease in substance P content of substantia nigra in Huntington's chorea. *Brain Res.* 120, 387–392.

Klawens, H. L. (1970) A pharmacologic analysis of Huntington's chorea. *Eur. Neurol.* 4, 148–163.

Lucas, D. R. & Newhouse, J. P. (1957) The toxic effect of sodium-L-glutamate on the inner layers of the retina. *Arch. Ophthal.* 58, 193–201.

McGeer, P. L. & McGeer, E. G. (1976) Enzymes associated with the metabolism of catecholamines, acetylcholine, and GABA in human controls and patients with Parkinson's disease and Huntington's chorea. *J. Neurochem.* 26, 65–76.

Nadler, V., Perry, B. W. & Cotman, C. W. (1978) Intraventricular kainic acid preferentially destroys hippocampal pyramidal cells. *Nature* 271, 676–677.

Olney, J. W., Ho, O. L. & Rhee, V. (1972) Cytotoxic effects of acidic and sulphur-containing amino acids on the infant mouse central nervous system. *Exp. Brain Res.* 14, 61–76.

Perez, V. J., Olney, J. W., Frolichstein, C. F., Martin, J. F. & Cannon, W. O. (1976) Regional uptake of neurotoxic and nontoxic amino acids *in vivo* by the infant mouse brain. *Biochem. Pharmacol.* 25, 1415–1419.

Perry, T. J., Hansen, S. & Kloster, M. (1973) Huntington's chorea – deficiency of γ-aminobutyric acid in brain. *N. Eng. J. Med.* 288, 337–342.

Schwarcz, R. & Coyle, J. T. (1977a) Neurochemical sequelae of kainate injections in corpus striatum and substantia nigra of the rat. *Life Sci.* 20, 431–436.

Schwarcz, R. & Coyle, J. T. (1977b) Striatal lesions with kainic acid: neurochemical characteristics. *Brain Res.* 127, 235–249.

Schwarcz, R. & Coyle, J. T. (1977c) Kainic acid: neurotoxic effects after intraocular injection. *Invest. Ophthal & Vis. Sci.* 16, 141–148.

Schwarcz, R., Bennett, J. P. & Coyle, J. T. (1977a) Loss of striatal serotonin synaptic binding induced by kainic acid lesion: correlations with Huntington's disease. *J. Neurochem.* 28, 867–870.

Schwarcz, R., Bennett, J. P. & Coyle, J. T. (1976b) Inhibitors of GABA metabolism: implications for Huntington's disease. *Ann. Neurol.* 2, 299–303.

Schwarcz, R., Creese, I., Coyle, J. T. & Snyder, S. H. (1978a) Dopamine receptors localized on cerebral cortical afferents to rat corpus striatum. *Nature* 271, 766–768.

Schwarcz, R., Scholz, D. & Coyle, J. T. (1978b) Structure-activity relations for the neurotoxicity of kainic acid derivatives and glutamate analogues. *Neuropharmacol.* 17, 145–151.

Simon, J. R., Contrera, J. F. & Kuhar, M. J. (1976) Binding of [^{3}H]kainic acid an analogue of L-glutamate to brain membranes. *J. Neurochem.* 26, 141–148.

Ungerstadt, U. (1971) Adipsia and aphagia after 6-hydroxydopamine-induced degeneration of the nigro-striatal dopamine system. *Acta. Physiol. Scand.* Suppl. 367, 95–122.

Walker, R. J. (1976) The action of kainic acid and quisqualic acid on glutamate receptors of three identified neurons from the brain of the snail; Helix Aspera. *Comp. Biochem. Physiol.* 55C, 61–67.

Zaczek, R., Schwarcz, R. & Coyle, J. T. (1978) Long-term sequelae of striatal kainate lesion. *Brain Res.* 152, 626–632.

GABA-Dopamine Interactions: Studies Using a New Enzyme-Activated Irreversible Inhibitor of GABA-Transaminase, γ-Acetylenic GABA

M. G. Palfreyman, Sylvie Huot, B. Lippert & P. J. Schechter

There is now considerable evidence for a descending striato-nigral pathway which uses GABA as a neurotransmitter and thereby modulates the activity of the ascending nigro-striatal dopamine pathway at the level of the substantia nigra (Tarsy *et al.* 1975, Dray & Straughan 1976). In addition, several experimental results suggest that GABA has a second action in the nigra that does not involve directly the ascending nigro-striatal dopamine pathway (Koob *et al.* 1976, Waddington 1976, 1977, 1978, Oberlander *et al.* 1977).

Of particular interest is the role of GABA in the limbic system, since this pathway has been implicated in the pathogenesis of schizophrenic states (see Baldessarini 1977 for recent review). It is known that GABA occurs in high concentrations in the limbic system (Fahn 1976) and it was therefore of interest to examine if GABA had any effect on limbic dopaminergic activity.

We have used an enzyme-activated irreversible inhibitor of 4-aminobutyrate: 2-oxoglutarate aminotransferase (E.C.2.6.1.19; GABA-T), namely γ-acetylenic GABA (4-aminohex-5-yonic acid; GAG) (Jung & Metcalf 1975, Metcalf, this conference), to elevate brain GABA concentrations and have examined the effect of these elevated GABA concentrations on central dopaminergic pathways by biochemical and pharmacological methods. Our results provide additional evidence for a complex inhibitory role of GABA in the substantia nigra and are consistent with inhibition of limbic dopamine pathways.

Centre de Recherche Merrell International, 16 rue d'Ankara, 67084 Strasbourg Cedex, France.

Table I
Effect of γ-acetylenic GABA (GAG) 100 mg/kg IP on GABA-transaminase activity of various regions of the rat brain 6 h after treatment

Region	GABA-T activity (nmoles/mg protein/hr ± SEM) Saline	GAG	% control
Substantia nigra	600±94 (5)	148±34 (4)*	25
Ventral tegmental area	903±206 (4)	140±11 (5)*	15
Caudata/Putamen	728±62 (5)	90±9 (5)**	12
Nucleus accumbens	787±76 (4)	109±6 (5)**	14
Olfactory tubercles	846±112 (4)	115±17 (5)**	14
Hypothalamus	744±94 (5)	134±20 (5)**	18

* $P<0.005$ compared to saline-injected
** $P<0.001$ compared to saline-injected
()=number of animals.

BIOCHEMICAL INVESTIGATIONS

As described by Metcalf (this conference) γ-acetylenic GABA (GAG) produces a profound and long lasting inhibition of GABA-T associated with a substantial increase in whole brain GABA concentrations. Since we were interested in various dopaminergic pathways in the brain, we verified that GABA-T inhibition occurred in these dopamine-containing regions. GABA-T activity was measured by the method used by Jung *et al.* (1977) in microdissected or micropunched samples from a large number of brain regions 6 h after an IP injection of 100 mg/kg of GAG. As can be seen from Table I, GABA-T activity was profoundly inhibited in all the dopamine-containing regions shown, as well as in all other parts of the brain examined.

It was reasoned that if GABA were inhibitory on dopaminergic neurons then by increasing GABA concentrations with GAG two possible effects might be seen: 1) an increase in steady state dopamine concentrations secondary to decreased impulse flow (Andén & Stock 1973, Stock *et al.* 1973), or 2) a decrease in the turnover of dopamine. Dopamine concentrations were therefore determined (Shellenberger & Gordon 1971) after GAG injections alone and following α- methyl-p-tyrosine (AMPT) treatment (Andén 1974). In the striatum and olfactory tubercles, but not the nucleus accumbens, GAG (100 mg/kg IP 4 h postdose) significantly elevated the steady state dopamine concentrations (Table II). When AMPT was administered 4 h before the rats were sacrificed, a significant decrease in dopamine concentrations was observed: 73% in the

Table II

Effect of γ-acetylenic GABA (GAG) (100 mg/kg IP) on α-methyl-p-tyrosine methyl ester (AMPT) (300 mg/kg IP)-induced disappearance of dopamine and on homovanillic acid concentrations in various brain regions of the rat 4 h after treatment (μg/g±SEM; n=6)

Dopamine	Treatment	Striatum	Olfactory tubercles	Nucleus accumbens
	Saline	2.92±0.35	1.96±0.23	1.24±0.06
	AMPT	0.79±0.38* (−73%)	0.75±0.14* (−62%)	0.60±0.07* (−52%)
	GAG	4.12±0.43*	2.96±0.39*	1.06±0.12
	GAG+AMPT	2.38±0.22 (−42%)	1.61±0.13 (−46%)	0.94±0.11* (−11%)
Homo-vanillic acid	Saline	0.55±0.08	0.32±0.02	-
	GAG	0.21±0.04 (−62%)	0.16±0.03* (−50%)	-

* $P<0.05$ compared to saline-injected.
Percent change in parenthesis.

striatum, 62% in the olfactory tubercles and 52% in the nucleus accumbens. When GAG was administered with AMPT, the decrease in dopamine was less marked: 42% in the striatum, 46% in the olfactory tubercles and 11% in the nucleus accumbens. Homovanillic acid concentrations (Murphy *et al.* 1969) 4 h after 100 mg/kg GAG showed a decrease in both the striatum and olfactory tubercles (Table II). These data suggest that GAG, and thus presumably GABA, are reducing dopamine turnover in both the extrapyramidal and limbic pathways.

Although a number of authors have suggested the existence of a descending striato-nigral pathway in which GABA is a neurotransmitter (Stock *et al.* 1973, Fonnum *et al.* 1974), a similar limbic ventral mesocephalic tegmental GABA-ergic descending pathway does not seem to exist (Fonnum *et al.* 1977). GABA is present, however, in reasonably high concentrations in the ventral mesocephalic tegmental area (VMA) or A10 region (Fahn 1976). In addition, the experiments reported by Stevens *et al.* (1974) suggest that in cats, bicuculline injections into the VMA, produce behavioral changes. We therefore investigated the effect of stereotaxically-placed unilateral injections of GAG into the VMA of rats on dopamine turnover by measuring the dopamine concentrations and AMPT-induced decrease of dopamine in the striatum and limbic system (olfactory tubercles and nucleus accumbens combined) of both sides of the brain (Fig. 1). Injection of 10 μg GAG into the right VMA markedly reduced the dopamine turnover in the right limbic forebrain (as compared to the left uninjected side). GAG injections, however, produced a small (not statistically significant)

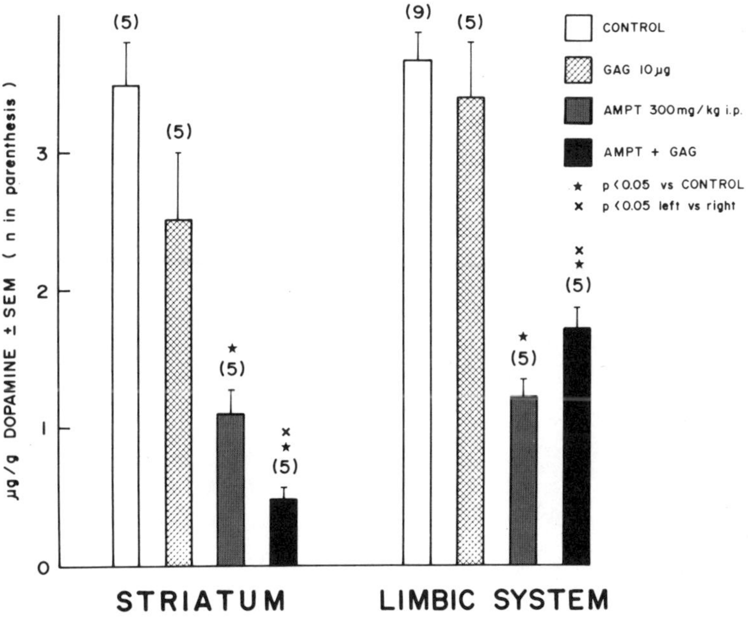

Fig. 1. Effect of γ-acetylenic GABA (GAG) injected into the right ventral tegmental area (A10) on dopamine turnover in the striatum and limbic system as estimated by dopamine disappearance induced by α-methyl-p-tyrosine methyl ester (AMPT). The results show the unilateral concentrations of dopamine in μg/g (mean ± SEM) in the striatum and in the nucleus accumbens and olfactory tubercle combined (limbic system) of the left side of control rats (left A10 uninjected), the right side 4 h after injection of GAG (10 μg in 1 μl saline) into the right A10 area, the left side 4 h after AMPT treatment, (300 mg/kg IP); and the right side 4 h after the combination of GAG injection into the right A10 area (10 μg in 1 μl saline) plus AMPT treatment (300 mg/kg IP). Numbers in parenthesis indicate number of rats used per determination.

decrease in the striatal dopamine content. The AMPT-induced decrease in striatal dopamine was significantly greater ($P<0.05$) in the GAG-injected animals although the absolute difference was similar to that seen following GAG injections alone. The results therefore suggest that GAG, presumably by increasing GABA, can inhibit limbic dopamine pathways at the level of the cell bodies of this system, but a possible influence on striatal dopamine pathways, perhaps resulting from limbic-striatal interactions, must also be considered. In contrast intranigral injections of GAG caused a reduction in dopamine turnover in the striatum without influencing limbic dopamine turnover (Data not shown).

PHARMACOLOGICAL AND BEHAVIORAL INVESTIGATIONS

In view of the biochemical evidence of reduced dopaminergic activity following

GAG injections we investigated several animal models to determine if this decrease in dopaminergic activity could be demonstrated in behavioral terms. Initially we examined the effect of unilateral intranigral injections of GAG on turning behavior to confirm what previous investigators had observed with other techniques designed to unilaterally alter the GABA-ergic system of the substantia nigra (Dray *et al.* 1975, Tarsy *et al.* 1975, Koob *et al.* 1976, Waddington 1976, 1977, Oberlander *et al.* 1977). It is believed that the direction of rotation is indicative of the relative balance between the two nigrostriatal pathways (Glick *et al.* 1977), although the original concept of turning behavior being an entirely dopamine-mediated phenomenon (Ungerstedt 1971) has been modified (Costall *et al.* 1976). In order to control for spread of injected material after intranigral injection, GABA-T activity was determined in micropunch samples from the substantia nigra and surrounding areas 5 h after unilateral intranigral injections of 20 μg GAG in 2 μl saline. The most prominent inhibition of GABA-T was seen in the nigra with gradually diminishing inhibition at more distal sites (Fig. 2a). No contralateral inhibition of GABA-T

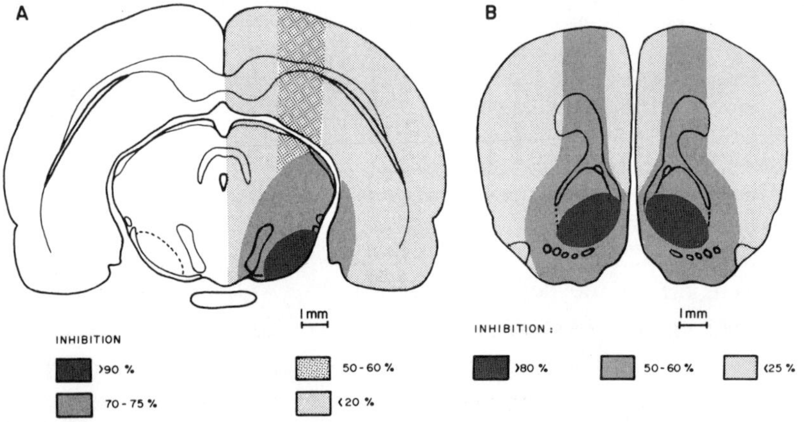

Fig. 2. Effect of intracranial injection of γ-acetylenic GABA (GAG) on GABA-transaminase activity of rat brain. The hatching on the diagram represents the mean percentage inhibition (mean of four rat brains)of GABA-transaminase of a 1-mm thick slice cut at (A) the level of the substantia nigra following 20μg GAG in 2 μl saline injected into the right substantia nigra and (B) following bilateral injections of 5 μg GAG/side in 2 μl saline into the nucleus accumbens. Four control rats were injected either unilaterally into the substantia nigra or bilaterally into the nucleus accumbens with 2 μl saline. Control values were taken as 100%. In the nigral slice control values ranged from 300–500 nmoles/mg protein/h and in the nucleus accumbens slice from 115–450 nmoles/mg protein/h. In the nigral slice the left uninjected side showed no inhibition of GABA-transaminase activity. Figures are taken from the atlas of Pelligrino & Cushman (1967) at the following levels (A) -3.8 (B) 4.0.

Table III

Effect of unilateral intranigral injections of γ-acetylenic GABA (GAG) on dexamphetamine and apomorphine-induced ipsilateral turning

	Ipsilateral turns/min±SEM*(n=8)		
	Dexamphetamine		Apomorphine
	3 mg/kg IP	6 mg/kg IP	6 mg/kg IP
GAG 20 μg	3±1	6±2	
GAG 40 μg	5±2	6±1	5±1

* determined over 2-h period, 5–7 h after GAG treatment.

was observed. The placement of the intranigral injections were also verified histologically.

Rats were prepared with unilateral indwelling cannulae aimed at the right substantia nigra. Two to 3 days later the rats were injected via the guide cannulae into the substantia nigra with 20 or 40 μg GAG in 2 μl saline and were then observed for the subsequent 5 h. Shortly after injection all the rats displayed marked *contralateral* torsion of the neck and trunk which, in approximately 50% of the animals, was superseded by contralateral turning (7±2 turns/min). This contralateral turning could not be modified by subcutaneous haloperidol (0.5 mg/kg) given 30 min after the GAG injections. *Contralateral* turning has been reported by several other authors (Koob *et al.* 1976, Waddington 1976, 1977, Oberlander *et al.* 1977) and has been interpreted as evidence for excitatory (or disinhibitory) effects of GABA in the nigra. It is believed that this contralateral turning does not involve GABA-dopamine interactions since it is not modified by haloperidol (Oberlander *et al.* 1977 and our experiments). The contralateral turning lasted approximately 4 h and had totally ceased by 5 h after GAG injection. Rats were then injected IP with various doses of amphetamine or apomorphine and observed for a further 2 hours. Both amphetamine and apomorphine induced strong *ipsilateral* turning (Table III) suggesting indirectly that GAG is able to modify ascending nigro-striatal dopamine pathways. Furthermore, 4 h after parenteral administration of GAG there is an attenuation of the ipsilateral turning provoked by amphetamine in striataly 6-hydroxydopamine-lesioned mice (S. D. Echols, personal communication). Injections of saline into the nigra or injections of saline IP into animals pretreated with intranigral GAG produced no *ipsilateral* turning. Rats injected with GAG more than 1 mm from the nigra were totally devoid of any postural asymmetry either before or after amphetamine. Whether the inhibitory effect of apomorphine on dopamine deamination as reported by Di Chiara *et al.* (1974) or the existence of other nondopaminergic pathways as suggested by Costall *et al.* (1976) are involved in the apomorphine-induced turning is at present unknown. Thus it would appear that there are two effects of GAG on nigral neurons, one of which appears to be inhibitory on ascending dopaminergic nigro-striatal nerves and the other which is excitatory, or disinhibitory, on nondopaminergic pathways.

For studies in the limbic system we initially chose the hypermotility model described by Costall & Naylor (1975) whereby bilateral injections of dopamine into the nucleus accumbens induce a strong locomotor stimulation of rats. Conscious hand-held rats with bilateral indwelling cannulae aimed at the nucleus accumbens were injected with 5 or 10 μg GAG in 2 μl saline/side 3 h before a bilateral injection of 25 μg dopamine in 2 μl saline side. All rats were dosed orally with 100 mg/kg isocarboxazid 2 h before dopamine injections. To

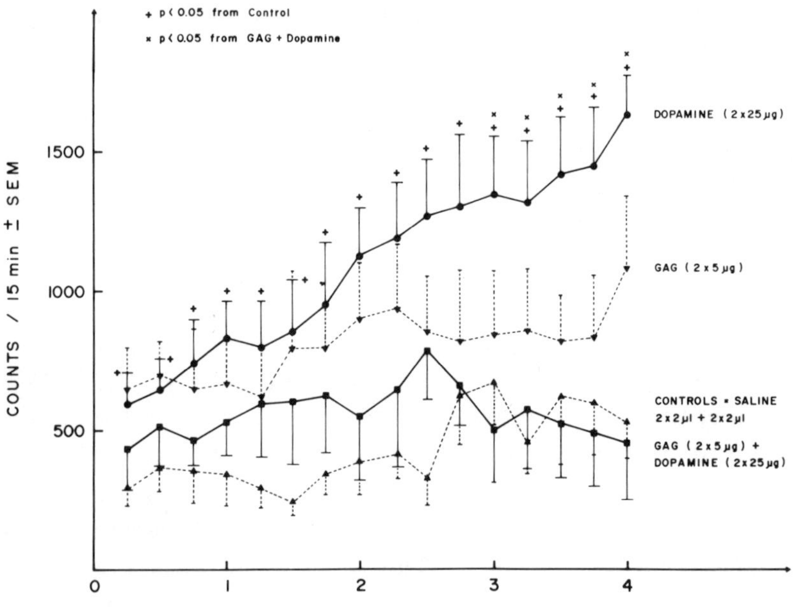

Fig. 3. Effect of intranucleus accumbens injection of γ-acetylenic GABA (GAG) on dopamine-induced locomotor activity. Groups of six rats were injected bilaterally into the nucleus accumbens with 2 μl saline/side 3 h before a bilateral injection of 2 μl/side saline (▲); with 5 μg GAG/side 3 h before a bilateral injection of 2 μl saline/side (▼); with 2 μl saline/side 3 h before a bilateral injection of 25 μg dopamine/side (●); or with 5 μg GAG/side 3 h before 25 μg dopamine/side (■). Locomotor activity is shown as counts/15 min (mean ± SEM) for the 4 h following the last injection.

verify the distribution of GAG after injections into the nucleus accumbens we determined GABA-T activity in various regions in and surrounding the nucleus accumbens 4 h after bilateral injections of 10 μg GAG in 2 μl saline/side. The enzyme inhibition was most prominent in the accumbens but limited diffusion to other more distal regions was indicated (Fig. 2b). Injection sites were also verified histologically. Locomotor activity was recorded automatically (Stoelting Activity Meter). Rats injected with dopamine alone showed a strong and longlasting increase in locomotor activity when compared to saline injected controls (Fig. 3). However, when GAG was injected prior to the dopamine it markedly attenuated the dopamine-induced increase in locomotor activity. In a similar experiment rats were injected into the nucleus accumbens with dopamine. Once the locomotor stimulation was clearly established, GAG was injected IP at 50 mg/kg and the locomotor activity recorded for a further 4 h. Again GAG significantly reversed the dopamine-induced locomotor stimulation. This dose of GAG was totally devoid of any locomotor inhibitory effect in animals injected into the nucleus accumbens with saline.

Although GAG administered systemically raises GABA throughout the brain the predominant effect on dopamine-stimulated locomotor activity is probably at the level of the limbic system, since we find that small amouts of GAG (5–10 μg) injected into the cerebral cortex lying just above the nucleus accumbens do not attenuate dopamine-induced hyperactivity. In fact, injections of GAG into the cortex produce excitation and locomotor stimulation. A similar stimulation is also seen after intraventricular (50–100 μg) or very large (~ 250 mg/kg) intraperitoneal injections of GAG.

Other authors have reported inhibition of dopamine-induced locomotor activity following either ethanolamine-O-sulphate (Pycock & Horton 1976) or muscimol injected into the nucleus accumbens (Scheel-Krüger *et al.* 1977). With the exception of the experiments reported by Stevens *et al.* (1974) little is known about the action of GABA in cell bodies of the limbic system. Although both GABA concentrations and GAD activity are fairly high in the ventral tegmental area (Fonnum *et al.* 1977), there does not appear to be a descending limbic ventral tegmental pathway using GABA as a neurotransmitter since hemisection did not alter GAD activity of the VMA (Fonnum *et al.* 1977) but significantly reduced nigral GAD (Fonnum *et al.* 1974). On the other hand, our results suggest that the injection of GAG into the VMA inhibits dopamine turnover in the limbic forebrain. This may be due to stimulation of GABA-ergic interneurons which lie in the VMA and which inhibit the dopaminergic cell

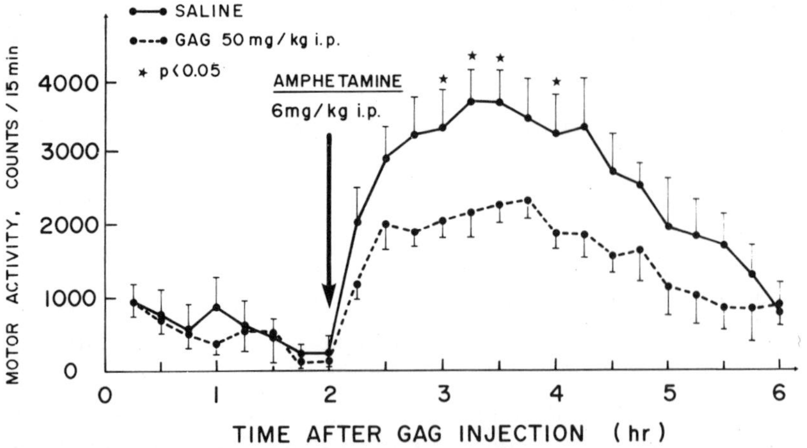

Fig. 4. Effect of γ-acetylenic GABA on amphetamine-induced locomotor activity in rats: Groups of six rats were injected IP with 50 mg/kg γ-acetylenic GABA or with saline and their locomotor activity automatically recorded at 15-min intervals for the next 2 h. All rats were then injected IP with 6 mg/kg dexamphetamine and their activity recorded for a further 4 h. The figure shows the locomotor activity (counts/15 min ± SEM). Statistical significance $P<0.05$ (Student's t-test – two tailed) is shown by the asterisks.

bodies in this region. Thus it would appear that GAG, presumably by elevating GABA, inhibits dopaminergic activity of the limbic system at at least two levels, i.e. the cell bodies and the nerve endings.

Since experiments in which injections of GAG into the nucleus accumbens, the ventral mesencephalic tegmental area and the peripheral circulation strongly suggested an inhibitory effect of GAG on limbic dopamine activity, it was of interest to validate these observations in various other animal models believed to involve limbic dopamine activity. It has been suggested that the locomotor stimulant effects of amphetamine are predominantly related to the release of dopamine in limbic structures (Iversen & Koob 1977). Rats were therefore injected IP with 50 mg/kg GAG or with saline 2 h before the IP injection of various doses of amphetamine (2–6 mg/kg). Locomotor activity was then recorded for the subsequent 4 h. This dose of GAG was totally devoid of effects on the locomotor activity of control rats but depressed the locomotor stimulant effects of amphetamine (Fig. 4). Over the dose range of amphetamine examined GAG displaced the dose-response curve of amphetamine to the right, again suggesting an inhibitory effect of GAG on the dopaminergic activity of the limbic system.

It is known that neuroleptic dopamine receptor blockers are very effective at inhibiting conditioned avoidance at doses which do not inhibit locomotor activity (Cook & Catania 1964). However, it is not known for certain if this behavior is entirely dependent on the activity of limbic dopamine receptors (Laverty & Taylor 1970), although this effect is certainly important (Cooper *et al.* 1972, 1973, Stern *et al.* 1972). Since we postulate that GAG can inhibit limbic dopaminergic activity, although probably not by a direct blockade of dopamine receptors, the conditioned avoidance model might provide additional information about limbic dopamine interactions. Rats were trained in a standard automated shuttle box (Tech. Serv. Inc., Maryland) until they achieved 90% or greater avoidance responding. Groups of rats were then injected with GAG 50 mg/kg IP or with saline 4 h prior to avoidance testing. This dose of GAG significantly reduced the percentage avoidance without significantly affecting avoidance or escape latency (Table IV).

A second behavioral model we have examined is the positive reinforcement responding model. Although positive reinforcement has been less well characterized in neurotransmitter terms, Schoenfeld & Seiden (1969) have emphasized the role of catecholamines in this behavior. Rats were trained to press a lever to obtain food pellets. Once a stable responding rate had been obtained, rats were injected with GAG, 50 mg/kg IP, and 4 h later their lever pressing rates recorded. This dose of GAG significantly reduced lever pressing for food reward (Table IV). The interpretation of this finding is circumstantial in terms of GABA-dopamine interactions and will need further investigation.

GENERAL DISCUSSION

γ-Acetylenic GABA inhibits GABA-T activity in all component parts of the dopaminergic systems examined and this inhibition is associated with a significant increase in GABA concentrations in these areas (unpublished observations). However, the cellular localization of this augmented GABA arising from treatment with γ-acetylenic GABA, or other GABA-T inhibitors, is not known. The characteristic pharmacological and behavioral effects following administration of potent GABA-T inhibitors (Schechter *et al.* 1977a, 1977b) indirectly suggest that at least some of the increased GABA may be involved with synaptic events in brain. Furthermore, the experimental data presented here also point to functional effects of elevated GABA concentrations.

The biochemical evidence we have presented suggests that elevated GABA

Table IV

Effect of γ-acetylenic GABA (GAG) on conditioned avoidance and positive reinforcement behavior

Treatment	Conditioned avoidance No. of avoidances in 100 trials (mean±SEM)	Positive reinforcement No. of lever presses in 10 min (mean±SEM)
Saline (0.5 ml/kg IP) 4-h postdose	94±1 (20)	91±7 (12)
GAG (50 mg/kg IP) 4-h postdose	75±4 (20)*	43±9 (12)*

* $P<0.001$ paired t-test.
Number of animals in parenthesis.

produced by GAG inhibits dopamine turnover in both the extrapyramidal and limbic systems. A similar inhibition of dopamine turnover following amino-oxyacetic acid has been reported by Andén (1974). In the striatum and olfactory tubercles GAG pretreatment causes a small increase in steady state concentrations of dopamine, while not affecting the dopamine content of the nucleus accumbens. This difference may reflect differences in intrinsic dopamine turnover in these areas. A similar increase in striatal dopamine has also been reported following γ-hydroxybutyrate treatment (Gessa *et al.* 1966, Andén & Stock 1973) and is presumably due to reduced impulse flow in nigro-striatal dopamine nerves (Stock *et al.* 1973).

Although the effects of GAG on the turnover of dopamine in the striatum are strongly indicative of an inhibitory role of GABA on ascending nigro-striatal dopamine neurons, the direct investigation of the phenomena by pharmacological means, i.e. rotational behavior, reveal that this pattern of inhibition is quite complex. Both inhibitory effects and excitatory (or disinhibitory) non-dopaminergic effects of elevated GABA in rotational behavior could be demonstrated.

In the limbic system, only inhibitory actions of GABA could be shown. However, none of the behavioral models so far examined distinguish between modification of dopaminergic activity in limbic nerve endings or cell bodies, nor do they exclude the possibility that GABA alters these behaviors by mechanisms that do not involve dopaminergic pathways. One model to assess the significance of the action of GABA at the level of the limbic cell bodies might be self-stimulation in the rat since electrodes placed in the ascending limbic dopamine pathway appear able to sustain self-stimulation (G. Anlezark, personal communication). Whether modulation of the cell bodies of the limbic dopamine pathway by GABA is as complex as the nigral effects of GABA therefore remains to be examined.

Our experiments with conditioned avoidance clearly indicate that elevation of brain GABA is associated with a significant decrement in avoidance responding at doses of GAG which cause no overt locomotor or behavioral deficit, an effect similar to the action of neuroleptic agents in this model. Since our data suggest that GABA inhibits dopamine pathways by a mechanism different from that of the neuroleptics, it will be interesting to see if GAG can potentiate the effects of neuroleptics on conditioned avoidance.

Our experiments on positive reinforcement indicate that elevated GABA concentrations are associated with a decreased lever pressing for food reward. We originally conceived this model as a way of examining the effect of GABA elevation on motivated behavior since it has been suggested that the limbic dopamine pathways might be involved in this behavior (Cook & Catania 1964, Kelleher & Morse 1964). However, on further examination it is clear that the model we examined is in fact extremely complex in its interplay of motivation, learning, memory and motor co-ordination. Since GABA may be inhibitory on one or all of these aspects of the rats behavior more selective behavioral paradigms will have to be developed.

Our results, using a relatively specific inhibitor of GABA-T, indicate that there is an interaction between GABA-ergic and dopaminergic pathways in the brain. In the extrapyramidal and limbic systems an increase in GABA concentrations produces a decrease in dopaminergic activity as determined both biochemically and pharmacologically. Such an inhibitory action on dopaminergic function, in addition to being theoretically important, may also have implications in clinical therapy. Tardive dyskinesia is believed to be a consequence of dopaminergic hyperactivity (Klawans & Weiner 1976, Tarsy & Baldessarini 1976). Hence elevations in brain GABA concentrations may be expected to ameliorate this syndrome. In addition, since dopaminergic blockage has been shown to be efficacious in the treatment of psychotic states, the neuroleptic-like effect of elevated brain GABA concentration we have demonstrated provides a rationale for the use of GABA-T inhibitors in schizophrenic therapy.

ACKNOWLEDGMENTS

The authors would like to thank Mrs. I. Fornieles and Mr. M. Robin for excellent technical assistance, Dr. M. J. Jung for stimulating discussions and Miss C. Schellenberger for typing the manuscript.

Footnote

Preliminary communications on portions of this work have been presented to the British Pharmacological Society (Huot *et al.* 1977) and as poster demonstrations at the 6th International Society of Neurochemistry Meeting, Copenhagen (Palfreyman *et al.* 1977a) and the Dopamine Satellite Symposium, Southampton (Palfreyman *et al.* 1977b). Tables I, II and III and Figs. 1, 2 and 3 are reproduced with the kind permission of the European Journal of Pharmacology from the article by Palfreyman *et al.* (1978).

REFERENCES

Andén, N.-E.& Stock, C. (1973) Inhibitory effect of gamma-hydroxybutyric acid on the dopamine cells in the substantia nigra. *Naunyn-Schmiedeberg's Arch. Phamacol.* 279, 89–92.

Andén, N.-E. (1974) Inhibition of the turnover of the brain dopamine after treatment with gamma-aminobutyrate: 2-oxyglutarate transaminase inhibitor aminooxyacetic acid. *Naunyn-Schmiedeberg's Arch. Pharmacol.* 283, 419–424.

Baldessarini, R. J. (1977) Schizophrenia. *New Engl. J. Med.* 297, 988–995.

Cook, L. & Catania, C. (1964) Effects of drugs on avoidance and escape behaviour. *Fed. Proc.* 23, 818–825.

Cooper, B. R., Breese, G. R., Howard, J. L. & Grant, L. A. (1972) Effect of central CA alterations by 6-OHDA on shuttle box avoidance acquisition. *Physiol. Behav.* 9, 727–731.

Cooper, B. R., Breese, G. R., Grant, L. D. & Howard, J. L. (1973) Effects of 6-OHDA treatments on active avoidance responding. Evidence for the involvement of brain dopamine. *J. Pharm. Exp. Therap.* 185, 358–370.

Costall, B. & Naylor, R. J. (1975) The behavioural effects of dopamine applied intracerebrally to areas of the mesolimbic system. *European J. Pharmacol.* 32, 87–92.

Costall, B., Marsden, C. D., Naylor, R. J. & Pycock, C. J. (1976) The relationship between striatal and mesolimbic dopamine dysfunction and the nature of circling responses following 6-hydroxydopamine and electrolytic lesions of the ascending dopamine systems of rat brain. *Brain Res.* 118, 87–113.

Di Chiara, G., Balakleevsky, A., Porceddu, M. L., Tagliamonte, A. & Gessa, G. L. (1974) Inhibition by apomorphine of dopamine deamination in the rat brain. *J. Neurochem.* 23, 1105–1108.

Dray, A., Oakley, N. R. & Simmonds, M. A. (1975) Rotational behaviour following inhibition of GABA metabolism unilaterally in the rat substantia nigra. *J. Pharm. Pharmacol.* 27, 627–629.

Dray, A. & Straughan, D. W. (1976) Synaptic mechanisms in the substantia nigra. *J. Pharm. Pharmacol.* 28, 400–405.

Fahn, S. (1976) Regional distribution studies of GABA and other putative neurotransmitters and their enzymes. In: *GABA in Nervous System Function,* ed. Roberts, E., Chase, T. N. & Tower, D. B., pp. 169-186. Raven Press, New York.

Fonnum, F., Grotova, I., Runvik, E., Storm-Mathiesen, J. & Walberg, F. (1974) Origin and distribution of glutamate decarboxylase in substantia nigra of the cat. *Brain Res.* 71, 77–92.

Fonnum, F., Iversen, E. & Walaas, I. (1977) Localization of glutamate decarboxylase choline acetyltransferase and DOPA decarboxylase in mesolimbic structures. In: *Advances in Biochem. Psychopharmacol.,* vol. 16, ed. Costa, E. & Gessa, G. L., pp. 417–421. Raven Press, New York.

Gessa, G. L., Vargiu, L., Crabai, F., Boero, G. C., Caboni, F. & Camba, R. (1966) Selective increase of brain dopamine induced by γ-hydroxybutyrate. *Life Sci.* 5, 1921–1930.

Glick, S. D., Jerussi, T. P. & Fleischer, L. N. (1977) Turning in circles: The neuropharmacology of rotation. *Life Sci.* 18, 889–896.

Huot, S., Lippert, B., Palfreyman, M. G. & Schechter, P. J. (1977) Inhibition of dopaminergic activity in the extrapyramidal and limbic systems by γ-acetylenic GABA. *Brit. J. Pharmac.* 60, 264–265P.

Iversen, S. D. & Koob, G. F. (1977) Behavioural implications of dopaminergic neurons in the mesolimbic system. In: *Advances in Biochem. Psychopharmacol., vol. 16, ed. Costa, E. & Gessa, G. L., pp. 209–214. Raven Press, New York.*

Jung, M. J. & Metcalf, B. W. (1975) Catalytic inhibition of γ-aminobutyric acid α-ketoglutarate transaminase of bacterial origin by 4-aminohex-5-ynoic acid, a substrate analog. *Biochem. Biophys. Res. Comm.* 67, 301–306.

Jung, M. J., Lippert, B., Metcalf, B. W., Schechter, P. J., Böhlen, P. & Sjoerdsma, A. (1977) The effect of 4-amino-hex-5-ynoic acid (γ-acetylenic GABA, γ-ethynyl GABA) a catalytic inhibitor of GABA transaminase on brain GABA metabolism *in vivo. J. Neurochem.* 28, 717–723.

Kelleher, R. T. & Morse, W. H. (1964) Escape behavior and punished behavior. *Fed. Proc.* 23, 808–817.

Klawans, H. L. & Weiner, W. J. (1976) The pharmacology of choreatic movement disorders. *Progress in Neurobiol.* 6, 49–80.

Koob, G. Del Fiaceo, M. & Iversen, S. D. (1976) The behavioural effects of EOS-induced changes in substantia nigra GABA levels. *Brit. J. Pharmacol.* 58, 454P.

Laverty, R. & Taylor, K. M. (1970) Effects of intraventricular 2,4,5 trihydroxyphenylethylamine (6-OHDA) on rat behaviour and brain CA metabolism. *Brit. J. Pharmac.* 40, 836–846.

Murphy, G. F., Robinson, D. & Sharman, D. F. (1969) The effect of tropolone on the formation of 3,4-dihydroxyphenylacetic acid and 4-hydroxy-3-methoxy phenylacetic acid in the brain of the mouse. *Brit. J. Pharmacol.* 36, 107–115.

Oberlander, C., Dumont, C. & Boissier, J. R. (1977) Rotational behaviour after unilateral intranigral injection of muscimol in rats. *European J. Pharmacol.* 43, 389–390.

Palfreyman, M. G., Huot, S. & Schechter, P. J. (1977a) The effect of γ-acetylenic GABA, a new inhibitor of GABA-transaminase, on catechol and indoleamine systems in rat brain. *Proc. of Int. Soc. Neurochem.* 6, 642.

Palfreyman, M. G., Huot, S., Lippert, B. & Schechter, P. J. (1977b) The effect of γ-acetylenic GABA, a new inhibitor of GABA-transaminase, on extrapyramidal and limbic dopaminergic activity. *Proc. of Int. Soc. Neurochem.,* Satellite Symposium on Dopamine, p. 7.

Palfreyman, M. G., Huot, S., Lippert, B. & Schechter, P. J. (1978) The effect of γ-acetylenic GABA, an irreversible catalytic inhibitor of GABA-transaminase on dopamine pathways of the extrapyramidal and limbic systems. *European J. Pharmacol.* 50, 325–336.

Pycock, C. J. & Horton, R. W. (1976) Possible GABA-mediated control of dopamine depressant behavioural effects from the nucleus accumbens of the rat. *Psychopharmacol.* 49, 173–178.

Schechter, P. J., Tranier, Y., Jung, M. J. & Sjoerdsma, A. (1977a) Antiseizure activity of γ-acetylenic γ-aminobutyric acid: A catalytic irreversible inhibitor of γ-aminobutyric acid transaminase. *J. Pharmacol. Exp. Ther.* 201, 606–612.

Schechter, P. J., Tranier, Y., Jung, M. J. & Böhlen, P. (1977b) Audiogenic seizure protection by elevated brain GABA concentration in mice: Effects of γ-acetylenic GABA and γ-vinyl GABA, two irreversible GABA-T inhibitors. *European J. Pharmacol.* 45, 319–328.

Scheel-Krüger, J., Cools, A. R. & Honig, W. (1977) Muscimol antagonises the ergometrine-induced locomotor activity in nucleus accumbens: Evidence for a GABA-dopaminergic interaction. *European J. Pharmacol.* 42, 311–313.

Schoenfeld, R. I. & Seiden, L. S. (1969) Effect of alpha-methyltyrosine on operant behaviour and brain catecholamine levels. *J. Pharmacol. Exp. Ther.* 167, 319–327.

Shellenberger, M. K. & Gordon, J. H. (1971) A rapid simplified procedure for simultaneous assay of norepinephrine, dopamine and 5-hydroxytryptamine from discrete brain areas. *Anal. Biochem.* 39, 356–372.

Stern, W. C., Hartman, E. L., Draskoczy, P. R. & Schildkraut, J. J. (1972) Behavioural effects of centrally administered 6-hydroxydopamine. *Psychol. Rep.* 30, 815–820.

Stevens, J., Wilson, K. & Foote, W. (1974) GABA blockade, dopamine and schizophrenia. Experimental studies in the cat. *Psychopharmacologia* 39, 105–119.

Stock, G., Magnusson, T. & Andén, N.-E. (1973) Increase in brain dopamine after axotomy or treatment with gamma-hydroxybutyric acid due to elimination of the nerve impulse flow. *Naunyn-Schmiedeberg's Arch. Pharmacol.* 278, 347–361.

Tarsy, D., Pycock, C., Meldrum, B. & Marsden, C. D. (1975) Rotational behaviour induced in rats by intranigral picrotoxin. *Brain Res.* 89, 160–165.

Tarsy, D. & Baldessarini, R. J. (1976) The tardive dyskinesia syndrome. In: *Clinical Neuropharmacol.*, Vol. I, ed. Klawans, H. L., pp. 29–61. Raven Press, New York.

Ungerstedt, U. (1971) Striatal dopamine release after amphetamine or nerve degenerated revealed by rotational behaviour. *Acta Physiol. Scand.*, Suppl. 367, 49–68.

Waddington, J. L. (1976) A behavioural model of the GABA-facilitating action of benzodiazepines: Rotational behaviour after unilateral intranigral injection of chlordiazepoxide. *Brit. J. Pharmacol.* 58, 453P.

Waddington, J. L. (1977) GABA-like properties of flurazepam and baclofen suggested by rotational behaviour following unilateral intranigral injection: A comparison with GABA agonist muscimol. *Brit. J. Pharmacol.* 60, 263P.

Waddington, J. L. (1978) Rotational behaviour and striatal dopamine metabolism following unilateral activation of nigral GABA mechanisms: GABA-like modulation of dopaminergic and non-dopaminergic neurons in rat substantia nigra. *Brit. J. Pharmacol.* 63, 384 P.

Development of New Animal Models for GABA-ergic Actions Using Muscimol as a Tool

J. Scheel-Krüger, J. Arnt[1], C. Bræstrup, A. V. Christensen[2] & G. Magelund

The purpose of the present study was to investigate the interaction between the GABA-dopamine systems in various biochemical and behavioral models, since these aspects are of interest for the possible medical treatment of various diseases: There is a severe deficit of GABA in the dopamine-containing basal ganglia system in both Huntington's and Parkinson's diseases. These two diseases can be differentiated in the alterations of dopaminergic and cholinergic systems. In Huntington's chorea there is a deficit in acetylcholine with normal dopamine levels, whereas the opposite occurs in Parkinsonism. For discussion see Coyle *et al.* 1977, Enna *et al.* 1976, 1977, Lloyd *et al.* 1975, 1977a, 1977b, McGeer & McGeer 1976a, b.

A dysfunction between dopamine and GABA may also exist in schizophrenia. Recently, Bird *et al.* (1977) reported on increased dopamine level and reduced glutamic acid decarboxylase (GAD) activity in schizophrenia in nucleus accumbens. Later this finding was questioned by observations on differences in GAD dependent on cause of death and postmortem effects (Iversen *et al.*, this symposium, Crow *et al.* 1978). No decrease of GABA was found by McGeer & McGeer (1977).

THE FUNCTIONAL ROLE OF GABA IN SUBSTANTIA NIGRA

We have been interested in substantia nigra (SN), since this area contains the

Psychopharmacological Research Laboratory Dept. E., Sct. Hans Mental Hospital, DK 4000 Roskilde, [1]Department of Pharmacology, The Royal Danish School of Pharmacy, Copenhagen, [2]Department of Pharmacology, H. Lundbeck & Co. A/S, Copenhagen, Denmark.

"GABA-NEUROTRANSMITTERS", Alfred Benzon Symposium 12, Munksgaard 1978

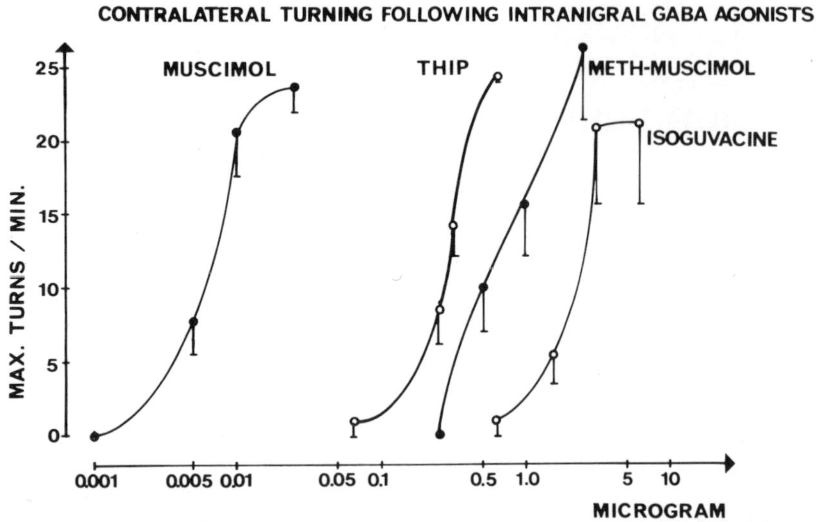

Fig. 1. The GABA agonists were injected into SNR at the coordinates A 1.2–2; L 1.7–2.4 and V−2.6–3, König & Klippel (1963). In the figure is shown the dose response curves after muscimol, THIP, 5′methylmuscimol and isoguvacine. The contralateral turning is shown as the maximum turns obtained after various doses of the compounds and was usually found within 1–20 min after the injection.

highest concentration of GABA and GAD compared to other brain regions (McGeer & McGeer 1976a, b, Tappaz *et al.* 1976, Fonnum *et al.* 1977, 1978). The GABA-ergic nerve terminals within SN arises mostly from the striatum and globus pallidus (Fonnum *et al.* 1978, McGeer & McGeer 1976b). The very low levels of GABA and GAD in SN of patients dying from Huntington's chorea and Parkinson's disease strongly suggest a role of GABA within this area for certain motor functions (Lloyd *et al.* 1975, 1977a, McGeer & McGeer 1976a, Enna *et al.* 1976).

Our behavioral studies have shown that the unilateral injection of muscimol and other GABA agonists into zona reticulata of substantia nigra (SNR) induced strong contralateral turning in the rats. The GABA antagonists picrotoxin and bicuculline methiodide induced ipsilateral turning within the same caudal area of SNR (Scheel-Krüger *et al.* 1977a). Similar results have also been found by other workers (Olianas *et al.* 1978b, Olpe *et al.* 1977, Oberlander *et al.* 1977, Waddington 1977). In fact this contralateral turning model was found useful for an *in vivo* evaluation of the potency of a large series of GABAergic drugs (Arnt *et al.*, in prep.) synthesized and supplied by Krogsgaard-

Larsen *et al.* (Fig. 1 and Table I). In general the rank order in potency corresponded to results obtained in ^{3}H-GABA receptor binding and found in microelectrophoretic studies (Krogsgaard-Larsen *et al.* 1975, 1978, and this symposium). It should be noted that the GABA uptake inhibitors nipecotic acid and guvacine only showed very weak and short lasting effects. The agonists thiomuscimol, isoguvacine and especially trans-aminocrotonic acid (t-ACA) and 3-aminopropane sulphonic acid (3-APS) showed all extraordinarily weak effects in the turning model, which today can not be explained satisfactorily.

The bilateral injection of muscimol in increasing doses (10–100 ng) induced increasingly amphetamine/apomorphine-like stereotyped behavior: nodding head movements, sniffing and gnawing. The contralateral turning and stereotyped behavior after muscimol was found independent of dopamine receptor activity, since high doses of haloperidol, perphenazine or reserpine plus *α*-methyltyrosine, did not antagonize. Muscimol bilaterally injected into the SNR (2×10 ng) immediately antagonized the neuroleptic catalepsy and induced

Table I
Comparison of different GABA-ergic compounds in different tests

GABA ergic compounds	SNR turning ED 50 (n Mol)	^{3}H-GABA binding IC 50 (μ Mol)	Micro-electro-phoresis relative potency
Muscimol	0.06	0.03	++++
THIP	2	3	+++
5′methylmuscimol	6	7	+++
5′ethylmuscimol	0	>100	++(?)
homomuscimol	7	10	+++
4-methylmuscimol	64	>100	+
thiomuscimol	28	0.10	++++
azamuscimol	36	>100	++
isomuscimol	280	380	+
isoguvacine	17	1.4	++++
isonipecotic acid	470	15	+++
guvacine	400	>100	0
nipecotic acid	280	>100	(+)
trans-amino-crotonic acid	560	0.2	+++
methyl-trans-amino-crotonic acid	66	4	?
3-amino propane-sulphonic acid	280	0.3	++++

The ED 50 value for contralateral turning after injection into the SNR is expressed in nanomoles inducing half-maximal turning rate. Maximum effect is considered as 25 turns/min.

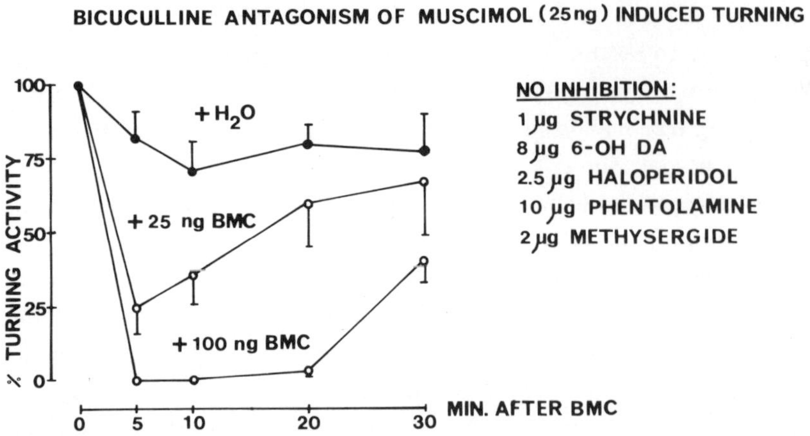

Fig. 2. Bicuculline methchloride (25 or 100 ng BMC) was injected into the SNR (through the chronically implanted guide cannula) 25 min after muscimol given in a maximum effective dose 25 ng. The figure shows that BMC when injected at the same site as muscimol dose-dependently antagonize the muscimol induced contralateral turning. Various other drugs summarized in the figure did not antagonize when injected after muscimol. However 6-OH-dopamine was injected in a dose of 8 μg 14 days before muscimol at the coordinates A 3, L 1.8, V−2.4.

stimulation and stereotyped behavior. A 6-OH-dopamine (8 μg in SN) lesion of the nigro-striatal dopamine pathway did not antagonize the contralateral turning either. However, local injection of picrotoxin (100–250 ng) or bicuculline methchloride (25 and 100 ng) antagonized the muscimol turning (Fig. 2). These data show that the behavioral effects seen after GABA receptor stimulation in the SNR are specific and mediated by neuronal systems independent of the nigro-striatal dopamine system (Scheel-Krüger *et al.* 1977a, and in prep.). Selective destruction of pars reticulata neurons after kainic acid induces a behavioral syndrome analogous to that induced by GABA-mimetics injected into the SNR: Chronic stereotypies in rats injected bilaterally and chronic contralateral turning following unilateral injection of kainic acid in the SNR. These symptoms are also independent of dopaminergic activity. (Di Chiara *et al.* 1977, Di Chiara *et al.,* this symposium, Olianas *et al.* 1978a and 1978b). This indicates that pars reticulata contains neurons controlling posture and behavioral stimulation in a manner opposite to the nigro-striatal dopamine neurons. These neurons are sensitive to inhibition by GABA or destruction by kainic acid. The function of dopamine receptors in striatum is probably to inhibit these neurons by activating a striato-nigral GABA-ergic pathway (Olianas *et al.* 1978b). The increase of GABA accumulation rate after inhibition of GABA-T in SN produced by apomorphine (Perez de La Mora *et al.* 1975) supports this hypothesis.

We have evidence that these pars reticulata neurons are cholinergic. In collaboration with Tagliamonte *et al.* was found that stimulation of these neurons by muscarinic stimulants induce catalepsia. Furthermore anti-cholinergics injected locally induce dopamine-like stereotypies independent of the dopamine system (De Montis *et al.* 1978), since the dopamine receptor step in striatum has been bypassed (Fig. 3). From this figure it also appears that the substantia nigra represents the major projection area for the striatal and pallidal efferent fibers (Carpenter 1976, Nieuwenhuys 1977). Therefore it is postulated

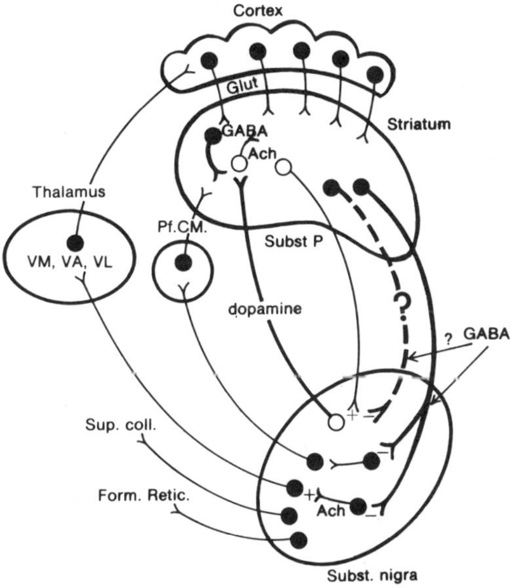

Fig. 3. A highly schematic model summarizing a neuronal model for recent findings made in collaboration with Tagliamonte *et al.* on the role of the descending striato-nigral GABA pathway(s) regulating posture and behavioral stimulation. In order to simplify the figure as much as possible we have not included the possible striato-pallidal, striato-entopenduncular, etc. GABA-ergic fibers (Fonnum *et al.* 1977, 1978) nor the other neurotransmitter candidates in substantia nigra, i.e. glycin, noradrenaline, serotonin, the enkephalins, etc. (Dray & Straughan 1976). According to this model stimulation of certain dopamine receptors in striatum (or other forebrain structures) stimulates the descending GABA fibers which inhibit certain cholinergic interneurons in SN zona reticulata. These cholinergic interneurons are considered inhibitory for the development of certain dopaminergic effects involved in posture and behavioral stimulation (De Montis *et al.* 1978). The neuronal pathways controlled by these cholinergic interneurons are presently unknown but may include thalamus (VM, VA, VL areas) the nucleus parafascicularis (Pf) and Center Median (CM) complex, the superior colliculus (Sup. coll) or the reticular formation (Form. Retic.).

that GABA in SNR acts as an important neurotransmitter in the dopamine striatal and /or forebrain output system (Garcia-Munoz *et al.* 1977). Several relevant brain areas receiving a projection from the nigra are known, i.e. the thalamus (VL and VM area), nucleus parafascicularis, superior colliculus and formatio reticularis (Carpenter 1976, Nieuwenhuys 1977, Ahlenius 1978, Di Chiara *et al.*,, this symposium).

THE GABA-DOPAMINE INTERACTION IN SUBSTANTIA NIGRA

Previously it has been suggested that GABA in SNR mainly inhibits the activity of the nigro-striatal dopamine pathway. This "feedback loop hypothesis" has undoubtly been inspired by the electrophysiological findings that activity of some nigral cells was inhibited by stimulation of neostriatum and this effect was antagonized by GABA antagonists. (Cheramy *et al.* 1978, Dray *et al.* 1976, 1977). However, the pars reticulata neurons are much more sensitive to the inhibitory effect of micro-iontophoretic applied GABA than the dopamine containing pars compacta neurons (Aghajanian & Bunney 1975, Dray *et al.* 1976, Walters & Lakoski 1978).

Recent electrophysiological studies using GABA-ergic drugs as muscimol, AOAA, valproate (Walters & Lakoski 1978, Walters *et al.*, this symposium) and EOS (Dray *et al.* 1977) found no inhibitory effects on the activity of substantia nigra dopamine neurons but in fact evidence for small increase in firing rate. Also, new biochemical data have shown that activation of GABA transmission by muscimol, GABA and other GABA-ergic compounds in SN induces release of dopamine in the nucleus caudatus (Cheramy *et al.* 1978, Dray *et al.* 1977). Even *in vitro* it has been shown that GABA stimulates dopamine release in slices of substantia nigra or corpus striatum (Giorguieff *et al.* 1978, Starr 1978, Stoof & Mulder 1977).

BIOCHEMICAL RESULTS WITH MUSCIMOL

The injection of muscimol into substantia nigra, zona reticulata showed results in agreement with the conclusions reached by Cheramy *et al.* 1978, since muscimol significantly increased the dopamine metabolites HVA and DOPAC measured in striatum 30 and 60 min after the SNR injection of muscimol (Table II). The dopamine synthesis was nearly doubled 5–35 min after muscimol. The dopamine level was not changed 30 min after the injection of muscimol. Taken

Table II

Striatal dopamine metabolism after injection of muscimol into the substantia nigra, zona reticulata (SNR)

Muscimol doses	Time interval	DA	L-DOPA	DOPAC	HVA
			% of saline injected site		
10 ng	60 min	–	–	166±10*	131±15*
25 ng	30 min	114±8	195±23*	182±13*	136±11*
25 ng	60 min	143±10*	–	195±19*	166±15*
100 ng	60 min	154±10*	–	208±24*	142±16*

Each value represents the mean±s.e.m. after six to eight rats. All rats were injected simultaneously into the right and left SNR with muscimol and saline 1 μl, respectively and analyzed for dopamine metabolism in striatum 30 or 60 min after the injections. NSD 1015 (100 mg/kg i.p.) was injected 5 min before muscimol and the accumulation of l-DOPA was measured 35 min later.
* $P<0.05$ difference from saline injected site.

together with the results on HVA, DOPAC and "l-DOPA" accumulation after decarboxylase inhibition this finding indicates that at this time muscimol increases the release of striatal dopamine. At 60 min the striatal dopamine level was found increased after muscimol 25 and 100 ng, which might indicate an interruption of dopamine neuron impulse flow and thus a biphasic influence of muscimol on the nigro-striatal dopamine system (For further discussion see Cheramy *et al.* 1978).

Following inhibition of tyrosine hydroxylase with α-methyl-p-tyrosine (H 44/68) (Costa 1971) muscimol 25 ng did not change the striatal dopamine disappearance rate. Muscimol 100 ng retarded the disappearance rate indicating a decreased dopamine utilization (Table III). The haloperidol (1 mg/kg) induced acceleration of striatal dopamine disappearance was not significantly changed by muscimol 25 ng injected into the SNR or SNC. However, an extremely high dose of muscimol 100 ng injected into the SNR and especially the SNC significantly retarded the dopamine disappearance rate. Gale & Guidotti (1976) found in agreement with our results that muscimol in high doses 25 ng and especially 50 ng injected into the SNC significantly antagonized the haloperidol activation of tyrosine hydroxylase. These high dose levels of muscimol may not be physiologically relevant, since muscimol 10 ng injected into the SNR is a sufficiently high dose for behavioral stimulation and antagonism of haloperidol catalepsy (Scheel-Krüger *et al.* 1977a, Olianas *et al.* 1978b, Olpe *et al.* 1977, Oberlander *et al.* 1977): Muscimol injected into the SNC

Table III

Effect of muscimol injected into subst.nigra on striatal dopamine disappearance after treatment with α-MT or α-MT+haloperidol

Treatments	Striatal dopamine % of saline site	
	+α-MT	α-MT+haloperidol
25 ng musc. in SNR	118±6	121±19
100 ng musc. in SNR	147±8*	145±10*
25 ng musc. in SNC	88±3	112±11
100 ng musc. in SNC	—	180±12*

Each value represents the mean±S.E.M. after five to six rats. All rats were injected simultaneously into the right and left SN with muscimol and saline 1 μl, respectively.

All rats received α-MT (H44/68 250 mg/kg i.p.) 2 hr before decapitation. Haloperidol (1 mg/kg s.c.) was injected simultaneously with α-MT. Control values of striatal dopamine from saline 1 μl injected site after α-MT, 4.3±0.02 μg/g and α-MT+haloperidol 2.9±0.02 μg/g.

* $P<0.025$ differences from saline injected site.

SNR=zona reticulata A 1.2–1.8, L 1.6–2.2, V–2.8 and

SNC=zona compacta A 1.2–1.8, L 1.6–2, V–2.2

Coordinates according to König & Klippel (1963).

induces no behavioral stimulation or antagonism of haloperidol-induced catalepsy (Arnt & ScheelKrüger, in prep.). The results obtained after systemic injection of muscimol provide an identical conclusion that muscimol only in extremely high dose may induce a retardation of the dopamine neuronal activity. Muscimol 20 mg/kg inducing loss of the righting reflex and anesthesia increased striatal dopamine (70±5%, $P<0.01$), whereas 10 mg/kg only moderately increased dopamine (30±4%, $P<0.01$) measured 90 min after the injection. Such effects are seen after various treatments blocking the dopamine neuronal impulse flow (Andén *et al.* 1972, Walters *et al.* 1973). In the α-MT turnover model the haloperidol (1 mg/kg) induced acceleration of striatal dopamine disappearance was only slightly retarded by a very high dose of muscimol 10 mg/kg (41±2%, $P<0.001$), whereas baclofen 10 mg/kg induced a stronger retardation of the haloperidol effect (70±9%, $P<0.001$). Muscimol 1, 2.5, 5 and 10 mg/kg *per se* did not in our schedule (i.e. muscimol and α-MT given simultaneously) significantly influence striatal dopamine disappearance rate. Muscimol in doses of 1 and especially 2 and 4 mg/kg s.c. induced dose-dependent increase of catalepsy in rats. We have found that 1 mg/kg muscimol increased the catalepsy after neuroleptics, but did not reduce the dopamine turnover nor the neuroleptic acceleration of dopamine turnover as measured by the α-MT technique (see also Walters *et al.,* this symposium). The increase of neuroleptic catalepsy caused by muscimol seems not dependent on a direct influence on dopamine, but on stimulation of GABA receptors beyond the dopamine neurons most likely localized in the ventro medial striatum (Magelund & Scheel-Krüger, in prep.).

GABA AND DOPAMINE DEPENDENT MOTILITY

The systemic injection of muscimol and other GABA agonists in non sedative doses strongly antagonized the locomotor stimulation of dopaminergic stimulants as apomorphine and cocaine (Scheel-Krüger *et al.* 1978). The morphine (50 mg/kg)-induced motility in mice was found even more sensitive to muscimol and THIP inhibition (Christensen *et al.* 1978, and in prep.). The direct injection of muscimol into nucleus accumbens strongly antagonized ergometrine or apomorphine motility in rats (Scheel-Krüger *et al.* 1977b, Scheel-Krüger *et al.* 1977c). These results have also been found by others using other GABA drugs and/or dopamine stimulants (Pycock & Horton 1976, Wachtel & Andén 1978). However, the GABA-dopamine interaction is complex also in nucleus accumbens, since the apomorphine stereotypy was increased. The stereotypy increased effects we interpreted as due to an interaction of GABA with different dopamine systems and /or dopamine receptors (Scheel-Krüger *et al.* 1977c).

ROLE OF GABA IN DOPAMINE-DEPENDENT STEREOTYPED BEHAVIOR

It is well established that DA agonists in the clinic can induce psychoses and exacerbate the symptoms in schizophrenic patients. In animal studies the amphetamines induce stereotyped behavior and the antagonism of stereotypy (including sniffing, licking and gnawing in mice and rats) is considered as a screening test for antipsychotic compounds with antidopaminergic effect (Randrup & Munkvad 1967, Munkvad *et al.* 1968, Fog 1972, Pedersen & Christensen 1972). Recently we found that muscimol *per se* induced no stereotypy, but strongly increased the stereotyped gnawing in mice after apomorphine, cocaine, and methylphenidate (Scheel-Krüger *et al.* 1978). In Fig. 4 is shown the dose response effect on methylphenidate gnawing after two established GABA agonists muscimol and THIP (Krogsgaard-Larsen *et al.* 1977, Curtis *et al.* 1971). In Table IV our results with other GABA related drugs are summarized. Stereotyped gnawing was increased by 5′-methyl-muscimol,

Table IV
Effect of various GABA-ergic and GABA-like compounds on methylphenidate-induced gnawing activity in mice

Drugs	Dose levels (mg/kg)	Gnawing activity
Muscimol	0.5−2	+++
THIP	5−10	+++
methylmuscimol	30−60	++
γ-acctylenic GABA	100	+++
benzodiazepines	0.5−10	+or++
barbiturates	10−40	+
baclofen	2.5−10	0
AOAA	12.5−25	(+)
Na-Valproate	100−400	(+)
Nipecotic acid	150	0
Guvacine	150−250	0
Saline	—	0

All mice received methylphenidate 10 mg/kg s.c. 15 min after pretreatment with the GABA-ergic compounds (given i.p.) summarized above. AOAA was, however, given 120 min and γ-acetylenic GABA 60 min before methylphenidate. Immediately after the methylphenidate injection the mice were placed for 1 h in gnawing cages, two mice in each. The cages consisted of 30 cm high perspex boxes (12×25 cm) without bottom. The cages were placed on corrugated paper, the corrugations facing upwards. For each drug combination was used at least five pairs of mice. After the experiments, the degree of gnawing activity seen on the corrugated paper was estimated semiquantitatively using the following 4-point scale: 0, +, ++, and +++.

the GABA-T inhibitor, γ-acetylenic GABA (GAG), the benzodiazepines and barbiturates. AOAA induced only a very weak increase of gnawing after 25 mg/kg, 2 h and similar weak response was found after valproate (sodium *di-n-propylacetate, 400 mg/*kg). The GABA uptake inhibitors nipecotic acid and guvacine (Krogsgaard-Larsen 1978) was found inactive. Baclofen (Lioresal), which is not a GABA agonist (Naik *et al.* 1976, Möhler & Okada 1977a), induced no increase in stereotyped gnawing (see also Delini-Stula, this symposium). This strong increase in methylphenidate (10 mg/kg) induced gnawing in mice seems characteristic for drugs known to increase GABA transmission. Among other drugs tested we found weaker effect after the anti-cholinergics atropine and scopolamine, but no increase following pretreatment with the noradrenaline antagonists phenoxybenzamine, aceperone or the serotonin antagonist methergoline.

In rats muscimol also strongly increased the apomorphine stereotyped gnawing activity or more precisely: the typical stereotyped behavior including sniffing, nodding head movements has a tendency to be decreased, whereas a typical oral "dyskinetic biting activity" is induced. A combined treatment with muscimol HBr, 1 and especially 2 mg/kg s.c. (30 min) apomorphine 0.5 mg/kg and especially 2 mg/kg s.c. induces a strong gnawing/biting activity on the wire nettings of the cages. This very pronounced oral dyskinetic biting activity is not seen after apomorphine given alone in even very high doses.

INHIBITION OF THE ANTISTEREOTYPIC EFFECT OF NEUROLEPTICS BY MUSCIMOL

Previously it has been suggested that GABA-ergic drugs in combination with neuroleptics may improve the medical treatment of schizophrenia (Fuxe *et al.* 1975), and reduce extrapyramidal side effects including tardive dyskinesias, which may appear after long-term treatment with neuroleptic drugs (Gerlach *et al.* 1974, Klawans 1973, Kobayashi 1977). This hypothesis was tested in acute experiments using the stereotyped gnawing induced by methylphenidate (60 mg/kg) in mice. In this model all classical neuroleptic drugs antagonize the

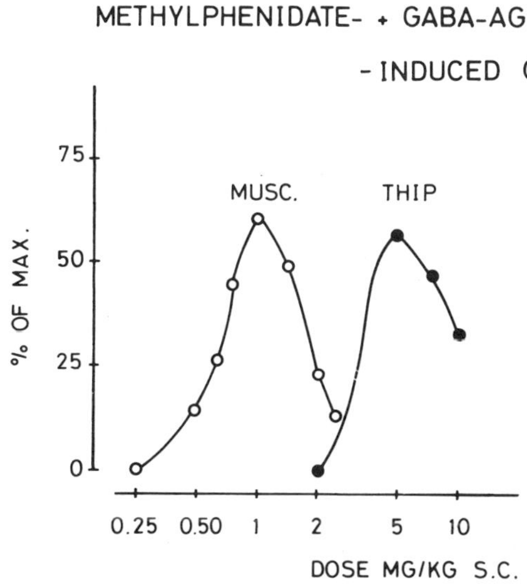

Fig. 4. Stereotyped gnawing in mice induced by methylphenidate (10 mg/kg s.c.) following pretreatment (15 min) with muscimol, HBr (s.c.) or THIP, HBr (s.c.). For further details see legend to Table IV.

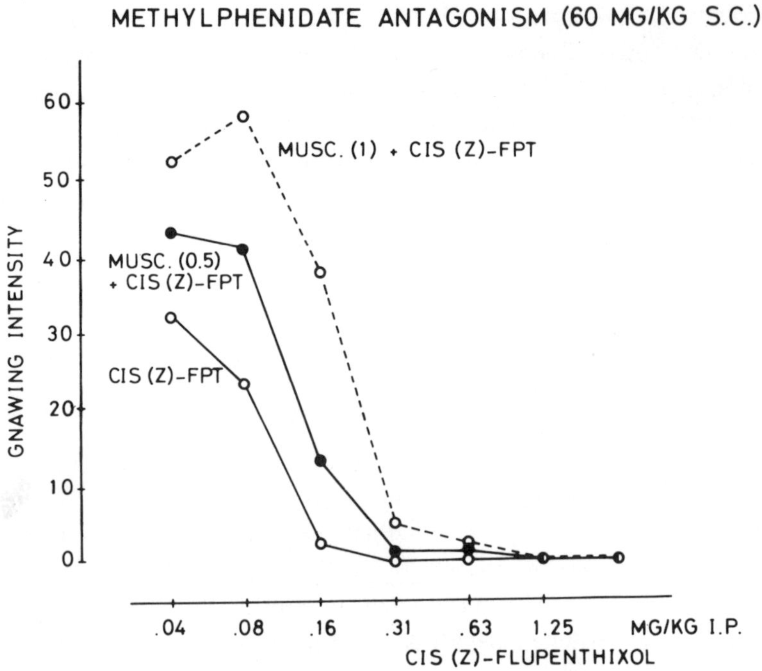

Fig. 5. Inhibition by muscimol (0.5 or 1 mg/kg s.c.) of the antistereotypic gnawing effect of cis-(z)-flupenthixol in mice. Flupenthixol in various doses was injected i.p. 90 min before muscimol HBr. Methylphenidate, 60 mg/kg s.c. was injected 15 min after muscimol.

compulsive gnawing syndrome induced by methylphenidate. The clinical most potent antipsychotic drugs are also most potent in this test (Pedersen & Christensen 1972). However, the addition of muscimol dose dependently antagonized the antistereotypic gnawing effect of neuroleptic drugs. In Fig. 5 is shown the dose-response effects by cis-(z)-flupenthixol and muscimol. Similar results have been obtained after other neuroleptic drugs, i.e. fluphenazine, haloperidol and pimozide. (Christensen *et al.,* in prep.). It seems therefore reasonable to suggest that a GABA agonist like muscimol will not improve the antipsychotic effect of neuroleptic drugs, if the traditional hypothesis still is to be maintained, i.e. antagonism of dopamine-dependent stereotypic gnawing correlates to the antipsychotic effect in the clinic.

Our results obtained after muscimol given alone or in combination with neuroleptic drugs raise also the question whether a GABA agonist like muscimol may improve the tardive-oral dyskinetic symptoms, which in the clinic are ameliorated by neuroleptic drugs with specific dopamine antagonistic properties (Gerlach *et al.* 1974, Klawans 1973, Kobayashi 1977).

BARBITURATES AND BENZODIAZEPINES INCREASE METHYLPHENIDATE GNAWING

The barbiturates and benzodiazepines facilitate GABA transmission (Haefely *et al.* and Guidotti, this symposium). These drugs tested in even extremely high doses induced a weaker gnawing activity after methylphenidate than seen after muscimol. Dependent on the drug, the gnawing activity reached between 20 and 50% of maximum score. The most effective doses to induce 40–50% of maximum gnawing score were as follows: clonazepam 0.50 mg/kg; lorazepam 1 mg/kg; estazolam and flurazepam 2.5 mg/kg; diazepam 5 mg/kg; chlordiazepoxide, chlorazepat and medazepam 40 mg/kg. Flunitrazepam (0.1–2.5 mg/kg) and nitrazepam (0.25–10 mg/kg) induced the weakest gnawing

Table V

Benzodiazepines and barbiturates potentiate methylphenidate-muscimol gnawing behavior in mice

		Gnawing Activity in % of Maximum Possible		
	Doses	Muscimol, mg/kg		
Drugs	mg/kg	0	0.25	0.50
Saline		0	0	11±4
Clonazepam	0.25	27±8	53±17	100
Lorazepam	0.25	3±3	40±12	100
Flunitrazepam	0.25	0	20±13	93±7
Diazepam	1	22±6	67±11	100
Estazolam	1	17±3	47±13	73±12
Nitrazepam	1.25	10±7	47±13	80±8
Flurazepam	1.25	10±9	47±13	60±19
Chlordiazepoxide	5	16±6	13±7	83±7
Chlorazepat	10	6±4	20±8	87±13
Medazepam	10	3±3	0	93±7
Pentobarbital	20	13±9	47±13	100
Phenobarbital	20−80	13−20	7−20	40−50

The benzodiazepines or barbiturates were given intraperitoneally simultaneously with saline or muscimol (0.25 or 0.50 mg/kg s.c.) 15 min before methylphenidate. The doses of benzodiazepines or barbiturates in the table indicate the minimal effective dose, which given in combination with muscimol (0.50 mg/kg) and methylpenidate (10 mg/kg s.c.) induce maximum possible gnawing score (data shown as % of max.±S.E.M.). For further details see legend to Table IV.

responses after methylphenidate reaching only 20% of maximum possible score. Phenobarbital and pentobarbital (10 and 40 mg/kg respectively) induced gnawing corresponding to 30–40% of maximum score.

POTENTIATION BY MUSCIMOL OF BENZODIAZEPINES AND BARBITURATES

The benzodiazepines and barbiturates in low doses potentiate the effect of muscimol on methylphenidate-induced stereotyped gnawing. In Table V the minimum effective doses of the benzodiazepines and barbiturates are summarized which in combination with an almost noneffective dose of muscimol (0.50 mg/kg) induced the maximum possible gnawing score. The rank order in potency of the benzodiazepines corresponds to their comparative affinity for the recently described benzodiazepine receptor in the CNS (Squires & Braestrup 1977, Möhler & Okada 1977b). The dose of muscimol used in this combined treatment was found important for induction of gnawing activity: Muscimol 0.25 mg/kg still induced gnawing (Table V), whereas muscimol (0.10 mg/kg) did not increase the gnawing activity induced by methylphenidate (10 mg/kg) and diazepam (1 and 5 mg/kg).

CONCLUSIONS

The results indicate that the connections between GABA and the dopamine systems are much more complex than previously considered. Data are presented, which make it doubtful whether GABA in substantia nigra under physiological conditions antagonizes the dopamine neuronal activity. It is much more likely that GABA in this area participates in the striato-pallidal forebrain output system controlling posture and behavioral stimulation.

Our data have also shown that certain dopaminergic effects are increased by GABA (stereotyped gnawing activity), whereas others contrastingly are decreased (locomotor activity). The neuroleptic-induced catalepsy is increased, whereas the neuroleptic-induced inhibition of stereotyped gnawing is antagonized by the GABA agonist muscimol. Muscimol strongly potentiates the effect of benzodiazepines and barbiturates on stereotyped gnawing induced by the dopamine stimulant methylphenidate. The profile of actions of GABA on behavior is thus unique and very complex.

In this symposium some very preliminary results about the effect of GABA mimetics in different diseases have been shown (Chase *et al.*, Bartholini *et al.*,

Palfreyman *et al.*) but still it is an open question, whether GABA agonists or GABA antagonists could be used in long-term therapeutic treatment in diseases like schizophrenia, tardive dyskinesia, parkinsonism or epilepsy. Elucidation of the effects of GABA agonists in animals and humans is in any case of great theoretical interest, since this may lead to a better understanding of the functional disturbances in various psychiatric disorders.

REFERENCES

Aghajanian, G. K. & Bunney, B. S. (1975) Dopaminergic and nondopaminergic neurons of the substantia nigra: differential responses to putative transmitters. In: *Neuropsychopharmacol.* ed. Boissier, J. R., Hippius, H. & Pichot, P., pp. 444–452. Excerpta Medica.

Ahlenius, S. (1978) Potentiation by haloperidol of the catalepsy produced by lesions in the parafascicular nucleus of the rat. *Brain Res.*, 150, 648–652.

Andén, N. E., Bédard, P., Fuxe, K. & Ungerstedt, U. (1972) Early and selective increase in brain dopamine levels after axotomy. *Experientia,* Basel, 28, 300–301.

Bird, E. D., Barnes, J., Iversen, L. L., Spokes, E. G., Mackay, A. V. & Shepherd, M. (1977) Increased brain dopamine and reduced glutamic acid decarboxylase and choline acetyl transferase activity in schizophrenia and related psychoses. *Lancet* 2, 1157–1159.

Carpenter, M. B. (1976) Anatomy of the basal ganglia and related nuclei: A review. *Adv. in Neurol.* 14, 7–48.

Cheramy, A., Nieoullon, A. & Glowinski, J. (1978) GABA-ergic processes involved in the control of dopamine release from nigrostriatal dopaminergic neurons in the cat. *Europ. J. Pharmacol.* 48, 281–295.

Christensen, A. V., Arnt, J. & Scheel-Krüger, J. (1978) Muscimol antagonizes morphine hypermotility without potentiation of analgesia. *Europ. J. Pharmacol.* 48, 459–462.

Costa, E. (1971) Methods for measuring indolealkylamine and catecholamine turnover rate *in vivo.* In: *Chemistry and brain development,* ed. Paoletti, R. & Davidson, A. N., pp. 157–174. Plenum Press.

Coyle, J. T., Schwarcz, R., Bennett, J. P. & Campochiaro, P. (1977) Clinical, neuropathologic and pharmacologic aspects of Huntington's disease: Correlates with a new animal model. *Prog. Neuro-psychopharmac.* 1, 13–30.

Crow, T. J., Owen, F., Cross, A. J., Lofthouse, R. & Longden, A. (1978) *Lancet* 1, 35–37.

Curtis, D. R., Duggan, A. W., Felix, D. & Johnston, G. A. R. (1971) Bicuculline, an antagonist of GABA and synaptic inhibition in the spinal cord of the cat. *Brain Res.* 32, 69–96.

De Montis, G. M., Olianas, M. C., Serra, G., Tagliamonte, A. & Scheel-Krüger, J. (1978) Evidence that a nigral GABA-ergic-cholinergic balance controls posture. *Europ. J. Pharmacol.,* submitted.

Di Chiara, G., Olianas, M., Del Fiacco, Spano, P. F. & Tagliamonte, A. (1977) Intranigral kainic acid is evidence that nigral nondopaminergic neurons control posture. *Nature* 268, 743–745.

Dray, A. & Straughan, D. W. (1976) Synaptic mechanisms in the substantia nigra. *J. Pharm. Pharmac.* 28, 400–405.

Dray, A., Gonye, T. F. & Oakley, N. R. (1976) Caudate stimulation and substantia nigra activity in the rat. J. Physiol., London, 259, 825–849.

Dray, A., Fowler, L. J., Oakley, N. R., Simmonds, M. A. & Tanner, T. (1977) Regulation of nigrostriatal dopaminergic neurotransmission in the rat. *Neuropharmacol.* 16, 511–518.

Enna, S. J., Bird, E. D., Bennett, J. P., Bylund, D. B., Yamamura, H. I., Iversen, L. L. & Snyder, S. H. (1976) Huntngton's chorea changes in neurotransmitter receptors in the brain. *New Engl. J. Med.* 294, 1305–1309.

Enna, S. J., Stern, L. Z., Wastek, G. J. & Yamamura, H. I. (1977) Neurobiology and pharmacology of Huntington's disease. *Life Sci.* 20, 205–212.

Fog, R. (1972) On stereotypy and catalepsy: Studies on the effect of amphetamines and neuroleptics in rats. *Acta Neurol. Scand.,* Suppl. 48, Suppl. 50, 1–64.

Fonnum, F., Walaas, I. & Iversen, E. (1977) Localization of GABA-ergic, cholinergic and aminergic structures in the mesolimbic system. *J. Neurochem.* 29, 221–230.

Fonnum, F., Gottesfeld, Z. & Grofova, I. (1978) Distribution of glutamic acid decarboxylase, choline acetyltransferase and aromatic amino acid decarboxylase in the basal ganglia of normal and operated rats. Evidence for striatopallidal, striatoentopeduncular and striatonigral GABA-ergic fibers. *Brain Res.* 143, 125–138.

Fuxe, K., Hökfelt, T., Ljungdahl, Å., Agnati, L., Johansson, O. & Perez de la Mora, M. (1975) Evidence for an inhibitory gabergic control of the mesolimbic dopamine neurons. Possibility of improving the treatment of schizophrenia by combined treatment with neuroleptic and gabergic drugs. *Med. Biol.* 53, 177–183.

Gale, K. & Guidotti, A., (1976) GABA-mediated control of rat neostriatal tyrosine hydroxylase revealed by intranigral muscimol. *Nature* 263, 691–693.

Garcia-Munoz, M., Nicolaou, N. M., Tulloch, I. F., Wright, A. K. & Arbuthnott, G. W. (1977) Feedback loop or output pathway in striato-nigral fibers. *Nature* 265, 363–365.

Gerlach, J., Reisby, N. & Randrup, A. (1974) Dopaminergic hypersensitivity and cholinergic hypofunction in the pathophysiology of tardive dyskinesia. *Psychopharmacol.* 34, 21–35.

Giorguieff, M. F., Kemel, M. L., Glowinski, J. & Besson, M. J. (1978) Stimulation of dopamine release by GABA in rat striatal slices. *Brain Res.* 139, 115–130.

Klawans, H. L. (1973) Pharmacology of extrapyramidal movements disorders Karger (Basel).

Kobayashi, R. M. (1977) Drug therapy of tardive dyskinesia. *N. Engl. J. Med.* 296, 257–260.

Krogsgaard-Larsen, P., Johnston, G. A. R., Curtis, D. R., Game, C. J. A. & McCulloch, R. M. (1975) Structure and biological activity of a series of conformationally restricted analogues of GABA. *J. Neurochem.* 25, 803–809.

Krogsgaard-Larsen, P., Johnston, G. A. R., Lodge, D. & Curtis, D. R. (1977) A new class of a GABA agonist. *Nature* 268, 53–55.

Krogsgaard-Larsen, P. (1978) GABA agonists and uptake inhibitors of restricted conformations: Structure-Activity Relations. In: *Amino Acids as Chemical Transmitters.* ed. Fonnum, F., Plenum Press. In press.

Lloyd, K. G., Möhler, H., Heitz, Ph. & Bartholini, G. (1975) Distribution of choline acetyltransferase and glutamate decarboxylase within substantia nigra and in other brain regions from control and parkinsonian patients. *J. Neurochem.* 25, 789–795.

Lloyd, K. G., Dreksler, S. & Bird, E. D. (1977a) Alterations in ^{3}H-GABA binding in Huntington's chorea. *Life Sci.* 21, 747–754.

Lloyd, K. G., Shemen, L. & Hornykiewicz, O. (1977b) Distribution of high affinity sodium independent ^{3}H-GABA binding in the human brain: Alterations in Parkinson's disease. *Brain Res.* 127, 269–278.

McGeer, P. L. & McGeer, E. G. (1976a) Enzymes associated with the metabolism of catecholamines acetylcholine and GABA in human controls and patients with Parkinson's disease and Huntington's chorea. *J. Neurochem.* 26, 65–76.

McGeer, P. L. & McGeer, E. G. (1976b) The GABA system and function of the basal ganglia:

Huntington's disease. In: *GABA in Nervous System Function.* ed. Roberts, E., Chase, T. N. & Tower, D. B., pp. 487–495. Raven Press.

McGeer, P. L. & McGeer, E. G. (1977) Possible changes in striatal and limbic cholinergic systems in schizophrenia. *Arch. Gen. Psychiatry* 34, 1319–1323.

Munkvad, I., Pakkenberg, H. & Randrup, A. (1968) Aminergic systems in basal ganglia associated with stereotyped hyperactive behaviour and catalepsy. *Brain Behav., Evol* (S. Karger, Basel) 1, 89–100.

Möhler, H. & Okada, T. (1977a) GABA receptor binding with ^{3}H(+) bicuculline-methiodide in rat CNS. *Nature* 267, 65–67.

Möhler, H. & Okada, T. (1977b) Benzodiazepine receptor: Demonstration in the central nervous system. *Science* 178, 849–851.

Naik, S. R., Guidotti, A. & Costa, E. (1976) Central GABA receptor agonists: comparison of muscimol and baclofen. *Neuropharmacol.* 15, 479–484.

Nieuwenhuys, R. (1977) Aspects of the morphology of the striatum. In: *Psychobiology of the Striatum.* ed. Cools, A. R., Lohman, A. H. M. & van den Bercken, J. H. L., pp. 1–19. North-Holland, Elsevier.

Oberlander, C., Dumont, C. & Boissier, J. R. (1977) Rotational behavior after unilateral intranigral injection of muscimol in rats. *Europ. J. Pharmacol* 43, 389–390.

Olianas, M. C., De Montis, G. M., Concu, A., Tagliamonte, A. & Di Chiara, G. (1978a) Intranigral kainic acid: evidence for nigral non-dopaminergic neurons controlling posture and behavior in a manner opposite to the dopaminergic ones. *Europ. J. Pharmacol.* 49, 223–232.

Olianas, M. C., De Montis, G. M., Mulas, G. & Tagliamonte, A. (1978b) The striatal dopaminergic function is mediated by the inhibition of a nigral non-dopaminergic neuronal system via a striato-nigral GABA-ergic pathway. *Europ. J. Pharmacol.* 49, 233–241.

Olpe, H.-R., Schellenberg, H. & Koella, W. P. (1977) Rotational behavior induced in rats by intra-nigral application of GABA-related drugs and GABA antagonists. *Europ. J. Pharmacol.* 45, 291–294.

Pedersen, V. & Christensen, A.V. (1972) Antagonism of methylphenidate-induced stereotyped gnawing in mice. *Acta Pharmacol. Toxicol.* 31, 488–496.

Perez de la Mora, M., Fuxe, K., Hökfelt, T. & Ljungdahl, Å. (1975) Effect of apomorphine on the GABA turnover in the DA cell group rich area of the mesencephalon. Evidence for an involvement of an inhibitory gabergic feedback control of the ascending DA neurons. *Neurosci. Lett.* 1, 109–114.

Pycock, C. J. & Horton, R. W. (1976) Possible GABA-mediated control of dopamine-dependent behavioural effects from the nucleus accumbens of the rat. *Psychopharmacol* 49, 173–178.

Randrup, A. & Munkvad, I. (1967) Stereotyped activities produced by amphetamine in several animal species and man. *Psychopharmacol.* 11, 300–310.

Scheel-Krüger, J., Arnt, J. & Magelund, G. (1977a) Behavioural stimulation induced by muscimol and other GABA antagonists injected into the substantia nigra. *Neurosci. Letters* 4, 351–356.

Scheel-Krüger, J., Cools, A. R. & Honig, W. M. M. (1977b) Muscimol antagonizes the ergometrine-induced locomotor activity in nucleus accumbens: Evidence for GABA-dopaminergic interactions. *Europ. J. Pharmacol.* 42, 311–313.

Scheel-Krüger, J., Cools, A. R. & van Wel, P. M. (1977c) Muscimol a GABA agonist injected into the nucleus accumbens increases apomorphine stereotypy and decreases the motility. *Life Sci.* 21, 1697–1702.

Scheel-Krüger, J., Christensen, A. V. & Arnt, J. (1978) Muscimol differentially facilitates stereotypy but antagonizes motility induced by dopaminergic drugs: A complex GABA-dopamine interaction. *Life Sci.* 22. 75–84.

Squires, R. F. & Bræstrup, C. (1977) Benzodiazepine receptors in rat brain. *Nature* 266, 732–734.

Starr, M. S. (1978) GABA potentiates potassium-stimulated ^{3}H-dopamine release from slices of rat substantia nigra and corpus striatum. *Europ. J. Pharmacol.* 48, 325–328.

Stoof, J. C. & Mulder, A. H.(1977) Increased dopamine release from rat striatal slices by inhibitors of GABA-aminotransferase. *Europ. J. Pharmacol.* 46, 177–180.

Tappaz, M. L., Brownstein, M. J. & Palkovits, M. (1976) Distribution of glutamate decarboxylase in discrete brain nuclei. *Brain Res.* 108, 371–380.

Wachtel, H. & Andén, N. E. (1978) Motor activity of rats following intracerebral injections of drugs influencing GABA mechanisms. *Naunyn-Schmiedeberg's Arch. Pharmacol.* 302, 133–139.

Waddington, J. L. (1977) GABA-like properties of fluazepam and baclofen suggested by rotational behavior following unilateral intranigral injection: a comparison with the GABA agonist muscimol. *Brit. J. Pharmacol.* 60, 263–264P.

Walters, J. & Lakoski, J. M. (1978) Effect of muscimol on single unit activity of substantia nigra dopamine neurons. *Europ. J. Pharmacol.* 47, 469–471.

Walters, J. R., Roth, R. H. & Aghajanian, G. K. (1973) Dopaminergic neurons: similar biochemical and histochemical effects of γ-hydroxy-butyrate and acute lesions of the nigro-neostriatal pathway. *J. Pharmacol. Exp. Ther.* 186, 630–639.

Strio-Nigral and Nigro-Thalamic GABA-ergic Neurons as Output Pathways for Striatal Responses

G. Di Chiara, M. L. Porceddu, M. Morelli, M. L. Mulas & G. L. Gessa

Dopaminergic drugs are known to produce stereotyped behavior, turning and catalepsy. These effects are due to an interaction with dopamine (DA) receptors located in the striatum (Fog *et al.* 1970, Asher & Aghajanian 1974, Kelly *et al.* 1975, Kelly 1975). In recent years much attention has been drawn to the neural pathways and to the neurotransmitters mediating these behavioral effects.

It is well known from anatomical studies that the striatum is provided of two main efferent pathways, the one terminating in the substantia nigra, the other in the globus pallidus (Mehler & Nauta 1974, Carpenter 1976a).

According to a view which has gained large consensus, strio-pallidal neurons are the major efferent route of the striatum, while strio-nigral neurons would be a feedback pathway regulating the activity of nigro-striatal DA neurons (Carpenter 1976b). This view derives in part from the notion that the main function of the substantia nigra is due to its DA neurons located in the pars compacta and that pars reticulata, traversed by the long DA dendrites, is essentially the receiving part, the "neuropil", of the compacta (Rinvik & Grofova 1970). With these premises, the discovery of GABA as a transmitter of the strio-nigral pathway has been taken to indicate that nigral GABA subserves the function of regulating DA neurons, probably by exerting an inhibitory influence on their activity (Gale & Guidotti 1976).

Recent studies, however, have suggested a rather different picture of the strio-nigral relationships and of the role of GABA in the nigra. Relevant to this has been the following evidence:

Institutes of pharmacology, University of Cagliari, Via Porcell 4, 09100 Cagliari, Italy.

"GABA-NEUROTRANSMITTERS", Alfred Benzon Symposium 12, Munksgaard 1978

1) Lesions of the strio-nigral pathway drastically reduce the contralateral turning elicited by apomorphine in rats bearing unilateral 6-0HDA-induced lesions of the nigro-striatal DA-neurons (Marshall & Ungerstedt 1977).
2) Unilateral or bilateral destruction of nigral perikaria by the local injection of kainic acid results in chronic contralateral turning and, respectively, in stereotyped behavior insensitive to blockade of DA receptors by neuroleptics and independent of the presence of DA neurons (Di Chiara *et al.* 1977, Olianas *et al.* 1978).
3) Intranigral administration of GABA receptor agonists elicits acute effects qualitatively similar to the chronic ones produced by the intranigral administration of kainic acid and, like them, insensitive to neuroleptics (Scheel-Krüger *et al.* 1977, Oberlander *et al.* 1977).

These results indicated the existence of nigral neurons different from the dopaminergic ones but capable of exerting a profound influence on behavior and posture (Di Chiara *et al.* 1977). Since destruction of nigral non-DA neurons elicited effects similar to those resulting from dopaminergic activation, these neurons appeared as functionally opposite to the dopaminergic ones.

These results also indicated that the strio-nigral pathway, being essential for the expression of the behavioral effects of striatal DA receptor stimulation, is not only a "feedback" pathway but also an efferent route for striatal impulses (Marshall & Ungerstedt 1977, Garcia-Munoz *et al.* 1977). Finally, these results showed that nigral non-DA neurons are very sensitive to stimulation of nigral GABA receptors and indirectly suggested that an important role of nigral GABA and of the strio-nigral pathway could be that of modulating the activity of nigral non-DA neurons.

THE NIGRA AS A STATION OF STRIATAL OUTPUT

If these hypotheses are correct, one should expect that the nigral non-DA neurons are, just like the strio-nigral path, essential for the expression of striatal dopaminergic behavioral responses. This, in fact, appears to be the case, since destruction of nigral neurons by intranigral injection of kainic acid (0.75 μg) on the same side previously denervated with 6-0HDA, results in drastic reduction of the contralateral turning elicited by periferal apomorphine administration (Table I). Moreover, if apomorphine is administered to rats bearing kainic-induced nigral lesions, it produces ipsilateral turning as a result of the prevalence of apomorphine action on the intact side (Di Chiara *et al.* 1978). Finally,

Table I

Reversal of contralateral turning in the 6OH-DA model by Kainic-induced nigral lesion

Intranigral injection	6-OHDA (MFB)	Apomorphine (0.5 mg/kg s.c.)	N	Turning Direction	Intensity (r.p.m.)
Saline	+	+	20	Contralateral	23±2.2
Kainic-acid (0.75 μg)	+	+	20	Ipsilateral	13±1.6
Kainic-acid	−	+	20	Ipsilateral	10±1.1

Rats were lesioned unilaterally with 6-OHDA (8 μg/1 μl/3 min) in the medial forebrain bundle at the level of the lateral hypothalamus and 7 days later were injected with kainic acid in the nigra of the side lesioned with 6-OHDA. 15 days later they were tested with apomorphine and turning was estimated by counting the number of turns made during each 5-min interval of a 30-min observation period. Turning intensity: turns made during the 5-min interval of maximal turning.

bilateral lesion of the nigra with kainic acid makes apomorphine and haloperidol incapable to elicit stereotypies and catalepsy, respectively (Olianas *et al.* 1978) (Table II).

The decreased effectiveness of dopaminergic drugs after kainic-induced lesions is not due to loss of striatal postsynaptic DA receptors since striatal DA-sensitive adenyl cyclase on the lesioned side is unchanged in respect to the normal one (see Table IV). Moreover, these effects of intranigral kainic acid cannot be explained as due to damage of the strio-nigral axons since nigral DA-sensitive adenylate cyclase, which has been shown to be associated to these axons, is also unchanged in respect to the normal side (Table IV). Finally, these effects of kainic acid do not appear to be due to an action on areas adjacent to the

Table II

Prevention of neuroleptic catalepsy by kainic-induced bilateral nigral lesions

Nigral injection (0.5 μl/3 min.)	Haloperidol (mg/kg i.p.)	N	Catalepsy (score) I	II	III
Saline	0.5	10	2	3	0
	2.5	10	1	3	6
	5.0	10	0	1	9
Kainic acid (0.75 μg)	0.5	10	0	0	0
	2.5	10	1	1	0
	5.0	10	2	1	0

Kainic-lesioned rats were selected on the basis of the presence of intense (score 4) spontaneous stereotypies (24 h after K. a.). Haloperidol was given 15 days after the intranigral injections when stereotypies had disappeared. Catalepsy was scored 1 h after haloperidol on the basis of the time they remained suspended on the vertical grid (I 15″; II: 30″; III: 60″).

Table III
Effect of picrotoxin, injected in the nigra of the side lesioned with 6-OHDA, on the turning behavior elicited by apomorphine

Intranigral injection (ng)	N	Turning behavior		
		n	Side	Intensity (rmp) (mean±S.E.M.)
Saline	38	24	C	18±3
Picrotoxin (5)	12	12	C	8±2
Picrotoxin (10)	16	9	C	6±1
Picrotoxin (20)	14	6	I	12±3
Bicuculline (20)	12	6	I	14±3
Strychnine (10)	8	8	C	16±3
Strychnine (100)	10	10	C	20±4
Atropine (20)	8	8	C	18±4
Atropine (200)	10	10	C	22±4

N=number of rats injected in the nigra
n =number of rats showing turning
C=turning contralateral to intranigral injection
I =turning ipsilateral to intranigral injection.

nigra since injection of kainic acid about 1 mm dorsal to the nigra fails to produce asymmetries in normal rats or to reduce contralateral turning in 6-0HDA-lesioned rats injected with apomorphine.

Therefore we conclude that the substantia nigra is essential for the expression of such behavioral effects of dopaminergic drugs as stereotyped and turning behavior and catalepsy, which are considered to result from an action on striatal DA receptors (Fog *et al.* 1970, Asher & Aghajanian 1974, Kelly *et al.* 1975, Kelly 1975). Taken together with those of Marshall & Ungerstedt (1977), our results suggest that striatal dopaminergic impulses are effected through an influence of the strio-nigral pathway on nigral non-DA neurons.

NIGRAL GABA AS A MEDIATOR OF STRIATAL OUTPUT

If we consider that destruction of nigral non-DA neurons or their probable depression by GABA receptor agonists results in behavioral effects similar to those elicited by activation of striatal DA receptors and in view of the massive contribution of GABA-ergic neurons to the strio-nigral pathway, we might postulate that the behavioral effects of striatal DA receptor stimulation are secondary to an activation of strio-nigral GABA-ergic neurons inhibitory to nigral non-DA neurons. In order to test this hypothesis we studied the effect of intranigral administration of GABA receptor antagonists on the turning elicited by apomorphine in rats bearing unilateral 6-0HDA lesions of nigro-striatal DA neurons.

Administration of 5–20 ng of picrotoxin on the side previously lesioned with 6-0HDA impaired the contralateral turning produced by the administration of 0.25 mg/kg of apomorphine given subcutaneously. While 10 ng of picrotoxin drastically reduced or abolished the contralateral turning, 20 ng of picrotoxin actually reversed it into an ipsilateral one in about 50% of the animals (Table III).

Similar results were obtained with the intra-nigral injection of 10–20 ng of bicuculline methiodide, another GABA receptor antagonist (Table III).

Intranigral injections of 10–100 ng of strychnine, a glycine-receptor antagonist, or of 20–200 ng of atropine, a muscarinic receptor antagonist, failed to reduce the intensity of the contralateral turning in respect to rats injected in the nigra with saline (Table III).

These results support the concept that striatal dopaminergic responses are mediated by a release of GABA within the nigra, possibly from the GABA-ergic strio-nigral pathway (Di Chiara *et al.* 1978b). Thus, stereotyped behavior and contralateral turning in response to DA receptor stimulation would be due to an increased release of GABA in the nigra, resulting in depression of non-DA pars reticulata neurons. Conversely, catalepsy in response to striatal DA receptor blockade would depend on a reduction of nigral GABA release with consequent activation of nigral non-DA neurons.

According to this hypothesis, stimulation of striatal DA receptors should increase the activity of nigral GABA-ergic synapses; moreover, facilitation of nigral GABA-ergic transmission should potentiate the behavioral effects of striatal dopaminergic stimulation. In agreement with these expectations, it has been reported that systemic administration of apomorphine stimulates GABA turnover in the nigra (Perez De La Mora *et al.* 1975), while the increase of nigral GABA levels by blockade of GABA transaminase with ethanolamine-O-sulphate, results in potentiation of the stereotypies induced by amphetamine (Koob *et al.* 1977).

According to our hypothesis an increased GABA-ergic transmission in the nigra should exert an anticataleptic effect. In agreement with this it has been reported that noncataleptogenic neuroleptics, in contrast to the cataleptogenic ones, stimulate nigral GABA turnover (Marco *et al.* 1976).

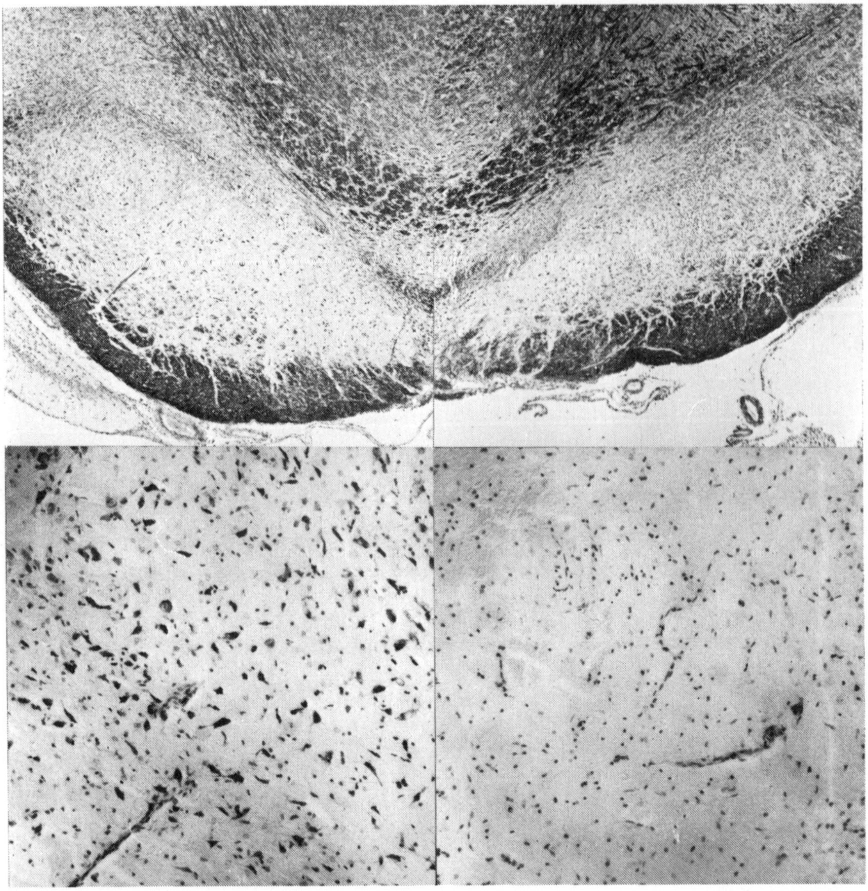

(a) (b) (c) (d)

Fig. 1. Histological effects of the unilateral intranigral injection of kainic acid (1.5 μg/0.5 μl/3 min). Pictures on the left refer to the control side, those on the right, to the lesioned side. A and B: 7 d. postkainic, Luxol fast-cresyl violet stain (2.5×). Note the complete loss of neuronal perikaria in the lateral half of the nigra. Within this area, pars compacta, reticulata and lateralis appear destroyed to a similar degree. Pars compacta and reticulata neurons located in the medial extremity of the nigra are spared. C and D: cresyl violet stain (10 ×) of pars reticulata. Notice the complete loss of neuronal perikaria in the kainic-injected side. 24 h postkainic.

HISTOLOGICAL CHANGES AFTER INTRANIGRAL KAINIC ACID

In the effort to clarify the nature of the nigral non-DA neurons lesioned by kainic acid, histological studies were performed using the cresylviolet stain alone or in conjunction with the Luxol fast blue stain for myelinated axons and the silver impregnation method of Fink-Heimer for terminal degeneration. Rats were injected with 0.75 μg or with 1.5 μg of kainic acid (0.5 μl/3 min) in one nigra

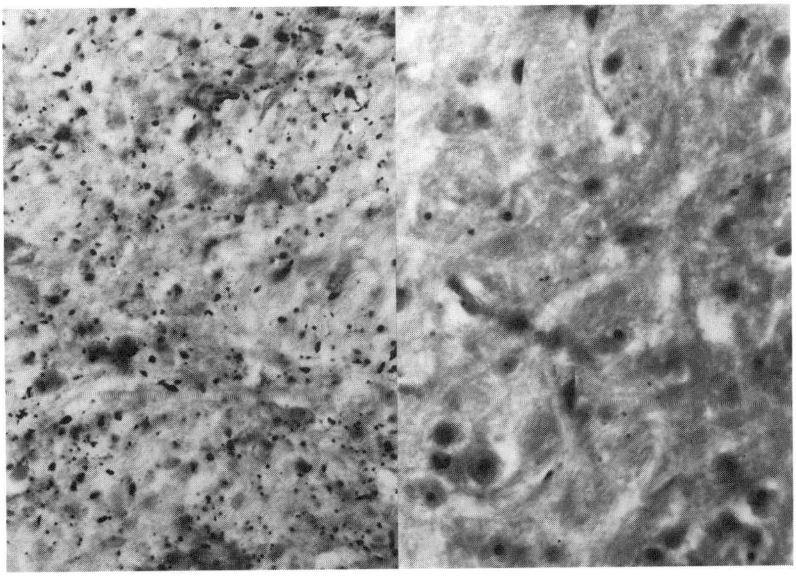

(*a*) (*b*)

Fig. 2. Terminal degeneration (Fink-Heimer stain) in the ventro-medial thalamus 3 days after injected side. B: control side.

and with saline in the contralateral one and were killed 12 h, 24 h and 1, 2, 3 and 7 days after kainic acid injection.

The lesion produced by kainic acid was localized to a spherical area of about 1.3–1.5 mm diameter and consisted of a loss of all neuronal perikaria (Fig. 1). Locations of the cannula tip in the ventral part of the pars reticulata resulted in less damage to the compacta than more medial locations. Nerve cells were replaced by glia, which 7 days after kainic acid produced an appearance of increased cellularity (Di Chiara *et al.* 1977). The most effective lesions for obtaining contralateral turning involved pars reticulata and pars lateralis and are shown in Fig. 1.

The fibers of mielinated tracts adjacent to the nigra (medial lemmiscus, cerebral peduncle) appeared normal (Fig. 1).

Three days after kainic acid (0.75 μg) injection in the pars reticulata, terminal degeneration was observed both in the compacta and in the reticulata, in the ventromedial (VM) thalamus (Fig. 2), superior colliculus, mesencephalic reticular formation and periventricular grey. In agreement with the only partial damage to the compacta, terminal degeneration in the caudate was scanty after injection of kainic acid in the center of pars reticulata.

Some degeneration was observed in the ventro-basal complex of the thalamus; however, it was present also on the control side injected with saline, and was probably due to mechanical damage of the lemmiscus medialis by the cannula.

These results indicate that kainic acid, at the doses effective for obtaining chronic contralateral turning, fails to produce degeneration of a specific neuronal type in the nigra. The relative involvement of the dopaminergic neurons of compacta versus those of the reticulata depends only on the actual location of the kainic acid injection.

Intranigral kainic acid resulted in terminal degeneration in the nigra as well as in areas which are known to receive nigral projection (Clavier *et al.* 1976, Jayaraman *et al.* 1977, Graybiel 1978, Hopkins & Nissen 1976). Therefore it appears that intranigral kainic acid produces degeneration of both intrinsic and extrinsic nigral neurons without damaging myelinated tracts adjacent to the nigra.

NEUROCHEMICAL CHANGES AFTER INTRANIGRAL KAINIC ACID

Since it appeared from the histological data that intranigral kainic acid was able to damage selectively the nigral neuronal perikaria, we studied its effect on some enzymatic markers of specific neurons in the nigra and in areas of projection of nigral neurons as the striatum and the VM thalamus, hoping that this study could shed some light on the nature of the nondopaminergic neurons of the nigra. Rats were injected in the nigra of one side with 1.5 μg of kainic acid and on the other side with saline; they were selected on the basis of the presence of continuous, obligated contralateral turning 24 h after the injections. Seven days after the injection the animals were sacrificed and the brains were cut by a coronal section which separated a cranial part, containing the caudates, from a caudal part containing the VM thalamus and the mesencephalon.

This caudal part was placed on a cryostat, frozen at $-10°$ and cut in serial 400 μm slices. From these slices samples of VM and ventrobasal (VB) thalamic nuclei and of nigra were punched out from each side using stainless steel cannulas.

The head of the caudate of each side and the samples of nigra were analyzed for tyrosine hydroxylase (TH), glutamic acid decarboxylase (GAD), choline acetyl transferase (CAT) and DA-sensitive adenylate cyclase, respectively the markers of dopaminergic, GABA-ergic and cholinergic neurons and of DA

Table IV

Pre- and postsynaptic enzymatic markers after intranigral kainic acid (1.5 μg)

Enzyme	N	Nigra Control	Nigra Lesioned	Striatum Control	Striatum Lesioned	VM-thalamus Control	VM-thalamus Lesioned	VB-thalamus Control	VB-thalamus Lesioned
GAD	7	930 ± 35	820 ± 38*	183 ± 9.3	174 ± 8.4^{ns}	352 ± 25	$210\pm20^{*1}$	150 ± 10	130 ± 9^{ns}
CAT	7	8.9 ± 0.9	7.7 ± 0.8^{ns}	320 ± 2.8	308 ± 2.5^{ns}	12.5 ± 0.7	11.3 ± 0.6^{ns}	9.2 ± 0.5	8.6 ± 0.5^{ns}
TH	7	1.1 ± 0.06	0.45 ± 0.03*	2.2 ± 0.12	2.0 ± 0.12^{ns}	—	—	—	—
DA-cyclase	7	127 ± 13	116 ± 12^{ns}	108 ± 11	145 ± 12^{ns}	—	—	—	—

Results are expressed in nmol/mg prot/hr (GAD, CAT and TH) or in pmol/mg prot/min (DA-sensitive adenylate cyclase). TH was assayed at 0.2 mM $DMPH_4$. DA-sensitive adenylate cyclase is the increase in c-AMP production over basal values in the presence of 1×10^{-4}M DA. Rats were killed 7 days after injection of kainic acid in the nigra of one side and of saline in the contralateral one (0.5 μl/3 min).

* $P<0.05$, us: not significantly different in respect to the control side.

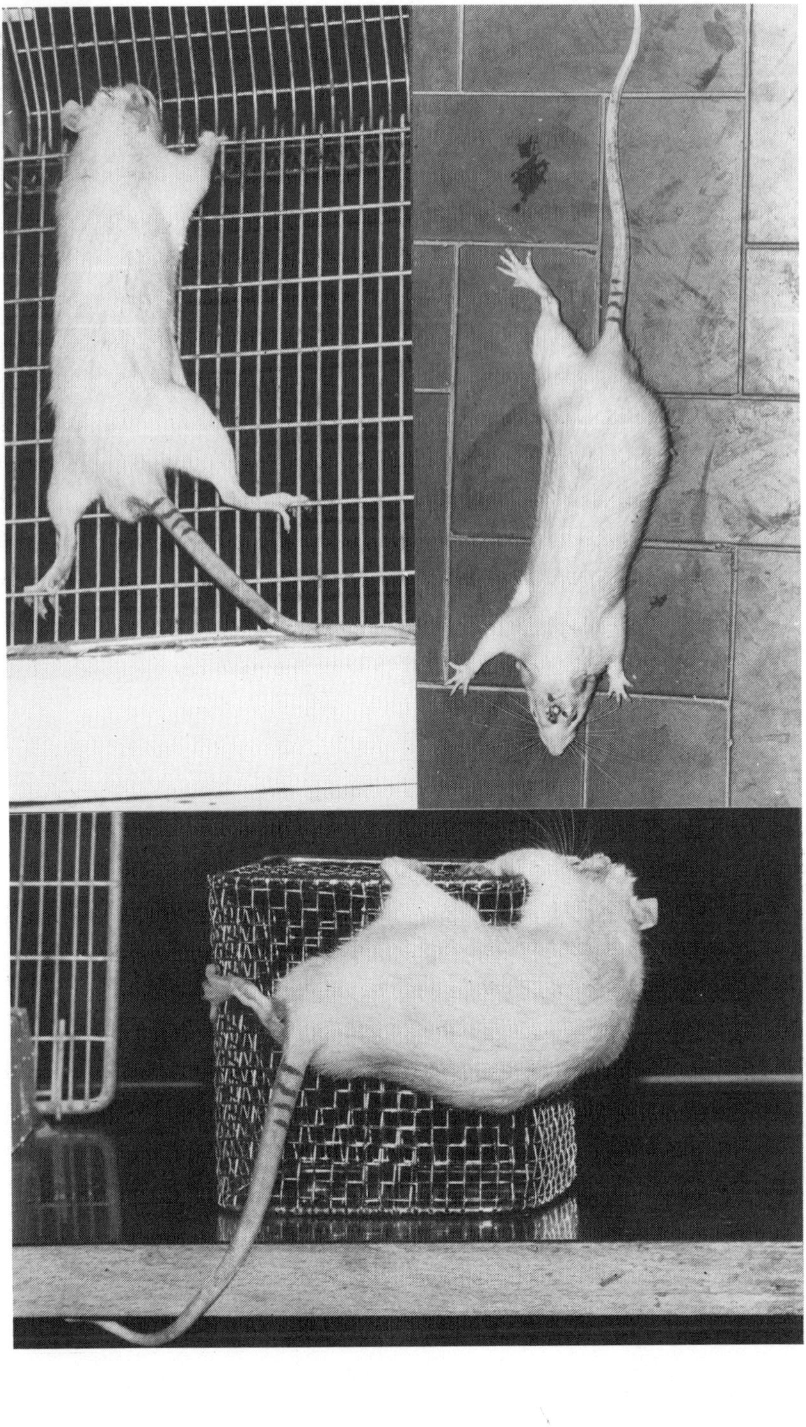

(a) (c)

(b)

receptors (Spano *et al.* 1977). The samples of VM and VB nuclei were analyzed only for GAD and CAT. Results were always expressed per mg of protein.

Table IV shows the results obtained. DA-sensitive adenylate cyclase and CAT resulted unchanged in all areas examined. TH was significantly reduced both in the nigra and in the striatum. GAD was unchanged in the striatum and in the VB thalamus but was significantly reduced in the VM thalamus and, although slightly, also in the nigra.

Since nigral DA-sensitive adenylate cyclase has been shown to be localized on strio-nigral neurons (Spano *et al.* 1977), the lack of change after kainic acid confirms the conclusions of the morphological studies that kainic acid fails to directly damage axonal structures.

Moreover, the lack of change of CAT, in spite of the neuronal loss and of the presence of terminal degeneration in the nigra, suggests that the perikaria of nigral cholinergic neurons are located outside the nigra. This conclusion is at variance with the current view, based on the lack of change of nigral CAT after hemitransections at the level of the lateral hypothalamus, that cholinergic neurons are intrinsic to the nigra (McGeer *et al.* 1973).

The specific decrease of GAD in the VM thalamus after nigral lesions with kainic acid suggests that nigro-thalamic neurons, which degenerate after these lesions, are, at least in part, GABA-ergic in nature. This finding provides an explanation for the inhibitory nature of the nigro-thalamic pathway as deduced from electrophysiological studies showing monosynaptic IPSPs in the VM thalamus after nigral stimulation (Ueki *et al.* 1977, Deniau *et al.* 1978).

POSSIBLE ROLE OF A GABA-ERGIC NIGRO-THALAMIC PATHWAY IN THE MEDIATION OF STRIATAL RESPONSES

The GABA-ergic nigro-thalamic pathway, being a non-DA-ergic pathway efferent from the nigra, is one of the candidates for the meditation of striatal efferent impulses beyond the nigra. We reasoned that if this GABA-ergic pathway had such a role, pharmacological manipulations of GABA-ergic mechanisms within the VM thalamus would have exerted some influence on

---

Fig. 3. Behavioral effects of muscimol (10 ng/0.5 μl/1.5 min) injected in the ventro-medial thalamus (coordinates: A−0.8; V 6.5; L 1.5 of Pellegrino & Cushman 1971).

A: vertical grid test for catalepsy

B: An "uncomfortable" posture

C: "Frozen posture" interrupting locomotion.

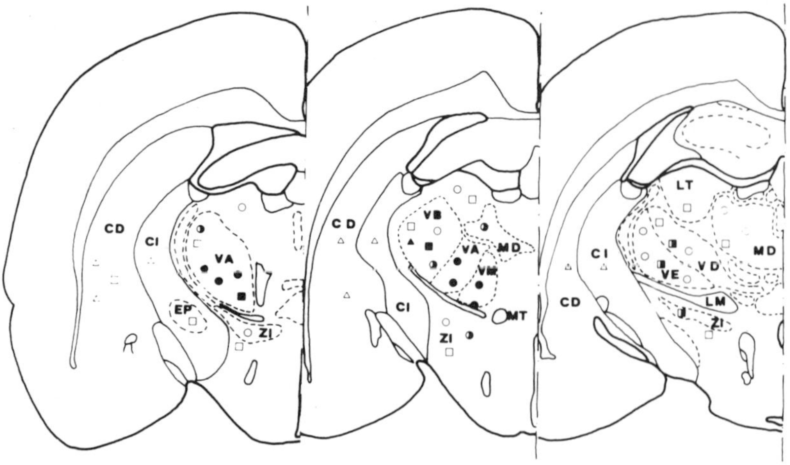

Fig. 4. Cerebral sites for muscimol-induced catalepsy. Rats were implanted stereotaxically with bilateral chronic guide cannulas and 2 days later drugs were injected by two injectors, protruding 1 mm from the guide cannula tip, each through connected polyethylene tubing to an hamilton syringe driven by an infusion pump. Coordinates and maps are taken from Pellegrino & Cushman (1971). Muscimol was dissolved in saline and injected at the doses of 10 ng (circles), 25 ng (squares) and 50 ng (triangles). Rats were tested for catalepsy on the vertical grid starting 15 min after the injection and every 15 min up 1 h postinjection. The test was considered positive if rats remained still on the vertical grid for at least 60 sec. Rats were injected only once and the same day were perfused with formalin. In order to ascertain the location of the injections, brains were cut by coronal sections along the plane of the atlas of Pellegrino & Cushman (1971) and the site of the injector tip was reported on maps of the atlas. This figure has been constructed on the basis of the results obtained in rats were the differences in location of the tips on the two sides were no larger than 0.2 mm. Each site represented in the figure corresponds to the actual location of the injector tip on the left side. Open symbols indicate negativity of all catalepsy tests. Filled symbols indicate positivity for catalepsy on at least two consecutive tests. Half-filled symbols indicate positivity for catalepsy on one or on more than one nonconsecutive tests.

motor and postural functions as well as on the behavioral effects of drugs acting on striatal DA receptors.

Therefore we studied the behavioral effects of local thalamic micro-injections of muscimol, a GABA receptor agonist, and of picrotoxin, a GABA receptor antagonist. Rats were implanted whith chronic intracerebral bilateral guide cannulas fixed to the skull with dental cement and screws and 2 days thereafter drugs were injected in 0.5 μl volumes by injectors inserted into the guides and connected through polyethylene tubing to an infusion pump delivering the solutions at a constant rate of 1 μl/6 min.

Muscimol was able to elicit a striking catalepsy when injected in nanogram amounts in the VM and adjacent ventral anterior (VA) nuclei of the thalamus. Ten nanograms of muscimol were effective in producing catalepsy in all rats within 10–15 min for about 90 min. Rigidity was prominent both in the trunk and in the limbs, particularly in the posterior ones. Rats maintained for long time most postures imposed to them, even the most unconfortable (Fig. 3). When tested on the vertical grid they could remain suspended to it, if undisturbed, for more than 30 min. Cataleptic postures could be broken by sensory stimuli such as pinching of the tail or handling. When placed on the floor, rats started walking but soon interrupted the movement during its execution to assume "frozen postures" (Fig. 3). Righting reflex was present and ptosis was absent. As shown in Fig. 4, the most sensitive area for muscimol-induced catalepsy was the VM and VA nuclei of the thalamus.

Doses of muscimol higher than 10 ng were able to elicit catalepsy also from other thalamic nuclei, but the shortest latencies were always observed after injections in the VM-VA nuclei (Fig. 4). Injection of up to 50 ng of muscimol in the adjacent caudate, in the globus pallidus, in the internal capsule or in the lateral hypothalamus failed to elicit catalepsy (Fig. 4). Therefore it is concluded that catalepsy obtained after intrathalamic injection of muscimol arises specifically from the VM-VA nuclei. Injection of picrotoxin (200 ng) in VM 30 min after the injection of 10 ng muscimol in the same area resulted in complete disappearance of catalepsy and "frozen postures" within 10–15 min.

The catalepsy produced by 10 ng muscimol injected in VM was not relieved by apomorphine (5 mg/kg s.c.) nor by intranigral muscimol (20 ng bilaterally).

However, intrathalamic muscimol (10 ng) failed to reduce the intensity of the stereotyped behavior produced by systemic apomorphine or by intranigral muscimol. Therefore in these animals catalepsy and stereotyped behavior were coexistent.

Injection of picrotoxin (100, 200 ng) in the VM nucleus resulted in hypermotility characterized by compulsive forward progression. This syndrome could not be elicited from any other thalamic areas. It should be noted that the hypermotility produced by intrathalamic picrotoxin did not take the form of stereotyped exploratory behavior such as that produced by dopaminergic stimulants. Moreover, stereotyped sniffing or gnawing was completely absent.

Injection of 200 ng of picrotoxin in the VM thalamus reversed the catalepsy produced by 2.0 mg/kg of haloperidol. Injection of the same dose of picrotoxin 1 mm dorsal to the VM site failed to affect the catalepsy induced by haloperidol.

These findings clearly indicate the existence in the VM thalamus of GABA-

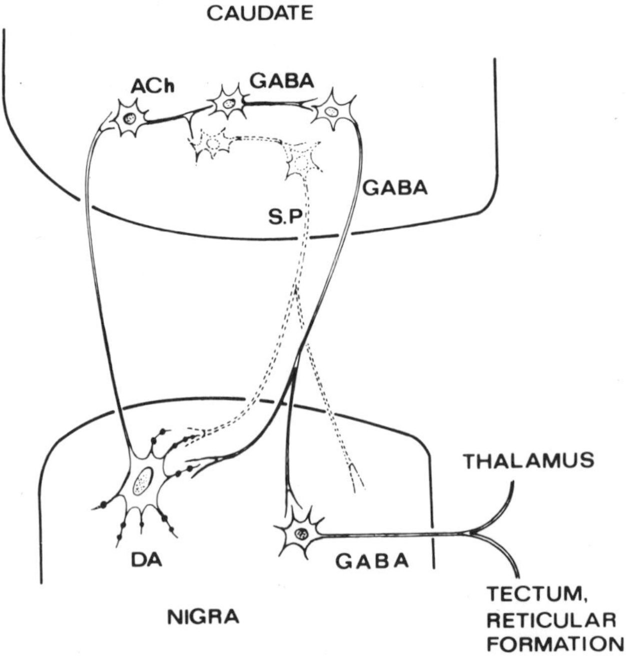

Fig. 5. Proposed pathways mediating dopaminergic behavioral responses arising from the striatum. The diagram shows that dopaminergic neurons influence the long strio-nigral GABA-ergic neurons by depressing striatal cholinergic interneurons excitatory to short GABA-ergic neurons. With this arrangement, stimulation of DA receptors would reduce the strong intrinsic inhibitory tone exerted on strio-nigral neurons by the coupling of excitatory and inhibitory interneurons. Therefore, stimulation of DA receptors would result in activation of GABA-ergic strio-nigral neurons and the resulting increased release of GABA in the nigra would depress nigral non-DA neurons effecting the behavior.

ergic mechanisms whose pharmacological manipulation has a profound influence on extrapyramidal functions and on the effects of drugs interacting with striatal DA receptors. The fact that the blockade of thalamic GABA receptors relieves the catalepsy produced by blockade of striatal DA receptors indicates that neuroleptic-induced catalepsy is mediated by release of GABA in the VM thalamus. The fact that the catalepsy elicited by stimulation of thalamic GABA receptors, is, in contrast to that produced by blockade of striatal DA receptors, resistant to apomorphine and to intranigral muscimol, suggests that the VM thalamus is located beyond the striatum and the nigra in the neuronal chain mediating some behavioral responses, such as neuroleptic catalepsy originating in the striatum.

In view of the GABA-ergic nature of the nigro-thalamic pathway, we suggest that the catalepsy produced by blockade of striatal DA receptors is due to activation of nigro-thalamic GABA-ergic neurons.

As suggested above, the catatonia produced by DA receptor blockers results from reduction of GABA-release from the strio-nigral neurons. Therefore, activation of nigro-thalamic neurons might be the consequence of a reduced inhibitory tone exerted by the strio-nigral pathway. Consistent with this hypothesis are electrophysiological studies of Deniau *et al.* (1976, 1978) showing that the strio-nigral neurons exert a potent inhibitory influence on nigro-thalamic neurons.

Thalamic GABA-ergic mechanisms, however, are not critical for all behavioral effects of striatal origin. In fact, the inability of intrathalamic picrotoxin to produce stereotyped behavior and of intrathalamic muscimol to block the stereotypies elicited by apomorphine or by intranigral muscimol, shows that, in contrast to catalepsy, stereotyped behavior is effected through pathways different from the nigro-thalamic ones. Possible candidates for this are the nigro-tectal or the nigro-reticular neurons.

Fig. 5 shows a diagram of the striatal output pathways according to the views exposed in the present article.

REFERENCES

Asher, I. M. & Aghajanian, G. K. (1974) 6-hydroxydopamine lesions of olfactory tubercles and caudate nuclei: effect on amphetamine-induced stereotyped behavior in rats. *Brain Res.* 82, 1–12.

Carpenter, M. B. (1976a) Anatomy of the basal ganglia and related nuclei: a review. In: *Advances in Neurology,* vol. 14, ed. Eldridge, R. & Fahn, S., pp. 7–47. Raven Press, New York.

Carpenter, M. B. (1976b) *Human Neuroanatomy,* pp. 513–514. The Williams & Wilkins Company, Baltimore.

Clavier, R. M., Atmajda, R. & Fibiger, H. C. (1976) Nigrothalamic projections in the rat as demonstrated by orthograde and retrograde tracing techniques. *Brain Res. Bull.* 1, 379–384.

Deniau, J. M., Feger, J. & Le Guyader, C. (1976) Striatal evoked inhibition of identified nigro-thalamic neurons. *Brain Res.* 104, 152–156.

Deniau, J. M., Lackner, D. & Feger, J. (1978) Effect of substantia nigra stimulation on identified neurons in the VL-VA thalamic complex: comparison between intact and chronically decorticated cats. *Brain Res.* 145, 27–35.

Di Chiara, G., Olianas, M., Del Fiacco, M., Spano, P.-F. & Tagliamonte, A. (1977) Intranigral kainic acid is evidence that nigral non-dopaminergic neurones control posture. *Nature* 268, 743–745.

Di Chiara, G., Porceddu, M. L., Morelli, M., Mulas, M. L. & Gessa, G. L. (1978a) Substantia nigra as an out-put station of striatal functions. *Naunyn-Schmiedeberg's Arch. Pharmacol.* In press.

Di Chiara, G., Morelli, M., Porceddu, M. L. & Gessa, G. L. (1978b) Evidence that nigral GABA mediates striatal dopaminergic responses. *Life Sci.* In press.

Fog, R., Randrup, A. & Pakkenberg, H. (1970) Lesions in corpus striatum and cortex of rat brains and the effect on pharmacologically induced stereotyped aggressive and cataleptic behaviour. *Psychopharmacologia* (Berl.) 18, 346–356.

Gale, K. N. & Guidotti, A. (1976) GABA-mediated control of rat neostriatal tyrosine hydroxylase revealed by intranigral muscimol. *Nature* 263, 691–693.

Garcia-Munoz, M., Nicolaou, N. M., Tulloch, I. F., Wright, A. K. & Arbuthnott, G. W. (1977) Feedback loop or out-put pathway in strio nigral fibers? *Nature* 265, 363–365.

Graybiel, A. M. (1978) Organization of the nigrotectal connection: an experimental tracer study in the cat. *Brain Res.* 143, 339–348.

Hopkins, D. A. & Niessen, L. W. (1976) Substantia nigra projections to the reticular formation, superior colliculus and central gray in the rat, cat, and monkey. *Neurosci. Lett.* 2, 253–259.

Jayaraman, A., Batton III, R. R. & Carpenter, M. B. (1977) Nigrotectal projections in the monkey: an autoradiographic study. *Brain Res.* 135, 147–152.

Kelly, P. H. (1975) Unilateral 6-hydroxydopamine lesions of nigrostriatal or mesolimbic dopamine-containing terminals and the drug-induced rotation of rats. *Brain Res.* 100, 163–169.

Kelly, P. H., Seviour, P. W. & Iversen, S. D. (1975) Amphetamine and apomorphine responses in the rat following 6-OHDA lesions of the nucleus accumbens septi and corpus striatum. *Brain Res.* 94, 507–522.

Koob, G., Del Fiacco, M. & Iversen, S. D. (1977) Dissociable properties of the DA-neurons in the nigro-striatal and mesolimbic DA-systems. In: *Non-Striatal Dopaminergic Neurons,* vol. 16, ed. Costa, E. & Gessa, G. L., pp. 352–356. Raven Press, New York.

Marco, E., Mao, C. C., Cheney, D. L., Revuelta, A. & Costa, E. (1976) The effects of anti-psychotics on the turnover rate of GABA and acetylcholine in rat brain nuclei. *Nature* 264, 363–365.

Marshall, J. F. & Ungerstedt, U. (1977) Striatal efferent fibers play a role in maintaining rotational behavior in the rat. *Sci.* 198, 62–64.

McGeer, E. G., Fibiger, H. C., McGeer, P. L. & Brooke, S. (1973) Temporal changes in amine synthesizing enzymes of rat extrapyramidal structures after hemitransections or 6-hydroxy-dopamine administration. *Brain Res.* 52, 289–300.

Mehler, W. R. & Nauta, W. J. H. (1974) Connections of the basal ganglia and of the cerebellum. In: *Confinia Neurologica,* vol. 36, ed. Spiegel, E. A., pp. 205–222. S. Karger, Basel.

Oberlander, C., Dumont, C. & Boissier, J. R. (1977) Rotational behaviour after unilateral intra-nigral injection of muscimol in rats. *Eur. J. Pharmacol.* 43, 389–390.

Olianas, M. C., De Montis, G. M., Concu, A., Tagliamonte, A. & Di Chiara, G. (1978) Intranigral kainic acid: evidence for nigral non-dopaminergic neurons controlling posture and behavior in a manner opposite to the dopaminergic ones. *Eur. J. Pharmacol.* 49, 223–232.

Pellegrino, L. J. & Cushman, A. J. (1971) *A Stereotaxic Atlas of the Rat Brain.* Meredith, New York.

Perez de la Mora, M., Fuxe, K., Hökfelt, T. & Ljungdahl, Å. (1975) Effect of apomorphine on the GABA turnover in the DA cell group rich area of the mesencephalon. Evidence for the involve-ment of an inhibitory GABA-ergic feedback control of the ascending DA neurons. *Neurosci. Lett.* 1, 109–114.

Rinvik, E. & Grofova, I. (1970) Observations on the fine structure of the substantia nigra in the cat. *Exp. Brain Res.* 11, 229–248.

Scheel-Krüger, J., Arnt, J. & Magelund, G. (1977) Behavioural stimulation induced by muscimol and other GABA agonists injected into the substantia nigra. *Neurosci. Lett.* 4, 351–356.

Spano, P. F., Trabucchi, M. & Di Chiara, G. (1977) Localization of DA-sensitive adenylate cyclase on neurons originating from the corpus striatum. *Sci.* 196, 1343–1344.

Ueki, A., Uno, M., Anderson, M. & Yoshida, M. (1977) Monosynaptic inhibition of thalamic neurons produced by stimulation of the substantia nigra. *Experientia* 15, 1480–1482.

Differential Effects of Baclofen and Muscimol on Behavioral Responses Implicating GABA-ergic Transmission

A. Delini-Stula

Since the preliminary report by Frederiksen (1975) that baclofen, a γ-amino butyric acid derivative, beneficially affects the symptoms of schizophrenia, there has been an explosion of research related to all aspects of baclofen action on the functional responses mediated by the nigro-striatal dopaminergic system. Because of its structural similarity with GABA, a natural inhibitory transmitter, speculations have been made that baclofen acts by mimicking GABA action on dopaminergic transmission and by virtue of this produces antipsychotic effects. The important aspects of this speculation was that it focused on a possible new approach to the treatment of schizophrenia by means of drugs which indirectly, through activation of inhibitory transmitter systems, reduce the excessive functioning of dopaminergic neurons.

Although an antipsychotic action of baclofen was not confirmed in subsequent controlled clinical trials, this compound has remained an interesting tool for psychopharmacological research of the complex transmitter interactions in the nigro-striatal system. However, it should be mentioned that the exact nature of the supraspinal central effects of baclofen is still an unresolved enigma.

Until now neurophysiological investigations have provided no evidence for a direct GABA agonistic action of baclofen (Curtis *et al.* 1974, Davies & Watkins 1974, Nistri 1975, Polc & Haefely 1976). Despite this fact, in many pharmacological and biochemical studies baclofen produced effects which were compatible with a GABA-like influence on in particular dopaminergic trans-

Research Department, Pharmaceuticals Division, CIBA–GEIGY Ltd., Basle, Switzerland.

"GABA-NEUROTRANSMITTERS", Alfred Benzon Symposium 12, Munksgaard 1978

mission (Bernard *et al.* 1975, Fuxe *et al.* 1975, Kääriäinen 1976, Waddington & Harrow 1977, Andén & Wachtel 1977).

The discrepancy between neurophysiological and psychopharmacological findings posed a question whether or not the manipulation of GABA-ergic transmission by drugs results in specific changes of behavioral responses and also whether or not behavioral manifestations discriminate the mode of action of GABA-like compounds. One possible approach to the resolution of these questions was to study in parallel the effects of baclofen and muscimol, a potent and selective GABA-agonist, on various behavioral responses believed to reflect the interference with GABA-ergic system.

ANTAGONISM OF IZONIAZID-INDUCED CONVULSIONS IN MICE

Izoniazid, a glutamic acid decarboxylase inhibitor, causes convulsions in rodents probably by virtue of its action in decreasing the levels of GABA in the brain (Naik *et al.* 1976, Löscher & Frey 1977). It has been suggested that selective antagonism of izoniazid induced convulsions may reflect a direct or indirect stimulation of GABA receptors (Costa *et al.* 1975, Haefely *et al.* 1975). Comparing the effects of baclofen and muscimol on izoniazid-induced seizures in mice we have found that both drugs significantly and in a dose-dependent fashion delay the onset of convulsive fits at doses which were below those inducing marked motor depression. The protective effects were selective in that neither baclofen (up to 100 mg/kg p.o.) nor muscimol prevented the convulsant action of strychnine (unpublished observation). As can be seen from Table I, baclofen showed, however, a pattern of action against izoniazid-induced effects which differed from that displayed by muscimol. In parallel with prolongation of latency, baclofen also decreased the lethal effects of izoniazid, whereas muscimol did not affect the mortality rate at any of the doses tested. It is interesting to note that agents which increase the content of GABA in the brain like amino-oxy-acetic acid (AOAA) (Wallach, 1961) or valproate sodium (Depakine) (Godin *et al.* 1969) showed effects which were comparable to those of baclofen. The biochemical investigations have provided no evidence that baclofen changes the level of GABA in the brain of either rats or mice (Naik *et al.* 1976, Bernasconi & Martin 1978). However, like muscimol and diazepam, baclofen decreased the rate of synthesis of GABA in mice in which the turnover was measured indirectly by determining the accumulation of GABA after maximal inhibition of GABA-T by gabaculine (Bernasconi & Martin 1978). These results, although providing no explanation for the mode of action, indicate that baclofen, like muscimol and diazepam, might interfere with the metabolism of GABA. The findings that baclofen afforded protection against izoniazid convulsions is at variance with observations in rats which were reported by Naik (Naik *et al.* 1976). The discrepancy between the observation of these authors and our own may indicate species-specific differences in the response of animals to the drugs, but the differences in the treatment schedules may have been also of importance.

The izoniazid model in mice appears to provide more or less general information of possible modulatory effect of drugs on the metabolism of GABA

Table I

Effect of baclofen and GABA-like drugs on izoniazid-induced convulsions in mice

Drug	Dose mg/kg i.p.	Izoniazid convulsions: mean latency±SEM	Izoniazid convulsions: % mortality	Dose mg/kg i.p.	Motility: counts/15 min mean±SEM
	0.3	39± 2.1	100	0.3	316±11
Baclofen	1.0	46± 6.3*	80	1.0	322±32
	3.0	81±13.4*	40	3.0	304±26
	0.1	38± 1.5*	100		
Muscimol	0.3	45± 2.7*	100	0.5	91±23
	1.0	69±12.1*	100	0.75	14±12
Diazepam	0.3	47± 5.3	60	2.0	160±13
	1.0	55± 5.2*	20	5.0	39± 5
AOAA	10	54± 0.2*	80		
	25	>+90	0		
Valproate sodium	300	42± 2.5*	100		
	400	70± 4.3*	60		
Controls	—	34± 1.1	100		345±49

Baclofen, muscimol and diazepam were administered 30 min, AOAA and Valproate sodium 60 min before 250 mg/kg i.p. izoniazid. The latency to the onset of seizures and mortality were recorded during an observation period of 3 h. Statistical significance was calculated by means of the t-test. Each dose was assayed in at least five mice. The control values are the mean of 50 mice.

Motility was measured by means of a photo-cell apparatus in groups of three to five mice during an interval of 15 min. Each dose was assayed in five groups. Control values are the mean±SEM of 15 groups. Drugs were administered 30 min before the test.

* $P<0.05$ (t-test).

(Löscher & Frey 1977). Although as such it can be used for a rather general screening of drugs, its validity seems to be limited by a lack of sufficient specificity. Unpublished results from this laboratory indicate that various pharmacologically distinct types of drugs may display protective effects against izoniazid induced seizures in mice (neuroleptics, β-receptor blocking agents). Furthermore, it does not reveal either the nature of possible GABA-mimetic action nor the relevance for the behavioral responses of animals.

ANTIEXCITATORY EFFECTS OF BACLOFEN AND MUSCIMOL

Gaba- mimetic agents seem to share a property of inhibiting hyperactive motor responses produced by various stimulating drugs. Cott & Engel (1977) suggested that this property may reflect a general nature of the inhibitory effect of GABA-mimetics on central nervous system, which would be in line with the widespread distribution of GABA neurons in the brain. In order to prove whether antiexcitatory effects of baclofen and muscimol are of a general nature, we have found it of interest to investigate their action in two distinctly different models of excitatory behaviour: on morphine-induced hyperactivity and on hyperactivity produced by combined treatment with MAO inhibitor,pargyline, and the CA-depletor reserpine. Morphine-induced excitation appears to be related primarily to dopamine (Kuschinski & Hornikiewicz 1974) and can be selectively antagonized by dopamine-receptor blocking drugs, or drugs which decrease the impulse flow in dopaminergic neurons (Cott & Engel 1977). Pargyline-reserpine-induced excitation appears in contrast to be mediated primarily by NA (Bapna & Dandiya 1972) and can be specifically inhibited by β-receptor blocking drugs (Delini-Stula & Meier 1976). Selective dopamine-receptor blocking agents antagonize this type of excitation only at doses which approach those inducing marked impairment of normal locomotion (Delini-Stula 1973). Baclofen and muscimol as well as diazepam suppressed strongly and in clearly dose-dependent fashion the hyperactivity induced by 25 mg/kg s.c. morphine in mice. In contrast, the pargyline-reserpine induced increase in locomotor activity was inhibited to maximally 45% or not at all (diazepam) irrespectively of the doses given. At the doses at which maximal degree of inhibition was achieved, normal locomotion of animals was also considerably diminished. It should be mentioned that β-receptor blocking drugs such as propranolol, inhibited pargyline-reserpine-induced hyperactivity at doses about 30–100 times lower than necessary to inhibit morphine-induced exaggerated motility in mice (Delini-Stula & Meier 1976, unpublished results).

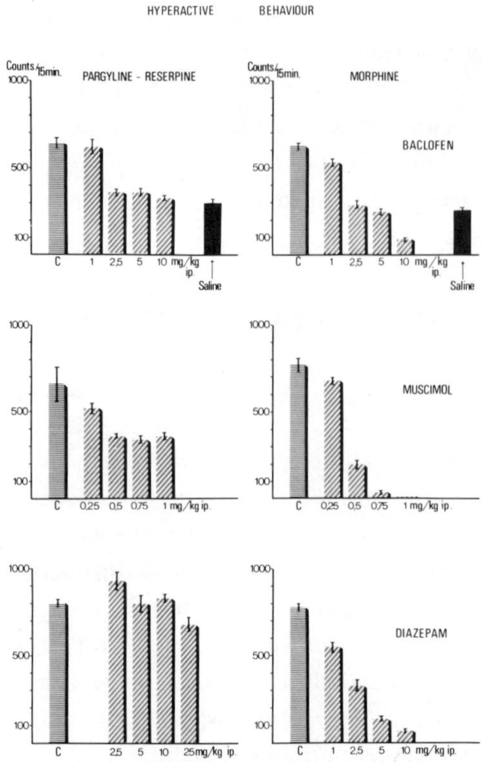

Fig. 1. Effects of baclofen, muscimol and diazepam on two types of excitatory behavior in the mouse. *Right panel:* Drugs were given i.p. 30 min before 25 mg/kg s.c. morphine. Motor activity was recorded 30 min after morphine injection during an interval of 15 min in a photo-cell apparatus. Each column represents the mean activity ± SEM of five groups consisting of five mice each. *Left panel:* Drugs were given 15 min before pargyline 75 mg/kg i.p. 30 min thereafter reserpine 5 mg/kg i.p. was administered. Motor activity was recorded 30 min after reserpine injection during a 15 min interval. Each column is the mean ± SEM of five groups consisting of five mice each. Details of the method and of the apparatus have been described previously (Delini-Stula & Meier 1976).

These findings suggest that drugs which may influence GABA-ergic transmission do not equally affect all types of hyperactive behavior. It seems that excitation resulting primarily from dopaminergic stimulation can be preferentially inhibited (Scheel-Krüger *et al.* 1977a, Cott & Engel 1977). Those hyperactivities resulting from the activation of other transmitter systems appear to respond to a lesser extent and in a non-specific manner.

Whereas investigations described hitherto have not pointed to any explicit differences between baclofen and muscimol, the studies of their effects on particular transmission systems in well-defined brain areas have provided more insight into the complex nature of their modulatory effects on behavior.

EFFECTS OF BACLOFEN AND MUSCIMOL ON BEHAVIORS RELATED TO NIGRO-STRIATAL DOPAMINE

The negative feedback hypothesis predicts that the increase in tonic inhibitory influence of GABA on dopaminergic nerve cells in the s. nigra will result in a decrease of axonal impulse flow in the dopaminergic neurons. An expected behavioral consequence of such an action would be the facilitation of responses reflecting postsynaptic dopamine receptor blockade. Several findings are compatible with the assumption that by activating the inhibitory input on dopaminergic neurons, baclofen and muscimol increase the effects due to the blockade of dopaminergic transmission.

We have reported previously (Delini-Stula 1977) that baclofen facilitates the blockade of conditioned avoidance response in rats pretreated with α-methyl-p-tyrosine, a catecholamine synthesis inhibitor. It was also found that it potentiates the cataleptic effects of haloperidol (Kääriäinen 1976) if administered 2 h prior to it. Furthermore it increased the antagonistic effect of haloperidol on amphetamine-induced stereotypies in the rat, although if administered alone it did not demonstrate any specific inhibition of this type of excitatory behavior.

A considerable number of biochemical findings support the view that these behavioral effects result from the cessation of the impulse flow in the striatal and mesolimbic dopaminergic neurons.

Like γ-butyrolactone, baclofen was found to increase the concentration of DA in the brain and this effect was antagonized with apomorphine (Gianutsos & Moore 1977). The increase in the DA content and its metabolites was parallel by a decrease in the DA turnover rate (Maitre & Waldmeier 1976, Waldmeier & Maitre 1978). Furthermore, baclofen inhibited the increase in the turnover of dopamine produced by neuroleptic drugs (Fuxe *et al.* 1975, Maitre & Waldmeier 1978). In line with these observations were also neurophysiological findings which have demonstrated that baclofen depresses the firing rate of dopaminergic neurons in the ventral tegementum (Bernard *et al.* 1975) and in the s. nigra (Olpe *et al.* 1977a).

Investigating the effects of muscimol on conditioned avoidance behavior in the rat, which is believed to be dependent on normal functioning of dopaminergic system (Lenard & Beer 1975a, 1975b) we have found that the pretreatment with α-methyl-p-tyrosine, (α-MT), like in the case of baclofen, markedly increased the suppressant effect of muscimol on conditioned behavioral responses. Furthermore, muscimol administered before haloperidol augmented the cataleptic effects of the latter and increaced its antagonistic action against

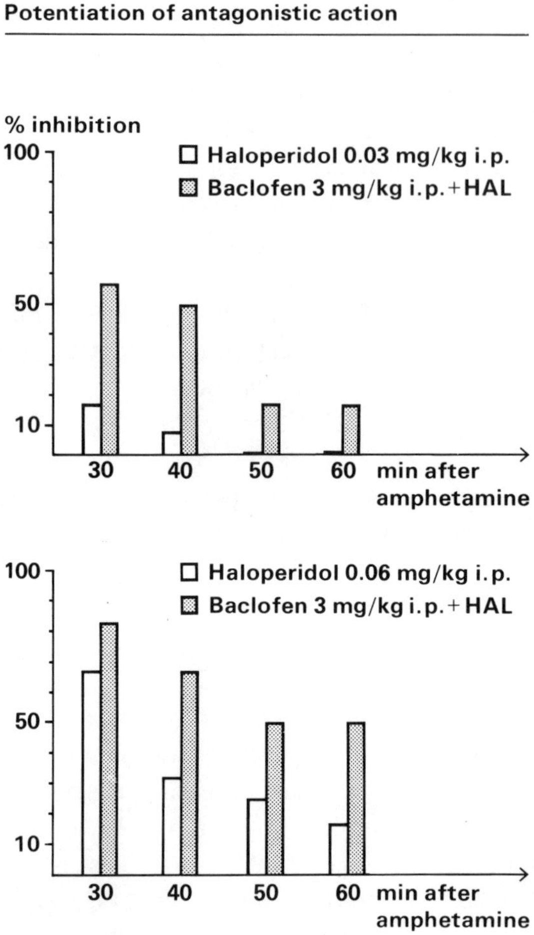

Fig. 2. Potentiation of the antagonistic action of haloperidol against amphetamine-induced stereotypies by baclofen.
Baclofen was given 2 h before threshold doses of haloperidol. A dose of 7.5 mg/kg s.c. d-amphetamine was administered 30 min after haloperidol. The number of rats showing stereotyped licking and gnawing was recorded at time intervals as indicated under the columns. The results are expressed as percentage inhibition in comparison to the controls receiving amphetamine alone. Each column is the average of 12 rats.

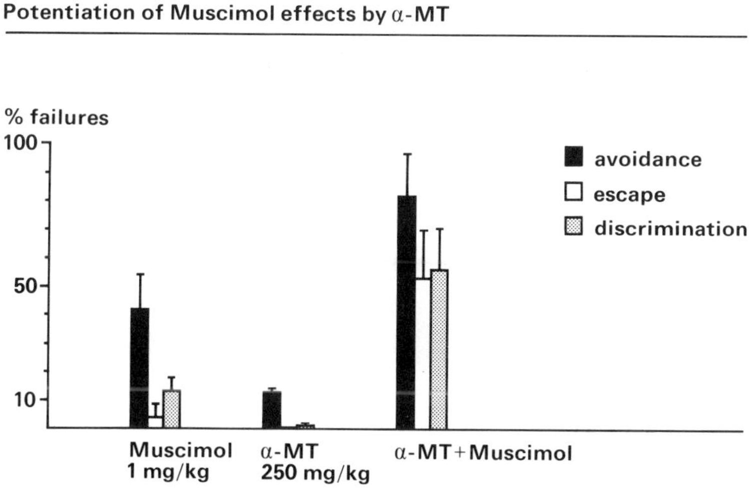

Fig. 3. Effect of the combination of muscimol and *α*-MT on the conditioned avoidance behavior in the rat.
Rats which have been trained to avoid electric shocks and to discriminate between the light and the dark compartment in a three-chambered apparatus (Delini-Stula 1977) were treated with i.p. muscimol 4 hours after 250 mg/kg i.p. *α*-MT. The number of performance errors during a 20-trial session was recorded 30 min after the administration of muscimol. Each column represents the mean number of response failures in percentages±SEM of 6 rats.
Muscimol alone was given 30 min before the start of the test and *α*-MT 4½ hours before.

amphetamine-induced stereotyped behavior. In line with these observations are also the findings that muscimol applied microiontophoretically onto nigral neurons, or given parenterally, inhibited the discharge rate of nigral cells (Olpe & Koella 1978).

Several other findings are, however, not consistent with the assumption that direct activation of the striato-nigral GABA-ergic pathway mainly results in the attenuation of the postsynaptic dopamine receptor stimulation. Direct administration of muscimol or other GABA-like compounds into s. nigra produced contraversive rotation in rats and this effect was not antagonized by haloperidol (Olpe *et al.* 1977b) or other neuroleptics (Scheel-Krüger *et al.* 1977b). Muscimol also greatly facilitated the stereotyped behavior induced by direct and indirect-acting dopaminergic stimulants like cocaine, methylphenidate or apomorphine in mice and produced stereotypies by itself if injected directly into s. nigra of rats. These effects were not antagonized either by pretreatment with catecholamine synthesis inhibitor *α*-MT nor by haloperidol (Scheel-Krüger *et al.* 1977a, 1977b).

Furthermore, muscimol administered 30 min before a low dose of amphet-

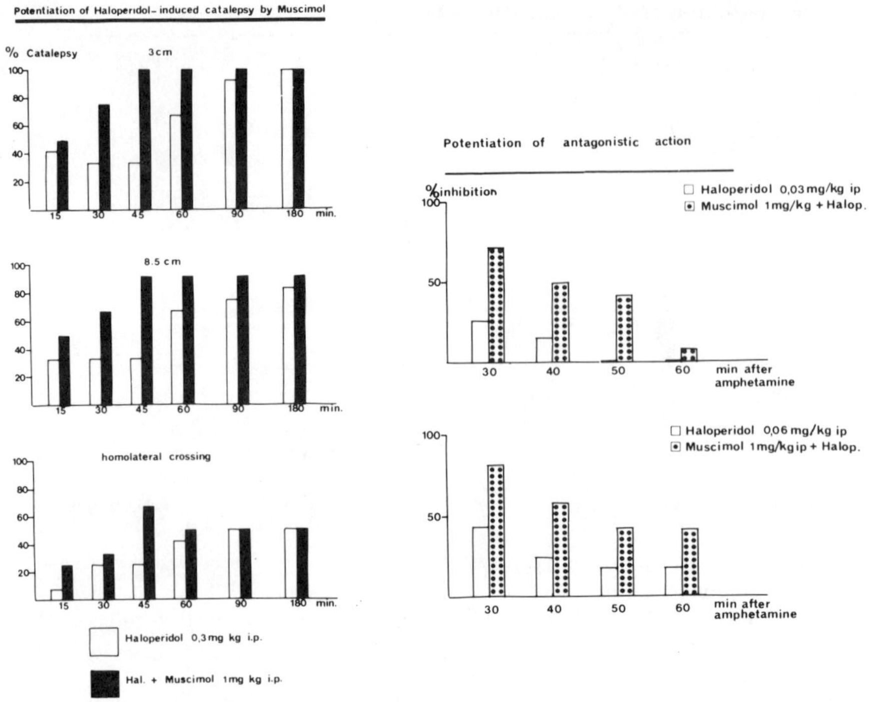

Fig. 4. A. Potentiation of cataleptic effects of haloperidol by muscimol.
Muscimol in a dose of 1 mg/kg was given immediately before haloperidol. Catalepsy was evaluated by placing each forepaw of a rat on a 3-cm and subsequently on a 8.5-cm high cork. In addition fore- and hind extremities were ipsilaterally crossed. The failure to correct the imposed potures of the body during 10–15 sec was scored as a positive cataleptic response. Each column represents the mean catalepsy in percentages of the maximal response (positiv score for each criterion) of six rats.
B. Potentiation of antagonistic action of haloperidol against amphetamine stereotypies. Muscimol was given 2 h before haloperidol. Other methodological details are the same as described under Fig. 2.

amine which produced only occasional licking and gnawing in a small percentage of animals, increased in a dose-dependent fashion the frequency and intensity of stereotyped behavior. The fact that this potentiation was attenuated by bicuculline strongly indicated that the effect was dependent on GABA-ergic mechanisms. It should be mentioned that baclofen did not increase the stereotyped responses produced by amphetamine or apomorphine to any appreciable extent although slight prolongation of their action may be seen at low doses of 0.5 and 1 mg/kg i.p. There was also no increase in the sensitivity to amphetamine after repeated administration of baclofen (5 and 10 mg/kg p.o.

daily for 10 days) but the initial depression of exploration was reversed and signs of hyperactive behavior were observed after the fourth treatment day (unpublished results).

An essential difference between baclofen and muscimol was also found in respect to their effects on the turning behavior induced by apomorphine in rats with unilateral 6-OHDA lesions of the s. nigra. Whereas baclofen markedly decreased the frequency of the turning episodes at doses which did not depress normal locomotion (Delini-Stula 1977), muscimol in contrast, increased the number of turns effected by rats after a challenge with 0.5 mg/kg i.p. apomorphine. The mean number of turns/5 min recorded over an interval of 1 h was significantly higher than in corresponding controls both after 0.5 mg/kg and 1 mg/kg i.p. of muscimol.

These findings, together with the observations of other authors (see before), strongly suggest that activation of the striato-nigral GABA-ergic pathway produces two distinctly different behavioral patterns. One of them apparently reflects tonic inhibition of the dopaminergic nigral neurons. The other one seems to be independent of the dopaminergic axonal inervation and reflects in all probability an indirect excitatory influence on postsynaptic dopamine receptors in the striatum. It is of interest to note that Walters & Lakoski (1978) recently found that muscimol significantly increased the firing rate of dopaminergic cells in the pars compacta of the s. nigra which is in contrast to its consistent depressing effect on the discharge rate of neurons localized in the pars reticulata (Olpe *et al.* 1977a, 1977b). Behavioral studies indicate that these excitatory effects may prevail over inhibitory ones, particularly under the conditions where increased dopamine receptor activity already exists. In clear distinction to muscimol, baclofen seems to possess predominant inhibitory actions on not only dopaminergic but also on other systems which modulate dopamine receptor activity. Recently Waldmeier & Fehr (1978) and Waldmeier *et al.* (1978) demonstrated that baclofen increases not only the content of DA in the striatum but also that of 5-HT and its metabolite 5-HIAA. This finding is consistent with the assumption that baclofen may also decrease the impulse flow in the serotoninergic neurons.

In support to this view is our observation that the depression of the apomorphine-induced turning in 6-OHDA lesioned rats, consistently observed after administration of 4 mg/kg i.p. of baclofen, could be prevented by 5-HT agonist quipazine but not by bicuculline.

Exitatory and inhibitory actions of 5-HT on the dopaminergic nigro-striatal

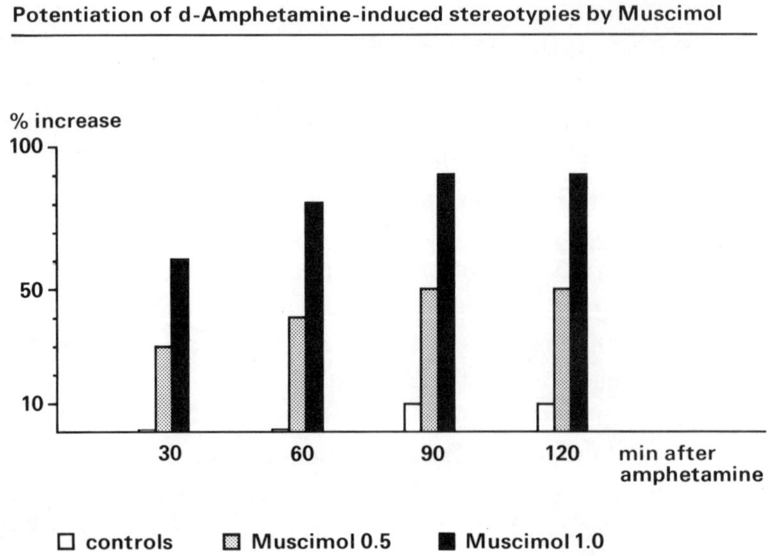

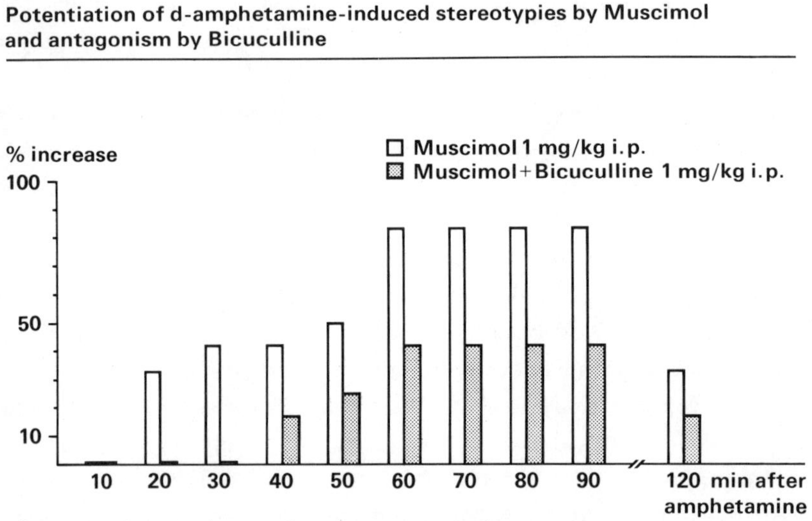

Fig. 5. Potentiation of d-amphetamine-induced stereotypies by muscimol and antagonism by bicuculline.

A. Muscimol was administered intraperitoneally (0.5 and 1.0 mg/kg) 30 min before 2.5 mg/kg s.c. d-amphetamine. The number of rats showing gnawing or licking response was recorded at time intervals as indicated under the columns. Each column represents the mean percentage of positive responses in 12 rats.

B. Muscimol 1 mg/kg i.p. was given 30 min before bicuculline and the latter immediately prior to 2.5 mg/kg s.c. d-amphetamine. The number of rats showing gnawing and licking responses were

Table II

Effects of baclofen and muscimol on apomorphine-induced turning behavior in rats with unilateral 6-OHDA lesions of the s.nigra

Drug	Dose mg/kg i.p.	Turns/5 min mean ± SEM	*P* (t-test)
Baclofen	4.0	21 ± 1.5	<0.001
Muscimol	0.5	82 ± 7.8	<0.001
	1.0	62 ± 2.6	<0.01
Quipazine	5.0	39 ± 2.9	N.S.
Bicuculline	0.25	63 ± 4.1	N.S.
Baclofen	4.0		
+		11 ± 1.7	<0.001
Bicuculline	0.25		
Baclofen	4.0		
+		45 ± 4.4	N.S.
Quipazine	5.0		
Controls	–	48 ± 2.8	–

6-OHDA lesions of the s. nigra were induced as previously described (Delini-Stula 1977). Rats were treated with drugs 1 h before 0.5 mg/kg i.p. apomorphine 6–8 weeks after the lesion. Each treated group served as its own control. The values in the table represent the mean number of turns/5 min ± SEM recorded simultaneously in six rats over a period of 1 h. Control values are the mean of 10 groups consisting of six rats each. Statistical significance was calculated in comparison to the corresponding controls by means of the t-test.

neurons have been described (Dray *et al.* 1976). Recently Tanner (1978) presented evidence suggesting that unlike GABA, 5-HT might have a direct inhibitory influence on the dopaminergic nigral cells. However, they indicated a possibility that GABA exerts a modulatory effect of these inhibitory serotoninergic pathway. The finding that the depressant action of baclofen on the turning behavior can be antagonized by quipazine and that these effects take place in animals in which dopaminergic terminals have been destroyed by 6-OHDA, strongly suggests that 5-HT-DA receptor interaction occurred at the level of striatum. It is possible and in line with other observations (Waldmeier & Delini-Stula, submitted for publication) that in contrast to the neurons in the s. nigra, striatal receptors receive an excitatory 5-HT input from the dorsal raphé (B7) fibers.

recorded at time intervals as indicated under the columns. Each column represents the mean percentage of positive responses of 12 rats. The parallel controls (d-amphetamine alone) showed no stereotypies.

The observations with baclofen fit the hypothesis that decrease of the excitatory influence of 5-HT neurons may change the functional state of the striatal dopaminergic receptors. Surprising, however, remains the fact that quipazine by itself failed to increase the effects of apomorphine in the 6-OHDA lesioned rats.

Although many questions related to the regulatory mechanisms controlling the function of the nigro-striatum still need to be answered, present investigations suggest an important fact. Selective activation of the GABA-ergic pathway does not lead to only inhibitory behavioral manifestations. Excitatory responses occur as well and may even prevail over the inhibitory ones. Baclofen seems to posses depressant action, which may simulate GABA effects but which possibly results from the influence on excitatory neurons which directly or indirectly modulate dopaminergic activity.

MODULATORY EFFECTS OF BACLOFEN AND MUSCIMOL ON MURICIDE BEHAVIOR IN THE RAT – ROLE OF GABA IN THE FUNCTION OF AMYGDALA

Whereas much emphasis has been given to the role of GABA in the modulation of the nigro-striatal functions, much less attention has been paid to its possible role in the control of behavioral responses which are dependent on other anatomical systems in the brain.

There is large experimental evidence supporting the view that muricide response which occurs spontaneously in a small population of normal albino rats (2–3%) involves *inter alia* disturbed functioning of the amygdala. Since nonkiller rats can be rendered aggressive against a mouse by ablation of the olfactory bulbs (Vergnes & Karli 1963) and on the other hand the muricide response can be abolished by bilateral destruction of the amygdala (Karli & Vergnes 1965), an inhibitory control of the olfactory bulbs over amygdala has been postulated. Recently Mack & Mandel (1976) suggested that an inhibitory pathway using GABA as transmitter and localized in the olfactory bulbs may be involved in the control of this interspecific aggressiveness. According to their findings, spontaneous killers show considerably lower concentrations of GABA in this brain region. Increase in GABA content by direct administration of GABA in the olfactory bulbs was found to inhibit spontaneous killer reaction, however, parenteral administration of sodium valproate in bulbectomized rats failed to attenuate their muricide behavior. In view of these findings it was of interest to investigate the effects of baclofen and muscimol in spontaneous and bulbectomized killer rats.

Table III

Effect of drugs on muricide response in spontaneous killer rats and killers after bulbectomy or kainic acid lesions

Drug	Dose mg/kg i.p.	Muricide response % inhibition					
		spontan.	N	bulbect.	N	kainic ac.	N
Baclofen	3.0	10	10	35	20	10	10
	6.0	60	10	40	10	30	10
	10.0	—	—	100	10	30	20
Muscimol	1.0	10	10	—	—	15	20
	1.5	70	10	10	10	40	10
GABA-cetylester	10	40	10	—	—	70	10
	20	—	—	—	—	70	10
	30	70	10	40	10	—	—
	50	83	12	50	12	—	—

Drugs were administered 30 min before placing a mouse in the home cage of a killer rat. The absence of killing reaction within 5 min was taken as criterion of inhibition. All killer rats used for the experiments consistently killed a mouse within 1–5 sec after its introduction into the cage. Spontaneous killers were selected from a population of normal albino laboratory rats (RAI: Tif, Sisseln Farm, Switzerland). Ablation of the olfactory bulbs was performed as described previously (Vassout & Delini-Stula 1977). Kainic acid dissolved in 0.9% NaCl and 0.2% ascorbic acid was introduced (2.5 μg/0.5 μl) bilaterally into the middle portion of the b. olfactorius (2-mm depth) by means of a Hamilton syringe. Killer reaction developed in about 60% of treated rats after a period of 10–15 days.

As can be seen from the Table III, baclofen, muscimol and GABA-cetylester inhibited the spontaneous muricide behavior. The effects were in a clear dependence of the given dose. In contrast, in rats in which consistent killing response was produced by ablation of the olfactory bulbs only baclofen retained its full activity (Delini-Stula & Vassout, in press). Muscimol was inactive at a dose of 1.5 mg/kg i.p. although the motor activity of these animals was reduced to about 45% in comparison to the predrug level (mean counts/15 min $\pm$ SEM: 1217 $\pm$ 194 after 1.5 mg/kg i.p., vs. 2090 $\pm$ 322 in untreated animals. Measurements were done by means of the Motron Motilitymeter apparatus). GABA-cetylester inhibited the mouse killing in a certain number of rats, but there was no increase of effect by increasing the dose and the inhibition coincided with depression of motor activity which exceeded 50% at a dose of 30 mg/kg i.p.

These results were not in disagreement with the view of Mack & Mandel that a GABA-ergic pathway intrinsic to the olfactory bulbs may control interspecific aggressiveness in rats. They suggested also that baclofen exerts an activity which may be independent of this pathway.

In order to further elucidate the importance of GABA in the elicitation of this type of behavior, we have found it of interest to study the effect of bilateral kainic acid lesions of the olfactory bulbs in rats. Kainic acid is a powerful neurotoxic agent (Olney *et al.* 1974) which has been shown to cause degeneration of GABA-ergic neurons intrinsic to the striatum while sparing the axons of extrinsic neurons terminating in or only passing through this region (Coyle & Schwarcz 1976, Campochiaro *et al.* 1977). In a total of 40 rats anesthetized with pentobarbitone sodium (Nembutal©, 40 mg/kg i.p.) 2.5 μg kainic acid dissolved in 0.9% NaCl and 0.2% ascorbic acid was injected bilaterally in a volume of 0.5 μl 2 mm below the surface of the olfactory bulbs by means of a Hamilton syringe. Ten days thereafter rats were tested for their killer reaction by placing a mouse in their homecage. Of the injected rats, 24 have shown an immediate killing response whereas neither of the sham-operated rats killed the mouse. This percentage of rats which developed mouse-killing response is roughly the same as that obtained after the ablation of the olfactory bulbs (Vassout & Delini-Stula 1977). Preliminary study of the effects of muscimol, baclofen and GABA-cetylester demonstrated surprising differences in their activity in these rats (Table III). Baclofen which at a dose of 10 mg/kg i.p. suppressed completely the muricide response in bulbectomized rats, failed to produce an inhibition in 14 out of 20 tested rats. Muscimol showed some effect, but GABA-cetylester was considerably more active than in either spontaneous or bulbectomized rats.

These differences cannot be explained at present and further investigations are needed in order to elucidate the type and extension of the damages in these rats. They may possibly shed more light on the site of neuronal action of baclofen.

CONCLUSIONS

Comparative investigations with baclofen and muscimol on various types of behavioral responses in mice and rats have demonstrated that baclofen exerts only in part an action on dopaminergic transmission system which could be considered as GABA-like. In all probability, however, it did not affect GABA system directly. Furthermore, selective stimulation of striato-nigral GABA-ergic pathway by muscimol produced both excitatory and inhibitory behavioral responses.

The excitatory effects seem to prevail over the inhibitory ones. The investigations of the muricide behavior in rats suggested also that GABA may participate in the control of emotionally-shaped behavioral responses which have their anatomical substrate in the amygdala.

REFERENCES

Andén, N. E. & Wachtel, H. (1977) Biochemical effects of baclofen (β-parachlorophenyl-GABA) on the dopamine and the noradrenaline in the rat brain. *Acta Pharmacol. Toxicol.* 40, 310–320.

Bapna, J. S. & Dandiya, P. C. (1972) The mechanism of excitation caused by reserpine in mice treated with pargyline. *Pharmakopsychiat.* 5, 241–248.

Bernard, P., Edwards, S. J., Fielding, S., Robson, R. D., Saelens, J. K., Simke, J. P. & Welch, J. (1975) Baclofen (Bf): unusual CNS active agent. *Pharmacologist* 17, 256.

Bernasconi, R. & Martin, P. (1978) Effects of diazepam and baclofen on the GABA turnover rate in various mouse brain regions. *Naunyn-Schmiedeberg's Arch. Pharmacol.* Suppl. 302, R58.

Campochiaro, P., Schwarcz, R., Coyle, J. T. (1977) GABA receptor binding in rat striatum: Localisation and effects of denervation. *Brain Res.* 136, 501–511.

Costa, E., Guidotti, A., Mao, C. C., Suria, A. (1975) New concepts on the mechanism of action of benzodiazepines. *Life Sci.* 17, 167–187.

Cott, J. & Engel, J. (1977) Suppression by GABA-ergic drugs of locomotor stimulation induced by morphine, amphetamine, and apomorphine: evidence for both pre- and post-synaptic inhibition of catecholamine systems. *J. Neural Transmission* 40, 253–268.

Coyle, J. T. & Schwarcz, R. (1976) Lesion of striatal neurones with kainic acid provides a model for Huntington's chorea. *Nature* 263, 244–246.

Curtis, D. R., Game, C. J. A., Johnston, G. A. R., McCulloch, R. M. (1974) Central effects of β-(p-chlorophenyl)-γ-aminobutyric acid. *Brain Res.* 70, 493–499.

Davies, J. & Watkins, J. C. (1974) The action of β-phenyl-GABA derivatives on neurones of the cat cerebral cortex. *Brain Res.* 70, 501–505.

Delini-Stula, A. (1973) Excitatory behaviour induced by combined pargyline-reserpine treatment. An experimental model of mania? *Psihofarmakologija 3,* Proc. 3rd. Yug. Psychopharmacol. Symp. Medicinska Naklada - Zagreb.

Delini-Stula, A. & Meier, M. (1976) Inhibitory effects of propranolol and oxprenolol on excitation induced by a MAO inhibitor and reserpine in the mouse. *Neuropharmacol.* 15, 383–388.

Delini-Stula, A. (1977) Baclofen-induced modification of conditioned discriminative avoidance behaviour and contraversive turning in the rat. *Eur. J. Pharmacol.* 46, 265–274.

Delini-Stula, A. & Vassout, A. Influence of baclofen and GABAmimetic agents on spontaneous and olfactory-bulb-ablation-induced muricidal behavior in the rat. *Drug Res.* In press.

Dray, A., Gonye, T. J., Oakley, N. R., Tanner, T. (1976) Evidence for the existence of a raphe projection to the substantia nigra in rat. *Brain Res.* 113, 45–57.

Frederiksen, P. K. (1975) Baclofen in the treatment of schizophrenia. *Lancet* 7908, 702–703.

Fuxe, K., Hökfelt, T., Ljungdahl, A., Agnati, L., Johansson, O. & Perez de la Mora, M. (1975) Evidence for an inhibitory gabergic control of the mesolimbic dopamine neurons. Possibility of improving the treatment of schizophrenia by combined treatment with neuroleptic and gabergic drugs. *Med. Biol.* 53, 177–183.

Gianutsos, G. & Moore, K. E. (1977) Increase in mouse brain dopamine content by baclofen: Effects of apomorphine and neuroleptics. *Psychopharmacol.* 52, 217–221.

Godin, Y., Heiner, L., Mark, J., Mandel, P. (1969) Effects of di-n-propylacetate, an anticonvulsive compound, on GABA metabolism. *J. Neurochem.* 16, 869–873.

Haefely, W., Kulisar, A., Mohler, H., Pieri, L., Polc, P. & Schaffner, R. (1975) Possible involvememt of GABA in the central actions of benzodiazepines. *Adv. Biochem. Psychopharmac.* 14, 131–151.

Kääriäinen, I. (1976) Effects of aminooxyacetic acid and baclofen on the catalepsy and on the increase of mesolimbic and striatal dopamine turnover induced by haloperidol in rats. *Acta pharmacol. Toxicol.* 39, 393–400.

Karli, P. & Vergnes, M. (1965) Analyse expérimentale de méchanismes de facilitation et d'inhibition de l'agressivité interspécifique du rat. *J. Physiol.* 57, 637–638.

Kuschinsky, K. & Hornykiewicz, O. (1974) Effects of morphine on striatal dopamine metabolism: Possible mechanism of its opposite effect on locomotor activity in rats and mice. *Eur. J. Pharmacol.* 26, 41–50.

Lenard, L. G. & Beer, B. (1975a) 6-Hydroxydopamine and avoidance: Possible role of response suppression. *Pharmacol. Biochem. Behav.* 3, 873–878.

Lenard, L. G. & Beer, B. (1975b) Modification of avoidance behavior in 6-Hydroxydopamine-treated rats by stimulation of central noradrenergic and dopaminergic receptors. *Pharmacol. Biochem. Behav.* 3, 887–893.

Löscher, W. & Frey, H. H. (1977) Effect of convulsant and anticonvulsant agents on level and metabolism of γ-aminobutyric acid in mouse brain. *Naunyn-Schmiedeberg's Arch. Pharmacol.* 296, 263–269.

Mack, G. & Mandel, P. (1976) Inhibition du comportement muricide du rat par la taurine, le GABA et ses analogues. *C. R. Acad. Sc. Paris* 283, Serie D, 361.

Maitre, L. & Waldmeier, P. (1976) Alteration of dopamine metabolism in the rat brain by baclofen (Lioresal). *Naunyn-Schmiedeberg's Arch. Pharmacol.* 293, (Suppl.) R9.

Naik, S. R., Guidotti, A. & Costa, E. (1976) Central GABA receptor agonists: Comparison of muscimol and baclofen. *Neuropharmacol.* 15, 479–484.

Nistri, A. (1975) Further investigations into the effects of baclofen (Lioresal) on the isolated spinal cord. *Experientia* 31, 1066.

Olney, J. W., Rhee, V. & Ho, O. L. (1974) Kainic acid: powerful neurotoxic analogue of glutamate. *Brain Res.* 77, 507–512.

Olpe, H. R., Koella, W. P., Wolf, P. & Haas, H. L. (1977a) the action of baclofen on neurons of the substantia nigra and of the ventral tegmental area. *Brain Res.* 134, 577–580.

Olpe, H. R., Schellenberg, H. & Koella, W. P. (1977b) Rotational behavior induced in rats by intranigral application of GABA-related drugs and GABA antagonists. *Eur. J. Pharmacol.* 45, 291–294.

Olpe, H. R. & Koella, W. P. (1978) The action of muscimol on neurons of the substantia nigra of the rat. *Experientia,* 34, 235.

Polc, P. & Haefely, W. (1976) Effects of two benzodiazepines, phenobarbitone and baclofen on synaptic transmission in the cat cuneate nucleus. *Naunyn-Schmiedeberg's Arch. Pharmacol.* 294, 121–131.

Scheel-Krüger, J., Christensen, A. V. & Arnt, J. (1977a) Muscimol differentially facilitates stereotypy but antagonizes motility induced by dopaminergic drugs: a complex GABA-dopamine interaction. *Life Sci.* 22, 75–84.

Scheel-Krüger, J., Arnt, J. & Magelund, G. (1977b) Behavioural stimulation induced by muscimol and other GABA agonists injected into the substantia nigra. *Neurosci. Letters,* 4, 351–356.

Tanner, T. (1978) Circling behaviour in the rat following unilateral injections of p-chlorophenylalanine and ethanolamine. O-sulphate into the substantia nigra. *J. Pharm. Pharmac.* 30, 158–161.

Vassout, A. & Delini-Stula, A. (1977) Effects de β-bloqueurs (propranolol et oxprénolol) et du diazépam sur différents modlles d'agressivité chez le rat. *J. Pharmacol.* (Paris) 8, 5–14.

Vergnes, M. & Karli, P. (1963) Déclenchement du comportement d'agression interspécifique Rat-Souris par ablation bilatéral des bulbes olfactifs. Action de l'hydroxyzine sur cette agressivité provoquée. *C. R. Soc. Biol.* 157, 1061–1063.

Waddington, J. L. & Harrow, U. K. (1977) Induction of rotational behaviour by intranigral baclofen suggests possible GABA-agonist activity. *Experientia* 33, 1345–1346.

Waldmeier, P. C. & Maitre, L. (1978) Effects of baclofen on dopamine metabolism and interaction with neuroleptic effects. *Eur. J. Pharmacol.* 47, 191–200.

Waldmeier, P. C., Feldtrauer, J. J., Kam, R. & Stöcklin, K. (1978) Effect of baclofen applied to the substantia nigra on striatal levels of dopamine, 5-HT and their metabolites. *Naunyn-Schmiedeberg's Arch. Pharmacol.* (Suppl.) 302, R58.

Waldmeier, P. C. & Fehr, B. Effects of baclofen and gamma-hydroxybutyrate on rat striatal and mesolimbic 5-HT metabolism. *Eur. J. Pharmacol.* In press.

Waldmeier, P. C. & Delini-Stula, A. Serotonergic modulation of haloperidol effects on behaviour and striatal dopamine turnover. Submitted

Wallach, D. P. (1961) Studies on GABA pathway. The inhibition of γ-aminobutyric acid – α-ketogluturic acid transaminase *in vitro* and *in vivo* by U-7524 (aminooxyacetic acid). *Biochem. Pharmac.* 5, 323–331.

Walters, J. R. & Lakoski, J. M. (1978) Effect of muscimol on single unit activity of substantia nigra dopamine neurons. *Eur. J. Pharmacol.* 47, 469–471.

GABA and Thalamo-Striatal Control of Apomorphine-like Effects

A. R. Cools

It is known that the substantia nigra forms a crucial link in the nigro-neostriato-nigral loop: dopaminergic, nigro-neostriatal fibers impinge upon cholinergic, intrastriatal neurons which, in turn, influence GABA-ergic, striato-nigral fibers (for reviews: Bartholini 1977, Butcher 1977, Cools 1977a, Wright *et al.* 1977). Evidence is available that the mentioned GABA-ergic neurons inhibit the impulse flow in the dopaminergic neurons arising from the substantia nigra (Aghajanian & Bunney 1973, Andén & Stock 1973, Yoshida & Precht 1971). Nevertheless, intranigral administration of the potent GABA-ergic agonist muscimol results in the elicitation of behavioral effects which are highly characteristic for an *increased* dopaminergic activity within the neostriatum and/or the N accumbens, i.e. head nodding, stereotyped sniffing, licking and gnawing (Scheel-Krüger *et al.* 1977a). As neither complete inhibition of the dopamine (DA) synthesis nor total blockade of DA receptors being sensitive to haloperidol attenuate the effects triggered by administration of muscimol into the substantia nigra, it has been concluded that nondopaminergic fibers arising from the substantia nigra are involved in the muscimol-induced behavioral phenomena (Scheel-Krüger *et al.* 1977a, Scheel-Krüger *et al.* 1978).

As a matter of fact, two hypotheses emerge. First, the neostriatum and/or the N accumbens are not at all implicated. Yet this is quite unlikely in view of the enormous amount of data that stress the involvement of these structures in the display of behavioral effects such as stereotyped sniffing, licking and gnawing (for reviews: Cools 1977a, Costall & Naylor 1977, Iversen 1977). And second, the neuronal activity within the neostriatum and/or the N accumbens that

Department og Pharmacology, University of Nijmegen, P.O.B. 9101, 6500 HB Nijmegen, The Netherlands.

"GABA-NEUROTRANSMITTERS", Alfred Benzon Symposium 12, Munksgaard 1978

mediates the muscimol-induced effects does not require a particular change in the impulse flow in the dopaminergic, nigro-neostriatal and/or mesolimbic pathways. The anatomical literature dealing with the hodology of the substantia nigra, indeed, shows that the substantia nigra can influence the mentioned telencephalic structures via a variety of polysynaptic pathways using transmitter substances of which the nature has yet to be established (for review: Nieuwenhuys 1977).

In the present study, the attention is focussed on the Center Median N parafascicularis complex (CM-Pf complex), because this complex not only receives afferents from the substantia nigra, but also projects on to the striatum (Ahlenius 1978, Carpenter & Peter 1972, Cowan & Powell 1955, Fibiger *et al.* 1972, Mehler 1966, Vogt & Vogt 1941). Apart from this, evidence has been collected that this complex can indeed modify the neostriatal, neuronal firing rates (Levine *et al.* 1977).

In general, the present study offers evidence that the CM-Pf complex is implicated in the elicitation of apomorphine-like effects, which are insensitive to blockade of the dopaminergic processes within the neostriatum and the N accumbens; nevertheless, the neostriatum and the N accumbens appear to be indispensable, because 1) activation of cholinergic or GABA-ergic processes within the *posterior part of the neostriatum* and 2) inhibition of α-noradrenergic processes within the *N accumbens* do attenuate the mentioned apomorphine-like effects.

METHODS AND MATERIALS

Male Wistar rats weighing 200 to 220 g were stereotaxically implanted with guide cannulas into a) CM-Pf complex (co-ordinates A 3.2–3.9, L 0.4–0.8 and H 0.0–0.8), b) neostriatum, posterior part (co-ordinates A 7.5, L 3.5 and H 4.7) c) neostriatum, anterior part (co-ordinates A 9.4, L 2.0 and H 1.0) and d) N accumbens (co-ordinates A 9.4, L 1.2 and H −0.6; König & Klippel atlas); the cannulas directed at the CM-Pf complex and the N accumbens were placed at an angle of 10° and 5° respectively in reference to the mid-sagittal plane. Injections were made by means of a 5 μl Hamilton syringe with a 31-gauge needle, which extended into the brain tissue 1.0–1.5 mm below the tip of the guide cannula; the injection volume was 0.5 μl (CM-Pf complex and N accumbens) or 1.0 μl (neostriatum) on each side (for details: Pijnenburg *et al.* 1976). All agents were bilaterally administered. The following drugs were used: saline, apomorphine hydrochloride, haloperidol (Serenase®), ergometrine maleate, (3,4-dihydroxy-phenylamino)-2-imidazoline hydrochloride (DPI), oxymetazoline hydrochloride, phentolamine methanesulphate (Regitine®), carbaminoylcholine chloride (carbachol), scopolamine hydrobromide, picrotoxin and muscimol hydrochloride. The solutions were freshly prepared before each experiment; the doses mentioned refer to the salts. All agents were dissolved in saline; in control experiments saline was used.

In addition, a number of rats were stereotaxically implanted with commercially available, twisted bipolar, stainless steel electrodes into the CM-Pf complex (Plastic Products Company; diameter of the electrode assembly 0.8 mm;

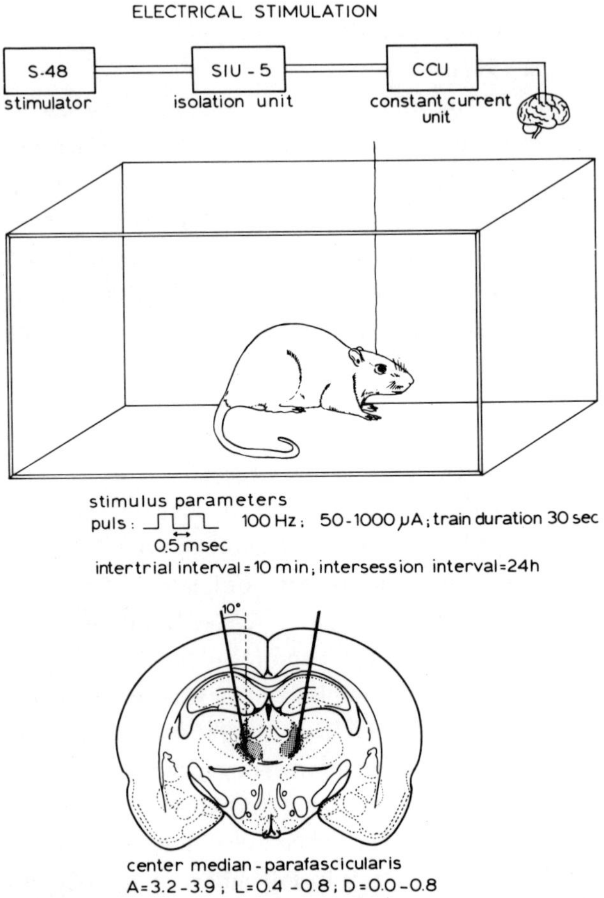

Fig. 1. Experimental set-up for electrical stimulation studies on the CM-Pf complex.

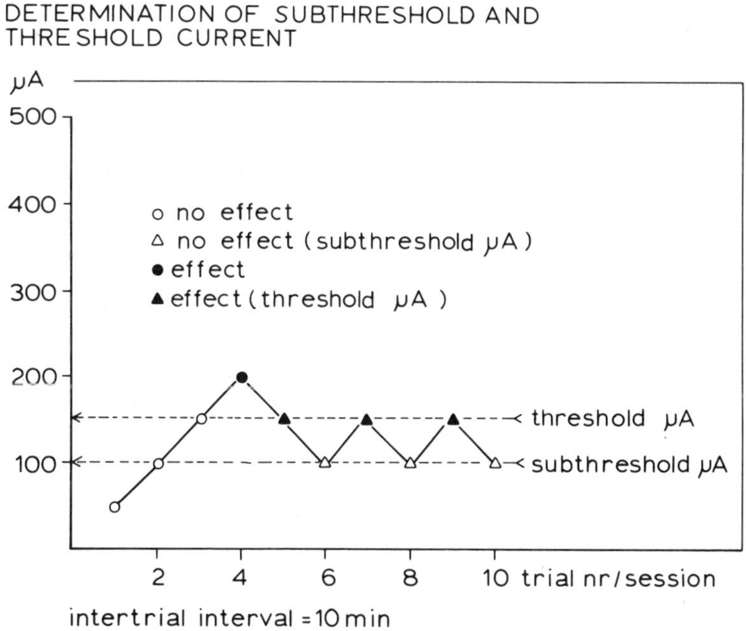

Fig. 2. Establishment of subthreshold and threshold current in rats equipped with electrodes directed at the CM-Pf complex.

diameter of the uninsulated tip 0.3 mm). The electrodes were stimulated with bipolar stimuli consisting of 30 sec trains of rectangular biphasic pulses (duration 0.5 msec; frequency 100 Hz); the intensity varied from 50–500 μA (Fig. 1). Per experiment, either the left or the right electrode assembly was used. Each trial was built up in four phases: a) habituation period of 30 min, restricted to the first trial of each series, b) pre-stimulus period of 1 min, c) electrical stimulation period of 30 sec, and d) post-stimulus period of 3 min. As long as continuous sitting was absent during the pre-stimulus period, no stimuli were delivered. As soon as the animal displayed motor phenomena such as turning or clonic movements, the rat was discarded. Subthreshold and threshold intensities were established as follows (Fig. 2). Once a behavioral change was produced, the chosen intensity was lowered step by step (50 μA) during the next trials (intertrial interval 10 min) until the stimulation became ineffective; subsequently, the intensity was increased step by step till the effects reappeared; this procedure was repeated three times. In this way, both threshold and subthreshold intensities were determined in two successive sessions (intersession interval 24 h): rats in which the effects could not be reproduced during the second session were discarded (±5%). The subthreshold current (threshold current minus 50 μA) was used for establishing the ability of drugs to potentiate the electrical stimulation effects, whereas the threshold current was used for establishing the ability of drugs to attenuate or inhibit the effects (Fig. 3).

All rats were habituated to the stimulation probe, the injection procedure and experimental cage in two 1-h sessions. Semi-circular, wooden cages with Plexiglass front (radius 40 cm; height 50 cm) were used. The behavior of each individually tested rat was recorded by means of the time-sample method: at the beginning of each 10 sec a written note was made of the behavior at that time using one of the following categories of each class: *class A,* sitting, walking running and rearing; *class B,* sniffing, licking, cleaning (self-licking or scratching) and grooming; and *class C,* teeth grinding, clonic movements, biting (gnawing) and head nodding. The observation period varied per experiment (see results). Only experiments in which the mentioned target areas were reached are discussed below.

CHEMICAL STIMULATION OF THE CM-Pf COMPLEX

In preliminary experiments, it turned out that the behavioral changes triggered by various drugs could be assessed by using a slightly modified rating scale indicating the presence of *continuous* or *discontinuous* display of sitting, walking, sniffing, head nodding and teeth grinding. As the changes elicited reached their optimum at about 15 min and/or 80 min after the intracerebral administration, the behavior was only observed between 10 and 20 min and between 70 and 90 min.

Apart from GABA (for review: Roberts 1974), the thalamus contains both noradrenaline and dopamine (Kizer *et al.* 1976, Lindvall & Björklund 1974, Lindvall *et al.* 1974, Swanson & Hartman 1975, cf. Glisson *et al.* 1976). Accordingly, only agents which are believed to interfere selectively with noradrenergic, dopaminergic and GABA-ergic processes were tested. Since the N parafascicularis in at least one species contains DA-loaded terminals and varicosities showing a remarkable morphological and histochemical resemblance to those found within the anterodorsal part of the neostriatum and the N accumbens of rats (cf. Ishikawa & Tanaka 1977, Olson *et al.* 1972, see also Cools 1977b), particular attention was paid to agents such as DPI and ergometrine, i.e. agents which stimulate and inhibit respectively DA receptors which normally occur within areas marked by the mentioned features (DA_i receptors); for a detailed discussion dealing with the difference between "dotted" and "diffuse" DA fluorescence on the one hand and the presence of different DA receptors on the other, see Cools & van Rossum 1976, Cools 1977b.

The outcome of the experiments is summarized in Table I. In contrast to the ineffectiveness of solvents in most experiments, saline applied into the CM-Pf complex resulted in effects which were highly characteristic for low doses of systemically given apomorphine: discontinuous display of stereotyped sniffing and walking; once elicited, the symptoms remained present for a period of about 20 min. Neither oxymetazoline (3 μg) nor phentolamine (2.5 μg) did produce effects different from those elicited by saline. As already expected on the basis of the absence of the delicate, weakly fluorescent DA varicosities in the CM-Pf complex (Ishikawa & Tanaka 1977), neither apomorphine nor haloperidol, i.e. agents that stimulate and inhibit respectively the DA receptors which normally occur within areas marked by such a DA fluorescence (DA_e receptors, Cools 1977b), altered the "placebo" effects. In contrast, ergometrine studied at a time that it inhibits the DA_i receptors, i.e. 60 min after its local administration, produced a clearcut shift from the *discontinuous* display of walking and sniffing towards the *continuous* display of walking and sniffing. In contrast, DPI attenuated the "placebo" effects as indicated by the shift towards the continuous display of sitting; this shift was accompanied by the appearance of teeth grinding. In about 50% of the tested rats (n=15) DPI also prevented the display of sniffing. Although we have not yet investigated whether the DPI-induced effects could be inhibited by ergometrine, the diametrically opposite nature of the mentioned effects strongly suggests that DA_i receptors were involved. This suggestion is strengthened by the fact that ergometrine exerted a biphasic effect: a) DPI-like effects during the first observation period, and b) diametrically opposite effects during the last observation period (Table I); this fits in very nicely with the recent finding that the DA_i receptors within the N accumbens are initially stimulated and, later on, inhibited by ergometrine (Cools 1978). As the thalamus not only contains DA, but also receives a dopaminergic, nigro-thalamic input (cf. Ahlenius 1978, Kizer *et al.* 1976), it is likely that this fiber system was affected.

Table I also shows that the GABA-ergic agonist muscimol mimicked the effects of DPI, whereas the GABA-ergic antagonist picrotoxin mimicked those elicited by ergometrine. Considering these data in view of the functional relationship between DA_i receptors and GABA-ergic mechanisms within telencephalic, dopaminergic structures (Cools & Janssen 1976, Cools 1977a, cf. Scheel-Krüger *et al.* 1977b), it appears that there is no fundamental difference between the thalamus and the striatal structures in this respect.

These experiments offer two important sets of data: A) the CM-Pf complex, or structures adjacent to it, is implicated in the elicitation of apomorphine-like effects and B) compounds such as DPI, ergometrine, picrotoxin and GABA can modify apomorphine-like effects both at the level of the neostriatum and the N accumbens (for review: Cools 1977a) *and* at the level of the thalamus.

ELECTRICAL STIMULATION OF THE CM-Pf COMPLEX

As shown in Fig. 3, electrical stimulation of electrodes which were correctly placed into the CM-Pf complex resulted in highly reproducible effects; the

Table I

Behavioral effects elicited by bilateral administration (0.5 µl per side) of various drugs into the CM-Pf complex. Note the effectiveness of saline

Drugs (µg)	Effects						Postdrug time	
	1	2	3	4	5	6	(min)	n
Saline	–	–	7	–	–	–	10–20	7
Saline	–	–	–	–	7	–	60–80	7
Apomorphine (0.5)	–	–	7	–	–	–	10–20	7
Haloperidol (2.5)	–	–	9	–	–	–	10–20	9
DPI[a] (1.0)	–	–	–	8	7	15	10–20	15
Ergometrine (1.0)	7	–	–	–	–	–	60–80	7
Muscimol (0.01)	–	–	–	–	15	11[b]	10–20	15
Picrotoxin (0.05)	7	–	–	–	–	–	10–20	7
Ergometrine (1.0)	–	–	–	–	7	6	10–20	7
Ergometrine (0.5)	7	–	–	–	–	–	60–80	7

1=continuous walking+continuous sniffing
2=discontinuous walking+continuous sniffing
3=discontinuous sniffing+discontinuous walking
4=continuous sitting+discontinuous sniffing
5=continuous sitting
6=teeth grinding
a=DPI=(3,4-dihydroxyphenylamine)-2-imidazoline
b=present during the first injection period of 1–7 min.

Determination of drug-induced effects upon electrical stimulation of Center median-parafascicularis complex

effects in control tests	test A	test B
a. continuous (sniffing+walking)	18.2	18.2
b. continuous sniffing; discontinuous walking	4.5	4.5
c. discontinuous (sniffing+walking)	0	0
d. continuous (sniffing+sitting)	38.2	40.0
e. discontinuous sniffing; continuous sitting	36.5	37.3
f. continuous sitting	2.6	0
	100%	100%

Test A

test B score	a	b	c	d	e	f	total
a	14	4	0	1	1	0	20
b	1	0	0	4	0	0	5
c	0	0	0	0	0	0	0
d	5	1	0	37	1	0	44
e	0	0	0	0	38	3	41
f	0	0	0	0	0	0	0
total	20	5	0	42	40	3	

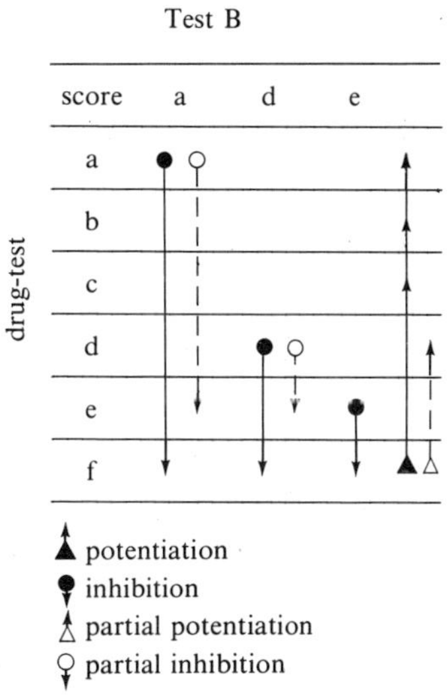

Fig. 3. Determination of drug-induced effects upon electrical stimulation of Center Median parafascicularis complex.

Upper part: effects elicited by stimulation in two successive control sessions using identical stimulus parameters (percentage of tested sites (n=110)); intersession interval = 24 h.

Lower part, left: correlation between the nature and number of effective sites in the first (A) and second (B) control session.

Lower part, right: determination of the nature of the drug-induced effects upon the behavior elicited by electrical stimulation.

effects themselves were identical to those described in the previous section. Remarkably, the effects were not always stimulus-bound as indicated by the fact that some rats (18.2%) continued to perform the elicited effects for a period of 10–60 sec following the discontinuation of the stimulation. From the anatomical point of view, it is of importance to note that stimulation was only effective on the condition that both the Center Median and the N parafascicularis were stimulated.

Effects of systemically applied drugs

The outcome of these experiments is summarized in Table II. Haloperidol (1 mg/kg, sc) did not affect the apomorphine-like effects triggered by electrical stimulation of the CM-Pf complex; in this respect, the CM-Pf effects resemble the effects elicited by intranigral administration of muscimol (Scheel-Krüger *et al.* 1977a). Apomorphine too remained ineffective. In contrast, muscimol and

Table II

Effects of systemic injections of various drugs upon electrical stimulation of Center Median parafascicularis complex

Drug (mg/kg)		Postdrug interval (min)	No effect	Potentiation[a]	Inhibition	n
Apomorphine	(0.05, sc)	15	100	0	0	6
Haloperidol	(0.05, sc)	30	100	0	0	13
	(0.05, sc)	45	100	0	0	13
	(1.0, sc)	45	100	0	0	12
Muscimol	(2.0[b], sc)	30	0	0	100	10
Picrotoxin	(1.0, ip)	10	14.3	85.7	0	7
DPI[c]	(1.0[d], ip)	10	100	0	0	2
	(2.0[d], ip)	10	0	100	0	4
	(3.0[d], ip)	10	0	100	0	4
Ergometrine	(8.0[d], ip)	25	0	100	0	7
	(8.0[d], ip)	135	0	100	0	7
Phentolamine	10.0[d], ip)	30	0	0	100	6

a=potentiation: 1) shift from sitting to walking; 2) shift from discontinuous to continuous sniffing
b="toxic" dose
c=DPI=(3,4-dihydroxyphenylamino)-2-imidazoline
d=absence of orientation reaction; particular lying posture.

phentolamine attenuated the CM-Pf effects, whereas picrotoxin, DPI and ergometrine potentiated them. Although the doses used have to be considered as "toxic" doses, the outcome of this series of experiments fully agrees with the outcome of the next series of experiments; the outcome, therefore, will be discussed below.

Role of the N accumbens

In view of the fact that the N accumbens contains a large number of DA_i receptors (Cools 1977b), DPI being an agonist of these receptors and ergometrine being an antagonist of these receptors were selected for investigating the role of mesolimbic DA. As shown in Table III, both drugs were able to potentiate the effects elicited by electrical stimulation of the CM-Pf complex; the same holds true for the outcome of the experiments in which these agents were systemically applied (see above). All these data together suggest that DA_i receptors were not implicated. As both DPI and ergometrine share the ability to interfere with α-noradrenergic receptors on the one hand (Struyker Boudier *et al.* 1975, Woodruff *et al.* 1969) and mesolimbic, α-noradrenergic receptors appear to be implicated in the CM-Pf effects on the other hand (see below), it is possible that the observed effects were due to interference with these receptors; future research is required to solve this. Apart from its ability to potentiate the electrical stimulation effects, DPI also resulted in the display of teeth grinding and head nodding, i.e. effects which are not elicited by the administration of DPI into the N accumbens of nonstimulated animals (Cools 1977b). Although it is yet impossible to ascribe the appearance of these effects to the involvement of a particular group of receptors, it is of importance to note that DPI or muscimol administered into the CM-Pf complex also elicits teeth grinding. This suggests that both brain structures may form part of the same functional circuit (see also below).

Considering the presence of α-noradrenaline-sensitive structures within the N accumbens (Blumberg *et al.* 1975, cf. Jackson *et al.* 1975, cf. Cools *et al.* 1978), it was of interest to investigate the role of mesolimbic, noradrenergic processes. As shown in Table III, oxymetazoline did potentiate the CM-Pf effects, whereas phentolamine attenuated them. From this point of view, it appears justified to suggest that α-noradrenergic receptors were involved. In this context it is of interest to note that the thalamus of man contains noradrenaline-rich cell bodies (Farley & Hornykiewicz 1977); this together with the fact that the thalamus innervates limbic structures (Van Buren & Borke 1974) opens the question

Table III

Effects of bilateral administration (0.5 μl per side) of various drugs into the N accumbens upon electrical stimulation of Center Median parafascicularis complex

		Drug-induced effects (%)					
			Inhibition[a]		Potentiation[b]		No.
Drug (μg)		No effect	partial	total	partial	total	tests
		A: postdrug interval: 10–20 min					
Saline		100	0	0	0	0	24
DPI	(5.0)	9.5	–	–	14.2[c]	76.3[c]	21
Ergometrine	(0.5)	62.5	–	–	20.8	16.7	24
Ergometrine	(1.0)	14.2	–	–	23.8	62.0	21
Oxymetazoline	(0.5)	23.8	–	–	0	76.2	21
Phentolamine	(2.5)	19.1	19.1	61.8	–	–	21
Haloperidol	(2.5)	35.6	42.2	22.2	–	–	18
Muscimol	(0.01)	50.0	44.4	5.6	–	–	18
Muscimol	(0.1)	6.7	26.7	66.6	–	–	15
Picrotoxin[d]	(0.02)	9.5	–	–	14.3	76.2	21
Carbachol	(0.2)	55.4	39.0	5.6	–	–	18
Scopolamine[e]	(5.0)	0	–	–	–	100	18
		B: postdrug interval: 25–35 min					
Saline		100	0	0	0	0	24
Oxymetazoline	(0.5)	90.5	–	–	9.5	0	21
Phentolamine	(2.5)	0	28.5	71.5	–	–	21
Muscimol	(0.01)	5.6	72.2	22.2	–	–	18
Muscimol	(0.1)	0	6.7	93.3	–	–	15
Picrotoxin[d]	(0.02)	9.5	–	–	14.3	76.2	21
Carbachol	(0.2)	22.2	50.0	27.8	–	–	18
Scopolamine[e]	(5.0)	0	–	–	0	100	18
		C: postdrug interval: 70–90 min					
Saline		100	0	0	0	0	18
Ergometrine	(0.5)	38.9	–	–	61.1	0	18
Ergometrine	(1.0)	47.6	–	–	28.4	24.0	21

a=effects measured during administration of threshold current; see Fig. 3.
b=effects measured during administration of subthreshold current; see Fig. 3.
c=teeth grinding and vertical head nodding.
d=picrotoxin (0.05 μg) alone, 1–35 min: continuous sniffing and walking.
e=scopolamine (5 μg) alone, 1–20 min: discontinuous sniffing.

whether there also exists a noradrenergic, thalamo-limbic input in rats. Till now, no evidence in this respect is available. Another explanation for the effectiveness of the noradrenergic agents might be that the mesolimbic output – which apparently plays a role in the CM-Pf effects – is influenced by a separate noradrenergic input, possibly originating from the locus coeruleus (Couch & Goldstein 1977).

The literature on the N accumbens also suggests that cholinergic processes can influence its neuronal activity (Koslow *et al.* 1974). As shown in Table III carbachol attenuated the CM-Pf effects, whereas scopolamine potentiated them. However, it is of importance to mention that both drugs reached their optimum effectiveness after a latency of about 20 min. Later on it will be seen that administration of these drugs into the posterior part of the neostriatum resulted in stronger effects. Accordingly, it seems likely that the effects were mediated by interference with cholinergic receptors outside the N accumbens rather than with cholinergic receptors inside this nucleus. This fits in with the finding that mesolimbic administration of 5 μg scopolamine in nonstimulated rats was less effective than the neostriatal administration of 2.5 μg scopolamine in non-stimulated rats (Tables III and V). The same holds true for the site of action of GABA-ergic drugs. Although both muscimol and picrotoxin administered into the N accumbens were able to inhibit and potentiate respectively the CM-Pf effects during the first part of the observation period, the effects reached their optimum during the second part of the observation period (Table III). In this case, too, the agents mentioned were more effective when applied into the posterior part of the neostriatum (Tables IV and V). Moreover, experiments in which picrotoxin was given to nonstimulated rats revealed that already a dose of 0.02 μg administered into the neostriatum elicited sniffing and walking (Table IV), whereas a dose of 0.05 μg had to be injected into the N accumbens in order to get comparable effects (Table III).

Considering the above-mentioned data, it becomes evident that only *a*-noradrenergic processes within the N accumbens could modify the CM-Pf effects.

Role of the neostriatum, posterior and anterior part

It is known that the neuronal activity within the neostriatum is regulated by acetylcholine, DA, GABA and serotonin (for reviews: Bartholini 1977, Butcher 1977, Cools 1977a). In the present study, the attention was focussed on acetylcholine, DA and GABA; as the majority of the DA receptors within the neostriatum are so-called DA_e receptors, which are stimulated by apomorphine and inhibited by haloperidol (Cools 1977b, Cools & Van Rossum 1976), only these agents were used for investigating the role of neostriatal DA.

Table IV
Effects of bilateral administration (1 μl per side) of various drugs into the neostriatum, anterior part upon electrical stimulation of Center Median parafascicularis complex

Drug (μg)		No effect	Drug-induced effect (%) Inhibition[a] partial	total	Potentiation[b] partial	total	No. tests
		A: postdrug interval: 10–25 min					
Saline		100	0	0	0	0	20
Apomorphine	(1.0)	100	–	–	0	0	18
Apomorphine	(5.0)	0	–	–	0	100	21
Haloperidol	(1.0)	100	0	0	–	–	18
Haloperidol	(2.5)	100	0	0	–	–	24
Muscimol	(0.01)	72.2	27.8	0	–	–	20
Muscimol	(0.1)	27.7	44.5	27.8	–	–	18
Picrotoxin[c]	(0.01)	0	–	–	4.8	95.2	21
		B: postdrug interval: 25–35 min					
Saline		100	0	0	0	0	20
Apomorphine	(1.0)	100	–	–	0	0	18
Apomorphine	(5.0)	38.1	–	–	0	61.9	21
Haloperidol	(1.0)	83.3	0	16.7	–	–	18
Haloperidol	(2.5)	100	0	0	–	–	24
Muscimol	(0.01)	5.5	66.7	27.8	–	–	21
Muscimol	(0.1)	0	27.8	72.2	–	–	18
Picrotoxin[c]	(0.01)	0	0	0	0	100	21

a=effects measured during administration of threshold current; see Fig. 3.
b=effects measured during administration of subthreshold current; see Fig. 3.
c=picrotoxin (0.02 μg) alone (10–35 min): continuous sniffing and walking.

As shown in Table IV, only a relatively high dose of apomorphine (5 μg) was able to potentiate the CM-Pf effects. Moreover, haloperidol (2.5 μg) did not really affect the CM-Pf effects. Taken these data together with the outcome of the experiments in which these drugs were systemically administered (Table II), it appears unlikely that DA_e receptors were implicated.

As shown in Tables IV and V, muscimol strongly attenuated the CM-Pf effects; on the other hand, picrotoxin potentiated them. Moreover, picrotoxin alone was able to elicit the display of sniffing and walking when a dose being slightly higher was given (Table IV). Considering the effectiveness of the administration of 0.01 and 0.1 μg muscimol into the *anterior* and *posterior* part of the neostriatum (Tables IV and V), it appears that the posterior part is the most effective site. Comparing the effectiveness of cholinergic drugs in the N

Table V

Effects of bilateral administration (1 μl per side) of various drugs into the neostriatum, posterior part upon electrical stimulation of Center Median parafascicularis complex

Drug (μg)		No effect	Drug-induced effects (%) Inhibition[a] partial	total	Potentiation[b] partial	total	No. tests
		A: Postdrug interval: 10–20 min					
Saline		100	0	0	0	0	21
Muscimol	(0.01)	75	8.3	16.7	–	–	18
Muscimol	(0.1)	0	16.7	83.3	–	–	18
Carbachol	(0.1)	100	0	0	–	–	12
Carbachol	(0.2)	14.3	85.7	0	–	–	21
Scopolamine[c]	(2.5)	83.3	–	–	0	16.7	18
		B: postdrug interval: 25–35 min					
Saline		100	0	0	0	0	24
Muscimol	(0.01)	0	27.8	72.2	–	–	18
Muscimol	(0.1)	0	16.7	83.3	–	–	18
Carbachol	(0.1)	100	0	0	–	–	12
Carbachol	(0.2)	0	33.3	66.7	–	–	21
Scopolamine[c]	(2.5)	0	–	–	27.8	72.2	18

a=effects measured during administration of threshold current; see Fig. 3.
b=effects measured during administration of subthreshold current; see Fig. 3.
c=scopolamine (2.5 μg) alone, 1–20 min: continuous sniffing and discontinuous walking.

accumbens with their effectiveness in the posterior part of the neostriatum, the same conclusion is reached (cf. Tables III and V). This conclusion is of utmost importance in view of the outcome of the anatomical studies, which were recently performed in our institute. These studies, in which the retrograde transport of micro-iontophoretically applied horseradish peroxidase (HRP) was investigated, showed that HRP injections into the neostriatum resulted in an extensive labeling of the Center Median, only on the condition that the injections were given at the level of A 6.9–7.5 (co-ordinates König & Klippel atlas); however, labeling of the N parafascicularis was rather independent of the chosen, neostriatal site (Cornelissen *et al.*, unpublished data).

In other words, our combined electrical and chemical stimulation studies together with the anatomical data point out that the neostriatal area that receives a monosynaptic input from the Center Median is the most effective target area for modulating the CM-Pf effects.

CONCLUSION AND SYNTHESIS

The present study offers evidence that the CM-Pf complex is implicated in the display of apomorphine-like effects such as stereotyped sniffing and walking. Although several studies have suggested that the CM-Pf complex fulfills a role in a) control of voluntary motricity, b) processing temporal pulse code for pain, and c) processing the temporal connections of instrumental conditioning (Delacour 1971, Emmers 1976, Lejeune 1977a, b, see also Grossman 1958, Hunter & Jasper 1949), its role in eliciting stereotyped behavior has not yet been reported. The mentioned effects are in fact elicited by a) intracerebral administration of ergometrine or picrotoxin into the CM-Pf complex, b) electrical stimulation of the CM-Pf complex, c) intracerebral administration of picrotoxin or scopolamine into the posterior part of the neostriatum, d) intracerebral administration of oxymetazoline into the N accumbens, and e) systemic administration of low doses of apomorphine; evidence in favor of a-d is presented in this report.

The present study also shows that the CM-Pf effects are not suppressed by systemically or intrastriatally applied haloperidol, although they are suppressed by intracerebral administration of a) DPI or muscimol into the CM-Pf complex, b) phentolamine into the N accumbens, and c) muscimol or carbachol into the posterior part of the neostriatum.

It is suggested on the basis of pharmacological and anatomical data presented in this article that there exists a close functional link between the CM-Pf complex and the neostriatum: *activation of this thalamo-striatal pathway results in apomorphine-like effects which are independent on changes in the dopaminergic activity within the neostriatum and the N accumbens.* As the substantia nigra *inter alia* projects onto the N parafascicularis (Ahlenius 1978), the present data make it possible to understand that apomorphine-like effects elicited by intranigral application of muscimol are not attenuated by a haloperidol-induced blockade of central dopaminergic processes: the display of effects mediated via a nigro-thalamo-neostriatal pathway is independent of dopaminergic processes which are inhibited by haloperidol.

The present study implies that effects elicited by intranigral administration of muscimol can be blocked by the same drug on the condition that it reaches either the CM-Pf complex or the posterior part of the neostriatum. From this point of view, it becomes important to realize that the increasing enthusiasm about the possible use of GABA-ergic drugs for the treatment of psychomotor diseases such as Huntington's chorea and schizophrenia has to be tempered.

REFERENCES

Ahlenius, S. (1978) Potentiation by haloperidol of the catalepsy produced by lesions in the parafascicular nucleus of the rat. *Brain Res.* 150, 648–652.

Aghajanian, G. K. & Bunney, B. S. (1973) Dopaminergic neurons: neurophysiological identification and responses to drugs. In: *Frontiers in Catecholamine Research,* ed. Usdin, E. & Snyder, S., pp. 643–649. Pergamon Press, New York.

Andén, N. E. & Stock, G. (1973) Inhibitory effect of γ-hydroxybutyric acid and γ-aminobutyric acid on the dopamine cells in the substantia nigra. *Naunyn-Schmiedeberg's Arch. Pharmacol.* 289, 89–92.

Bartholini, G. (1977) Interaction of dopaminergic and other transmitter systems in the brain: relation to the action mechanism of neuroleptic drugs. In: *Neurotransmission and Disturbed Behavior,* ed. Van Praag, H. M. & Bruinvels, J., pp. 103–112. Bohn, Scheltema & Holkema, Utrecht.

Blumberg, J. B., Taylor, R. & Sulser, F. (1975) Blockade by pimozide of a noradrenaline sensitive adenylate cyclase in the limbic forebrain: possible role of limbic noradrenergic mechanisms in the mode of action of antipsychotics. *J. Pharm. Pharmac.* 27, 125–128.

Butcher, L. L. (1977) Nature and mechanisms of cholinergic-monoaminergic interactions in the brain. *Life Sci.* 21, 1207–1226.

Carpenter, M. B. & Peter, P. (1972) Nigrostriatal and nigrothalamic fibers in the rhesus monkey. *J. Comp. Neurol.* 144, 93–116.

Cools, A. R. (1977a) Basic considerations on the role of concertedly working dopaminergic, GABA-ergic, cholinergic and serotonergic mechanisms within the neostriatum and nucleus accumbens in locomotor activity, stereotyped gnawing, turning and dyskinetic activities. In: *Advances in Behavioral Biology,*vol. 21, ed. Ellinwood, E. E. & Kilbey, M. M., pp. 97–141. Plenum Press, New York.

Cools, A. R. (1977b) Two functionally and pharmacologically distinct dopamine receptors in the rat brain. In: *Advances in Biochemical Psychopharmacology,* vol. 16, ed. Costa, E. & Gessa, G. L., pp. 215–225. Raven Press, New York.

Cools, A. R. (1978) Ergometrine and its biphasic action at dopaminergic receptors in the nucleus accumbens of rats. *Pharmacology* 16, suppl. 1, 93–98.

Cools, A. R. & Janssen, H.-J. (1976) γ-Aminobutyric acid: the essential mediator of behaviour triggered by neostriatally applied apomorphine and haloperidol. *J. Pharm. Pharmac.* 28, 70–74.

Cools, A. R. & Van Rossum, J. M. (1976) Excitation-mediating and inhibition-mediating dopamine-receptors: a new concept towards a better understanding of electrophysiological, biochemical, pharmacological, functional and clinical data. *Psychopharmacologia* (Berl.) 45, 243–254.

Cools, A. R., Van Dongen, P., Janssen, H.-J. & Megens, A. (1978) Functional antagonism between dopamine and noradrenaline within the caudate nucleus of cats: a phenomenon of rhythmically changing susceptibility. *Psychopharmacologia* (Berl.). In press.

Costall, B. & Naylor, R. J. (1977) Mesolimbic and extrapyramidal sites for the mediation of stereotyped behaviour patterns and hyperactivity by amphetamine and apomorphine in the rat. In: *Advances in Behavioral Biology,* vol. 21, ed. Ellinwood, E. E. & Kilbey, M. M. pp. 47–76. Plenum Press, New York.

Couch, J. R. & Goldstein, G. (1977) Projections of locus coeruleus and raphe nuclei to neostriatum. In: Abstracts, vol. III, 7th Annual Meeting Society for Neuroscinces, abstract no. 102, pp. 39.

Cowan, W. M. & Powell, T. P. S. (1955) The projection of the midline and intralaminar nuclei of the thalamus of the rabbit. *J. Neurol. Neurosurg. Psychiat.* 18, 266–279.

Delacour, J. (1971) Effects of medial thalamic lesions in the rat: a review and an interpretation. *Neuropsychologia* 9, 157–174.

Emmers, R. (1976) Thalamic mechanisms that process a temporal pulse for pain. *Brain Res.* 103, 425–441.

Farley, I. R. & Hornykiewicz, O. (1977) Noradrenaline distribution in subcortical areas of the human brain. *Brain Res.* 126, 53–62.

Fibiger, H. C., Pudritz, R. E., McGeer, P. L. & McGeer, E. G. (1972) Axonal transport in nigro-striatal and nigro-thalamic neurons; effects of medial forebrain bundle lesions and 6-hydroxy-dopamine. *J. Neurochem.* 19, 1697–1708.

Glisson, S. N., El-Etr, A. A. & Bloor, B. C. (1976) The effect of ketamine upon norepinephrine and dopamine levels in rabbit brain parts. *Naunyn-Schmiedeberg's Arch. Pharmacol.* 295, 149–152.

Grossman, R. (1958) Effects of stimulation of non-specific thalamic systems on locomotor movements in cat. *J. Neurophysiol.* 21, 85–93.

Hunter, J. & Jasper, H. (1949) Effects of thalamic stimulation in unanaesthetized animals. *E.E.G. Clin. Neurophysiol.* 1, 305–323.

Ishikawa, M. & Tanaka, C. (1977) Morphological organization of catecholamine terminals in the diencephalon of the rhesus monkey. *Brain Res.* 119, 43–55.

Iversen, S. (1977) Striatal function and stereotyped behaviour. In: *Psychobiology of the Striatum,* ed. Cools, A. R., Lohman, A. H. M. & Van den Bercken, J. H. L., pp. 99–118. North Holland Biomedical Press, Amsterdam.

Jackson, D. M., Andén, N. E. & Dahlström, A. (1975) A functional effect of dopamine in the nucleus accumbens and in some other dopamine-rich parts of the rat brain. *Psychopharmacologia* (Berl.) 45, 139–149.

Kizer, J. S., Palkovits, M. & Brownstein, M. J. (1976) The projections of the A8, A9 and A10 dopaminergic cell bodies: evidence for a nigral-hypothalamic-median eminence dopaminergic pathway. *Brain Res.* 108, 363–370.

Koslow, S. H., Racagni, G. & Costa, E. (1974) Mass fragmentographic measurements of nor-epinephrine, dopamine, serotonin and acetylcholine in seven discrete nuclei of the rat tel-diencephalon. *Neuropharmacol.* 13, 1123–1130.

Lejeune, H. (1977a) Lesions thalamiques médianes et effets différentiels dans les apprentissages operants. *Physiol. Behav.* 18, 349–356.

Lejeune, H. (1977b) Type de réponse operante et lésions thalamique médianes. *Physiol. Beh.* 18, 357–359.

Levine, M. S., Hull, C. D., Buchwald, N. A., Garcia-Rill, E., Heller, A. & Erinhoff, L. (1977) The spontaneous firing patterns of forebrain neurons III. Prevention of induced asymmetries in caudate neuronal firing rats by unilateral thalamic lesions. *Brain Res.* 131, 215–225.

Lindvall, O. & Björklund, A. (1974) The organization of the ascending catecholamine neuron systems in the rat brain. *Acta Physiol. Scand.,* suppl. 412, 1–48.

Lindvall, O., Björklund, A., Nobin, A. & Steveni, U. (1974) The adrenergic innervation of the rat thalamus as revealed by the glyoxylic acid fluorescence method. *J. Comp. Neurol.* 154, 317–348.

Mehler, W. R. (1966) Further notes on the center median nucleus of Luys. In: *The Thalamus,* ed. Purpura, P. P. & Yahr, M. D., pp. 109–122. Columbia University Press, New York.

Nieuwenhuys, R. (1977) Aspects of the morphology of the striatum. In: *Psychobiology of the Striatum,* ed. Cools, A. R., Lohman, A. H. M. & Van den Bercken, J. H. L., pp. 1–19. North Holland Biomedical Press, Amsterdam.

Olson, L., Seiger, A. & Fuxe, K. (1972) Heterogeneity of striatal and limbic dopamine innervation: highly fluorescent islands in developing and adult rats. *Brain Res.* 44, 283–288.

Pijnenburg, A. J. J., Honig, W. M. M., Struyker Boudier, H. A. J., Cools, A. R., Van der Heyden, J. A. M. & Van Rossum, J. M. (1976) Further investigations on the effects of ergometrine and other ergot derivatives following injection into the nucleus accumbens of the rat. *Arch. Int. Pharmacodyn.* 222, 103–115.

Roberts, E. (1974) Disinhibition as an organizing principle in the nervous system – the role of gamma-aminobutyric acid. In: *Advances in Neurology,* vol. 5, pp. 127–143. Raven Press, New York.

Scheel-Krüger, J., Arnt, J. & Magelund, G. (1977a) Behavioral stimulation induced by muscimol and other GABA agonists injected into the substantia nigra. *Neurosci. Letters* 4, 351–356.

Scheel-Krüger, J., Cools, A. & Honig, W. (1977b) Muscimol antagonizes the ergometrine-induced locomotor activity in nucleus accumbens: evidence for a GABA-dopaminergic interaction. *Europ. J. Pharmacol.* 42, 311–319.

Scheel-Krüger, J., Arnt, J., Braestrup, C., Christensen, A. V., Cools, A. R. & Magelund, G. (1978) The GABA-dopamine interaction in substantia nigra and nucleus accumbens – the relevance to behavioral stimulation and stereotyped behaviour. *Proceedings Southampton Meeting.* Raven Press, to be published.

Struyker Boudier, H. A. J., De Boer, J., Smeets, G., Lien, E. & Van Rossum, J. M. (1975) Structure-activity relationships for central and peripheral α-adrenactivity of imidazoline derivatives. *Life Sci.* 17, 377–386.

Swanson, L. W. & Hartman, B. K. (1975) The central adrenergic system. An immunofluorescence study of the location of cell bodies and their efferent connections in the rat utilizing dopamine-β-hydroxylase as a marker. *J. Comp. Neurol.* 163, 467–506.

Van Buren, G. & Borke, A. (1974) Nucleus dorsalis superficialis (lateralis dorsalis) of the thalamus and the limbic system in man. *J. Neurol. Neurosurg. Psychiat.* 37, 765–789.

Vogt, C. & Vogt, O. (1941) Thalamusstudien. *J. Physiol. Neurol.* 50, 32–154.

Woodruff, G. N., Agar, J., Albani, M., Allen, K. & Folkard, J. (1969) Observations on some actions of ergometrine, noradrenaline and dopamine on the guinea pig vas deferens and on the rabbit jejunum. *J. Pharm. Pharmac.* 21, 860–861.

Wright, A. K., Arbuthnott, G. W., Tulloch, I. F., Garcia-Munoz, M. & Nicalaou, N. M. (1977) Are the striatonigral fibres the feedback pathway? In: *Psychobiology of the Striatum,* ed. Cools, A. R., Lohman, A. H. M. & Van den Bercken, J. H. L., pp. 31–50. North Holland Biomedical Press, Amsterdam.

Yoshida, M. & Precht, W. (1971) Monosynaptic inhibition of neurons of the substantia nigra by caudato-nigral fibres. *Brain Res.* 32, 225–231.

GABA-ergic Neurotransmission and the Secretion of Prolactin in the Rat

*E. E. Müller, **D. Cocchi, **V. Locatelli, ***P. Krogsgaard-Larsen, *F. Bruno & *G. Racagni*

INTRODUCTION

A conspicuous literature has appeared in the last few years on the neuroendocrine control of prolactin (PRL) secretion in mammals. The mammalian hypothalamus exerts a tonic inhibitory action on PRL release. Removal of hypothalamic influences by placement of lesions in the median eminence (ME), or by section of the pituitary stalk, results in enhanced release of PRL. The agents in the hypothalamus responsible for inhibition of PRL release comprise a presumed polypeptide PRL-inhibiting factor (PIF), whose nature still remains elusive, dopamine (DA) which can also act directly on the anterior pituitary (AP), acetylcholine, and histamine (H) acting at the level of H_2 receptors. The hypothalamus also contains substances which can promote the release of PRL; they comprise an alleged polypeptide PRL, releasing factor (PRF), whose structure is as yet undetermined, serotonin (5-HT) and melatonin which may act by increasing PRF or by decreasing PIF activity, TRH which can release PRL by direct action on the AP, and prostaglandins which likely act on hypothalamic centers. All exteroceptive stimuli that alter PRL secretion presumably act via the central nervous system (CNS) (Fig. 1).

The evidence relating other proven or putative neurotransmitters to the control of PRL secretion is still scarce and contradictory findings have been reported at times (Müller *et al.* 1978). For gamma-aminobutyric acid (GABA), evidence although inferential for its participation in the mechanism(s) control-

Institute of Pharmacology and Pharmacognosy, University of Cagliari and Milan* (Italy), ** Department of Pharmacology, University of Milan (Italy) & ***Department of Chemistry BC, Royal Danish School of Pharmacy, Copenhagen (Denmark).

"GABA-NEUROTRANSMITTERS", Alfred Benzon Symposium 12, Munksgaard 1978

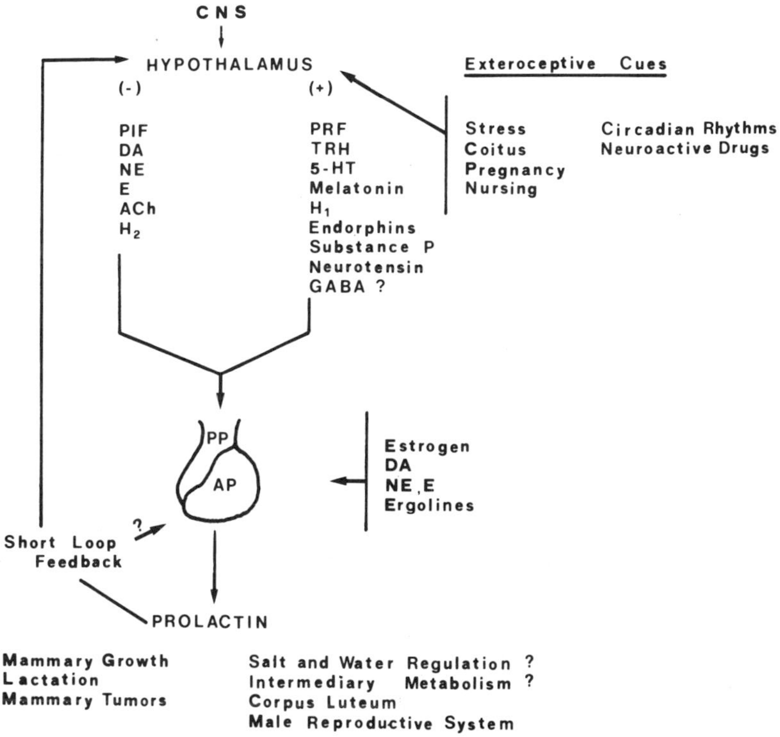

Fig. 1. Factors or conditions which influence prolactin secretion in mammals. Modified from Meites (1977) by courtesy of Raven Press.

ling PRL secretion was derived from the observation that the release of PRL induced by ovarian steroids in spayed female rats was inhibited by picrotoxin (PICRO), an antagonist of GABA receptors (Bruggencate & Engberg 1971). In addition 5-HT-induced PRL release was blocked by PICRO whereas stimulation induced by TRH or α-metyl-p-tyrosine (α-MpT) was unaffected (Caligaris & Talesnik 1974).

The data suggested that inhibition of PRL release by the GABA antagonists took place at the CNS rather than at the AP level, a view supported by the findings that huge doses of GABA administered intraventricularly (IVT) induced PRL release in proestrus or ovariectomized female (Mioduszewski *et al.* 1976) or intact male rats (Ondo & Pass 1976, Pass & Ondo 1977) but were ineffective when injected systemically into hypophysectomized (hypox) rats bearing an AP transplant (Mioduszewski *et al.* 1976). In contrast to these findings which indicated a PRL-releasing activity of the amino acid, Schally *et al.* (1977) recently purified and isolated from pig hypothalami a neutral fraction chromatographically distinct from catecholamines (CA's), which exhibited PIF activity in many *in vivo* and *in vitro* systems.The PIF active substance was identified as GABA.

Based on these controversial findings, the present study was undertaken to determine either the effect of functional activation of GABA-ergic neurotransmission, induced by highly potent and specific GABA-mimetic drugs, or the effect of antagonists of GABA receptors, on basal and stimulated PRL release in the rat. In addition, some interactions between GABA and CA systems with respect to PRL release were evaluated.

Details on materials and methods have been incorporated into the Results section. Double antibody radioimmunoassay for rat PRL (rPRL) was used to measure plasma PRL in rats (Niswender *et al.* 1969).

Effect of GABA-mimetic drugs on plasma PRL in unanesthetized male rats

For these experiments male Sprague-Dawley (S.D.) rats (300–350 g BW) were housed in temperature and humidity-controlled rooms with 14:10 h light-dark cycle (lights on at 06.00 h). The animals were given free access to water and laboratory food. Rats were prepared with chronic indwelling jugular cannulae inserted into the right atrium, and blood samples were taken from rats housed in small isolation cages, using a procedure previously described (Cocchi *et al.* 1976).

Table I shows the effect on plasma PRL levels of muscimol (M), a psychotomimetic compound (Waser 1967), which is a powerful GABA agonist with respect to bicuculline-sensitive postsynaptic receptors (Curtis *et al.* 1971). M administered at 11.30 h induced a clear-cut reduction of plasma PRL starting 30 min after injection and still present at 210 min. Similar results were obtained when M was administered at 15.30 h; its administration was followed by a decrease in plasma PRL, which was evident at 30 min postinjection. A comparison with plasma PRL values of control rats showed the presence of significantly lower PRL levels in M-treated rats at 30, 45, 60 and 90 min postinjection.

In a second series of experiments, the effect was tested of ethanolamine-O-sulphate (EOS), a specific catalytic inhibitor of GABA transaminase (Fowler & John 1972), which is the enzyme responsible for catabolism of GABA (Baxter 1976). IVT injection of EOS (300 μg/ 10 μl) induced a significant reduction in plasma PRL at 4.0 and 4.5 h postinjection, while PRL levels were not

Table I

Effect of iv administration of muscimol on plasma PRL levels in intact male rats[a]

	Plasma PRL (ng/ml)								
Treatment	t-60 min (No. of rats)	t_0	$t_{15\ min}$	$t_{30\ min}$	$t_{45\ min}$	$t_{60\ min}$	$t_{90\ min}$	$t_{105\ min}$	$t_{210\ min}$
I Experiment Muscimol (2 mg/kg iv)	51.0±10.2 (7)	20.9± 2.1	20.0±2.5	12.5±0.8***	—	9.5±1.5**	7.5±1.8**	—	13.0±1.6*
II Experiment Saline	45.6±16.4 (3)	35.6±14.1	25.3±9.3	27.3±8.4	21.6±5.3	20.3±6.1	16.0±3.1	18.0±2.0	—
Muscimol (2 mg/kg iv)	28.8± 9.3 (4)	19.8± 4.3	19.1±6.0	6.8±1.2†	9.7±0.7†	10.4±1.9†	6.9±2.1†	11.5±7.4	—

* $P<0.05$ vs t_0

** $P<0.005$ vs t_0

*** $P<0.001$ vs t_0

† $P<0.05$ vs saline-injected rats.

[a] From Locatelli *et al.*, *Brain Res.* (1978), by courtesy of Elsevier-North-Holland Biochemical Press.

significantly altered after IVT administration of saline. In EOS-treated rats plasma PRL was significantly lower than in control rats at 4.5 h postinjection (Locatelli *et al.* 1978). Administration of EOS elicited an almost twofold increase of GABA levels in the hypothalamus-determined with a mass fragmentographic method (Cattabeni *et al.* 1976).

Like EOS and M, also iv administration of guvacine (40 mg/kg), a potent substrate-competitive inhibitor of GABA uptake (Johnston *et al.* 1975), caused a short-lived inhibition of plasma PRL-levels at times (30–45 min) when reduction of spontaneous activity, attributable to hyperfunctioning of the GABA-ergic system was present (Locatelli *et al.* 1978).

Collectively, these data were in essence in keeping with the findings of Schally *et al.* (1977) and contrasted those studies reporting a stimulatory effect of IVT-injected GABA on PRL release (see above).

Effect of GABA-antagonists on basal or stimulated PRL release and Muscimol-induced PRL suppression

The observation that activation of GABA-ergic neurotransmission by GABA-mimetic compounds had induced in our experimental model suppression of basal PRL levels, led to investigate the effect of GABA antagonists alone or in combination with one of the GABA-mimetic compounds previously used. Were the reported effect of the latter on PRL release specific, it had to be counteracted by treating animals with GABA antagonists.

In a preliminary experiment, freely behaving male rats, cannulated in the jugular vein, as previously described, were given either PICRO or M alone or their combination. It is evident from Table II that a subconvulsive dose of PICRO (1 mg/kg iv) induced 15 min later a clear-cut plasma PRL rise, followed at 30 min by a striking lowering of PRL levels; 45 min after injection the effect of PICRO on plasma PRL had vanished. As already noticed, (data not reported), M (2 mg/kg iv) induced a short-lived rise in plasma PRL at 15 min, followed by an inhibition at later time intervals. PICRO was unable to counteract the PRL-inhibiting effect of M; if any, following combined treatment, plasma PRL levels were even lower than those present after administration of M alone. Similar results were obtained when bicuculline (BIC) (0.4 mg/kg iv, 2 hrs before) was used with the aim of counteracting the effect of M; the drug by itself decreased baseline PRL levels evaluated 2.5 and 3 h after injection and did not antagonize, but even potentiated, the PRL lowering-effect of M (data not shown).

The unexpected failure of GABA antagonists to counteract the PRL-lowering

Table II

Effect of muscimol and picrotoxin on plasma PRL levels in male rats

	Plasma PRL (ng/ml)						
Treatment[a]	$t_{-30\ min}$	t_0	$t_{15\ min}$	$t_{30\ min}$	$t_{45\ min}$	$t_{60\ min}$	$t_{90\ min}$
Saline	5.0±1.1[b]	15.9±8.5	24.2±12.8	17.2±4.7	26.0±8.0	17.2±1.8	13.5±2.3
Picrotoxin	9.3±2.7	10.1±2.9	13.4± 4.2	8.3±3.7↓	67.2±17.9[c]	0.17±0.1[c]	7.2±2.7
Muscimol	11.7±3.2	8.0±2.3↓	27.7±2.7[c]	8.8±0.8	3.2±0.4	1.5±0.4[c]	2.2±0.6
Muscimol+picrotoxin	5.0±1.4	6.2±0.7↓	15.7±1.6[c]	6.1±1.3↓	3.0± 0.9[c]	0.7±0.2[c]	1.3±0.3[c]

[a] muscimol, 2 mg/kg iv; picrotoxin, 1 mg/kg iv 30 min after muscimol.
[b] mean±SE of 4–5 determinations.
[c] $P<0.05$ vs baseline.
↓ indicates time at which drug was administered.

effect of M and their ability to lower baseline PRL levels suggested their use in an animal model in which baseline PRL levels had been artificially increased.

Female S.D. rats (170–180 g BW) were bilaterally ovariectomized (OVX) and were primed 10 days after surgery with a single subcutaneous injection of 0.5 mg of polyestradiol phosphate (PEP; 1 mg of Estradurin, Ayerst Labs., Inc.). Experiments were performed 6–7 days after PEP injection at 15.00 h, when the rhythmic rise in plasma PRL induced by estrogens is evident (Lawson & Gala 1974).

Fig. 2 shows that PICRO alone (1.0 mg/kg ip) elicited a striking decline of the elevated basal PRL levels; the PRL-lowering effect of M alone (2 mg/kg ip) was even greater than that of PICRO and was almost unaffected by administration of the antagonist drug, 30 min after M. Similar results were obtained in the experiments with BIC (0.4 mg/kg ip), which was administered either alone or 2 h before M (data not shown).

Effect of IVT-injected Muscimol on plasma PRL release

Failure of antagonists of GABA receptors to antagonize the M-induced inhibition of PRL release could be conceivably ascribed either to the non-specificity of the drugs used with respect to GABA-ergic neurotransmission and PRL release, or alternatively, to different site(s) and, likely, mechanism(s) of action. For instance, a blockade of PRL release exerted by M directly at the AP level coupled to blockade of GABA-ergic receptors by PICRO or BIC in the CNS might have explained both the profound inhibition of PRL release observed during combined treatment and the ability of PICRO and BIC *per se* to lower either basal or stimulated PRL release. With this in mind, an experiment was devised aimed at investigating the effect of IVT-injected M.

Male S.D. rats, (250–300 g BW), bearing a polyethylene cannula (PE-10) permanently implanted into the right lateral ventricle were given acutely M (250 or 500 ng/20 μl) through the implanted cannula and were sampled by the orbital route 30 and 60 min later. Fig. 3 shows that M induced at the higher dose a clear cut rise in plasma PRL evident at both time intervals; the lower dose of the compound was ineffective.

In a following experiment M (500 ng/20 μl) was injected IVT into male rats which had received 1 h before an iv injection of BIC (0.4 mg/kg). Blood samples were obtained through cannulae implanted into the jugular vein. Administration of BIC induced again a decrease in baseline PRL levels and suppressed the rise in plasma PRL evoked by M at 30 and 45 min (data not shown).

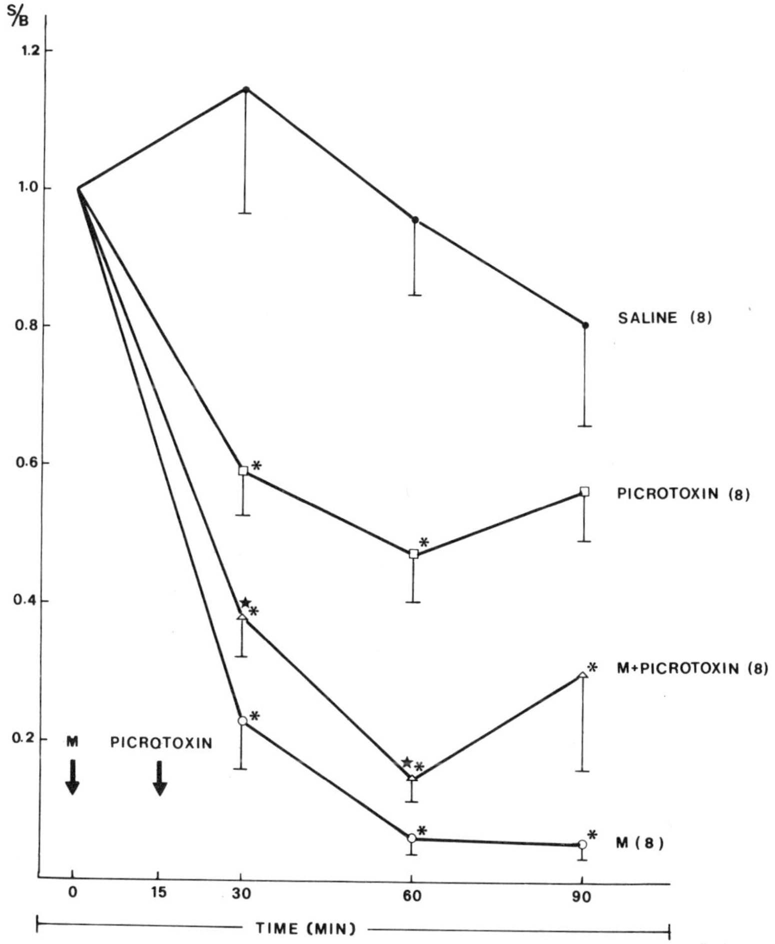

Fig. 2. Effect of ip administration of Muscimol (2.0 mg/kg) or Picrotoxin (1.0 mg/kg) alone or associated on plasma PRL levels in OVX-rats primed with polyestradiol phosphate. Values are expressed as ratio of suppressed (S) to baseline (B)±SE. Number of rats in parenthesis. Baseline PRL levels in OVX-PEP treated rats were 1343±159.3 ng/ml*=$P<.05$ vs corresponding time of saline-treated rats. ★=$P<.05$ vs corresponding time of Picrotoxin-treated rats. For further details see text.

The ability of centrally administered M to elicit stimulation of PRL release in the male rat was reminiscent of the stimulatory effect on PRL release previously reported after IVT administration of huge doses of GABA (see Introduction). These findings, when viewed together with the ability of M (this study) or GABA itself (Schally *et al.* 1977) to lower plasma PRL levels after systemic administration, might suggest for the latter effect an extra-CNS, likely, an AP site of action.

Effect of GABA and Muscimol on PRL release from anterior pituitaries disconnected from the CNS

The postulated inhibitory action on PRL release of M and GABA exerted at AP level, was investigated both in *in vivo* and *in vitro* experiments.

Female S.D. rats (130–140 g BW), 10 days after hypophysectomy, received under the kidney capsule an entire AP gland. One week following transplantation, rats were given an iv injection of M (2.0 mg/kg) and were sampled by orbital route 60 and 90 min later. From Fig. 4 it is apparent that M lowered plasma PRL levels in the hypox-transplanted rats at both time intervals; its effect attained statistical significance only at 90 min.

The *in vitro* experiments were performed on hemipituitaries obtained from S.D. male rats (200 g BW). Four hemipituitaries were placed in 2 ml of medium TC 199 (Difco Labs., Detroit, Mich., U.S.A.). Incubation was carried out in a

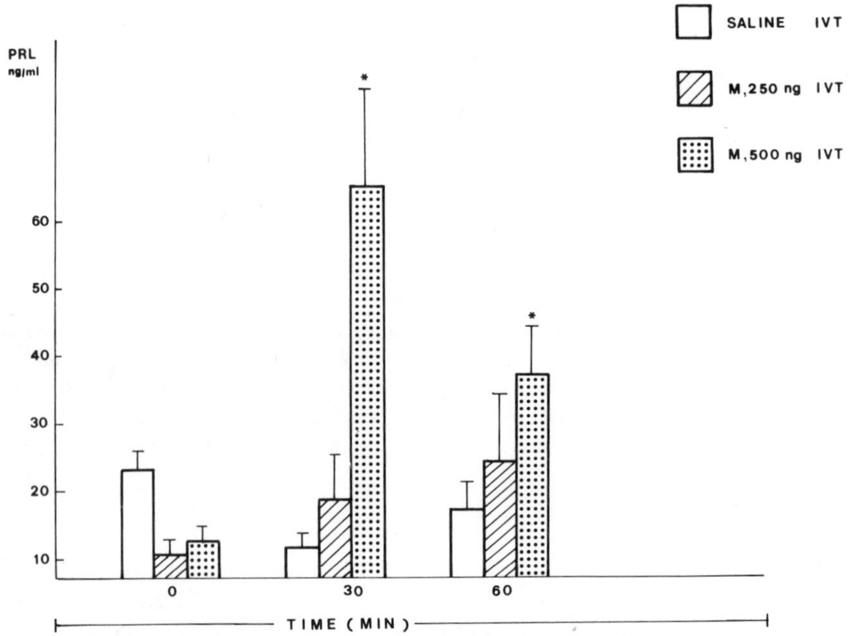

Fig. 3. Effect of Muscimol injected into the right lateral ventricle of unanesthetized male rats on plasma PRL levels. Means±SE of 5 to 6 determinations for each point are shown. $* = P < .01$ vs saline-treated rats. For further details see text.

Dubnoff metabolic shaker under constant gassing with 95% O_2–5% CO_2 at 37° C. After 30 min of preincubation, the medium was removed and pituitary tissue was placed in 2 ml of fresh medium containing either diluent or drugs. After incubation for 4 h each AP fragment was blotted on filter paper and weighed. GABA at 0.5 and 2.5 μg/ml did not lower PRL release from AP glands *in vitro* whereas the higher dose of M (2.5 μg) was effective in this context (data not shown).

Interaction between GABA-ergic and dopaminergic neurotransmission on PRL release.

If, as suggested by the last experiments, there exists the possibility for GABA-mimetic drugs to modulate directly in an inhibitory fashion PRL release from the AP, stimuli capable of eliciting a rise in plasma PRL through a

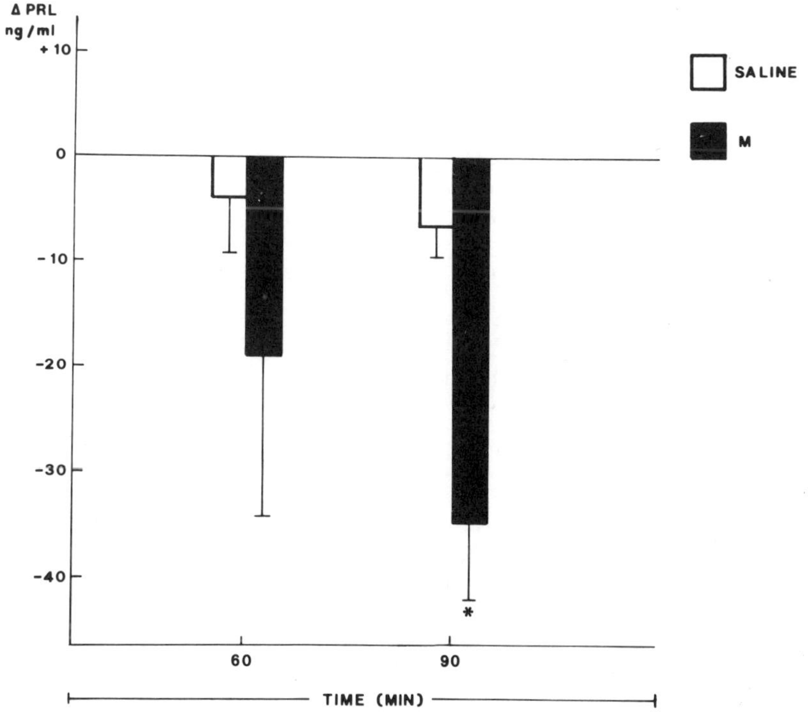

Fig. 4. Effect of iv administration of Muscimol (2.0 mg/kg) on plasma PRL levels in hypophysectomized-transplanted rats. Values are expressed as Δ from baseline. Means±SE of 6–7 determinations for each point are shown. *=$P<.01$ vs saline-treated rats.

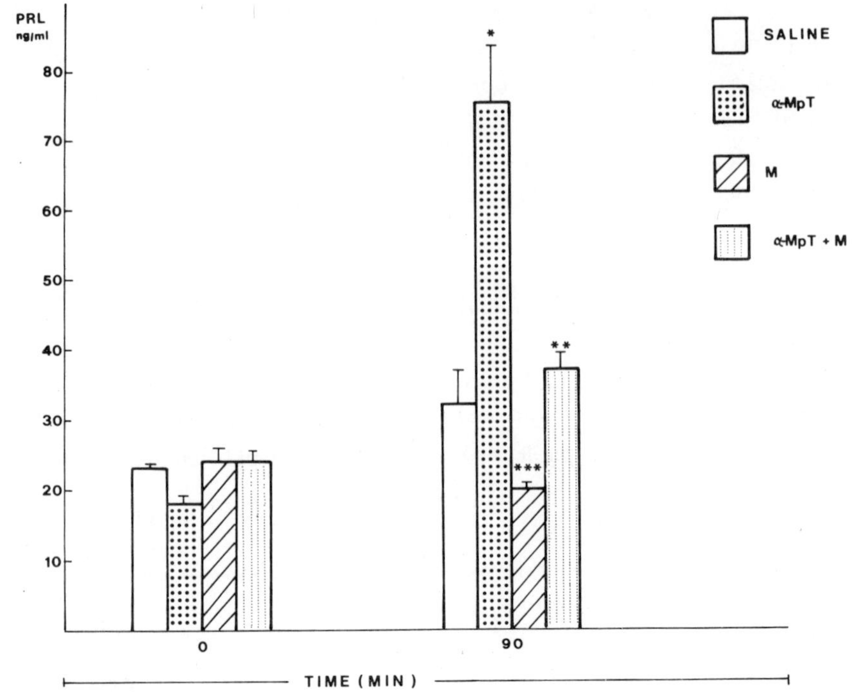

Fig. 5. Effect of ip administration of Muscimol (2.0 mg/kg) in male rats pretreated with α-methyl-p-tyrosine (200 mg/kg ip). α-MpT was administered at time 0; M 30 min later. Means $\pm$SE of 5–7 determinations for each point are shown. * $= P < .01$ vs saline-treated rats. ** $= P < 0.001$ vs α-MpT-treated rats. *** $= P < .01$ vs α-MpT+M-treated rats.

CNS-mediated mechanism, when given in association with systemically-injected GABA-mimetic drugs would be ineffective.

For these experiments, male S.D. rats (250 g BW) received at time 0, saline or α-MpT (200 mg/kg ip) and 30 min later an ip injection of either saline or M (2.0 mg/kg). Blood samples were taken by orbital route at time 0 or 90 min later. As it appears from Fig. 5, the striking PRL rise elicited by α-MpT was almost completely abolished in the animals which had received 30 min later administration of M. In line with these results were those obtained in rats which had received 1 week before 250 μg of 6-hydroxydopamine (6-OHDA) or vehicle into the third brain ventricle preceded or not by desmethylimipramine (DMI, 25 mg/kg ip), a drug which protects norepinephrine nerve terminals by 6-OHDA-induced depletion (Breese & Traylor 1971). Administration of M (2.0 mg/kg ip) caused 30, 60 and 90 min later, a decrease in plasma PRL of similar entity in all groups, irrespective of treatment with 6-OHDA alone or plus DMI (data not shown).

DISCUSSION

The reported results underline both the complexity of GABA involvement in PRL regulation and our present paucity of knowledge. The series of data obtained following peripheral administration of M and guvacine or IVT injection of EOS favored the existence of an inhibitory role for GABA-ergic neurotransmission on PRL release. The effectiveness of EOS injected by IVT route, and of guvacine, a drug whose mechanism of action relies on blockade of GABA reuptake (Johnston *et al.* 1975), standing the observation that no evidence exists for the presence of GABA-ergic nerve terminals in the AP (Saavedra *et al.* 1975), suggested for these drugs a CNS rather than a direct action at AP level.

Of difficult interpretation and, apparently paradoxical, were the findings that antagonists of GABA receptors such as PICRO and BIC, which easily cross the blood brain barrier (BBB) (Straughan *et al.* 1971) far from antagonizing the PRL-lowering effect of M induced *per se* inhibition of both tonic and stimulated PRL release. This fact, coupled to detection of abrupt and transient elevations in baseline PRL levels following both M and guvacine administration, and the reported ability of IVT-injected GABA to raise plasma PRL levels (Mioduszewski *et al.* 1976, Ondo & Pass 1976), led to hypothesize that a stimulatory component, likely of central nature, had to be considered in the action of GABA on PRL release. Such a component, in the experiments in which M and guvacine were injected peripherally, due to a poor penetrability of the BBB, might have been masked. Interestingly, centrally administered M increases food consumption in satiated rats, but is ineffective by systemic route (Grandison & Guidotti 1977).

Proof for the existence of a central GABA-ergic component stimulatory to PRL release was given in our experiments with the observation that M, at nanogram doses, induced a short-lived rise in plasma PRL, which was antagonized by BIC. In view of the ability of the latter to lower *per se* both tonic and stimulated PRL release, it would appear that the central component of GABA action plays a functional role in PRL secretion.

The reported dissociation of M effects on PRL release according to the route of administration and the different ability of BIC to antagonize such effect, suggested for GABA two different mechanism(s) and, likely, sites of action. Experiments performed with M *in vivo* on ectopic AP or on hemipituitaries incubated *in vitro* would favor the existence, in accordance with the conclusions of Schally *et al.* (1977), of a direct inhibitory effect of GABA at AP level. It must be noticed, however, that: 1) GABA, at the doses found active to inhibit PRL release from *in vitro* AP glands by Schally *et al.* (1977), in our hands was ineffective and 2) M was ineffective to inhibit release of PRL from ectopic AP when administered by intraperitoneal route (Locatelli *et al.* 1978), so that these points necessitate clarification.

That M, administered peripherally, may act directly at AP level, would be also supported by its ability to antagonize the PRL rise induced by α-MpT, a drug which impairs DA neurotransmission in the CNS. This finding is reminiscent of those of Rivier & Vale (1977), reporting in estrogen-progesterone-primed male rats blockade of a series of PRL-releasing stimuli which act at CNS level by systemic administration of high doses of GABA.

Information concerning the organization of the GABA-ergic fiber system in the hypothalamus is quite scarce (Tappaz *et al.* 1976). Nevertheless, the neuroanatomical substrate for a GABA mediated-mechanism involved in PRL secretion is offered by the detection of GABA-ergic terminals on the arcuate and ventromedial nuclei (Tappaz & Brownstein 1977), areas which give rise to the tubero-infundibular DA (TIDA) pathways, inhibitory to PRL secretion (Meites 1977). Inhibition of the DA system by GABA-ergic neurons, likely projecting from lateral and posterior hypothalamus (Tappaz & Brownstein 1977), would result in stimulation of PRL release. In addition, proof has been given for the existence of an intrahypothalamic (tuberoinfundibular?) GABA-ergic pathway which projects to the ME (Tappaz & Brownstein 1977). The possible functional analogy between this pathway and the TIDA pathway with regard to PRL control does not escape attention; as the latter, this GABA-ergic intrahypothalamic pathway might provide a direct inhibitory control over PRL secretion at the level of the anterior pituitary.

REFERENCES

Baxter, C. F. (1976) Some recent advances in studies on GABA metabolism and compartmentation. In: *GABA in Nervous System Function,* eds. Roberts, E., Chase, T. N. & Tower, D. B., pp. 61–88. Raven Press, New York.

Breese, G. R. & Traylor, T. D. (1971) Depletion of brain noradrenaline and dopamine by 6-hydroxydopamine. *Br. J. Pharmacol.* 42, 88–99.

Bruggencate, G. T. & Engberg, I. (1971) Iontophoretic studies in Deiter's nucleus of the inhibitory actions of GABA and related amino acids and the interactions of strychnine and picrotoxin. *Brain Res.* 25, 431–448.

Caligaris, L. & Taleisnik, S. (1974) Involvement of neurones containing 5-hydroxytryptamine in the mechanism of prolactin release induced by estrogen. *J. Endocrinol.* 62, 25–33.

Cattabeni, F., Galli, G. & Eros, T. (1976) A simple and highly sensitive mass fragmentographic procedure for GABA determinations. *Anal. Biochem.* 72, 1–7.

Cocchi, D., Gil-Ad, I., Panerai, A. E., Locatelli, V. & Müller, E. E. (1976) Circadian variations in plasma growth hormone and prolactin in the infant rat: comparison with the adult pattern. *Life Sci.* 19, 825–836.

Fowler, L. J. & John, R. A. (1972) Active-site-directed irreversible inhibition of rat brain4-amino-butyrate aminotransferase by ethanolamine-O-sulphate *in vivi. Biochem. J.* 130, 569–573.

Grandison, L. & Guidotti, A. (1977) Stimulation of food-intake by muscimol and B-endorphin. *Neuropharmacology* 16, 533–536.

Johnston, G. A. R., Krogsgaard-Larsen, P. & Stephanson, A. (1975) Betel nut constituents as inhibitors of γ-aminobutyric acid uptake. *Nature* (London) 258, 627–628.

Lawson, D. M. & Gala, R. R. (1974) The influence of surgery, time of day, blood volume reduction and anaesthetics on plasma prolactin in ovariectomized rats. *J. Endocrinol.* 62, 75–83.

Locatelli, V., Cocchi, D., Racagni, G., Cattabeni, F., Maggi, A., Krogsgaard-Larsen, P. & Müller, E. E. (1978) Prolactin-inhibiting activity of gamma-aminobutyric acid-mimetic drugs in the male rat. *Brain Res.* 145, 173–179.

Meites, J. (1977) Catecholamines and prolactin secretion. In: *Nonstriatal dopaminergic neurons,* Vol. 16, eds. Costa, E. & Gessa, G. L., Adv. in Biochem. Psychopharmacol. pp. 139–146. Raven Press, New York.

Mioduszewski, R., Grandison, L. & Meites, J. (1977) Stimulation of prolactin release in rats by GABA. *Proc. Soc. Exp. Biol. Med.* 151, 44–47.

Müller, E. E., Nisticò, G. & Scapagnini, U. (1978). *Neurotransmitters and Anterior Pituitary Function.* Academic Press, New York.

Niswender, G. D., Chen, C. L., Midgley, A. R. Jr., Meites, J. & Ellis, S. (1969) Radioimmunoassay for rat prolactin. *Proc. Soc. Exp. Biol. Med.* 130, 793–797.

Ondo, J. G. & Pass, K. A. (1976) The effect of neurally active amino acids on prolactin. *Endocrinology* 9, 1248–1252.

Pass, K. A. & Ondo, J. G. (1977) The effect of γ-aminobutyric acid on prolactin and gonadotropin secretion in the unanesthetized rat. *Endocrinology* 100, 1437–1442.

Rivier, C. & Vale, W. (1977) Effect of γ-aminobutyric acid and histamine on prolactin secretion in the rat. *Endocrinology* 101, 506–511.

Saavedra, J. M., Palkovits, M., Kizer, J. S., Brownstein, M. J. & Zivin, J. A. (1975) Distribution of biogenic amines and related enzymes in the rat pituitary gland. *J. Neurochem.* 25, 257–260.

Schally, A. V., Redding, T. W., Arimura, A., Dupont, A. & Linthicum, G. L. (1977) Isolation of gamma-aminobutyric acid from pig hypothalami and demonstration of its prolactin release-inhibiting (PIF) activity *in vivo* and *in vitro. Endocrinology* 100, 681–691.

Straughan, D. W., Neal, M. J., Simmonds, M. A., Collins, G. G. S. & Hill, R. G. (1971) Evaluation of bicuculline as a GABA antagonist. *Nature* 233, 352–354.

Tappaz, M. L. & Brownstein, M. J. (1977) Origin of glutamate-decarboxylase (GAD)-containing cells in discrete hypothalamic nuclei. *Brain Res.* 132, 95–106.

Tappaz, M. L., Brownstein, M. J. & Palkovits, M. (1976) Distribution of glutamate decarboxylase in discrete brain nuclei. *Brain Res.* 108, 371–379.

Waser, P. G. (1967) The pharmacology of Amanita muscaria. In: *Ethnopharmacologic Search for Psychoactive Drugs,* eds. Efron, D. H., Holmsted, B. & Kline, N. S., pp. 419–439. Public Health Service Publ. No. 1645, Washington.

Status and Perspective

Eugene Roberts

A former American president, Harry Truman, had a sign of his desk that said: "The buck stops here". For a number of years I have felt that such a sign also has a place in my laboratory and that of other neuroscientists. Too often data about nervous systems are produced and floated out onto an ever-expanding sea of undigested information with the implicit hope that some friendly theoretician will attempt to fit the data into a framework that is relevant to the main business of nervous systems, information processing. In reality the frenetic search for "facts" and fear of criticism too often preclude a neuroscientist from making his own integrative efforts. I believe that in order eventually to achieve an integrated understanding of normal and abnormal nervous system function it is necessary to attempt to construct progressively more adequate frameworks to help organize and keep track of the detailed information coming at an ever-accelerating rate from the various pertinent disciplines. Information about the GABA system and other transmitters and modulators would then find its place in larger schemata. I have made several such attempts and hope to continue to make them (Roberts 1966a, 1966b, 1972, 1976, 1977, 1978; Roberts & Kuriyama 1968, Roberts & Matthysse 1970, Roberts *et al.* 1964)

GABA NEURONS PARTICIPATE IN NUMEROUS AND COMPLEX RELATIONS

Those of us who are concerned with the GABA story are involved in

---

Division of Neurosciences, City of Hope National Medical Center, Duarte, Ca, USA.

This work was supported in part by USPHS Grants NSO1615 and NS12116 from the National Institute of Neurological and Communicative Disorders and Stroke, and Grant MH22438 awarded by the National Institute of Mental Health, DHEW. This paper was written while the author was a Fellow at the Center for Advanced Study in the Behavioral Sciences, Stanford, and supported in part by grant BNS–76–22943 from the National Science Foundation.

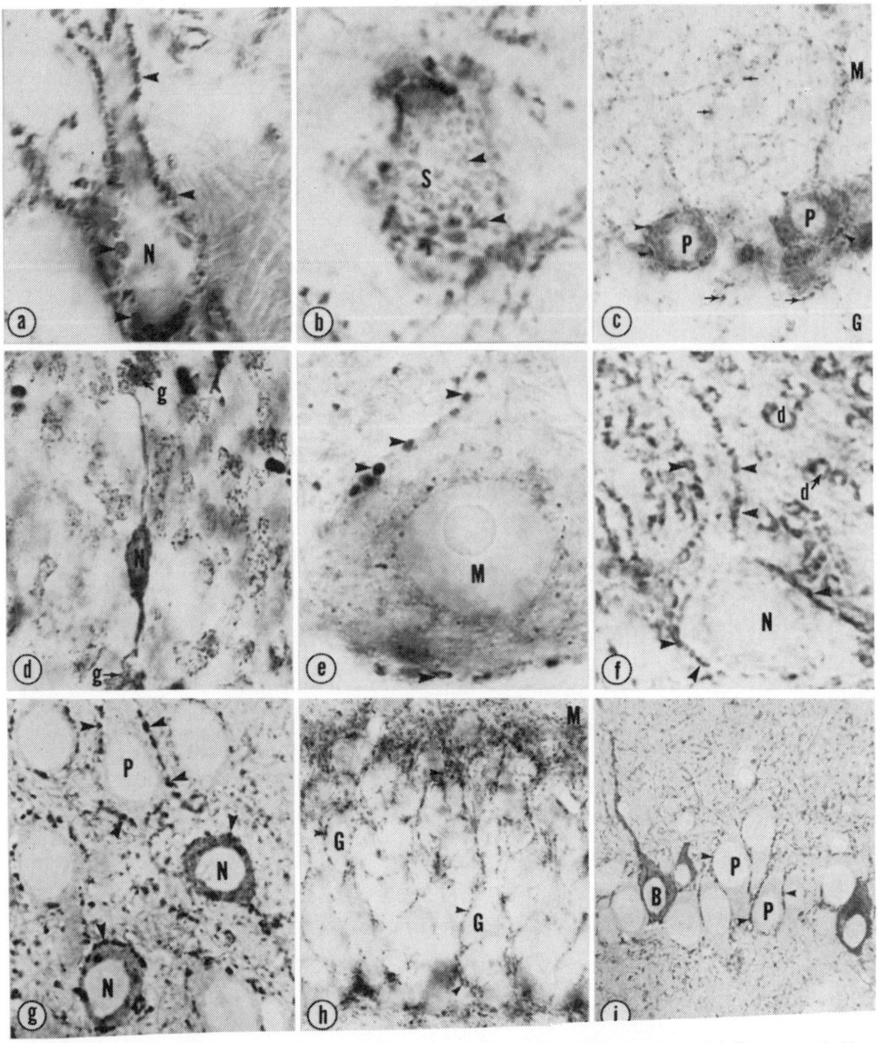

Photomicrographs of GAD-positive terminals in rat central nervous system. (a) Deep cerebellar nucleus (nucleus interpositus). A neuron (N) is shown studded by round, GAD-positive terminals (arrow heads) which are probably Purkinje cell axonal terminals (X 1590). (b) Deep cerebellar nucleus (nucleus interpositus). A grazed neuronal soma (S) showing numerous GAD-positive terminals (arrow heads) on the somal surface (X 1590). (c) Cerebellar cortex. The Purkinje cell somata are studded with GAD-positive terminals (arrow heads) which may be basket cell terminals. In the molecular layer (M), there are numerous GAD-positive punctate structures (arrows), and in the granular layer (G), GAD-positive punctute structures (Golgi II axonal terminals) are associated with glomeruli (X 660). (d) Granular layer of the cerebellum from tissue treated with colchicine to block axon flow. The Golgi II neuronal soma (N) has GAD-positive cytoplasm and two of its processes are seen to terminate on glumeruli (G) (X 614). (e) Ventral horn of the spinal cord. A

problems of neural inhibition (Roberts *et al.* 1960, Roberts *et al.* 1976). But it is necessary to remember that neither inhibition nor the GABA system *per se* is the main issue. The question for those of us interested in the rôles of GABA-releasing neurons is how the GABA neurons, wherever they are demonstrated to be present, participate in information processing in such a way that it is possible for particular organisms to respond adaptively to their environments in such a manner that they can survive and minimally reproduce their numbers. The ubiquity and extent of presynaptic endings of GABA neurons on various structures in the vertebrate nervous system is illustrated by the light micrographs of sections of rat CNS immunocytochemically stained for GAD shown in Fig. 1. The extensive studding by such endings on neuronal postsynaptic surfaces in the nucleus interpositus (Figs. 1a, b), globus pallidus (Fig. 1f), cortex (Fig. 1g), and hippocampus (Figs. 1h, 1i) is particularly striking. Similar observations have been made in the substantia gelatinosa of the spinal cord, olfactory bulb, substantia nigra, and other regions. After examining many such pictures, one really gains the impression that one is looking at a highly restrained nervous system, the inhibitory neurons acting like reins that serve to keep the neuronal "horses" from running away. Elsewhere, I have cited evidence supporting the view that disinhibition may be one of the major principles of nervous system function (Roberts 1972, 1976, 1977, 1978; see also Fentress 1976). A major tenet of this hypothesis is that in behavioral sequences, innate or learned, genetically preprogrammed circuits are *released* to function at varying rates and in various combinations largely by the *disinhibition* of pacemaker neurons whose activities are under the control of tonically active inhibitory command neurons, many of

---

single motoneuron (M) exhibits several GAD-positive terminals (arrow heads) on the somal membranes (X 1571). (f) Globus pallidus. A neuronal profile (N) is shown which has numerous GAD-positive terminals (arrow heads) studding its surface. Several dendritic cross sectional profiles (D) also are covered by punctate, GAD-positive terminals (X 1575). (g) Visual cortex from tissue treated with colchicine. Two neurons (N) have GAD-positive products in their cytoplasm, while pyramidal cells (P) in layer V have clear cytoplasm. There are some GAD-positive terminals (arrow heads) on the somal surface of all of the neurons shown here (X 940). (h) Dentate gyrus (Ammon's horn). Numerous GAD-positive terminals (arrow heads) stud the profiles of granule cells (G). In the molecular layer (M), there is a heavier investment of GAD-positive terminals around apical dendrites of the granule cells (X 630). (i) Ammon's horn, treated with colchicine. A basket cell soma (B) exhibits cytoplasmic GAD-positive product, while pyramidal cell somata (P) do not. GAD-positive punctate structures (arrow heads) presumably basket cell terminals, cover the pyramidal cell somal profiles (X 560). (I am indebted to my colleagues, Robert Barber and Charles Ribak, for the preparation of this figure.)

which may use GABA as a transmitter. According to this view, excitatory input to pacemaker neurons would have largely a modulatory rôle.

Immediately after the transduction event in a particular sensory receptor, there is a surprising amount of information processing, consisting of a coordinated interplay of excitation and inhibition. Two general aspects of sensory inhibition have emerged. Units in receptor systems inhibit their nearest neighbors via interneurons (intrasystem), causing enhancement of contrast and sharpening of input signals; and inhibitory and disinhibitory influences from higher relay centers (intersystem) may impinge on the receptors to set their gain. In the case of the retina, some of the amacrine cells, believed to be intraretinal inhibitory neurons, have been shown to be GABA-ergic (Vaughn *et al.* 1978). Thus, even close to the place and time of entry of environmental information, the organism abstracts those aspects which are most essential for adaptation. Subsequently, the neural signals carrying the information from the sensory receptors enter the CNS. Many variable sources of excitatory sensory inputs constantly are competing for the attention of the organism. It would be asking a great deal of a central neural element to adjudicate all of the competing claims. Nature has devised ways for resolving such conflicts. A great deal of information processing also occurs even at the most peripheral levels of the CNS with the aid of networks of closely-lying indigenous neurons, many of which appear to be GABA neurons. The latter are postsynaptic to primary afferent terminals and, in turn, are presynaptic to axon terminals of the primary afferent neurons and to each other's processes as well to those of central neural elements (see Barber *et al.* 1978, and references cited therein for relevant information on spinal cord). GABA depolarizes the primary afferent endings and, therefore, less excitatory transmitter is liberated from these endings by a given amount of stimulation when they receive an input from GABA neurons than when they do not. GABA neurons also may hyperpolarize (inhibit) each other and the other types of neurons upon which they impinge. In addition to liberating GABA phasically in amounts related to the extent of their depolarization by presynaptic excitatory inputs, GABA neurons also may liberate GABA tonically onto their postsynapticc sites (Parnas *et al.* 1975). Increases or decreases in the extent of release of

---

"Thus, disinhibition, acting in conjunction with intrinsic pacemaker activity and often with modulatory excitatory input, appears to be one of the major organizing principles in nervous system function. Disinhibition may act as a switch, turning on a specific coherent neuronal pattern which is otherwise actively and continuously inhibited, as well as play a rôle in the organization of sequential and alternating discharges among separate groups of elements" (Maynard 1972).

GABA by GABA-ergic neurons may be regulated by other intra-, inter-, and supra-segmental neural influences (Castiglioni *et al.* 1978), as well as by hormonal and metabolic factors. Thus, the main receiving neurons in the spinal cord, cuneate nucleus, and probably other regions of the nervous system get highly processed information with which to make further computations, as a result of which there is selective release of some central pacemaker neurons that begin to activate motor and secretory activities appropriately in response to the environmental needs as well as to signal other neural stations. Communication between neural stations and substations, I believe, takes place largely by the throwing of disinhibitory "switches", and the activities within them takes place largely through preprogrammed, hard-wired circuitry (see Roberts 1976 for further details).

INTERACTIONS AMONG NEUROTRANSMITTER SYSTEMS

GABA neurons obviously are in constant interaction with neurons liberating other transmitters or neuro-modulators (see Garattini *et al.* 1978). One of the major objectives of current neurobiological research is to delineate the relationships of various neuronal cell types to each other. Our work in tracing the complexities of the synaptic relationships of GABA neurons has raised serious questions about the conceptual utility of formulating detailed hypotheses about information processing in the whole brain or in specific regions strictly on the basis of "classical" biochemical analytical approaches, by observing behavioral changes produced by lesions or pharmacological manipulations, or even by combinations of approaches. Just as intracellular physiologic recordings from neurons must be carried out in morphologically characterized regions before they can reveal secrets of information processing, so now it is necessary to begin to perform chemical studies in more adequately described settings. It seems obvious to me that it is necessary to begin to develop detailed chemomorphologic maps of various brain regions in order to understand how neurons liberating the various putative transmitters, known and *still unknown,* are related to each other. Further refinement of immunocytochemical techniques, which are still in their infancy, will be required. It will be necessary to develop procedures that can be applied to ultrathin sections and which can visualize two or more antigens on one electronmicroscopic section, so that three-dimensional reconstructions eventually will be possible.

In this connection it seems advisable for conceptual purposes to make a distinction between at least two major classes of neurons in the vertebrate central nervous system. It appears that some neurons, such as those that may release GABA, acetylcholine, glutamate, aspartate, and glycine, probably largely are involved in direct point-to-point information transmittal. In other words, release of transmitter from the presynaptic endings of such neurons affects postsynaptic sites in such a way that in a fraction of a millisecond excitatory or inhibitory information is transmitted, recognized, and the signalling substance removed. There are other groups of neurons, such as those which release catecholamines, serotonin, peptides, prostaglandins, and possibly other substances. Current evidence suggests to me that in most instances these latter neurons may act by liberating their transmitter more generally into whole regions which contain various neuronal elements, as well as glial cells and blood vessels, where they may exert relatively long lasting effects on blood flow and capillary permeability as well as more direct metabolic and trophic effects on the cellular elements. Of course, some of these substances also may set the gain on the efficacy of individual synapses, on specific types or all of the synapses in a given region, etc. The effects may be exerted at many functional loci, from transmitter synthesis to the postsynaptic control of the length of time of ion channel opening resulting from transmitter impingement; and the effects could be exerted by a large variety of molecular mechanisms. Such neurons may furnish the "oil" required for the neuronal machinery to function smoothly. That is, the effects of the neurons releasing such substances may be analogous to that of squirting oil into inadequately lubricated, but intact machinery, the parts of which will not function properly if sufficient oil is not furnished. However, the oil is not part of the actual machinery. I would like to suggest that in many instances in which they act in the CNS, the catecholamines, serotonin, neurally released peptides, and prostaglandins may serve to optimize regional nervous system function in relation to environmental demands without themselves being involved in specific information transmittal. Roger Guillemin has called such substances cybernenes. For example, immunocytochemical, isotope labelling, and physiologic experiments are compatible with the suggestion that norepinephrine neurons in rat brain largely perform global, hormone-like functions, although occasionally they also may participate in typical synaptic relationships (Pickel *et al.* 1976, Amaral & Sinnamon 1977, Hoffer *et al.* 1978, Cimarusti *et al.* 1978).

BARRIERS TO FURTHER PROGRESS

The work described on the immunocytochemical localization of GABA neurons has allowed us to begin to study the biology of identified inhibitory local circuit neurons in various parts of the vertebrate central nervous system. However, this is only one small part of the story. Work with this information alone would be like trying to play the piano with one finger of each hand using only the pedals and the black keys. One immediately urgent task is to be able to trace the connectivities of the mainline neurons that excite the local circuit neurons and whose activities the latter serve to regulate. Glutamate and aspartate may be major excitatory transmitters in vertebrate and invertebrate nervous systems (Takeuchi & Takeuchi 1964, Graham *et al.* 1967, Curtis & Johnston 1974, Johnston 1972). It seems to me that eventually it will be necessary to identify the relationships of the neurons liberating these substances by techniques similar to those developed for GABA neurons. Currently what is lacking is the knowledge of the enzymes that are rate-limiting in the biosynthesis of these amino acids in the presynaptic endings of the neurons that may liberate them. Once these enzymes are identified with certainty, their purification, development of antisera to them, and application of immunocytochemical procedures to CNS tissue for their visualization probably could be achieved rapidly. The major difficulty for the biochemist lies in the multiplicity of metabolic pathways in which these ubiquitously occurring amino acids participate. Although the strategy is not yet clear as to how to approach this problem, it seems more likely to me that in the case of glutamate, for example, less common metabolic pathways, such as arginine→ornithine→glutamate or proline→Δ'-pyrroline-5-carboxylate→ glutamate would be more likely to be used for transmitter synthesis than would the various transaminases or glutaminase. This would be in keeping with the need for specificity of control and sequestration that seem to be part of neurotransmitter logistics. Of course, a variant of one of the more generally occurring enzymes with unique control properties also might possess suitable characteristics. At this point, it seems that a systematic search for such enzymes would yield rich scientific dividends.

What are the fundamental functional units of nervous system function?

When one seeks to understand how nervous systems process information, one always is faced with the problem as to whether or not meaningful units have been chosen for study. Certainly the activities of neurons, parts of neurons, synapses,glial cells, capillaries, or aggregates of them all are legitimate objects of investigation by the numerous techniques available. However, one must be careful that the approach to the problem of information processing should not be comparable to dissolving a magnetic tape in strong acid and performing elemental analysis on it in an attempt to discern the message that it carries.

In recent years, as a result of a confluence of morphologic and physiologic observations, the concept has arisen that there may be aggregates of mutually interrelated neurons, perhaps several thousand in number, in the cortex and elsewhere in the CNS that may serve as "power packs" (PPs) (Woolsey & Van Der Loos 1970, Feldman & Peters 1974, Szentagothai & Arbib 1974, Szentagothai 1975). I would like to speculate that at each level, from receptor to cortex and from cortex to effector, there are redundant, functionally similar (but not identical) groups of neural PPs. At each function level I presume there to be classes of PPs that respond to a given input which is first determined at the level of receptor transduction and first-order neurons. In turn these PPs signal the frequency and intensity of input received by them in a manner interpretable by related PPs in other sectors. The PPs are presumed to send collaterals to inhibitory neurons, so that after the onset of activity each PP would have a tendency to create an inhibitory surround in which other closely-lying PPs would be held in a state of inactivity. Units for different, or even antagonistic, functions frequently might be located side by side, exerting influence upon one another. Thus, the activities of PPs subserving a particular function not only could inhibit some functionally redundant PPs but also those involved in incompatible responses. A scheme will be presented elsewhere by which a combination of lateral inhibition of closely-lying PPs by the active ones and disinhibition of more distant ones would give a system of PPs at each neural level in which the number of pertinent units activated would bear a quantitative relationship to the amount of input coming into that level. The operational microstructure within each individual PP would be similar in principle. Redundant mainline neurons would be interlaced with tonically and phasically active inhibitory local circuit neurons. The information entering the PP would largely impinge on the dendrites of the large mainline neurons and phasically active inhibitory local circuit neurons that inhibit the tonically active ones so that, with sufficient input, disinhibition of the activity of some of the mainline neurons would take place. I believe that in this context disinhibition largely would be permissive and excitation would be modulatory. Activity of collaterals of excitatory mainline neurons could result in depolarization of phasically active inhibitory neurons creating inhibitory surrounds in the immediate vicinity of active neurons, disinhibitory recruitment of somewhat more distant ones, and a decrement in excitatory input to the PP through presynaptic inhibition. If the mainline neurons are inhibitory, as is the case in the cerebellar cortex and possibly other coordinative regions, they could inhibit each other directly via axon collaterals, in this way creating inhibitory surrounds. The results of the activities of the PPs largely would be communicated via the axons of the mainline neurons, and could be either excitatory or inhibitory.

Where do we go with a hypothesis such as that presented above? A good first approach might be to apply immunocytochemical techniques for localization of GABA neurons and the neurons liberating the major excitatory transmitter (probably glutamate) to the columnar organizations already identified in the somesthetic and primary visual cortex and studied in considerable detail at the light and electron microscopic levels (see Szentagothai & Arbib 1974, Szentagothai 1975 for references). Cells belonging to a particular column could be identified by physiological techniques and marked prior to fixation for microscopy. In this way one might begin to gain the specificity necessary to decide whether or not units, with relationships such as those postulated above, actually might exist in the cortex. If they do, it would be worthwhile to extend the work to other levels in the CNS.

Neurophysiologic and morphologic analyses of the cerebellum have shown that the Purkinje, basket, stellate, and Golgi type II cells of the cerebellar cortex all are inhibitory; and the basic communication patterns among the above cell types and the excitatory mossy and climbing fiber inputs and the excitatory, indigenously occurring, parallel fiber systems of granule cell origin have been thoroughly explored (Eccles *et al.* 1967). On the basis of the above observations several theoretical formulations of cerebellar functions have been made (Marr 1969, Pellionisz & Szentagothai 1973, Pellionisz & Szentagothai 1974, Gilbert 1974, Eccles 1977). In none of these treatments has it been necessary for the authors to go beyond the physiologic and morphologic data and to consider that all of the above inhibitory cells in the cerebellum use GABA as transmitter and that the excitatory ones may use glutamate (Young *et al.* 1974). The question arises as to whether the latter type of information will add any essential features to the understanding of the principles of information processing in the cerebellum and whether even three-dimensional reconstruction with transmitter type identification would add significantly to the interpretations. One discouraging possibility is that the chemical data will not add any more to the effort than the knowledge of the kind of solder employed does to the understanding of electrical circuitry. However, it is hard for me to believe that the ebbs and flows of transmitters and their physiologic and biochemical consequences are not a part of a hitherto unsuspected superdimensionality which holds important keys to the understanding of the function of the cerebellum and other neural structures.

HISTORICAL PERSPECTIVE

To my knowledge, the current meeting on the GABA system is the third international symposium devoted entirely to the subject since the initial report of the presence of GABA in mouse brain (Roberts & Frankel 1950). The intervening period of 28 years has seen the flowering of most of modern neurosciences. There has been a great development of instrumental and intellectual technologies during that period, and it has become more fashionable to participate in interdisciplinary experimentation and conferences than was the case at that time. The first conference (Roberts *et al.* 1960) was the greatest learning experience in my life. From having spent most of my scientific career in the rather narrow confines of classical biochemistry and the bare beginnings of molecular biology, I was thrust into the world of EEG, membranes, electrodes, voltage clamps, neuroanatomy, clinical seizures, and animal behavior. I had the privilege of meeting a number of the world's greatest neuroscientists among the participants, many of whom are still active scientifically and have remained close personal friends. During the planning of the meeting the Killams. Eva and Keith, kindly introduced me to the mysteries of an oscilloscope; E. Roy John demonstrated to me the technique of continuous multiple recordings from the brain of a conscious behaving cat; C. A. G. Wiersma showed me how to dissect out a crayfish stretch receptor; A. van Harreveld demonstrated cats with cerebellar lesions and had just discovered the specific excitatory effects of L-glutamate on crustacean muscle; W. Ross Adey was applying ever more sophisticated computer techniques to analysis of physiological data; C. Terzuolo introduced me to the excitement attendant upon the penetration of a cat spinal motoneuron with a microelectrode; H. W. Magoun impressed me with his deep sense of history in the neurosciences and his overall view of the structure of the field. What a mind-boggling intellectual feast!

The meeting, itself, was overwhelming to a number of us. The sense of excitement was pervasive because we all sensed that a new era was beginning. The subject of neuronal inhibition finally had returned to front stage and center after many years of languishing in the wings. It was obvious that future progress would have to be interdisciplinary and that we all would have to begin to learn each other's languages and ways of thinking. It is true that at times the proceedings resembled what one imagines may have taken place at the Tower of Babel. However, we all shared the optimistic feeling that we could help each other learn enough so that effective communication soon would take place. For must of us this turned out to be true, and many students in the laboratories of the participants reaped the benefit of the "new enlightenment". It was a particularly heartening social occasion because individuals from Australia, Canada, England, France, Hungary, Japan, United States, and the Soviet Union met in enthusiastic amity and forged longlasting scientific and personal links.

In the years that followed there were good times and fallow periods. For some years many doubted that GABA is a truc neurotransmitter. These doubts now have been laid to rest. Great advances in our understanding of neural circuitry based on neuroanatomic and physiologic observations gave us chemists the opportunities and incentives to follow with more specific ways of localizing GABA neurons *in situ,* eventually leading to the development of immunocytochemical tools. Advances in techniques of cell fractionation, autoradiography, nerve tracing techniques with isotopes and peroxidase, lesioning procedures, and clinical neurology led to the convocation of the second GABA meeting seventeen years after the first one (Roberts *et al.* 1976). Now rapid developments in the studies of general membrane and specific receptor properties and of the effects of drugs on these properties and on ionic movements have led to the organization of the present meeting at which are present two individuals, D. R. Curtis and myself, who attended the first meeting and a number of individuals who either attended the second one or have worked with the attendees of the first two conferences.

I have tried to indicate in my contributions to this volume what directions my own work now is taking and have listened eagerly to the advances made by others. I have gotten the feeling that we have more than scratched the surface of the function of GABA in nervous system function, but that many advances remaining to be made in this field will have to take place hand in hand in a contingent fashion with other types of progress. A case in point is the necessity for definitive characterization of the major excitatory transmitters and visualization of the neurons using them.

All of the participants join me in thanking the Organizing Committee for making possible this wonderful occasion.

Index of Authors

REFERENCES

Amaral, D. G. & Sinnamon, H. M. (1977) The locus coeruleus: neurobiology of a central noradrenergic nucleus. *Progress in Neurobiol.* 9, 147–196.

Barber, R. P., Vaughn, J. E., Saito, K., McLaughlin, B. J. & Roberts, E. (1978) GABA-ergic terminals are presynaptic to primary afferent terminals in the substantia gelatinosa of the rat spinal cord. *Brain Res.* 141, 35–55.

Castiglioni, A. J., Gallaway, M. C. & Coulter, J. D. (1978) Spinal projections from the midbrain in monkey. *J. Comp. Neur.* 178, 329–346.

Cimarusti, D. L., Saito, K., Vaughn, J. E., Barber, R. P., Roberts, E. & Thomas, P. E. (1978) Immunocytochemical localization of dopamine-β-hydroxylase in rat locus coeruleus and hypothalamus. *Brain Res.* In press.

Curtis, D. R. & Johnston, G. A. R. (1974) Amino acid transmitters in the mammalian central nervous system. *Ergebn. Physiol.* 69, 97–188.

Eccles, J. C. (1977) An instruction-selection theory of learning in the cerebellar cortex. *Brain Res.* 127, 327–352.

Eccles, J. C., Ito, M. & Szentagothai, J. (1967) *The Cerebellum as a Neuronal Machine.* Springer, Berlin.

Feldman, M. & Peters, A. (1974) A study of barrels and pyramidal dendritic clusters in the cerebral cortex. *Brain Res.* 77, 55–76.

Fentress, J. C. (1976) *Simpler Networks and Behavior,* 403 pp. Sinauer Associates, Inc., Sunderland, Mass.

Garattini, S., Pujol, J. F. & Samanin, R. (1978) *Interactions Between Putative Neurotransmitters in the Brain,* 415 pp. Raven Press, New York.

Gilbert, P. F. C. (1974) A theory of memory that explains the function and structure of the cerebellum. *Brain Res.* 70, 1–18.

Graham, L. T., Shank, R. P. Werman, R. & Aprison, M. H. (1967) Distribution of some transmitter suspects in cat spinal cord: glutamic acid, aspartic acid, γ-aminobutyric acid, glycine and glutamine. *J. Neurochem.* 14, 465–472.

Hoffer, B. J., Freedman, R., Woodward, D. J., Puro, D. & Moises, H. (1978) A functional role for adrenergic input to the cerebellar cortex: interaction of norepinephrine with mossy and climbing fiber excitation and GABA-mediated inhibition. In: *Interactions Between Putative Neurotransmitters in the Brain,* ed. Garattini, S., Pujol, J. F. & Samanin, R., pp. 231–243. Raven Press, N. Y.

Johnson, J. L. (1972) Glutamic acid as a synaptic transmitter in the nervous system: a review. *Brain Res.* 37, 1–19.

Marr, D. (1969) A theory of cerebellar cortex. *J. Physiol.* (Lond.) 202, 437–470.

Maynard, D. M. (1972) Simpler networks. *Ann. N. Y. Acad. Sci.* 193, 59–72.

Parnas, I., Rahamimoff, R. & Sarne, Y. (1975) Tonic release of transmitter at the neuromuscular junction of the crab. *J. Physiol.* (Lond.) 250, 275–286.

Pellionisz, A. & Szentagothai, J. (1973) Dynamic single unit simulation of a realistic cerebellar network model. *Brain Res.* 49, 83–99.

Pellionisz, A. & Szentagothai, J. (1974) Dynamic single unit simulation of a realistic cerebellar network model. II. Purkinje cell activity within the basic circuit and modified by inhibitory systems. *Brain Res.* 68, 19–40.

Pickel, V. M., Joh, T. H. & Reis, D. J. (1976) Monoamine-synthesizing enzymes in central dopaminergic, noradrenergic and serotonergic neurons. Immunocytochemical localization by light and electron microscopy. *J. Histochem. Cytochem.* 24, 792–806.

Roberts, E. (1966a) The synapse as a biochemical self-organizing microcybernetic unit. *Brain Res.* 1, 117–166.

Roberts, E. (1966b) Models for correlative thinking about brain, behavior, and biochemistry. *Brain Res.* 2, 109–144.

Roberts, E. (1972) A hypothesis suggesting that there is a defect in the GABA system in schizophrenia. *Neurosci. Res. Program Bull.* 10, 468–482.

Roberts, E. (1976) Disinhibition as an organizing principle in the nervous system – the rôle of the GABA system. Application to neurologic and psychiatric disorders. In: *GABA in Nervous System Function,* ed. Roberts, E., Chase, T. N. & Tower, D. B., pp. 515–539. Raven Press, New York.

Roberts, E. (1977) The γ-aminobutyric acid system and schizophrenia. In: *Neuroregulators and Psychiatric Disorders,* ed. Usdin, E., Hamburg, D. A. & Barchas, J. D., pp. 347–357. Oxford University Press, New York.

Roberts, E. (1978) Roles of GABA neurons in information processing in the vertebrate CNS. In: *Neuronal Information Transfer,* ed. pp. 213–239. Academic Press, Inc., New York.

Roberts, E., Baxter, C. F., Van Harreveld, A., Wiersma, C. A. G., Adey, W. R. & Killam, K. F. (1960) *Inhibition in the Nervous System and γ-Aminobutyric Acid,* 591 pp. Pergamon Press, Oxford.

Roberts, E., Chase, T. N. & Tower, D. B. (1976) *Gaba in Nervous System Function,* 554 pp. Raven Press, New York.

Roberts, E. & Frankel, S. (1950) γ-Aminobutyric acid in brain. *Fed. Proc.* 9, 219.

Roberts, E. & Kuriyama, K. (1968) Biochemical-physiological correlations in studies of the γ-aminobutyric acid system. *Brain Res.* 8, 1–35.

Roberts, E. & Matthysse, S. (1970) Neurochemistry: At the crossroads of neurobiology. *Ann. Rev. Biochem.* 39, 777–820.

Roberts, E., Wein, J. & Simonsen, D. G. (1964) γ-Aminobutyric acid (GABA), vitamin B_6, and neuronal function – a speculative synthesis. *Vitam. Horm.* 22, 503–559.

Szentagothai, J. (1975) The 'module-concept' in cerebral cortex architecture. *Brain Res.* 95, 475–496.

Szentagothai, J. & Arbib, M. A. (1974) Conceptual models of neural organization. *Neurosci. Res. Prog. Bull.* 12, 310–510.

Takeuchi, A. & Takeuchi, N. (1964) The effect on crayfish muscle of iontophoretically applied glutamate. *J. Physiol.* 170, 296–317.

Vaughn, J. E., Barber, R. P., Saito, K., Roberts, E. & Famiglietti, Jr., E. V. (1978) Immunocytochemical identification of GABA-ergic neurons in rat retina. *Anat. Rec.* 190, 571–572.

Woolsey, T. A. & Van Der Loos, H. (1970) The structural organization of layer IV in the somatosensory regions (sl) of mouse cerebral cortex. The description of a cortical field composed of discrete cytoarchitectonic units. *Brain Res.* 17, 205–242.

Young, A. B., Oster-Granite, M. L., Herndon, R. M. & Snyder, S. H. (1974) Glutamic acid: selective depletion by viral-induced granule cell loss in hamster cerebellum. *Brain Res.* 73, 1–13.

Subject Index